de Gruchy's
Clinical Haematology in
Medical Practice

de Gruchy's

Clinical Haematology in Medical Practice

EDITED BY

FRANK FIRKIN
PhD, FRACP, FRCPA
First Assistant
St Vincent's Hospital, Melbourne

COLIN CHESTERMAN
DPhil, FRACP, FRCPA
Professor of Medicine
University of New South Wales

DAVID PENINGTON
DM, FRCP, FRACP, FRCPA
Professor of Medicine
University of Melbourne

BRYAN RUSH
FRACP, FRCPA
Director of Haematology
St Vincent's Hospital, Melbourne

FIFTH EDITION

Blackwell
Science

Editorial Offices:
Osney Mead, Oxford OX2 0EL
25 John Street, London WC1N 2BL
23 Ainslie Place, Edinburgh EH3 6AJ
238 Main Street, Cambridge
Massachusetts 02142, USA
54 University Street, Carlton
Victoria 3053, Australia

Other Editorial Offices:
Arnette Blackwell SA
1, rue de Lille, 75007 Paris
France

Blackwell Wissenschafts-Verlag GmbH
Kurfürstendamm 57
10707 Berlin, Germany

Feldgasse 13, A-1238 Wien
Austria

First published 1958
Reprinted 1960, 1962
Second edition 1964
Reprinted 1966, 1967, 1968
Third edition 1970
Reprinted 1972, 1973, 1976
Fourth edition 1978
Reprinted 1981
Fifth edition 1989
Four Dragons edition 1989
Japanese edition 1974

Special reprint for India 1997

ISBN 0-632-01715-5

For sale in India, Nepal, Bangladesh,
Myanmar, Bhutan and Sri Lanka

Printed and bound by Thomson Press (India) Ltd.

DISTRIBUTORS
Marston Book Services Ltd
PO Box 87
Oxford OX2 0DT
(*Orders*: Tel : 01865 791155
Fax: 01865 791927
Telex: 837515)

North America
Blackwell Science, Inc.
238 Main Street
Cambridge, MA 02142
(*Orders*: Tel: 800 215-1000
617 876-7000
Fax: 617 492-5263)

Australia
Blackwell Science Pty Ltd
54 University Street
Carlton, Victoria 3053
(*Orders*: Tel: 03 9347-0300
Fax: 03 9349-3016)

Contents

Preface to Fifth Edition

The present edition of *Clinical Haematology in Medical Practice* is the second revision of Professor de Gruchy's book since his untimely death in 1974. This book has acquired an outstanding reputation as a clear and authoritative introduction to haematology for undergraduates as well as graduates in training for higher degrees, and as a companion for the general physician. Its strengths are that it describes haematological disorders in a clinical context in a highly readable and readily comprehensible style. The objective was to provide a balanced view of clinical features, laboratory diagnosis and management of blood conditions in a manner which did not require the reader to have a specialist background.

The demand for a work of this kind remains as great as ever, in view of the needs of medical and nursing professionals to have access to an authoritative but easily comprehensible coverage of this rapidly expanding field. The large number of developments that have taken place since the publication of the previous edition have made it necessary to incorporate an extensie amount of new information, which has resulted in comprehensive revision of the entire work, Emphasis on the clinical aspects of blood disease has been maintained, although new concepts of pathophysiology have received appropriate attention. Revisions have been carried out in a manner which adheres to the style of former editions, and the volume of the text has likewise been maintained within practicable limits.

We wish to thank our many colleagues for their advice and assistance in the preparation of this edition. We are indebted to Miss Joan Osbourne for her zeal in the preparation of the manuscript, and to Mr Mark Robertson, and Mr Per Saugman of Blackwell Scientific Publications for their encouragement.

F.C. FIRKIN
C.N. CHESTERMAN
D.G. PENINGTON
B.M. RUSH

Preface to First Edition

The aim of this book is to present an account of clinical haematology which is helpful to the general physician. It is hoped that the book will also be of use to the senior and post-graduate student. Emphasis is laid throughout on diagnosis and management, with particular stress on clinical problems as they are met by the practitioner. Essential details of normal and pathological physiology are briefly discussed. In general, morbid anatomical findings are not given; however, a description of the bone marrow as seen at autopsy is given in some disorders in which the bone marrow findings have a direct relation to diagnosis. Haematological techniques are not discussed.

Chapters 2 to 7 give an account of the anaemias. In Chapter 2 the general principles of the diagnosis and management of a patient with anaemia are discussed. The succeeding chapters describe the various types of anaemia; at the end of each of these chapters, a method of investigation of a patient who presents with the type of anaemia described in the chapter is summarized. It should be realized that these summaries are only a guide, designed to include the clinical features and special investigations pointing to the more important causes of the type of anaemia under investigation, and that they are necessarily incomplete.

With a few exceptions, references have not been included in the text. However, a list of references suitable for further reading is given at the end of each chapter. Certain articles which are particularly helpful are listed in bold type; most are either general reviews or key papers.

I wish to express my thanks to the many colleagues and friends who, in various ways, have helped and advised me. I am particularly grateful to Dr T.A.F. Heale, Dr M. Verso, Dr G. Hale and Dr G. Crock who read the manuscript and proofs and who made many valuable suggestions and criticisms. Dr J. Niall, Dr P. Cosgriff, Dr J. Murphy, Dr E. Seal, Dr J. Madigan, Miss Hal Crawford and Mr I. Parsons have greatly assisted me by reading parts of the manuscript. I am most indebted to Dr R. Sawers who kindly consented to write the section on coagulation disorders; his authoritative account is based on an extensive personal experience in the investigation and management of these disorders. It is with pleasure that I express my indebtedness to Professor J. Hayden, Professor R. Wright, Dr A. Brenan, Dr R.M. Biggins, Dr W. Keane and Mr C. Osborn for the help they gave me in establishing the Haematology Clinical Research Unit. To my friend and teacher, Professor John Dacie, I cannot adequately express my thanks for the help, advice and encouragement he has always given me.

I wish to thank those authors who have given me permission to reproduce illustrations; detailed acknowledgments are given in the text. I also wish to thank the following publishers for permission to include illustrations; J. & A. Churchill Ltd, Blackwell Scientific Publications and the Australasian Medical Publishing Co., and the Editors of the following Journals: *Practitioner* and *Australasian Annals of Medicine*. Dr R. Walsh and Professor H.K. Ward have allowed me to quote extensively, in Chapter 15, from their book *A Guide to Blood Transfusion*. I am most grateful to Mr P. Sullivan who took most of the photographs, for his patient co-operation and skill. I am also indebted to Mr J. Smith who took a number of the photomicrographs, and who gave special help with those of the red cells. Mr T. O'Connor contributed the photographs of Figures 13.7 and 13.8. Figure 3.3 is reproduced by courtesy of Dr F. McCoy. The black and white figures were drawn by Miss P. Simms, Miss J. Nichols and Miss L. Hogg; I am very grateful to them for their careful and skilful work. Miss J. Chirnside kindly assisted in typing the manuscript. It is with pleasure that I acknowledge the efficient and willing co-operation of Mrs S. Luttrell in typing and retyping the manuscript and in proof-reading. I deeply appreciate the helpful and patient collaboration of Mr Per Saugman of Blackwell Scientific Publications. Finally, I wish to acknowledge my debt to my mother for her constant help, not only during the writing of this book, but throughout my medical studies.

G.C. DE GRUCHY
Melbourne

Chapter 1
Formation of Blood Cells; Bone Marrow Biopsy

General aspects of blood cell formation

Red cells, leucocytes and platelets constitute the essential cellular components of the blood. The rates at which these cells are produced are regulated in healthy individuals to match the rates at which they leave the circulation. The concentration of each cell type is consequently maintained in the blood within well-defined limits, unless the balance between production and elimination is disturbed by pathological processes.

Sites of blood formation

Formation of blood cells occurs at different anatomical sites during the course of development from embryonic to adult life (Metcalf & Moore 1971). Production of blood cells commences in the yolk sac of the embryo, but then shifts to the liver, and to a lesser extent to the spleen, so that these organs become the dominant sites of production between the second and seventh month of gestation. The liver and spleen are then superseded by the bone marrow, which serves as the only important site of blood cell production after birth. An exception is lymphocyte production, which occurs substantially in other organs, in addition to the bone marrow, in adult life.

Haemopoietic tissue fills all of the cavities within the bones of the newborn, but with increasing age, becomes localized in the cavities of the upper shafts of the femur and the humerus, the pelvis, spine, skull, and bones of the thorax. The total volume of haemopoietic tissue in adults is 1–2 litres. This tissue is referred to as *red marrow* because of its macroscopic appearance; the remaining bone marrow in the more peripheral regions of the skeleton contains predominantly fat, and is termed *yellow marrow*. Yellow marrow also occupies a volume of 1–2 litres, and serves as a reserve space into which haemopoietic tissue can expand in response to an increased demand for blood cell production. Only in pathological situations does significant haemopoietic activity occur in the liver, spleen and other sites during adult life, when it is referred to as extramedullary haemopoiesis.

Development of blood cells

Stem cells

The most commonly accepted view is that blood cells develop from a small population of stem cells, which maintain their numbers by self-replication and also give rise to precursors of one or other of the various blood cell series. Cells of the immune system are also derived from these primordial stem cells, which are referred to as *totipotential haemopoietic stem cells* in view of the wide range of haemopoietic cell series to which they can give rise. A schematic view of the sequence of events in the differentiation of totipotential stem cells is shown in Fig. 1.1.

Proliferative activity increases from a low level at the totipotential stem cell stage, to a relatively high level in progenitor cells that are restricted to differentiating into only one, or a limited number, of the blood cell series. Proliferative activity of the immature, morphologically identifiable blood cell precursors is also high, but ceases at later stages in

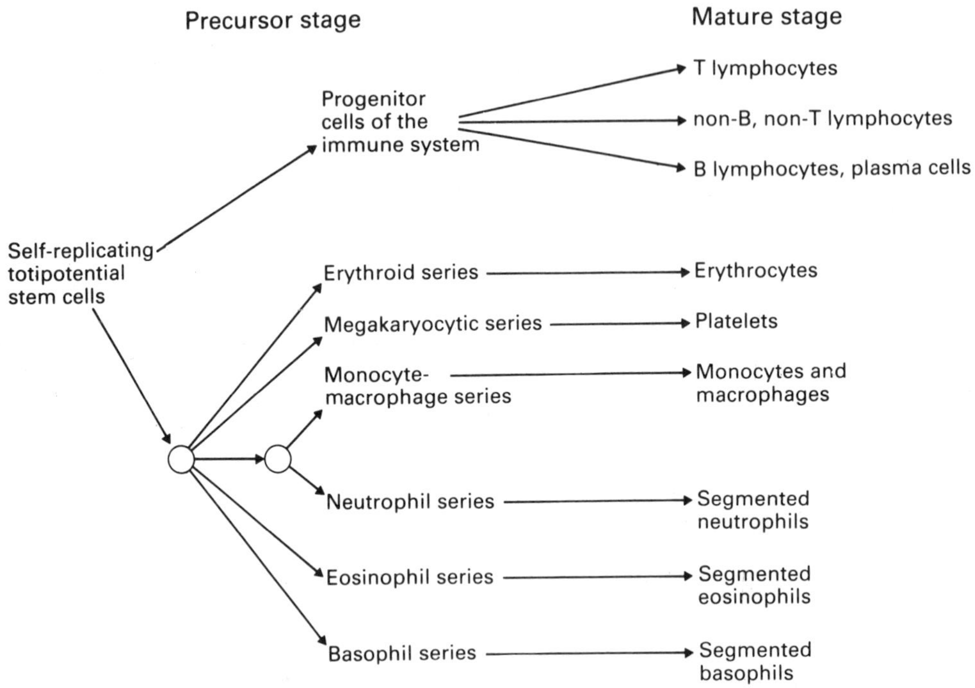

Fig. 1.1. *An overview of the process of differentiation from the totipotential stem cell to the mature blood cell. Progression through a greater number of stages in the maturation sequence is involved in vivo than in the abbreviated scheme depicted here.*

the differentiation pathway. The cells have then reached what is termed the *maturation compartment*, in which a sequence of morphological changes takes place in the absence of cell division to yield the mature end cell. The range of different blood cell series which can develop from a particular precursor progressively declines as the precursor acquires a greater degree of differentiation.

STEM CELL ASSAYS

Certain cells in human blood and bone marrow can be identified with the aid of specialized tissue-culture techniques as possessing the capacity to produce clones of cells belonging to one or more blood cell series. Such cells are often referred to as *progenitor cells* with capacity to differentiate along one or more maturation pathways. The most commonly employed technique enables a group of daughter cells to be produced from a single progenitor in cultures with a gel-like matrix, initially formed with agar (Bradley & Metcalf 1966, Pluznik & Sachs 1965), and more recently with methylcellulose or fibrin. The gel-like matrix ensures that the progeny are retained at a focus, which is defined as a colony if the number of cells exceeds about 40, and a cluster if the number is between 4 and 40.

Assays of this type have been devised to identify different types of progenitor cells. The *colony-forming units*, or progenitor cells, which generate only neutrophil granulocytic series (CFU_{-G}), or only monocytes and macrophages (CFU_{-M}), exist in bone marrow and blood, along with colony-forming units capable of forming colonies containing both cell series (CFU_{-GM}). This co-existence suggests that neutrophil and monocyte macrophage series share a common progenitor.

Approximately 1 in every 1000 bone marrow cells in the human acts as a progenitor of one or other type of myeloid colony in currently employed culture procedures. Colonies do not develop unless their formation is stimulated by added material, referred to by a variety of terms such as *myeloid colony-stimulating activity* (G-CSF, M-CSF, GM-CSF). Such material is derived from various tissues, and it has been proposed, but not conclusively proven, that colony-stimulating activity released by monocytes and macrophages serves as the physiologically relevant stimulus for granulocyte production *in vivo*.

A somewhat greater proportion of cells in bone marrow gives rise to small colonies of eight or more red cell precursors, when stimulated in the culture by erythropoietin at a concentration which corresponds to that in the blood of subjects with moderate anaemia. This *erythroid colony-forming unit* (CFU_{-E}) possesses relatively limited proliferative potential *in vitro*, which approximates that of the pro-erythroblast *in vivo*. Colony-forming units committed to eosinophil production (CFU_{-EO}), or to megakaryocyte production (CFU_{-MEGA}), are also present in human bone marrow, and yield progeny under culture conditions only in the presence of certain stimulatory substances. The role of these stimulators in the *in vivo* production of these cell series is unclear.

A considerably smaller population of cells in bone marrow generates colonies that are relatively large and can contain several different blood cell series. The *erythroid burst-forming unit* (BFU_{-E}) is one example of this type of progenitor cell. It produces foci of up to thousands of cells when subjected to a stimulator, previously referred to as burst-promoting activity, in addition to erythropoietin. The BFU_{-E} is considered to be less mature than the CFU_{-GM} or CFU_{-E} in the hierarchy of blood cell development, and responds to burst-promoting activity (interleukin-3) by producing daughter cells which are in turn stimulated by erythropoietin to produce an agglomeration of erythroblast colonies. Net proliferative potential is considerably greater than in the case of the CFU_{-GM}, and it is evident at the termination of growth and maturation *in vitro* that haemopoietic cells other than erythroblasts are present.

It remains to be clarified whether erythroid burst-forming units differ fundamentally from other progenitors that possess a degree of multipotentiality, as indicated by their capacity to yield neutrophils, eosinophils, macrophages and erythroblasts when exposed to erythropoietin in addition to stimulators in conditioned medium derived from mitogen-stimulated lymphocytes. It does appear, however, on the basis of studies in mice, that progenitors of this type do not possess the essential property of the totipotential haemopoietic stem cell of being able to effect permanent reconstitution of haemopoietic tissue (Hodgson & Bradley 1979).

Progenitor cells are present in blood, but the site at which they undergo differentiation to produce blood cells in adults is normally limited to the micro-environment within the cavities of the bones. The induction of haemopoietic differentiation is understood to be mediated by specialized cells which are part of the stroma of the bone marrow (Lichtman 1981). Progenitor cells are located among

Table 1.1. *Cell composition of aspirated normal adult bone marrow*

Cell classification	Percentage of total cells
Granulocytic series	
Myeloblasts	0.1–3.5
Promyelocytes	0.5–5
Myelocytes	5–23
Metamyelocytes	7–27
Band forms	9–18
Segmented forms	4–28
Erythroid series	
Pro-erythroblasts	0.1–1.1
Basophilic	0.4–2.4
Polychromatic	2–30
Orthochromatic	2–10
Lymphocytes	5–24
Plasma cells	0–3.5
Monocytes	0–0.6
Macrophages	0–2
Megakaryocytes	0–0.5

Values are the *extremes* of ranges from various published sources reported by Dacie & Lewis (1984) and by Wintrobe *et al.* (1981). The mean percentage of granulocytic series is about 55 per cent, and erythroid series about 25 per cent. The ratio of granulocytic to erythroid series is usually between 2 and 4:1. Neutrophil series constitute approximately 90–95 per cent of the total granulocyte series, and eosinophils make up virtually all of the remainder.

low-density cells isolated by density-gradient separation of peripheral blood leucocytes, and cannot be distinguished on morphological criteria from lymphocytes. The proportion of progenitors is very low in peripheral blood leucocytes, and is less than one per cent of cells in bone marrow, which consists predominantly of differentiated cells with relatively low or absent proliferative capacity. Most of the cells in bone marrow can be reliably identified by their morphological features; the distribution of the various cell types in adult human bone marrow is shown in Table 1.1.

Morphology

The described appearance of cells in blood and bone marrow normally refers to cells spread flat on a plane glass surface during the spreading of a thin film of blood or bone marrow aspirate. The diameter of cells is consequently greater than in fixed tissue sections. Thin films can be more rapidly prepared for examination than tissue sections, and the flattened nature of cells in thin films permits greater resolution of the features of the cytoplasm and nucleus. Fixation of the cells is normally carried out by immersion of the air-dried film in methanol, and the staining of the cells by one of the Romanovsky dye preparations such as Giemsa, May–Grunwald–Giemsa, Leishman, Wright etc. These are metachromatic stains which develop a bluish colour in contact with acidic cellular components, and an orange–red colour when in contact with basic constituents. Nucleic acids, for example, are described as basophilic because of their affinity for the blue form of the dye.

Erythropoiesis

Red cells are produced by proliferation and differentiation of precursors whose dominant representatives in the bone marrow are the erythroblasts. Erythroblasts are referred to as normoblasts when their morphological features are within normal limits. During the course of differentiation, the size of erythroblasts progressively decreases, and the character of the nucleus and cytoplasm changes as the cells proceed toward the point where proliferative capacity is lost and haemoglobin becomes the predominant protein in the cytoplasm.

THE ERYTHROID SERIES

The *pro-erythroblast* is the least mature of the morphologically identifiable members of the erythroid series. It has a diameter of 14–20 μm, and a basically round outline with minor peripheral protruberances. There are several nucleoli in the nucleus, which is round and occupies most of the cell. The chromatin in the nucleus consists of a network of fine red–purple strands. A characteristic feature is that the peripheral cytoplasm is more basophilic than in the myeloblast, which is the corresponding member in the maturation sequence of the granulocytic series. Pro-erythroblasts undergo rapid division and give rise to basophil erythroblasts.

The *basophil erythroblast* is a round cell with a diameter of 12–16 μm, and more basophilic cytoplasm than the pro-erythroblast. It also undergoes rapid proliferation. The nucleus occupies a relatively large proportion of the cell, but differs from the nucleus of the pro-erythroblast by having coarser and more basophilic chromatin strands.

The *polychromatic erythroblast* is a round cell between 12 and 14 μm in diameter, and is the next stage in the maturation sequence after the basophil erythroblast. The characteristic polychromatic appearance of the cytoplasm is derived from the mixture of the basophilic ribonucleic acid (RNA) and acidophilic haemoglobin. Nuclear chromatin is in coarse, deeply basophilic clumps, and proliferative activity ceases after this stage. The polychromatic erythroblast occupies a position in the pathway of maturation between the early, immature stages characterized by active proliferation, and the later stages characterized by absence of proliferative activity and predominance of haemoglobin in the cytoplasm of the cell. For this reason these cells are frequently referred to as *intermediate erythroblasts*.

Orthochromatic erythroblasts constitute the next and final stage of maturation of the nucleated red cell series. They are smaller than their predecessors, and have a diameter between 8 and 12 μm. The nucleus is relatively small and pyknotic, with a homogeneous blue–black appearance. Active haemoglobin synthesis occurs in the cytoplasm, which contains mitochondria and ribosomes. The ribosomal RNA imparts a basophilic tint to the cytoplasm, although the cytoplasm is predominantly acidophilic due to the presence of large amounts of haemoglobin. Terms such as *pyknotic* or *late* are employed as alternatives to *orthochromatic* to describe this stage of erythroblast maturation.

The nucleus is extruded from the orthochromatic erythroblast to form the *reticulocyte*. Reticulocytes have the same biconcave discoid shape as mature red cells, although they have a slightly greater volume and diameter than the latter. Consequently, when the percentage of reticulocytes in the blood is abnormally high, the mean corpuscular volume of the overall red cell population in blood increases, and can rise above normal. Reticulocyte cytoplasm is similar in staining characteristics to that of orthochromatic erythroblasts, which are distinguished from mature red cells by a diffuse basophilic hue. Vital staining with dyes such as new methylene blue reveals deeply stained granules or chains of granules in reticulocytes, and this method is employed in the laboratory to identify reticulocytes in the determination of the reticulocyte count. Reticulocytes lose their mitochondria and ribosomes over the course of a few days, and in doing so, lose the basophilic tint and evolve into the *mature erythrocyte*. A detailed description of the properties of the mature erythrocyte is given in Chapter 2.

Red cells normally enter the blood at the stage of the reticulocyte or of the mature erythrocyte. It is currently not understood how these non-motile cells pass from the extravascular space into the blood within the sinusoids of the bone marrow, in view of the remarkable consistency with which red cells subsequently remain within the vascular compartment during their lifespan of approximately 120 days.

Granulopoiesis

The predominant white blood cell, or leucocyte, in the circulation is the mature granulocyte. The colour of the numerous granules in the cytoplasm after staining with Romanovsky stains is the basis of the classification of granulocytes into neutrophil, eosinophil and basophil series. This distinction is important, as the mature forms of the different granulocyte series perform different roles. Neutrophils are by far the most common circulating form of granulocyte, and play an essential role in phagocytosing and killing invading microorganisms. Eosinophils and basophils perform separate functions in inflammatory processes.

Mature granulocytes are produced by the proliferation and maturation of precursors from the earliest recognizable stage, the myeloblast, through the promyelocyte, myelocyte, metamyelocyte and stab-form stage, until the mature segmented stage is reached. Development of the neutrophil, eosinophil and basophil series follows a similar pattern, except that the characteristic distinction between the colour of the granules becomes obvious at the myelocyte stage.

THE GRANULOCYTE SERIES

The *myeloblast* is a relatively large cell, 15–20 μm in diameter, with a round to oval nucleus which occupies a large proportion of the cell. There are no typical granules in the moderately basophilic cytoplasm. Nuclear chromatin is arranged in a fine network of red–purple strands with occasional small aggregates. Nucleoli are typically prominent; while two or three is the usual number, there may be up to six nucleoli.

The following stage in the maturation sequence is the *promyelocyte*. The features of this cell are similar to those of the myeloblast, except for the development of some cytoplasmic granules and a slightly more coarse appearance of the chromatin. Nucleoli are still present.

The *myelocyte* is the next stage in the maturation sequence. It has prominent cytoplasmic granules, and the area of cytoplasm relative to the nucleus is greater than in the promyelocyte. The cytoplasm is also less basophilic, nucleoli are no longer present, and the chromatin appears more aggregated than in the promyelocyte. Granulocyte precursors undergo active proliferation until after the myelocyte stage.

Subsequent steps in the maturation process consequently occur in non-dividing cells, and in particular, involve progressive changes in the conformation of the nucleus from round in the myelocyte to segmented in the mature form.

The nucleus becomes indented and assumes a kidney-shaped appearance in the *metamyelocyte*. Granules are prominent in the cytoplasm.

When the degree of indentation of the nucleus is greater than 50 per cent of the nuclear diameter, the precursor has reached the *band* or *stab-form* stage. Cytoplasmic granules are identical to those in the mature segmented form.

The terminal stage of development is a cell 12–14 μm in diameter, characterized by a lobulated nucleus with two to five lobes of clumped chromatin, each linked by a thin chromatin strand. Such segmentation of the nucleus gives rise to the designation of these cells as *segmented* or *polymorphonuclear* granulocytes. An abnormally high number of nuclear lobes is indicative of disordered granulopoiesis. Approximately 1–3 per cent of segmented neutrophils in females have clearly defined drumstick-like appendages protruding from one of the nuclear lobes (Davidson & Smith 1954). Drumsticks are not present in males, and are thought to reflect the presence of the condensed chromatin of the inactivated X-chromosome in female cells, equivalent to the Barr body in buccal mucosal cells.

Polymorphonuclear eosinophils are slightly larger than segmented neutrophils and have a diameter of up to 16 μm. The number of nuclear lobes is usually two. The cytoplasm has a pale hue similar to that of the segmented neutrophil, and contains many granules which are larger than those in the segmented neutrophil. These granules stain bright orange with Romanovsky stains. They also stain with eosin, which is employed to identify eosinophils in the more accurate direct eosinophil count. Granules in eosinophil series stain more intensely with histochemical stains for peroxidase than granules in the neutrophil series.

Polymorphonuclear basophils are similar to the mature eosinophil, with the characteristic distinction that the granules are intensely basophilic, and tend to overlie and obscure the nucleus.

Stab and segmented granulocytes are motile, and thus possess the capacity to migrate into the blood passing through bone marrow sinusoids.

Formation of monocytes and macrophages

The monocyte–macrophage and granulocytic series collectively constitute the myeloid series, whose mature forms are the most important mobile phagocytic cells involved in host defence against infection. Mature monocytes have less vigorous phagocytic capacity and a longer lifespan than segmented neutrophils. They are able to re-enter the circulation, but are primarily distributed in the extravascular space. The macrophages, and the multi-nucleated giant cells to which they give rise, are distributed in the extravascular space. Macrophages located in lymph nodes, liver, spleen and bone marrow are an integral part of the reticuloendothelial system, which ingests and degrades both foreign and damaged autologous material.

THE MONOCYTE–MACROPHAGE SERIES

Monoblasts are the least mature of the morphologically recognizable members of the monocyte–macrophage series, and are very similar in appearance to myeloblasts. They are located predominantly in the bone marrow, which is the major site of monocyte production.

The *promonocyte* is the next stage in the differentiation pathway. It is similar in size to the promyelocyte, but has a more irregularly shaped, and often deeply cleft, nucleus containing nucleoli. The cytoplasm contains granules often arranged in a localized region, and the granules are larger and more basophilic than in the mature monocyte.

The mature *monocyte* is slightly larger than the segmented granulocyte. It has an irregularly shaped nucleus with a relatively fine chromatin pattern. The shape of the nucleus ranges from almost round to sufficiently indented to produce a lobulated appearance. Cytoplasm is abundant, and of a pale grey-blue tint. It contains some small neutrophilic or basophilic granules, which are less common than in granulocytes. Monocytes are motile cells and are thus capable of migrating into the blood passing through bone marrow sinusoids.

Macrophages range from 15 to 80 μm in diameter. They have one or more oval nuclei, and an irregular or oval cytoplasmic outline. Cytoplasm in larger macrophages is particularly abundant, and contains granules and, in some instances, vacuoles which may contain phagocytosed material. Giant cells have comparable features apart from the greater size of the cell and number of nuclei.

Distinction between the granulocyte and monocyte–macrophage series can be facilitated by a number of differences in histochemical properties. The monocyte–macrophage series tends to contain high levels of non-specific esterase, and low levels of peroxidase, relative to cells of the granulocytic series.

Lymphopoiesis

Production of lymphocytes has been much more extensively studied in experimental animals than in humans. Animal studies indicate that the lymphocytes which are present in foci in the bone marrow and in the thymus are engaged in particularly rapid proliferation which is not specifically related to antigenic stimulation. Lymphocytes migrate from these sites to other locations in the body. Germinal centres in other lymphoid tissues, such as lymph nodes and spleen, also actively produce lymphocytes, but do so to a greater extent as a response to antigenic stimulation.

Lymphocytes pass through a series of developmental changes in the course of evolving into various lymphocyte subpopulations, or subsets, yielding a complex interacting system which carries out immune responses. The developmental process in certain instances involves migration of immature precursors to other organs such as the thymus, where inductive effects on differentiation are mediated via locally produced factors.

Mature lymphocytes are engaged in extensive recirculation through the extravascular and vascular compartments. This is important in facilitating the recognition of foreign antigens by lymphocytes, and it naturally assists the recognition by lymphocytes of foreign antigens to which the individual has been previously exposed. Such immunological memory can persist for many years in circulating lymphocytes which have remained dormant in terms of immunological activity.

Cell-mediated and antibody-mediated immune responses involve a complex sequence of events in which lymphocyte subsets interact with other subsets of lymphocytes, as well as the macrophages which play a role in the processing of foreign antigens. The net result of these interactions is the generation of a population of cells with immunological reactivity directed towards the relevant antigen. Mature plasma cells represent the culmination of the processes involved in the antibody response, as these cells are particularly effectively in antibody production.

THE LYMPHOID SERIES

Lymphoblasts are slightly smaller than the myeloblasts which they resemble, except that the ratio of the diameter of the nucleus to that of the cell tends to be greater, and the number of nucleoli per nucleus tends to be fewer than in the myeloblast. Lymphoblasts are actively dividing cells. There is no readily detectable difference in appearance between actively dividing lymphoid cells in normal germinal centres and small lymphocytes which have been induced to divide *in vitro* by exposure to specific antigen or non-specific mitogens such as phytohaemagglutinin. Differentiation into mature forms does not proceed along such morphologically well-demarcated steps as with the other blood cell series, and the morphological features largely reflect whether the cell is engaged in proliferative activity or is in the dormant state.

The *large lymphocyte* is between 12 and 16 μm in diameter, and is round in outline. The nucleus is round or slightly indented, and its chromatin is more clumped than in the lymphoblast. The cytoplasm is more abundant than in the lymphoblast, and is usually pale blue, although it can extend to intense basophilia, particularly in certain inflammatory states. Some granules may be present in the cytoplasm, but are fewer than in granulocytes. Atypical large lymphocytes may be the predominant leucocyte in the circulation in viral infections such as infectious mononucleosis.

Small lymphocytes are between 9 and 12 μm in diameter, and are thus smaller than segmented granulocytes. The cytoplasm usually forms only a thin, medium to deeply basophilic rim encircling a round or marginally indented nucleus which contains deeply staining, heavily clumped chromatin.

Plasma cells at the most immature stage of development resemble lymphoblasts, except for possessing more basophilic cytoplasm. In the next stage of development, the nucleus is smaller, and the chromatin is more clumped. The nucleus at this intermediate stage has assumed the eccentric location at the periphery of the cell which is characteristic of the mature plasma cell. Nuclei of mature forms are round or oval with coarsely clumped chromatin. The ratio of the diameter of the cell to that of the nucleus is large, and the cytoplasm is basophilic, in keeping with its large content of RNA-laden ribosomes engaged in antibody synthesis.

T AND B LYMPHOCYTES

Morphological features do not provide an adequate index of the functional properties of lymphocytes. Human lymphocytes perform roles which can be broadly grouped into those that correspond in animal studies to thymus-derived lymphocytes (T cells) and bursa-derived lymphocytes (B cells). While some T cells contain occasional cytoplasmic granules, this criterion is not adequate to distinguish between T and B cells reliably.

T cells are characterized by the receptors on their surface which attach to sheep red cells at 4°C to form sheep red cell rosettes. This receptor for sheep red cells correlates with the CD2 surface antigen which is identified by its reactivity with specific monoclonal antibody. The CD2 surface antigen is one of the earliest specific surface antigens to appear during the process of T cell development. It is followed at a slightly later stage by the CD3 surface antigen, a molecule associated with the receptor on the T cell which binds to foreign antigen. This antigen-binding receptor is constructed of two distinct molecules whose genes have undergone rearrangement in a manner similar to that by which the immunoglobulin molecule attains its specificity to foreign antigen. At a somewhat later stage, the majority of T cells become committed to either helper cell or cytotoxic–suppressor cell status (Roitt *et al.* 1985).

T cells exert a wide variety of effects, including stimulatory and inhibitory regulatory action on immune responses, as well as cytotoxicity in the absence of specific antibody (*natural killer cells*) or in its presence (*antibody-dependent cytotoxic cells*). The T cells that stimulate immune responses and are known as helper cells possess a surface antigen (CD4) which can be identified by a specific monoclonal antibody. These T cells constitute a larger subset of the lymphocytes in peripheral blood than the subset which exerts suppressor action on immune responses. The latter subset can be identified by monoclonal antibody to a specific surface antigen (CD8).

B cells are usually identified in the diagnostic laboratory by detection of immunoglobulin on their surface with immunofluorescent procedures. The B cell population is derived from precursor cells in which rearrangement has taken place of the genes encoding the variable regions of the light and heavy chains of the immunoglobulin molecule. The specific nature of the rearrangement serves as the basis of the specificity of the antibody produced by the clone of cells generated from each precursor. In the next phase of development, μ chains appear in the cytoplasm before any immunoglobulin appears on the cell surface, a step described as the *pre-B cell* phase of differentiation. Development then proceeds through the *immature B cell* phase in which antibody of the IgM class alone appears on the cell surface. This is in turn followed by progression to the *mature B cell*, which possesses various immunoglobulin classes on its surface. Further exposure to specific antigen promotes the formation of the *plasma cell* which, in addition to possessing surface immunoglobulin, generates large amounts of immunoglobulin in its cytoplasm for secretion to the exterior.

B cells possess receptors which attach to the complement-binding (Fc) region of immunoglobulin heavy chains, and also to activated complement itself, but these receptors are present on other cell types and are therefore not specific.

NULL LYMPHOCYTES

A small proportion of lymphocytes in the circulation lacks the characteristic surface markers of either T or B cells, and these lymphocytes are consequently designated as *null cells*. Null cells are predominantly members of the immune system, but cannot be readily distinguished by simple procedures from the small proportion of other mononuclear cell types, such as progenitor cells.

LYMPHOCYTE PROLIFERATION

Small lymphocytes that are not in cell cycle can be stimulated to undergo mitosis. T cells respond in such a manner during the immune response *in vivo*, as well as after exposure to the non-specific mitogen, phytohaemagglutinin, *in vitro*. B cell proliferation occurs in response to antigenic stimulation, leading to the production of antibody *in vivo*, as well after exposure to bacterial lipopolysaccharide *in vitro*. Cells at all stages of the cell cycle can be identified as T or B cells by the previously described methods, and even immature malignant forms can be classified by these means in lymphoproliferative disorders. The basic features of T and B cells are summarized in Table 1.2.

Thrombopoiesis

Platelets are formed in the bone marrow by megakaryocytes, and are subsequently released into the vascular compartment where they play an essential role in haemostasis.

THE MEGAKARYOCYTIC SERIES

The most immature stage of platelet development is the *megakaryoblast*, which resembles the myeloblast in its basic features. These cells amount to less than eight per cent of the total megakaryocyte population.

The *promegakaryocyte* is the next stage in the sequence of maturation, and is larger than its precursor because it has undergone endoreduplication. *Endoreduplication* is nuclear replication without division of the cell, and is a characteristic feature of the more mature members of the megakaryocytic series. Such replication leads ultimately to the formation of very large cells containing up to 32 times the normal diploid content of deoxyribonucleic acid (DNA). Promegakaryocytes make up about 25 per cent of megakaryocytes, and have deeply basophilic cytoplasm containing some basophilic granules. The nucleus may be lobulated, and the chromatin is more deeply basophilic than in the megakaryoblast.

Mature *megakaryocytes* range from 30 to 90 μm in diameter, and contain 4 to 16 nuclear lobes with coarsely clumped chromatin. The larger expanse of cytoplasm stains light blue and contains many small red-purple granules. Platelets appear to be formed by protrusion into the bone marrow sinusoids of pseudopods of megakaryocyte cytoplasm, which detach into the bloodstream and fragment to yield small discoid platelets (Bessis 1950). Such a process

Table 1.2. *Properties of normal adult T and B cells*

	T cells	B cells
Percentage of peripheral blood lymphocytes*	42–74	16–28
Possession of immunological memory	+	+
Helper and suppressor capability	+	–
Effectors of cell-mediated immunity	+	–
Antibody-producing capability	–	+
Localization in lymph nodes	Paracortical regions	Germinal centres and medullary cords

*Uhr & Molle (1968).

would explain how the non-motile platelet enters the circulation (p. 374).

Platelets are the small, anucleate, terminal stage of development of the megakaryocytic series. They are discoid and have a diameter of 1–4 μm. The cytoplasm stains light blue and contains small red–purple granules which are centrally located in platelets in blood films. Clumping, or aggregation of platelets, occurs readily, and is particularly prevalent in inadequately anticoagulated blood, where it can cause spurious lowering of the platelet count.

Regulation of haemopoiesis

Erythropoiesis

A critical factor in the control of red cell production is the effective oxygen-carrying capacity of arterial blood. A decrease in the partial pressure of oxygen or oxygen-carrying capacity of arterial blood results in decreased oxygen delivery to specialized sensor organs, which respond by increasing the production of the erythropoietic stimulatory hormone *erythropoietin*. This causes an increase in red cell production, which in turn raises the arterial haemoglobin concentration in the course of correcting the deficit in oxygen delivery.

A decrease in erythropoietin production occurs when tissue oxygen delivery exceeds a certain threshold. This feedback system maintains a relatively constant blood haemoglobin concentration under normal circumstances, by matching the rate at which red cells are produced with the rate at which they are removed from the circulation. The sequence of events which occurs as a compensatory response to acute blood loss is summarized in Fig. 1.2.

Transfusion of blood sufficient to raise the haemoglobin concentration above normal, or prolonged inhalation of elevated partial pressures of oxygen, results in depression of erythropoiesis in keeping with the expected consequences of such a feedback system on erythropoietic regulation (Lawrence *et al.* 1952).

ERYTHROPOIETIN

Erythropoietin production in the human increases in response to a reduction in the oxygen-carrying

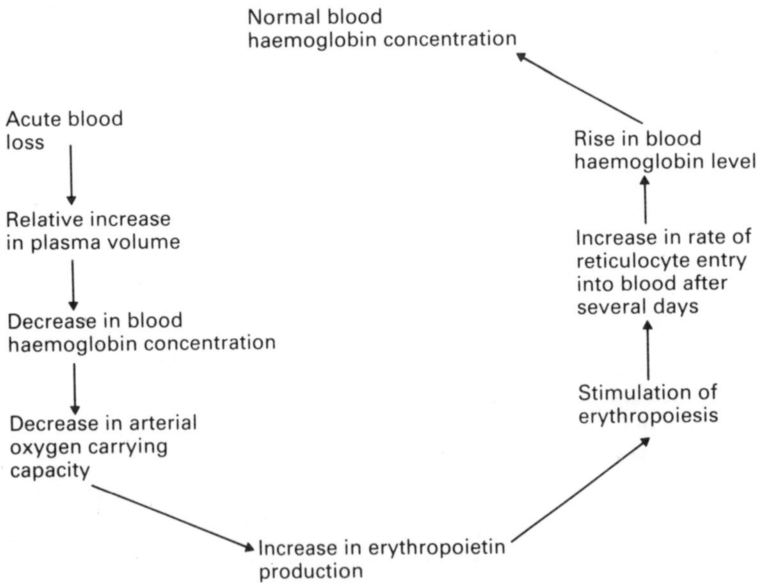

Fig. 1.2. *Overview of the mechanisms that lead to restoration of a normal blood haemoglobin concentration after haemorrhage.*

capacity of blood in the descending aorta, and the kidney appears to be the most important organ involved in this response to reduced tissue oxygen supply.

Erythropoietin is a glycoprotein, and when purified to homogeneity from human urine has a molecular weight of appoximately 70 000 (Miyake *et al.* 1977). Its concentration has traditionally been estimated by bioassay, but genetically engineered homogeneous material has been employed to develop a radioimmunoassay which will hopefully become available for routine diagnostic purposes.

The reference method for estimation of the biological activity of erythropoietin is based on determination of erythropoietic stimulation induced by injection of material into mice in which a low background level of erythropoietic activity has been induced by starvation, or by elevation of the blood haemoglobin concentration above the normal range. The amount of erythropoietin is then extrapolated from the extent to which erythropoiesis is stimulated, which is most commonly determined by measurement of radioactive iron incorporation into red blood cells after a period of several days. Measurement of erythropoietic stimulation in cultured erythropoietin-responsive tissues has more recently been employed in the hope that this would provide a more simple and sensitive procedure for determination of biological activity than intact animal procedures. The reliability of *in vitro* bioassays is, however, dependent on compensating for the considerable modifying influences of other human serum components on erythropoietic activity when *in vitro* procedures are employed to measure erythropoietin in human serum (de Kerk *et al.* 1978, Firkin & Russell 1983).

The concentration of erythropoietin in normal human serum is sufficiently low to be difficult to quantitate by bioassay, but rises substantially in almost all forms of anaemia. An important exception is anaemia secondary to loss of renal tissue.

The cell populations that respond to erythropoietin in the intact individual include morphologically unidentifiable erythroid precursors in the bone marrow, which produce pro-erythroblasts, and immature morphologically identifiable members of the erythroid series.

INFLUENCE OF ENDOCRINE HORMONES

Androgens stimulate red cell production to a considerable extent by enhancing the formation and release of erythropoietin, and are responsible for the relatively higher post-pubertal haemoglobin concentration in the male than the female. Orchidectomy in adult males results in a fall in haemoglobin concentration which can be corrected by androgen replacement therapy. Androgens act both by enhancing erythropoietin production and by exerting a direct stimulatory effect on the proliferation of erythroid precursors.

Hypophysectomy and hypothyroidism are associated with anaemia. The anaemia in hypothyroidism is largely caused by haemodilution due to expansion of the plasma volume, although some decrease does occur in erythropoietic activity (Finch *et al.* 1970).

Regulation of granulopoiesis

The mechanism by which neutrophil production is regulated is unclear, although it is recognized that tissue invasion by micro-organisms is accompanied by substantial stimulation of neutrophil granulopoiesis. Studies in subjects with subacute or chronic infection indicate that production of neutrophils increases up to 12 times the mean rate in healthy individuals (Athens *et al.* 1965). The extent to which the neutrophil count increases in the blood may approximate only roughly to the increase in the rate of production in subacute or chronic infection, and may fail to correlate with the extent of increased production in severe infection, when migration of neutrophils from the bloodstream is accelerated.

A mechanism proposed to explain the means by which neutrophil granulopoiesis is stimulated is that a variety of cells, such as the monocyte, after contact with invading bacteria release material that is transported in the blood to the bone marrow, where it stimulates the proliferative activity of the neutrophil granulocyte series.

Regulation of eosinophil granulopoiesis also remains to be clarified. Production of eosinophils increases substantially in the allergic response, and studies in animals indicate that interaction between lymphocytes and eosinophil granulocyte precursors accounts for the link between the recognition of the allergen and the increase in production of eosinophils (Basten & Beeson 1970).

Regulation of thrombopoiesis

Platelets normally circulate in the vascular compartment at a concentration that is regulated by a feedback mechanism: production is increased in response to accelerated removal of platelets, and decreased in response to infusion of platelets (de Gabriele & Penington 1967). The means by which the concentration of circulating platelets is sensed, and the various mechanisms responsible for the increase in production that occurs in accelerated platelet destruction, or in inflammation, remain to be clarified.

Haemopoietic reserve capacity

Erythroid precursors are required to produce about 2×10^{11} red blood cells per day to maintain a steady-state haemoglobin concentration in the blood of the normal adult. The most immature of the morphologically identifiable members of the erythroid series take approximately seven days to undergo maturation to the point where the reticulocyte enters the peripheral blood, but this interval decreases under conditions of increased demand for red blood cells (Finch *et al.* 1970). The extent to which the rate of production can increase in response to demand is estimated to be four to six times the mean normal value (Finch *et al.* 1970). Such increased production is achieved not only by acceleration of differentiation from the pro-erythroblast to the reticulocyte stage, but also by expansion of the total mass of erythroblasts in the body. This expansion results in an increase in the proportion of erythroblasts in the bone marrow, and in the amount of red marrow in regions normally occupied by yellow marrow.

Under conditions of extreme demand for red cells in severe anaemia, the time for transit from the pro-erythroblast to the reticulocyte stage is appreciably shortened. This is achieved in part by reduction in the number of cell divisions that occur during the maturation of the erythroid series, with elimination of the nucleus at an earlier stage to yield a relatively large *'stress'* red cell. The number of mature red blood cells contained within the bone marrow and spleen is relatively small in comparison with the amount in the circulation, and thus affords *relatively little reserve capacity* to cope immediately with increased demands for red blood cells.

Neutrophil granulopoietic precursors, as noted previously, are able to increase the production of segmented neutrophils up to about 12 times the normal rate when evaluated in adults with chronic infection. *Capacity to respond in this manner is reduced in young infants, and can compromise their ability to cope with infection.* The number of segmented neutrophils contained within the bone marrow is approximately three times that in the vascular compartment, and thus provides a reserve pool of cells which can be rapidly released into the circulation in response to increased demand for neutrophils.

Platelet production can also increase substantially in response to increased demand for platelets. Studies by Harker & Finch (1969) indicate that capacity to increase production is up to about eight times the normal value when evaluated in adults with increased rates of platelet destruction.

The bone marrow

Examination of the structure and cellular composition of bone marrow in the marrow aspirate and trephine biopsy is essential for diagnostic purposes in a wide variety of disorders affecting the haemopoietic system.

Normal bone marrow structure

The red marrow interspersed between the trabeculae of bone within the bony cavity contains specialized connective tissue cells, reticulin fibrils, blood vessels, fat cells, nerves and macrophages, in addition to cells of the lymphoid and haemopoietic series. The architecture of this tissue is illustrated in Fig. 1.3.

A supportive framework for the components of

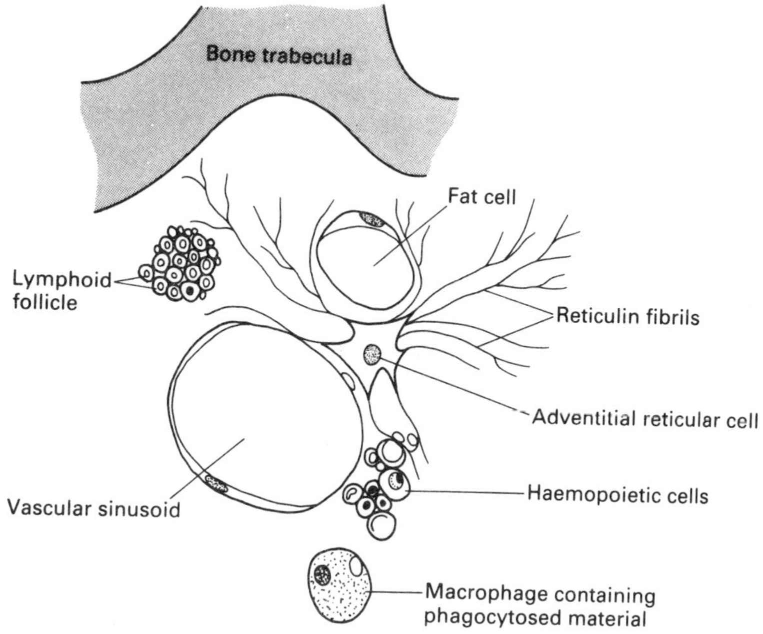

Fig. 1.3. *Schematic view of the architecture of red bone marrow.*

the bone marrow is provided by a network of fine *reticulin fibrils*. These fibrils stretch from the endosteum of the bony trabeculae to the vascular sinusoids and appear to be produced by the *adventitial reticular cell*, which is a different entity from the macrophage. Reticulin is delineated by silver staining, and is present in the form of very fine fibrils in normal subjects, although the amount is *greatly increased and accompanied by formation of collagen in pathological conditions such as myelofibrosis*.

Arteriolar blood passes into the relatively large lumen of *sinusoids* lined by a single layer of endothelial cells. Entry of newly formed blood cells into the circulation occurs at this site.

Fat cells make up approximately half the extravascular volume of red marrow, and nearly all of the extravascular volume of yellow marrow in the more peripheral parts of the long bones. Distribution of fat cells is irregular in red marrow, and an adequate sample size is necessary in order to obtain a reliable indication of the cellularity of haemopoietic tissue. Fat cells can be rapidly replaced by haemopoietic elements under conditions of increased demand for blood cell production. Lymphocytic and other blood cell precursors, as well as the macrophages which constitute the remaining important cellular components of the bone marrow, have been previously described.

Bone marrow biopsy

Aspiration of particles of bone marrow by suction via a wide-bore needle inserted into the bone marrow cavity is usually the method of choice for obtaining bone marrow for diagnostic purposes.

The advantages of this type of approach are that films prepared from aspirated material can be examined almost immediately, and the morphological detail is superior to that in histological sections of core biopsies obtained by the trephine procedure. The bone marrow trephine, on the other hand, provides a more reliable index of the cellularity of haemopoietic elements, and reveals certain abnormalities such as neoplastic cells or fibrotic material which may not be dislodged from the marrow cavity by suction. The information obtained by each procedure is therefore additive, so that the combined data is of greater diagnostic value than that provided by either procedure alone.

Bone marrow aspiration

Several types of aspiration biopsy needle are available. They consist in general of a strong, wide-bore, short-bevelled needle fitted with a stilette and an adjustable guard to prevent over-penetration.

The iliac crest and the body of the sternum are the most common sites for aspiration biopsy in adults, while the medial aspect of the proximal part of the tibia is preferred in children under the age of one year; in older children, the iliac crest should be used. Details of the procedure are described by Dacie & Lewis (1984). The choice of site in adults varies with the operator, and while sternal bone marrow is considered by some to be more cellular, the iliac crest procedure cannot be viewed by the patient and is thus less likely to provoke anxiety.

Sedation is usually employed, and general anaesthesia may be necessary with young children. The procedure is performed in a sterile manner. Local anaesthetic is infiltrated into the periosteum, before the needle is introduced into the bony cavity by pressure associated with to-and-fro rotation. After the cavity is penetrated, the stilette is withdrawn and a tightly fitting syringe is attached. Strong but brief suction yields about 0.2 ml of bone marrow tissue and contaminating peripheral blood. Successful aspiration is accompanied by transient pain.

Films are prepared immediately by placing the aspirated material on a glass slide, sucking off most of the blood, and preparing a film where the particles are drawn along by a spreader to leave trails of dislodged bone marrow cells (Fig. 1.4). Particles may also be added to fixatives for preparation of fixed-tissue sections.

The air-dried films are then fixed in the manner appropriate for the desired staining procedure. One of the Romanovsky stains employed for the staining of blood films is used for assessment of cellularity and morphology. Other histochemical stains include stains for iron and, particularly in the classification of acute leukaemia, stains for peroxidase, acid phosphatase, naphthyl acetate or butyrate esterase, and periodic acid-Schiff and Sudan black-reacting material.

Assessment of cellularity is attempted when the films preferably contain at least several particles. It may be difficult to visualize the haemopoietic cell content in large particles because of the overlap of cells. The number of cells in the trail is also employed as a guide to the degree of cellularity, but the results are less reliable than estimates based on examination of sections of bone marrow trephine biopsies. Serious interpretative errors can occur when particles are absent from the aspirate. It is incorrect to conclude that a bone marrow is hypocellular when few haemopoietic cells are present under such circumstances, as the sample may consist primarily of peripheral blood due to failure to retrieve bone marrow tissue in the aspirate.

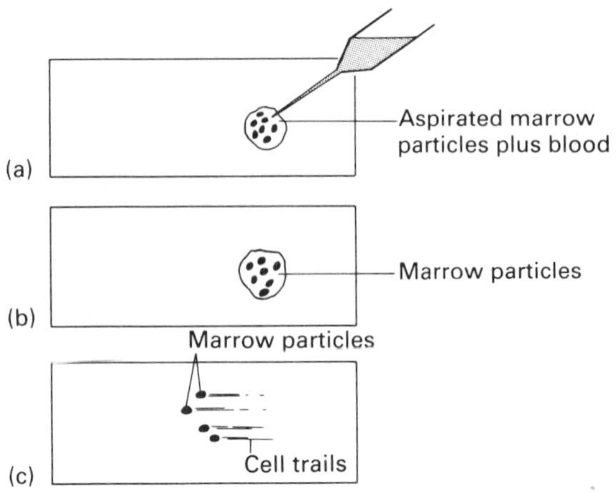

Fig. 1.4. *Preparation of films of aspirated bone marrow. (a) A drop of aspirated marrow is placed on one end of a glass slide. (b) The blood is sucked off with a Pasteur pipette to leave the marrow particles. (c) A film is made with a spreader, which leaves trails of marrow cells behind the marrow particles.*

Estimation of the proportion of individual cellular components of the bone marrow is relatively unreliable unless determined by differential counts of 500 or more cells. This enables the ratio of myeloid to erythroblast series to be calculated in order to estimate whether there is a *relative* abundance of either cell series. In the relevant circumstances, particular efforts are made to detect neoplastic cells infiltrating the bone marrow, abnormal macrophages in storage diseases, microorganisms such as acid-fast bacilli, fungi or protozoa in macrophages and, of course, atypical features in red cell and leucocyte precursors.

Failed aspiration

Failure to aspirate any material at all is referred to as a *dry tap*, while aspiration of blood without particles is referred to as a *blood tap*. Such inadequate results can be due to *technical factors* such as failure to site the tip of the needle in the bone marrow or to apply sufficient suction, or to *pathological factors* which prevent the disruption of the bone marrow into particles of suitable size for aspiration.

Pathological processes that interfere with aspiration include *increased connective tissue* in the bone marrow, which occurs classically in *myelofibrosis* and *hairy cell leukaemia*, and to a lesser extent in other disorders such as leukaemia, other myeloproliferative disorders, lymphoma, metastatic carcinoma and tuberculosis involving the bone marrow. Other causes are densely *hypercellular bone marrow*, and localization of the needle tip in *neoplastic tissue* such as metastatic carcinoma, lymphoma, or multiple myeloma. Occassionally, no obvious cause can be established for failure to aspirate particles, and thus *a dry or blood tap is not specifically diagnostic of any particular disease process.*

Bone marrow trephine biopsy

Trephine biopsy is performed by rotating a specialized biopsy needle under pressure, usually into the iliac crest, to obtain a core extending from the periosteum into the interstices of the bone marrow cavity. Various types of needles are available, but the needle devised by Jamshidi & Swain (1971) generally produces little disruption of the bone marrow architecture. Certain methods of fixation and embedding, such as in methacrylate, yield good structural definition in histological sections (Green 1970), and optimally prepared specimens provide an excellent index of the overall architecture, including the bone and connective tissue, the cellularity of haemopoietic elements, and the presence of lymphoid follicles, granulomas or infiltrating neoplastic cells.

Trephine biopsy is more suited than aspiration for detection of foci of certain types of neoplastic cells, and the likelihood of success is increased by obtaining the biopsy from potentially involved sites, such as areas of tenderness or of abnormality on X-ray or isotope scan. Foci of lymphoma can be detected by trephine biopsy in the absence of clinical or radiological abnormality of the bone, and the procedure is consequently widely employed in the *staging of patients with lymphoma*. Neoplastic cell foci, and even significant regions of hypoplasia, may be unevenly distributed and thus may not be revealed by a single trephine biopsy.

References and further reading

Athens, J.W., Haab, O.P., Raab, S.O., Boggs, D.R., Ashenbrucker, H., Cartwright, G.E. & Wintrobe, M.M. (1965) Leukokinetic studies XI. Blood granulocyte kinetics in polycythemia vera, infection and myelofibrosis. *J. Clin. Invest.* **44**, 778.

Basten, A.R. & Beeson, P.B. (1970) Mechanism of eosinophilia II. Role of the lymphocyte. *J. Exp. Med.* **131**, 1288.

Bessis, M. (1950) Studies in electron microscopy of blood cells. *Blood*, **5**, 1083.

Bradley, T.R. & Metcalf, D. (1966) The growth of mouse bone marrow cells in vitro. *Aust. J. Exp. Biol. Med. Sci.* **44**, 287.

Dacie, J.V. & Lewis, S.M. (1984) *Practical Haematology*, 6th Ed., Churchill Livingstone, London.

Davidson, W.M. & Smith, D.R. (1954) A morphological sex difference in the polymorphonuclear neutrophil leucocytes. *Brit. Med. J.* **2**, 6.

De Gabriele, G. & Penington, D.G. (1967) Physiology of the regulation of platelet production. *Brit. J. Haemat.* **13**, 202.

de Klerk, G., Hart, A., Kruiswijk, C. & Goudsmit, R. (1978) Modified method of erythropoietin (ESF) bioassay in vitro using mouse fetal liver cells II. Measurement of ESF in human serum. *Blood*, **52**, 569.

Finch, C.A., Deubelbeiss, K., Cook, J.D., Eschbach, J.W., Harker, L., Funk, D.D., Marsaglia, G., Hillman, R.S., Slichter, S., Adamson, J.W., Ganzoni, A. & Giblett, E. (1970) Ferrokinetics in man. *Medicine*, **49**, 17.

Finch, C.A., Harker, L.A. & Cook, J.D. (1977) Kinetics of the formed elements of human blood. *Blood*, **50**, 699.

Firkin, F.C. & Russell, S.H. (1983) Influence of human serum components on measurement of erythropoietin biological activity in vitro. *Scand. J. Haemat.* **31**, 349.

Goldwasser, E. (1984) Erythropoietin and its mode of action. *Blood Cells*, **10**, 147.

Green, G.H. (1970) A simple method for histological examination of bone marrow particles using hydroxyethyl methacrylate embedding. *J. Clin. Path.* **23**, 640.

Harker, L.A. & Finch, C.A. (1969) Thrombokinetics in man. *J. Clin. Invest.* **48**, 963.

Hodgson, G.S. & Bradley, T.R. (1979) Properties of haemopoietic stem cells surviving 5-fluorouracil treatment: evidence for a pre-CFU-s cell? *Nature*, **281**, 381.

Jamshidi, H. & Swain, W.R. (1971) Bone marrow biopsy with unaltered architecture: a new biopsy device. *J. Lab. Clin. Med.* **77**, 335.

Lawrence, J.H., Elmlinger, P.J. & Fulton, G. (1952) Oxygen and the control of red cell production in primary and secondary polycythemia. *Cardiology*, **21**, 337.

Lichtman, M. (1981) The ultrastructure of the hemopoietic environment of the marrow: A review. *Exp. Hematol.* **9**, 391.

Metcalf, D. & Moore, M.A.S. (1971) Haemopoietic cells. *Frontiers of Biology* 24, North-Holland, Amsterdam.

Miyake, T., Kung, G.K.H. & Goldwasser, E. (1977) Purification of erythropoietin. *J. Biol. Chem.* **252**, 5558.

Pluznik, D.H. & Sachs, L. (1965) The cloning of normal "mast" cells in tissue culture. *J. Cell. Comp. Physiol.* **66**, 319.

Quesenberry, P. & Levitt, L. (1979) Hematopoietic stem cells. *New Engl. J. Med.* **301**, 755.

Roitt, I.V., Brostoff, J. & Male, D.K. (1985) *Immunology*, Churchill Livingstone, Edinburgh.

Tavassoli, M. (1979) The marrow–blood barrier. *Brit. J. Haemat.* **41**, 297.

Uhr, J.W. & Moller, G. (1968) Regulatory effect of antibody on the immune response. *Adv. Immunol.* **8**, 81.

Wintrobe, M.M., Lee, G.R., Boggs, D.R., Bithell, T.C., Foerster, J., Athens, J.W. & Lukens, J.N. (1981) *Clinical Hematology*, 8th Ed. Lea & Febiger, Philadelphia

Chapter 2
The Red Cell;
Basic Aspects of Anaemia

Structure and metabolism of the red cell

Structure

Mature erythrocytes are unique among the cells of human tissues in that they normally lack nuclei and cytoplasmic structures such as lysosomes, endoplasmic reticulum and mitochondria. They exist in large blood vessels as biconcave discs, but their shape changes to a parachute-like conformation in the capillaries, which have a diameter less than that of erythrocytes in the biconcave disc form. The membranes of red cells are elastic and thus rapidly resume the biconcave disc form after the red cells re-enter larger vessels. Loss of flexibility or elasticity leads to membrane damage and shape change which is accompanied by diminished lifespan of the red cell in many different forms of anaemia.

MEMBRANE AND CYTOSKELETON

The membrane and cytoskeleton of the erythrocyte have in the past been collectively referred to as *stroma*. The membrane is normally a highly deformable, but non-expansile or contractile, structure. It is fragile, but its integrity is firmly maintained by the attachment of its inner surface to a lattice-like structure of specialized cytoskeletal proteins which supports the membrane and dictates the shape of the erythrocyte (Cohen 1983). The membrane is composed of certain specific proteins and lipids as outlined in Fig. 2.1.

The major protein component of the membrane is designated *band 3 protein*. It spans the full width of the membrane, and is understood to encase the channels through which the facilitated transport of anions and glucose takes place. The derivation of the term band 3 protein is based on the order in which this particular protein migrates during polyacrylamide gel electrophoresis of membrane proteins.

Another important transmembrane protein is *glycophorin*. The section protruding into the exterior is so heavily substituted with sugars that they comprise nearly two-thirds of the mass of the molecule, and contain most of the sialic acid which contributes to the negative charge of the outer surface of the red cell at physiological pH. Glycolipids in the outer leaflet of the membrane contain specific oligosaccharide sequences which constitute the *ABO blood group substances*. Phospholipid and, to a lesser extent, cholesterol are the dominant lipid components of the matrix of the membrane.

The most important constituent of the cytoskeleton is the protein *spectrin*. Intertwined spectrin molecules are linked together by a specific protein and actin to form a lattice-like network which is attached to the internal surface of the membrane. This network is a resilient structure, which normally causes red cells to resume the biconcave disc form after forces causing distortion have been removed. Specific sites on spectrin serve as points of attachment to molecules that protrude from the membrane (band 4.1 protein), and to the protein ankyrin which links spectrin to the internal pole of band 3 protein.

A heterogeneous group of abnormalities results from inherited defects in cytoskeletal components. Those that primarily cause defective binding of

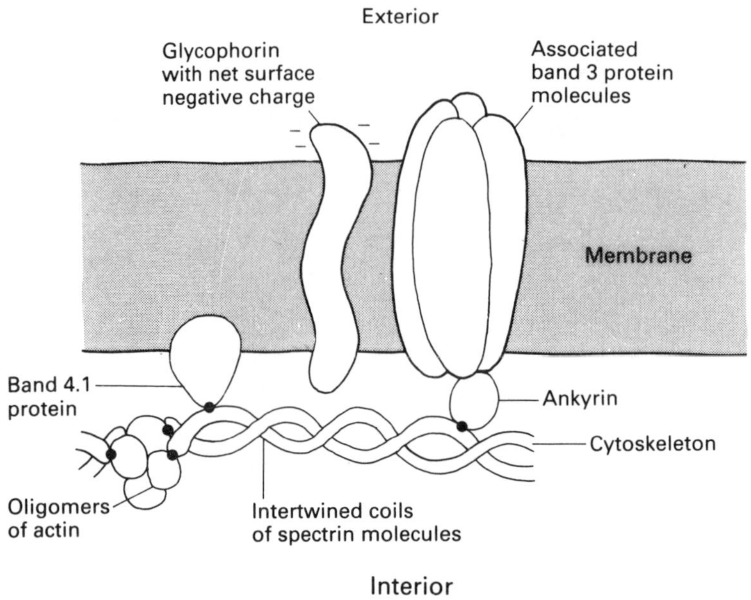

Fig. 2.1. *A simplified view of the current concept of the structure of the erythrocyte cytoskeleton and membrane.*

spectrin to the membrane impart fragility to the membrane, which leads to loss of part of the membrane and assumption of the *spherocytic* shape. Others that primarily cause loss of elastic resilience of the cytoskeleton lead to failure of the erythrocyte rapidly to resume the discoid shape, and this results in assumption of the *ovalocytic* shape.

Transformation of the shape of the red cell occurs under metabolic stresses to yield either *echinocytes,* characterized by protrusion of spiny processes of membrane from the external surface, or *stomatocytes,* characterized by a bowl-like appearance, as illustrated in Fig. 2.2.

Both types of change are reversible when the underlying derangement, such as an inadequacy of adenosine triphosphate (ATP) causing echinocyte formation, is corrected at an early stage. If not corrected, the processes proceed to acquisition of the spherocytic conformation, and ultimately lysis of the red cell.

CYTOPLASM

The cytoplasm of the red cell is made up overwhelmingly of haemoglobin. Haemoglobin makes up about 90 per cent of the dry weight of the erythrocyte, and is present in an amount about 30 times greater than that of the next most common cytoplasmic protein, the enzyme carbonic anhydrase. Confinement of haemoglobin within erythrocytes vastly reduces the viscosity that would prevail in the bloodstream if haemoglobin circulated as a solution in the plasma.

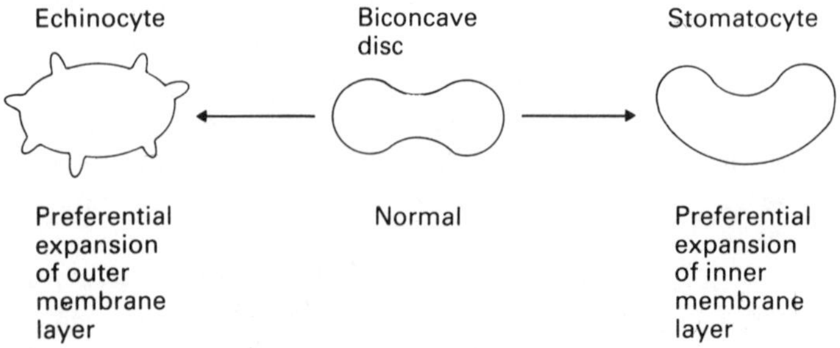

Fig. 2.2. *Echinocytic and stomatocytic transformation of the erythrocyte.*

HAEMOGLOBIN

Haemoglobin molecules consist of two pairs of polypeptide globin chains. Each globin chain bears a haem group whose central iron atom is the site at which oxygen attaches to haemoglobin. The type of globin chain synthesized by erythroid precursors undergoes progressive change with time after conception, and the nature of the globin chains dictates the oxygen-binding properties of the haem. Embryonic haemoglobins predominate until about the third month of gestation, after which fetal haemoglobin becomes the major form. Fetal haemoglobin consists of two α and two γ globin chains.

Adult haemoglobin A_1 consists of two α and two β globin chains, and the formation of significant amounts of haemoglobin A_1 commences just before the beginning of the third trimester. The proportion of haemoglobin A_1 then progressively increases to make up about 25 per cent of the total haemoglobin at birth, and about 97 per cent 12 months later. Fetal haemoglobin makes up less than two per cent of the total haemoglobin after the first year of life, and the small remaining portion consists of HbA_2. This minor form of adult haemoglobin consists of two α and two δ globin chains. It is present in only trace amounts in the fetus, and does not exceed 3–4 per cent of the total haemoglobin in normal adults.

The β globin chain confers different oxygen-binding characteristics on the haemoglobin molecule than are conferred by the α globin chain. Receptors are present on β but not on γ globin chains for 2,3-diphosphoglycerate. Attachment of 2,3-diphosphoglycerate to these receptors on adult haemoglobin A_1 decreases affinity for oxygen, and largely accounts for its lower oxygen affinity than fetal haemoglobin.

Glycosylation of haemoglobin

Several substances undergo non-enzymatic linkage to haemoglobin in circulating erythrocytes. The most important is glucose, which becomes covalently bound to haemoglobin in amounts that parallel the blood glucose concentration. The proportion of haemoglobin present as *glycosylated haemoglobin* A_{1c} can consequently be employed as an index of the average blood glucose level over the preceding few weeks in patients with diabetes mellitus (Koenig *et al.* 1976).

Metabolic processes

The survival of normal red cells is dependent in particular on their capacity to generate high-energy molecules in the form of *adenosine triphosphate* (ATP), and to generate the *reduced dinucleotides*, nicotinamide adenine dinucleotide (NADH) and nicotinamide adenine dinucleotide phosphate (NADPH).

ATP is produced by the relatively inefficient anaerobic glycolytic (Embden–Meyerhoff) pathway, as mitochondria are not present in the mature erythrocyte. About 90 per cent of the glucose entering the red cell is utilized for this purpose under normal conditions. Each glucose molecule is phosphorylated and then converted by a series of enzymatic steps to pyruvate or lactate, with the net production of two molecules of ATP as illustrated in Fig. 2.3.

A constant supply of ATP is necessary to drive the *cation pump*, which expels Na^+ and results in the acquisition of K^+ against the concentration gradients of both electrolytes. This removes excess Na^+ which has leaked into the erythrocyte, and thereby helps to prevent the electrolyte concentration from altering to the point where haemolysis takes place.

Large amounts of *2,3-diphosphoglycerate* are present in erythrocytes, and the molecule is produced by diversion of 1,3-diphosphoglycerate from the anaerobic glycolytic pathway, as shown in Fig. 2.3. Its level is regulated by the balance between the rates of synthesis and degradation in what is described as the *Rapoport–Luebering shunt* and, as previously described, is important in regulating the oxygen affinity of haemoglobin A_1. Storage of red cells in phosphate-free media is accompanied by a progressive decline in the content of 2,3-diphosphoglycerate, and this can lead to undesirably high oxygen affinity of haemoglobin in banked blood stored under such conditions.

The remaining ten per cent of the glucose entering the erythrocyte is utilized by the hexose

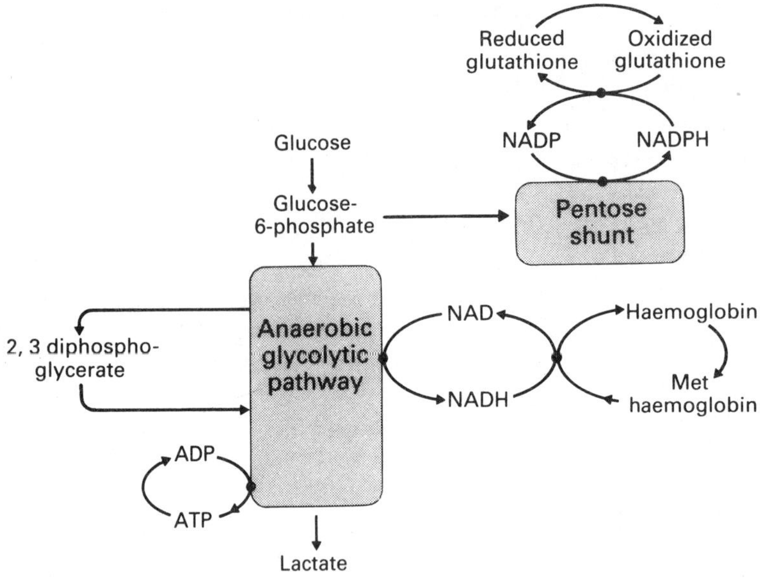

Fig. 2.3. *Inter-relationships between metabolism of glucose and key metabolic processes in the red cell.*

monophosphate pathway, or *pentose shunt*, under normal conditions. Reduced NADP is the most important product of this metabolic pathway in terms of the requirements of the erythrocyte, as it is the major source of the hydrogen atoms required to reduce oxidized *glutathione*. A constant supply of reduced glutathione is necessary to repair the effects of spontaneous oxidation of sulphydryl groups which leads to damage to the membrane and to the haemoglobin molecule.

Spontaneous oxidation of the *ferrous* iron in haem occurs in up to several per cent of the haemoglobin in red cells each day. The product is *methaemoglobin*, which contains iron in the *ferric* state and does not function in the body as an oxygen carrier. Methaemoglobin is converted back to haemoglobin by enzymatic reduction of the ferric iron, predominantly with NADH generated by anaerobic glycolysis, and to a lesser extent with NADPH generated by the pentose shunt. An increase in the rate of oxidation of haem is met by an increase in the activity of the pentose shunt, which can extend up to 20 times that of the normal value. Inability to increase the rate of reduction of NADP under such circumstances in subjects with an inherited deficiency of the first enzyme of the pentose pathway, *glucose-6-phosphate dehydrogenase*, leads to oxidant damage of erythrocyte components and haemolysis. Products of oxidant damage can form aggregates attached to the membrane and are referred to as *Heinz bodies*, which are visualized after supravital staining with dyes such as crystal violet, or less well with brilliant cresyl blue.

Carbonic anhydrase

This enzyme constitutes almost four per cent of the red cell protein, and catalyzes the reaction of carbon dioxide with water to form carbonic acid. The physiological role of this enzyme is uncertain, but a suggestion has been made that it enables the subsequent dissociation of carbonic acid into hydrogen and bicarbonate ions to occur at a rate sufficient to keep pace with other acid–base reactions in the erythrocyte.

Nutritional requirements for red cell production

Iron is essential for red cell production because it is part of the haem molecule in haemoglobin. The iron in haemoglobin normally makes up about two-thirds or more of the iron in the body. *Copper* plays an indirect role in red cell production: copper-containing macromolecules are believed to facilitate iron turnover in the body, as well as the incorporation of iron into protoporphyrin during the final stages of the synthesis of haem.

Vitamin B_{12} and *folic acid* play an interconnected role in the biosynthesis of the nucleotide precursors of nucleic acids. Defective formation of nucleic acids due to deficiency of either of these vitamins produces toxic changes in erythroblasts earlier than in almost all other tissues, presumably because of the need for active nucleic acid synthesis in the rapidly proliferating erythroid precursors.

Ascorbic acid (vitamin C) is believed to play an indirect role in erythropoiesis by facilitating the turnover of iron in the body, and also by maintaining certain folate intermediates in the functional state.

Pyridoxine (vitamin B_6) is important because pyridoxal-6-phosphate is a co-enzyme in the synthesis of δ-aminolevulinic acid. This is the first step in the biosynthesis of the protoporphyrin rings, of which four combine to form the porphyrin molecule. *Vitamin E* deficiency can lead to reduced resistance of the erythrocyte to oxidative stress, which is believed to reflect the lack of the antioxidant effect of this vitamin.

Severe amino-acid deficiency due to protein deprivation results in depression of red cell production, which appears to be mediated to a significant extent by decreased formation of erythropoietin.

Function of the red cell

The biconcave structure of the red cell provides a large surface area, which facilitates the entrance and exit of oxygen from the red cell in the course of its role as the major vehicle for oxygen transport in the blood. The presence of erythrocytes enables the blood to carry about 100 times the amount of oxygen than can be carried in plasma alone.

About one-third of the oxygen-binding sites in haemoglobin of erythrocytes in venous blood returning to the lungs is not combined with oxygen, and is thus in the 'deoxy' state. The relatively high partial pressure of oxygen in pulmonary capillaries leads to virtual saturation of available oxygen-

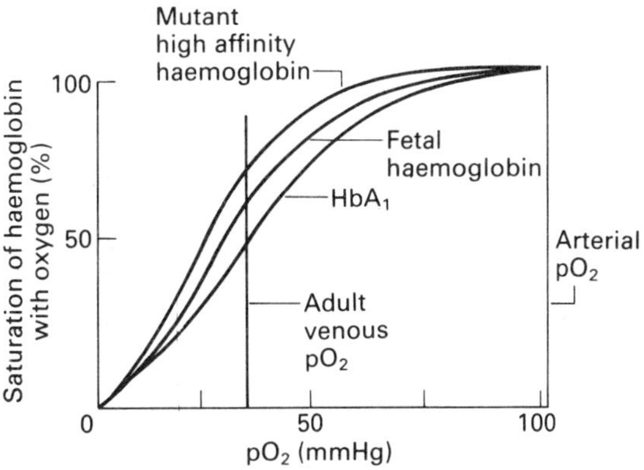

Fig. 2.4. *Oxygen dissociation curve of human haemoglobins at pH 7.4; pO_2 = partial pressure of oxygen.*

combining sites on haemoglobin as illustrated in Fig. 2.4. The erythrocytes then travel to tissue capillaries, where the prevailing partial pressure of oxygen is relatively low, and, as a result, release oxygen to an extent illustrated by the oxygen dissociation curve of haemoglobin in Fig. 2.4.

Reversible attachment of oxygen to form 'oxy' haemoglobin is mediated by non-covalent bonding of oxygen to the iron atoms in haem. The extent to which oxygen is released from haemoglobin at the partial pressue of oxygen in tissue capillaries is influenced to a physiologically significant extent by the *nature of the globin chain*, the pH, and the *concentration of 2,3-diphosphoglycerate* within the erythrocyte. Normal adult haemoglobin A_1 has lower affinity for oxygen than fetal haemoglobin, and thus releases a greater proportion of bound oxygen at the partial pressure of oxygen of tissue capillaries. Certain mutant haemoglobins also release less oxygen when the change in the composition of the globin chain has increased the affinity for oxygen.

A fall in pH increases oxygen dissociation by reducing the affinity of oxyhaemoglobin for oxygen, and this phenomenon, known as the *Bohr effect*, enhances the release of oxygen from erythrocytes at the lower pH existing in tissue capillaries where oxygen is required. The affinity for oxygen of adult haemoglobin A_1 also decreases with increasing concentration of intracellular 2,3-diphosphoglycerate. A rise in 2,3-diphosphoglycerate concentration occurs in anaemia and hypoxia, and thereby enhances the delivery of oxygen to the tissues (Oski *et al.* 1969).

Erythrocytes also perform a key role in *carbon dioxide transport* in the body. Carbon dioxide at the relatively high partial pressure in tissue capillaries diffuses into erythrocytes where most of it (about 70 per cent) is converted to bicarbonate ions, much of which re-enters the plasma. The process is reversed in the pulmonary capillaries by conversion of bicarbonate to carbon dioxide, which diffuses into the alveoli of the lungs and is exhaled.

About one-third of the carbon dioxide produced by the tissues forms a chemical compound with deoxyhaemoglobin known as *carbaminohaemoglobin*. This compound breaks down and releases carbon dioxide when the erythrocyte is exposed to the lower partial pressure of carbon dioxide in the pulmonary capillaries.

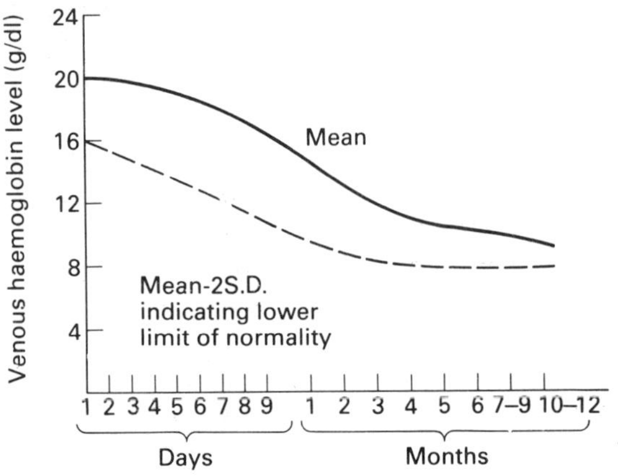

Fig. 2.5. *Haemoglobin level in the first year of life. (Walsh & Ward 1969)*

Red cell values

There has been a progression in most countries towards acceptance of the International System of Units (SI) for expression of haematological indices. Values are now determined in many countries largely by electronic means, although such devices do not produce a result for the haematocrit as defined by the proportion of packed red cells obtained by centrifugation of the blood.

Normal red cell values depicted in Table 2.1 refer to northern European Anglo-Saxon populations, and are expressed as means ± two standard deviations. These include values for most normal people: the mode in which they are expressed encompasses about 95 per cent of individuals in a so-called normally distributed population. Values outside this range are for practical purposes considered abnormal, although it is evident that a few per cent of normal people will have values just above or below this range.

Blood haemoglobin level

The level of haemoglobin in blood is normally determined in the laboratory by spectrophotometric measurement of the concentration of the cyanmethaemoglobin derivative of haemoglobin after lysis of the red cells (Dacie & Lewis 1984).

INFLUENCE OF AGE AND SEX

The mean haemoglobin level at the time of delivery in full-term infants is 16.5 ± 3.0 g/dl in cord blood. The haemoglobin level rises in the subsequent 24 hours due to transfusion of placental blood into the infant, followed by a compensatory reduction in plasma volume. After several days, the haemoglobin level begins a progressive fall, which continues (as shown in Fig. 2.5) to a nadir of about 12.0 ± 1.0 g/dl at the 12th month of life. The

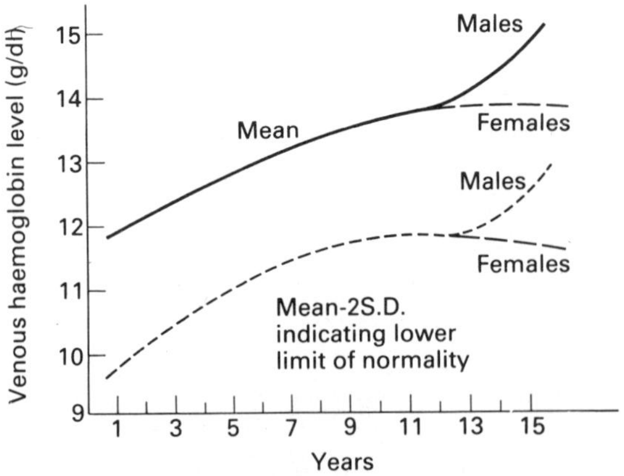

Fig. 2.6. *Haemoglobin levels in childhood and adolescence. (Walsh & Ward 1969)*

level then rises progressively until the beginning of puberty, when the adult value for the female is established. The level rises further in the male until a plateau about 1.5 g/dl higher than in the female is reached (Fig. 2.6).

Mean values then remain essentially constant until the age of about 70 years, when they fall progressively by approximately 0.5 g/dl per decade.

PHYSIOLOGICAL VARIATION

A minor degree of diurnal variation occurs: the haemoglobin level is slightly higher in the morning than in the evening. Such variation in any one individual is usually considerably less than 1.0 g/dl. Assumption of the horizontal posture is associated with a relatively rapid fall in haemoglobin level of comparable magnitude, thought to

Table 2.1. *Normal* red cell values (mean ± 2s.d.) (Dacie & Lewis 1984)*

Red cell count	
Men	$5.5 \pm 1.0 \times 10^{12}$/l
Women	$4.8 \pm 1.0 \times 10^{12}$/l
Full-term/cord blood	$5.0 \pm 1.0 \times 10^{12}$/l
Children, 1 year	$4.4 \pm 0.8 \times 10^{12}$/l
Children, 10–12 years	$4.7 \pm 0.7 \times 10^{12}$/l
Haemoglobin	
Men	15.5 ± 2.5 g/dl
Women	14.0 ± 2.5 g/dl
Full-term/cord blood	16.5 ± 3.0 g/dl
Children, 1 year	12.0 ± 1.0 g/dl
Children, 10–12 years	13.0 ± 1.5 g/dl
Packed cell volume (PCV; haematocrit)	
Men	0.47 ± 0.07 (l/l)
Women	0.42 ± 0.05 (l/l)
Full-term/cord blood	0.54 ± 0.10 (l/l)
Children, 3 months	0.38 ± 0.06 (l/l)
Children, 10–12 years	0.41 ± 0.04 (l/l)
Mean corpuscular volume (MCV)	
Adults	85 ± 9 fl
Full-term/cord blood	106 fl (mean)
Children, 1 year	78 ± 8 fl
Children, 10–12 years	84 ± 7 fl
Mean corpuscular haemoglobin (MCH)	
Adults	29.5 ± 2.5 pg
Mean corpuscular haemoglobin concentration (MCHC)	
Adults and children	33 ± 2 g/dl
Mean corpuscular diameter in dry films	
Adults	6.7–7.7 μm
Reticulocytes	
Adults and children	0.2–2.0 % or 2–16 $\times 10^{10}$/l
Full-term/cord blood	2–6 %

*Normal for northern European Anglo-Saxon populations; $\mu = 10^{-6}$, $p = 10^{-12}$, $f = 10^{-15}$.

reflect a relative increase in plasma volume due to redistribution of tissue fluid. The opposite trend occurs soon after assuming the erect posture (Fawcett & Wynn 1960).

Day-to-day variation occurs to a greater degree, and is most pronounced in women. The range is 0.8–3.0 g/dl, and a factor postulated to contribute to the reduced level is a relative increase in plasma volume in the premenstrual phase (Cotter *et al.* 1953).

The influence of factors such as these should be considered before the diagnosis of anaemia is made on the result of a single haemoglobin estimation. Variability also hampers assessment of the trend in the haemoglobin level in disorders of the blood, and the overall pattern in more than two estimations provides a more reliable indication of the course of events.

PREGNANCY

Plasma volume increases by a mean of 43 per cent in pregnancy, which produces a fall in haemoglobin level despite a mean increase of 25 per cent in the total volume of circulating red cells (Low *et al.* 1965). The haemodilutory effect commences in the first trimester. The lower limit of the haemoglobin level in normal pregnant women is about 10.5 g/dl, and is thus less than in the non-pregnant state.

Red cell count

Before the advent of reliable, automated electronic counting devices in the routine diagnostic laboratory, the red cell count was estimated visually in a haemocytometer on diluted samples of blood. The number of red cells that it is feasible to count under diagnostic laboratory conditions by the latter method is insufficient to yield a highly reproducible value (Dacie & Lewis 1984). For this reason, the red cell count was formerly rarely employed in clinical practice as an index of the adequacy, or otherwise, of red cells in the blood. Vastly greater numbers of red cells can be counted in a brief interval by currently available electronic devices, and the error in the red cell count is consequently reduced to an order comparable to, or even less than, that of the haemoglobin level.

Haematocrit

The haematocrit or packed red cell volume (PCV) refers to the *proportion of the volume of red cells relative to the total volume of the blood.* High-speed centrifugation in the microhaematocrit procedure used to sediment the red cells yields highly reproducible results. The values do not correspond strictly to those obtained by electronic automated devices which derive a result from a formula which involves multiplying the red cell count by the mean red cell volume. The microhaematocrit procedure is of value in providing a reliable and simple means for rapid determination by the clinician of the red cell content of the blood.

Red cell indices

Mean corpuscular volume

The mean volume of red cells (MCV) was formerly determined by dividing the total volume of red cells (derived from the packed cell volume, PCV) by the number of red cells in that particular sample of blood. The accuracy of the total volume determination by the manual haematocrit method provided little difficulty, but manual estimation of the red cell count was laborious and unreliable, so that determination of MCV, like the red cell count, was formerly rarely performed in the routine diagnostic laboratory.

Automated electronic-particle counting devices have revolutionized the estimation of the MCV. Most devices measure the electrical impedance caused by each red cell as it passes through the counting mechanism, and the extent of the impedance provides an accurate indication of the volume of each cell. Such machines not only indicate the profile of the distribution of the volume of red cells, but also provide a highly reproducible value for the MCV. The MCV derived by this means therefore provides a reliable index of the average size of red cells, which is a guide of considerable importance to the nature of the disorder underlying an abnormality in the haemoglobin level. A subnormal MCV is indicative of microcytosis, and an elevated MCV indicative of macrocytosis.

Mean corpuscular haemoglobin

The mean amount of haemoglobin per red cell (MCH) is also rapidly and reliably estimated by automated electronic counting devices by dividing the total amount of haemoglobin by the number of red cells in a sample of blood. A subnormal MCH occurs in microcytosis, but is even lower when microcytosis occurs in conjunction with a subnormal concentration of haemoglobin in the red cell, as in thalassaemia minor or iron deficiency.

Mean corpuscular haemoglobin concentration

The mean concentration of haemoglobin within red cell (MCHC) reflects an entirely different parameter than the MCH. It is derived by dividing the concentration of haemoglobin in g/dl by the volume of red cells in ml/dl. Both measurements are readily and reliably obtained by manual methods, and the result is expressed in g haemoglobin/dl packed red cells.

A subnormal MCHC is usually indicative of an abnormality where interference with the synthesis of haemoglobin is greater than that of other constituents of the red cells, as in thalassaemia or iron deficiency. Elevated values reflect dehydration of the erythrocyte, and one of the relatively few important clinical causes of this phenomenon is *spherocytosis*. Values obtained by automated electronic counting devices are indirectly determined, and not only fail to correspond strictly to those obtained when the microhaematocrit method is employed to estimate the PCV, but also fail to display a shift to the same extent in abnormal states as values determined by the traditional method.

Definition of anaemia

Anaemia is present when the haemoglobin level in the blood is below the lower extreme of the normal range for the age and sex of the individual. The lower limit of normality is reduced during pregnancy.

A common error leading to misdiagnosis of anaemia is failure to refer to the normal range appropriate for the age and sex of the individual, as an acceptable level in a one-year-old child could represent moderately severe anaemia in an adult male. The haemoglobin level is employed as the prime arbiter in the diagnosis of anaemia. The red cell count does provide an alternative means of assessment, but it can be in the normal range in people who are anaemic on the basis of the haemoglobin level when the red cells are microcytic, as in thalassaemia minor or iron deficiency.

Abnormal red cell indices can exist in subjects even where the underlying disorder is not sufficiently severe to cause anaemia. This is not uncommon in thalassaemia minor or iron deficiency, where the MCV, MCH and MCHC can be low, and in megaloblastosis, where the MCV and MCH are elevated.

Physiological adaptations in anaemia

Tissue hypoxia develops when compensatory physiological adjustments that enhance release of oxygen from haemoglobin, and increase the flow of blood to the tissues, fail to counteract the effects of the decreased oxygen-carrying capacity of the blood caused by the subnormal level of haemoglobin. Hypoxia causes impairment of function in many tissues, and the symptoms and signs of anaemia are therefore referred to many systems. The degree of functional impairment of individual tissues depends largely on their oxygen requirements, and thus symptoms referable to systems with high requirements, such as the skeletal musculature during activity, the heart and the central nervous system, are particularly prominent.

Several mechanisms are brought into play in anaemia to make more effective use of the available haemoglobin for delivery of oxygen to the tissues.

Increased release of oxygen from red cells. A greater proportion of the oxygen attached to haemoglobin is released when the red cell passes through the tissues in anaemic subjects. This results from the increase in concentration of 2,3-diphosphoglycerate which takes place in the red cell in anaemia; the oxygen dissociation curve (see Fig. 2.4) is shifted to the right, and a greater proportion of the oxygen on the haemoglobin molecule is released at the partial pressure of oxygen of venous blood. It has been calculated that the extent of the change in the oxygen dissociation curve that occurs at a haemoglobin level of 5 g/dl is accompanied by release of a further 90 per cent of the oxygen attached to the haemoglobin of the red cell (Huehns 1971).

Increased blood flow. Cardiac output increases in anaemia, mainly as a consequence of increased stroke volume. This *high output state* increases oxygen delivery to tissues by increasing the flow of blood through them, and tends to occur to a progressively increasing extent in resting, otherwise fit individuals as the level of haemoglobin falls below 7 g/dl.

Maintenance of blood volume. The volume of the blood is maintained within approximately normal limits by an increase in the volume of the plasma to counteract the decrease in the volume of red cells. A relatively rapid flow of fluid from the extravascular to the intravascular space occurs after acute blood loss, and along with other changes, results in restoration of the circulatory volume after 48–72 hours (Walsh & Ward 1969). Adjustment occurs insidiously in more slowly developing forms of anaemia.

Redistribution of blood flow. Some deviation of blood flow occurs from tissues with lesser oxygen requirements to those with greater requirements. Thus, skin blood flow is reduced, while cerebral and muscle blood flow are increased.

Clinical features of anaemia

The symptoms and signs in an anaemic patient are due to:

the anaemia itself;

the disorder causing the anaemia.

The relative prominence of each of these groups of symptoms varies in the individual patient, depending on the degree of anaemia and the nature and severity of the causative disorder. Frequently, the manifestations of the causative disorder are mild or absent, and the symptoms of anaemia dominate the clinical picture.

The haemoglobin level at which symptoms of anaemia develop depends on two main factors: the rate of development of the anaemia, and the age and state of the cardiovascular system of the patient.

In general, symptoms occur at a higher haemoglobin level with rapidly developing anaemias, e.g. anaemia due to acute haemorrhage, than in a slowly developing anaemia. Children and younger adults can tolerate a much greater degree of chronic anaemia than older patients, due largely to the fact that, with advancing age, the cardiovascular system is unable to compensate as efficiently. In some adults, symptoms, e.g. tiredness and lassitude, develop when the haemoglobin value falls to between 10 and 11 g/dl, but care should be taken not to confuse these symptoms with those of an underlying disease which, in turn, is causing the anaemia. It is not uncommon for the haemoglobin level to drop to much lower values before symptoms occur, and then the symptomatology is largely that of limitation of exercise tolerance. With a slowly developing anaemia, such as that due to chronic gastrointestinal bleeding, the haemoglobin level may fall to 6 g/dl or less without the patient having any significant disability. Children with moderately severe congenital haemolytic anaemia, and haemoglobin levels of 8–9 g/dl, often lead a normally active life.

The age of the patient also influences the nature of the symptoms; cardiac and cerebral symptoms are more prominent in the older age group because of the association of degenerative cardiovascular disease with age.

Symptoms and signs of anaemia are now considered in detail.

Fatigue and weakness

Tiredness, lassitude, easy fatiguability, and generalized muscular weakness are the most common, and often the earliest, symptoms of anaemia. However, many individuals with these symptoms are not anaemic. Such symptoms occur in other conditions, and are especially prominent in neurotic disorders.

Pallor

Pallor is the most prominent and characteristic sign. It may be seen in the skin, nail beds, mucous membranes and conjunctivae. Skin pallor, particularly of the face, is a sign that must be interpreted with caution. The colour of the skin depends not only on the haemoglobin level in the blood, but also on the state of the blood vessels, the amount of fluid in the subcutaneous tissues, and the degree of skin pigmentation. Pallor is commonly seen in persons who are not anaemic, such as those who remain indoors, and patients with nephritis or myxoedema. Furthermore, patients with mild anaemia, and some with moderate anaemia, show no pallor of the face. Marked dilatation of the small vessels of the cheeks, which occurs in some people, especially middle-aged males, may mask the presence of anaemia. Pallor of the palms of the hands, particularly of the skin creases, is more reliable than pallor of the skin elsewhere, provided the hands are examined while warm.

Pallor of the nail beds, mucous membranes of the mouth, and conjunctivae is a more reliable indication of anaemia than is pallor of the skin. Pallor in these sites should be looked for in any patient suspected of being anaemic. Conjunctival pallor is sought by turning down the lower eyelid.

The character of the pallor may be influenced by the nature of the disorder causing the anaemia. After severe acute blood loss, superficial skin vessels are constricted and the skin becomes dead white in colour. In acute leukaemia, pallor is often pronounced and may be associated with an ashen tint of the skin. In advanced pernicious anaemia, the skin may have a lemon or pale yellowish tint.

Cardiovascular system

Clinical manifestations in the cardiovascular system may result from three factors: (i) the effect of hypoxaemia on the myocardium; (ii) pre-existing heart disease; and (iii) the high cardiac output state.

Dyspnoea on exertion and palpitation are common symptoms. Dyspnoea usually occurs only on exertion or with emotional stress, but in very severe anaemia (e.g. 3 g/dl or less), and in patients with cardiac failure, dyspnoea may occur at rest.

Angina pectoris can occur in older patients. Most anaemic patients who develop angina have some degree of coronary artery stenosis which may not, in the absence of anaemia, be sufficiently severe to cause ischaemic heart pain. The haemoglobin level at which angina occurs varies with the extent of the stenosis. The haemoglobin level should thus be determined in patients suffering from angina, as anaemia represents a treatable factor that can contribute to myocardial ischaemia.

Intermittent claudication may be precipitated by anaemia, typically in patients with atherosclerotic vascular disease.

Murmurs are relatively common, and become more prominent as the degree of anaemia increases. They may be caused entirely by the haemodynamic changes secondary to the anaemia itself (haemic murmurs), by underlying heart disease, or by a combination of both factors. Haemic murmurs are nearly always mid-systolic 'flow' murmurs, reflecting the increased velocity of blood passing through the valves. They are common in the pulmonary area, but can be heard in areas corresponding to any of the heart valves. Diastolic flow murmurs occur, but are uncommon. Severe anaemia, especially in the older patient, may provoke ventricular dilatation and cardiac failure. The dilatation may be sufficient to cause secondary regurgitant murmurs. Very severe anaemia in its own right can precipitate cardiac failure in individuals with a normal cardiovascular system. Systolic bruits may also be heard over the peripheral arteries as a consequence of the increase in blood flow.

Many of the abnormal cardiovascular features, such as angina pectoris, flow murmurs, and cardiac failure, disappear after restoration of the haemoglobin level to normal. Such correction is obviously more likely to occur in individuals who have no significant underlying myocardial, atherosclerotic or valvular lesions.

The *high output state* in severe anaemia is characterized by a high pulse pressure with a 'collapsing' character to the pulse, and features of increased stroke volume on palpation over the apex of the heart. Sometimes the jugular venous pressure is elevated, although this and the mild oedema that occurs in otherwise fit individuals with severe anaemia are not usually the consequences of cardiac failure.

Electrocardiographic changes are found in approximately 30 per cent of patients with a haemoglobin value of less than about 6 g/dl. The usual findings are normal QRS waves, depression of the

S–T segments, and flattening or inversion of T waves. In the absence of pre-existing heart disease, these changes disappear when the anaemia is corrected.

Central nervous system

Symptoms referable to the nervous system are common in severe anaemia, particularly in older patients who have some degree of cerebrovascular disease. Symptoms include faintness, giddiness, headache, roaring and banging in the ears, tinnitus, spots before the eyes, lack of concentration and drowsiness, and, with severe anaemia, clouding of consciousness.

Numbness, coldness, and sometimes tingling of the hands and feet may be complaints in severe anaemia.

Fundi

Abnormalities in the fundi due to anaemia are essentially restricted to severe anaemia. The retina may appear pale, but this change is relatively difficult to assess. Haemorrhages are more common when vascular disease is also present, and particularly when there is an associated bleeding diathesis due to thrombocytopenia. Papilloedema has been reported as a rare consequence of severe anaemia.

Reproductive system

Menstrual disturbances are often associated with anaemia. Amenorrhoea is the most common sequel of anaemia, and is sometimes the presenting symptom. Menorrhagia, on the other hand, is more usually a cause of anaemia, although rarely it appears to result from anaemia. In disorders causing both anaemia and thrombocytopenia, e.g. acute leukaemia, menorrhagia is common because of the severe bleeding diathesis. Loss of libido may occur in the anaemic male.

Renal system

Slight proteinuria and some impairment of the concentrating power of the kidney can occur in severe anaemia. Although anaemia does not cause significant renal failure in individuals with previously normal kidneys, it may reduce renal function in individuals with renal impairment to a point at which uraemia develops. In such patients, correction of the anaemia is usually followed by a fall in blood urea.

Gastrointestinal system

Symptoms referable to the alimentary tract are common in anaemic subjects, but are usually due to the causative disorder rather than the anaemia itself. Anorexia is the commonest symptom due to anaemia *per se*, but flatulence, nausea and constipation may also occur. Weight loss is not usually caused by anaemia alone and, when marked, suggests that an underlying or complicating disorder is present.

Pyrexia

Mild pyrexia may occur in severe anaemia with a hyperplastic bone marrow, but marked fever is due either to a causative disorder or to a complicating factor.

Recognition and investigation of the anaemic patient

The basic questions to be considered are:

1 Is the patient anaemic?

2 If this is the case, what is the type of anaemia indicated by examination of the blood?

3 What is the cause of the anaemia?

Is the patient anaemic?

The symptoms that point to the possibility of anaemia are, in particular, lethargy, easy fatiguability, tiredness and effort intolerance (Table 2.2). These symptoms are obviously not specific for anaemia and can easily be misinterpreted as symptoms of emotional, respiratory or cardiovascular disorders. They are also less prominent in anaemia of insidious onset, and in otherwise fit individuals. A *high index of suspicion* must therefore be main-

Table 2.2. *Clinical manifestations of anaemia*

Symptoms	
Common	Fatigue, tiredness, effort intolerance, effort dyspnoea, palpitations
Less common	Faintness, giddiness, pounding in the ears, effort angina*
Signs	
Common	Pallor
Less common	High cardiac output state, congestive cardiac failure*

*More likely in elderly subjects.

tained in order to avoid overlooking the presence of anaemia. The most important physical sign is *pallor*, and the best single site to assess pallor due to a subnormal haemoglobin level is the *conjunctivae* on the turned down lower eyelid. Unequivocal *conjunctival pallor is not inevitably present in all patients with anaemia.* It is often absent in anaemia when the haemoglobin level is greater than 9 g/dl, although it is usually present when the haemoglobin level is less than 6 g/dl. The presence of anaemia is established by laboratory confirmation of a subnormal haemoglobin level.

What is the type of anaemia?

The type of anaemia is generally indicated by the features of the red cells, leucocytes and platelets noted in the examination of the blood. It is now common practice to employ automated electronic devices to establish the level of haemoglobin, red cell count, mean red cell volume, mean corpuscular haemoglobin, mean corpuscular haemoglobin concentration, leucocyte count, and platelet count. *Examination of the blood film* constitutes a particularly important part of establishing the cause of anaemia, as it remains the best method for detecting aberrations in red cells indicative of specific pathological entities, and of associated abnormalities in leucocytes. In appropriate circumstances, these tests are supplemented by determination of the erythrocyte sedimentation rate and the reticulocyte count. The information obtained by such investigations can serve in turn as the basis for further, more specialized, tests for establishing the nature of the particular pathological process responsible for the anaemia.

MORPHOLOGICAL CLASSIFICATION OF ANAEMIA

Three main types of anaemia are recognized on the basis of the mean volume (MCV), mean haemoglobin content (MCH), and mean haemoglobin concentration (MCHC) of the red cells.

Hypochromic microcytic anaemias

The MCV is subnormal (< approx. 80 fl), as is the MCH (< approx. 27 pg) and MCHC (< approx. 30 g/dl). Such abnormal red cell indices correspond to microcytosis and hypochromia, respectively, of red cells in the blood film. This particular type of anomaly can, for convenience, be viewed as the result of a defect in red cell formation in which haemoglobin synthesis is impaired to a greater extent than that of other cellular components. The most important examples are *iron deficiency*, in which there is inadequate iron for formation of the haem component of haemoglobin, and the *thalassaemias*, in which the formation of the globin components of haemoglobin is defective.

Normochromic normocytic anaemias

The MCV, MCH, and MCHC are within the normal range, corresponding to normal size and haemoglobinization of red cells in the blood film. Many different disorders produce an anaemia of this type. It can, for example, occur following loss of substantial volumes of blood, or in haemolysis, where the rate of red cell destruction is accelerated. It also occurs when red cell production is impaired by bone marrow failure, when bone marrow is replaced by infiltrating neoplastic tissue, and as a result of the effects of renal failure and chronic inflammation or infection.

Macrocytic anaemias

The MCV is above the upper limit of normal (> approx. 96 fl), corresponding to macrocytosis of red cells in the blood film. The red cells are usually normochromic. Macrocytic anaemia can be due to a number of different underlying disorders, the most important of which is *megaloblastosis* of the bone marrow due to vitamin B_{12} or folic acid deficiency. *A significant elevation in the proportion of reticulocytes, which are larger than mature red cells, can also produce elevation of the MCV.*

POINTS OF IMPORTANCE IN THE BLOOD FILM

The morphological features of the blood film are best evaluated in the region where cells are closely associated but do not overlap (Dacie & Lewis 1984). Initial examination with low-power magnification provides a guide to the number and type of leucocytes present. High-power dry-lens inspection is most suitable for evaluating deviation of red cell morphology from normal, and for locating atypical cells of diagnostic significance. Oil-immersion lens inspection is employed to provide the high magnification required for examination of fine detail of abnormal red cells and leucocytes. Key features are summarized in Table 2.3.

Red cell size and shape

There is normally some variation in diameter about the mean value of 7.2 μm, with most red cells being 6.7–7.7 μm in diameter. There is also some deviation from a round profile, but this occurs only to a minor degree.

Increased variation in the size of red cells is referred to as *anisocytosis*. This condition may be due to an increase in the proportion of microcytes, or macrocytes, or both.

Increased variation in shape is referred to as *poikilocytosis*, and the nature of the abnormal shape may point to the cause of the anaemia. Extensively fragmented cells of reduced size are, for example, seen in micro-angiopathic haemolysis due to mechanical trauma to red cells in the circulation.

Table 2.3. *Key features in the blood film*

Red cells	
Size	Microcytes, normal-sized cells, macrocytes (a lymphocyte or segmented neutrophil can be employed for reference). Anisocytosis
Shape	Variation from the normal round profile, e.g. oval, pencil, tear, sickle, fragmented, crenated, burr cells and acanthocytes. Poikilocytosis. Abnormality of overall configuration, e.g. spherocytes, target cells, stomatocytes
Pattern of staining	Normal intensity of haemoglobin staining, or subnormal hypochromic cells with characteristically increased central pallor. Increased purple hue in polychromatic cells
Inclusions	Basophilic stippling, Howell–Jolly bodies, malarial parasites, Pappenheimer bodies, areas of deficient staining referred to as blisters
Association	Clumping of red cells to form aggregates or rouleaux
White cells	
Relative number	Decreased, normal, or increased
Morphology	Lymphocytes, monocytes and segmented granulocytes present in normal or abnormal ratios Presence of cells normally absent, e.g. erythroblasts, immature myeloid or lymphoid cells, atypical lymphocytes, hypersegmented neutrophils, or increased proportions of band neutrophils
Platelets	
Relative number	Decreased, normal, or increased
Morphology	Normal or enlarged forms

Red cell staining

The intensity of the orange–pink colour of haemoglobin in Romanovsky-stained red cells gradually decreases from the periphery to the centre of the cell. The internal paler area, known as the zone of central pallor, normally occupies less than one-third of the cell diameter. Deviation from the pattern of staining in normochromic cells towards less intense staining, with a greater region of central pallor, is described as *hypochromia*. This tends to correlate in the uncomplicated situation with a low MCHC, and is a feature of iron deficiency and thalassaemia. A *dimorphic* blood film is one in which populations of normochromic and hypochromic red cells co-exist. Such a situation is seen, for example, after a patient with iron deficiency anaemia is transfused with normal red cells, or after administration of iron to an iron-deficient patient has resulted in partial replacement of pre-existing hypochromic red cells with newly formed normochromic red cells. A dimorphic blood film is commonly seen in *sideroblastic* anaemia.

Polychromasia refers to the presence of a diffuse basophilic hue in the red cell. Polychromatic red cells are present in increased proportions in the blood when the rate of red cell production is increased, and correlates with an increased percentage of reticulocytes (normally <2%). A reticulocyte count should be performed to establish a more accurate index of the percentage of newly formed erythrocytes when polychromasia is noted in the blood film. Reticulocytes are slightly larger than mature red cells, so that marked polychromasia can be associated with an abnormally elevated MCV.

Deviations from the normal staining pattern which indicate particular types of underlying causative factors include *spherocytosis. Spherocytes have abnormally increased central staining, and are usually associated with certain specific types of haemolytic processes.* Spherocytosis is one of the few states associated with an abnormally elevated MCHC.

Target cells have a small, normally stained centre surrounded by a hypochromic ring, and finally a normally stained rim. Target cells are present in iron deficiency, thalassaemia and liver disease, but also become evident in otherwise normal individuals after splenectomy. *Stomatocytes* have an oval rather than circular zone of central pallor.

Inclusions

Small discrete dots in *basophilic stippling* occur in red cell cytoplasm in many haemopoietic disorders such as *lead poisoning*, aplastic anaemia, thalassaemia, myelodysplasia, and megaloblastosis.

Howell–Jolly bodies are purple–black, usually round, chromatin fragments. They are usually single, and are larger and more deeply stained than the granules in basophilic stippling. Howell–Jolly bodies are seen in disorders such as megaloblastic anaemia, but appear in red cells after splenectomy in otherwise normal individuals because the function of the spleen is to remove inclusions of this type from red cells, as well as to remove abnormal red cells such as spherocytes from the circulation.

Pappenheimer bodies resemble large versions of the granules in basophilic stippling, but contain iron which can be identified by a positive Prussian blue reaction.

Blister cells contain small clear areas, apparently lacking haemoglobin. This is due to displacement of haemoglobin by inclusions such as Heinz bodies, which do not react with Romanovsky stains, but can be identified with certain supravital stains.

Cell types involved

One of the fundamental questions in the evaluation of the cause of an anaemia is whether the underlying disorder is selectively involving red cells or involving more than one blood cell series, as in leukaemia. Distinction between these can often be made on the examination of the blood film, as this provides an indication of the status of leucocytes and platelets in the blood.

The *reticulocyte count* may provide useful information about the type of anaemia, as it is elevated in conditions in which erythroid precursors can increase the production of red cells in response to an increase in demand. This is commonly seen in *haemolysis* when erythropoietic activity is unimpaired. An increase also occurs in response to *haemorrhage* in patients with adequate iron stores, and in those whose deficiency of iron, folic acid or vitamin B_{12} has been corrected by appropriate replacement therapy.

Erythrocyte sedimentation rate

The ESR is a non-specific phenomenon reflecting mainly changes in plasma proteins, but it is useful as a screening test (Dacie & Lewis 1984). In an anaemic patient, the ESR can sometimes give a lead to the underlying causative disorder. A normal ESR cannot be taken to exclude organic disease, but nevertheless in the majority of acute and chronic infections, and in many neoplasms and other diseases, e.g. collagen diseases and renal insufficiency, the ESR is raised. It is often markedly raised in paraprotein-producing disorders such as macroglobulinaemia and multiple myeloma. It should be noted that the ESR increases with age, and in both men and women over the age of 60 years an ESR of 30 mm/hour or more may be present without any obvious cause (Miller *et al.* 1983). Anaemia itself may cause some increase in ESR, and formulae to correct for the effect of anaemia have been devised, but as the changes produced by anaemia are irregular, corrective attempts are generally considered not worthwhile (Dacie & Lewis 1984).

What is the cause of the anaemia?

Anaemia can be generally regarded to result from:
- blood loss;
- impaired red cell production;
- excessively rapid red cell destruction.

More than one of these processes can contribute to the genesis of anaemia. Accelerated red cell destruction, for example, can substantially aggravate the degree of anaemia resulting from impaired red cell production. The categories of anaemia based on underlying pathophysiological processes are summarized in Table 2.4.

The cause of anaemia in a particular patient is determined from consideration of:
- the type of anaemia indicated by examination of the blood;
- the clinical features; and
- results of further investigations when these are necessary.

Table 2.4. *Basic pathophysiological categories of anaemia*

Blood loss
Impaired red cell production
Inadequate supply of nutrients essential for eythropoiesis, such as:
iron deficiency
vitamin B_{12} deficiency
folic acid deficiency
protein-calorie malnutrition
other less common deficiencies
Depression of erythropoietic activity
Anaemia associated with chronic disorders, such as:
infection
connective tissue disorders
inflammatory disorders
disseminated malignancy
Anaemia associated with renal failure
Aplastic anaemia
Anaemia due to replacement of normal bone marrow by:
leukaemia
lymphoma
myeloproliferative disorders
myeloma
myelodysplastic disorders
Anaemia due to inherited disorders, such as thalassaemia
Excessive red cell destruction
Due to intrinsic defects in red cells
Due to extrinsic effects on red cells

Often, the clinical picture and the results of the blood examination are sufficient. For example, a recent episode of major blood loss reasonably explains the presence of normochromic normocytic anaemia. However, more insidious recurring losses of small amounts of blood can lead to iron deficiency, in which the blood film indicates the anaemia is hypochromic and microcytic in type. When the source of blood loss is not evident under such circumstances, thorough evaluation must be carried out to establish the source of the occult bleeding, as this lesion is the basic cause of the anaemia, and is the logical focus of the management of the patient—it could, for example, be a resectable neoplasm.

Clinical features that are of particular value in indicating the primary cause of anaemia are summarized in Table 2.5. This list is by necessity only a guide to some of the more important features.

CAUSES OF ANAEMIA

Overt blood loss is an important cause of anaemia, and a thorough history should be taken to establish whether *epistaxis, rectal bleeding, menorrhagia* or *recurrent bleeding from other sites* has occured.

Occult bleeding from the gastrointestinal tract is an important cause of iron deficiency anaemia, and care should be taken to elicit whether the patient has had symptoms consistent with erosive or ulcerative disorders, such as *heartburn, altered bowel habit, abdominal pain, abdominal discomfort,* or *diarrhoea.*

A bleeding tendency is suggested by easy bruising or petechiae, prolonged bleeding after trivial injuries, or bleeding from more than one site. However, a history of easy bruising is common in women, and so this symptom must be interpreted with caution. A definite bleeding tendency suggests that the anaemia is due to a disorder causing thrombocytopenia, a coagulation defect, or to renal insufficiency.

Central nervous system. Megaloblastic anaemia due to vitamin B_{12} deficiency may be accompanied by peripheral neuritis and subacute combined degeneration of the spinal cord. The paraesthesiae, of which numbness and tingling are the commonest, are characteristically bilateral and symmetrical, and occur first in the hands and feet. Difficulty in walking and disturbances of micturition may also occur.

Skeletal system. Bone pain may occur in the anaemias due to marrow infiltration or replacement, such as multiple myeloma, acute leukaemia, lymphoma, and myelofibrosis.

Diet. Inadequate diet can contribute to iron deficiency anaemia, and is generally the basis of megaloblastic anaemia due to folic acid deficiency.

Social history. Alcoholism is increasingly recognized as associated with nutritional folic acid deficiency.

Family history. A family history of anaemia or jaundice can *sometimes* be elicited in congenital haemolytic anaemias.

Fever. Night sweats occur in lymphomas, especially Hodgkin's disease, and in leukaemia, but occasionally are due to other disorders causing anaemia, e.g. chronic infections or collagen diseases. Fever due to anaemia *per se* is rare, although mild pyrexia occasionally occurs in severe anaemia. Significant fever is therefore due either to the causative disorder or to some complicating factor, such as infection due to neutropenia or responses of the body to acute intravascular haemolysis.

Drug ingestion. A history of drug ingestion over the preceding year should always be obtained. Occult gastric bleeding is very common with persistent analgesic intake, and inquiry should be made about the ingestion of such tablets and the symptoms of headache or arthritis for which such medication is commonly taken. (Some patients may be unaware of the nature of medication taken for these conditions.) When blood examination reveals pancytopenia, detailed and repeated inquiry may be necessary.

Occupation. Inquiry about exposure to toxic chemicals, metal dust, paint or to radiation is appropriate in individuals with pancytopenia, haemolysis and lead poisoning.

EXAMINATION OF THE ANAEMIC PATIENT

Particular emphasis should be placed during *examination of the patient* on the search for mucocutaneous features of iron deficiency, petechial haemorrhages suggestive of concurrent thrombocytopenia, and features suggestive of proliferative disorders of the lymphoid or myeloid series, such as enlargement of lymph glands, liver or spleen.

Skin. The colour and texture of skin should be noted, and petechiae and ecchymoses looked for. In severe pernicious anaemia, the skin may have a lemon-yellow tint. In myxoedema, the skin is coarse and dry. Petechiae in anaemic patients are usually due to thrombocytopenia, but may be due to decreased platelet function, such as in renal insufficiency. Ecchymoses occur most commonly in

Table 2.5. *Key points in the clinical evaluation of the anaemic patient*

History	
Full medical history with special emphasis on the following points:	
Age, sex	
Rate of onset	Rapid or slow
Blood loss	Haematemesis, melaena, bleeding from haemorrhoids, menorrhagia, metrorrhagia, epistaxis, haematuria, haemoptysis
Alimentary system	Appetite, weight loss, dysphagia, regurgitation, dyspepsia, abdominal pain, diarrhoea, constipation, jaundice, soreness of the tongue, previous abdominal operations
Reproductive system	Menstrual history in detail, number and intervals of pregnancies, miscarriages
Urinary system	Nocturnal polyuria
Central nervous system	Paraesthesiae, difficulty in walking
Bleeding tendency	Easy bruising, prolonged bleeding after trivial injuries, bleeding from more than one site
Skeletal system	Bone pain, arthritis, arthralgia
Temperature	Fever, night sweats
Drug ingestion	Previous and current
Occupation	Metal dusts, solvent fumes, lead
Diet	
Social history	Alcoholism
Past history	Previous anaemia—diagnosis, treatment, response to treatment
Family history	Anaemia, recurrent jaundice, intra-uterine and childhood deaths
Examination	
Complete physical examination with special emphasis on the following features:	
Skin	Colour, texture, petechiae, ecchymoses, scratch marks
Nails	Brittleness, longitudinal ridging, koilonychia
Conjunctiva & sclera	Pallor, icterus, haemorrhage
Retina	Haemorrhages, hypertensive or renal failure, retinal changes
Mouth	Mucous membranes—pallor, petechiae Gums—bleeding or hypertrophy Tongue—redness or atrophy of papillae
Abdomen	Hepatomegaly, splenomegaly, tenderness, mass, ascites
CVS	Blood pressure, valvular or vascular prostheses
CNS	Peripheral neuritis, subacute combined degeneration of spinal cord
Superficial lymph nodes	Enlargement of cervical, axillary, inguinal or epitrochlear nodes
Bones	Tenderness, especially of sternum, tumour
Legs	Ulcers or scars of healed ulcers
Rectal examination	Haemorrhoids, carcinoma of the rectum
Pelvic examination	Menorrhagia or metrorrhagia
Tourniquet test	
Urine	Protein, urobilinogen, bilirubin

anaemias associated with either thrombocytopenia or a disturbance of coagulation.

Nails. Brittleness, flattening and longitudinal ridging are common in chronic iron deficiency anaemia, and occasionally spoon-shaped nails (koilonychia) are seen. However, brittleness with breaking of the nail edges is not uncommon in women in the absence of iron deficiency, and koilonychia may occur as a congenital phenomenon.

Conjunctiva and sclera. The conjunctiva may reveal pallor due to the presence of anaemia. Icterus is more easily appreciated in the sclera than in the skin. Icterus is relatively uncommon in anaemia, but when present suggests haemolytic anaemia or hepatic disease. However, the absence of icterus does not exclude a haemolytic anaemia.

Retina. Changes in the retina, particularly haemorrhages, are not uncommon in severe anaemia, but are not diagnostic. When thrombocytopenia co-exists with anaemia, haemorrhages are common and may be large.

Mouth. Atrophy of the papillae of the tongue can occur in chronic deficiency of iron, vitamin B_{12}, or folic acid. The mucous membranes may appear inflamed in vitamin B_{12} or folic acid deficiency. Hypertrophy of gums is occasionally observed in myelomonocytic leukaemia. Acute inflammatory changes and ulceration in the mouth and pharynx can occur as a primary feature of disorders affecting haemopoiesis, such as infectious mononucleosis, or as a secondary feature of disorders that have suppressed the capacity of the host to resist infection, such as agranulocytosis or haematological neoplasia.

Splenomegaly. It is doubtful if anaemia *per se* causes clinical enlargement of the spleen. Thus splenomegaly in the anaemic patient is related to the cause of the anaemia, and its degree varies with the nature of the causative disorder and its duration. The causes of splenomegaly are listed on p. 351.

Hepatomegaly. When present, hepatomegaly is usually due to the causative disorder. The physical character of the liver may give a lead to the cause, e.g. the liver is firm and has a sharp border in cirrhosis, or may be nodular in secondary carcinoma. When hepatomegaly is due to anaemia, the liver is smooth, slightly to moderately enlarged, and sometimes tender, especially in the presence of congestive cardiac failure.

Abdominal mass. A mass may give a clue to the cause of the anaemia. There may be an epigastric mass in carcinoma of the stomach, a mass in the right iliac fossa in carcinoma of the caecum, or a retroperitoneal mass of nodes in secondary carcinoma, chronic lymphatic leukaemia or lymphoma. Localized tenderness may be present over a peptic ulcer.

Superficial lymph nodes. These may be significantly enlarged in leukaemia, lymphomas, and secondary carcinoma. Slight enlargement of the tonsillar and inguinal nodes is not uncommon in normal persons as a result of infection of the throat, feet, groin or perineal region. However, in the absence of infection of the scalp, enlargement of the occipital and posterior triangle nodes is uncommon, and these should always be carefully palpated when any disease causing lymph node enlargement is suspected.

Bone tenderness. In marrow infiltrative disorders, bone tenderness may be present in the abence of bone pain. It occurs in acute leukaemia, metastatic bone carcinoma, multiple myeloma, chronic leukaemia, myelofibrosis and lymphoma. In disorders characterized by focal involvement, e.g. secondary carcinoma, tenderness may be localized, and systematic palpation may be necessary before a tender spot is found. Bone tenderness is most often demonstrated in the sternum, particularly over the lower end, but it may occur in the ribs, clavicles, vertebrae, pelvic bones, or skull, which should therefore be palpated.

Rectal examination is necessary in patients with symptoms suggestive of haemorrhoids or rectal bleeding, and in patients in whom occult gastrointestinal bleeding is suspected.

Tourniquet test. This is a bedside test which should be performed in patients with signs or symptoms suggestive of a bleeding tendency, or in whom there is a possibility of thrombocytopenia.

Urine. Minor degrees of proteinuria may occur in severe anaemia, but marked proteinuria suggests a renal disorder or multiple myeloma. Urobilinogen and bilirubin should be tested for in jaundiced patients, and in non-jaundiced patients in whom liver disease or haemolysis is suspected.

References and further reading

Bellingham, A.J. (1974) The red cell in adaptation to anaemic hypoxia. *Clin. Haemat.* **3**, 577.

Bessis, M. (1974) *Living Blood Cells and their Ultrastructure.* Springer, New York.

Bessis, M. & Mohandas, N. (1975) Red cell structure, shapes and deformability. *Brit. J. Haemat.* **31**, Suppl.5.

Bessis, M. & Weed, R.I. (1973) The structure of normal and pathological erythrocytes. *Adv. Biol. Med. Physics* **14**, 35.

Beutler, E. (1975) *Red Cell Metabolism*, 2nd Ed., Grune & Stratton, New York.

Cohen, C.M. (1983) The molecular organisation of the red cell membrane skeleton. *Semin. Hematol.* **20**, 141.

Cooper, R.A. (1970) Lipids of human red cell membrane: normal composition and variability in disease. *Semin. Haemat.* **7**, 296.

Cotter, H., Lancaster, H.O. & Walsh, R.J. (1953) The variation from day to day in the haemoglobin value of young women. *Austr. Ann. Med.* **2**, 99.

Dacie, J.V. & Lewis, S.M. (1984) *Practical Haematology*, 6th Ed., Churchill Livingstone, London.

Dawson, A.A. & Palmer, K.N.U. (1966) The significance of cardiac murmurs in anaemia. *Am. J. Med. Sci.* **252**, 5.

Duke, M. & Abelmann, W.H. (1969) The haemodynamic response to chronic anaemia. *Circulation*, **39**, 503.

Elwood, P.C., Waters, W.E., Greene, W.J.W. *et al.* (1969) Symptoms and circulatory haemoglobin level. *J. Chron. Dis.* **21**, 615.

Fawcett, J.K. & Wynn, V. (1960) Effects of posture on plasma volume and some blood constituents. *J. Clin. Path.* **13**, 304.

Greenwalt, T.J. & Jamieson, G.A. (1976) *The Human Red Cell in vitro*, Grune & Stratton, New York.

Huehns, E.R. (1971) Biochemical compensation in anaemia. *Sci. Basis Med. Ann. Rev.* 216.

Koenig, R.J., Peterson, C.M., Jones, R.L. *et al.* (1976) Correlation of glucose regulation and haemoglobin A_{1c} in diabetes mellitus. *New Engl. J. Med.* **295**, 417.

Low, J.A., Johnston, E.E. & McBride, R.L. (1965) Blood volume adjustments in normal obstetric patients with particular reference to the third trimester. *Am. J. Obstet. Gynecol.* **91**, 356.

Miller, A., Green, M. & Robinson, D. (1983) Simple rule for calculating normal erythrocyte sedimentation rate. *Brit. Med. J.* **286**, 266.

Oski, F.A., Gottlieb, A.J., Delivoria-Paradopoulos, M. *et al.* (1969) Red cell 2,3 DPG levels in subjects with hypoxemia. *New Engl. J. Med.* **280**, 1165.

Silber, R. & Goldstein, B.D. (1970) Vitamin E and the haematopoietic system. *Semin. Haemat.* **7**, 40.

Surgenor, D.M. The Red Blood Cell, 2nd Ed., Vol.1 (1974) and Vol.2 (1975), Academic Press, New York.

Torrance, J., Jacobs, P., Restrepo, A., Eschbach, J., Lenfant, C. & Finch, C.A. (1970) Intraerythrocyte adaptation to anaemia. *New Engl. J. Med.* **283**, 165.

Walsh, R.J. & Ward, H.K. (1969) *A Guide to Blood Transfusion*, 3rd Ed., Australian Medical Publication Company, Sydney.

Weed, R.I. (1970) Disorders of red cell membrane: history and perspectives. *Semin. Haemat.* **7**, 249.

Yoshikawa, H. & Rapaport, S.M. (Eds) (1975) *Cellular and Molecular Biology of Erythrocytes.* University Park Press, Baltimore.

Chapter 3
Hypochromic Anaemia: Iron Deficiency and Sideroblastic Anaemia

Blood loss is the most common cause of anaemia in clinical practice. The blood loss may be either acute or chronic. With anaemia due to acute haemorrhage, there is seldom a diagnostic problem. However, in patients with anaemia due to chronic blood loss, especially those with occult gastrointestinal bleeding, diagnosis of the cause of the anaemia may be difficult. It is not always easy to establish that blood loss is taking place, and even when this is established, it can be difficult to determine the precise source of bleeding.

Chronic blood loss is the principal cause of iron deficiency in industrialized society. This chapter opens with a discussion of iron metabolism, as an understanding of the physiology of iron absorption, storage, and excretion provides a basis for the interpretation of the hypochromic anaemias.

Iron metabolism

Amount and distribution

The total body iron content of the normal adult varies from 3 to 5 g, depending on the sex and weight of the individual. It is greater in males than in females, and it increases roughly in proportion to body weight. Iron is distributed in the body in several distinct forms as illustrated in Table 3.1.

HAEMOGLOBIN IRON

Haemoglobin iron constitutes approximately 60–70 per cent of the total body iron, the absolute amount varying from 1.5 to 3.0 g. At the end of their lifespan, aged red cells are phagocytosed by cells of the reticulo-endothelial system. Nearly all the iron derived from the breakdown of haemoglobin is released into the circulation bound to the iron-binding protein, transferrin, and is re-utilized by marrow erythroblasts for haemoglobin synthesis.

TISSUE IRON

From the standpoint of blood formation, tissue iron may be subdivided into: (a) *storage or available iron*, i.e. tissue iron that, when needed, can be readily mobilized from the body tissues for haemoglobin synthesis; and (b) *non-available iron*, which in general is not available for haemoglobin synthesis.

Storage iron

The amount of storage iron has been estimated to be about 1000–2000 mg in the healthy adult male, and less in the female. Iron stores are slowly accumulated during childhood and adolescence, due to a

Table 3.1. *Distribution of body iron in the average adult male (after Bothwell et al. 1979)*

Haemoglobin	2.3 g
Storage (available) tissue iron (ferritin and haemosiderin)	1.0 g*
Essential (non-available) tissue iron (myoglobin and enzymes of cellular respiration)	0.5 g†
Plasma (transport) iron	3–4 mg
Total	3.8 g

*This amount is sufficient to replace between one-third and one-half of the circulating haemoglobin. Storage tissue iron is substantially less in women.
†Mainly myoglobin.

slight excess of absorption over loss from the body. Storage iron is depleted in iron deficiency anaemia, and is increased in conditions of excessive iron storage, e.g. transfusion haemosiderosis and haemochromatosis.

Storage iron occurs in two forms—ferritin and haemosiderin. Ferritin is normally predominant. In the normal person, storage iron is divided about equally between the reticulo-endothelial cells (mainly in spleen, liver, and bone marrow), hepatic parenchymal cells, and skeletal muscle. Haemosiderin, the main storage form in reticulo-endothelial cells, is more stable and less readily mobilized for haemoglobin formation than ferritin, which predominates in hepatocytes. In states of iron overload, haemosiderin increases to a greater degree than ferritin and becomes the dominant storage form.

Ferritin is colourless and is finely dispersed in tissues, where it is not ordinarily visible microscopically. However, when present in large quantities, it gives a faint bluish tint to tissues stained for iron by the ferrocyanide method. It is composed of a spherical outer shell of an iron-free protein, *apoferritin*, and an inner core of trivalent iron as illustrated schematically in Fig. 3.1. Apoferritin has a molecular weight of about 450 000 and is made up of 24 subunits, each of a molecular weight of approximately 18 500. Iron passes in and out of the shell through six channels, and each molecule of apoferritin binds a variable number of iron atoms, ranging up to about 4500. The iron, which represents up to 23 per cent of the total dry weight of the molecule, is present as complexes of hydrous ferric oxide phosphate. Ferritin from any one tissue is not homogeneous, but consists of a range of different isomers, which may be separated on the basis of electrophoretic mobility. Isomers of ferritin, or *isoferritins*, are hybrid molecules composed of varying proportions of two types of subunits called H and L. Heart and red cell ferritin contain largely acidic (H subunit-rich) isoferritins, and the basic (L subunit-rich) type predominates in liver, spleen and serum ferritin (Drysdale *et al.* 1977).

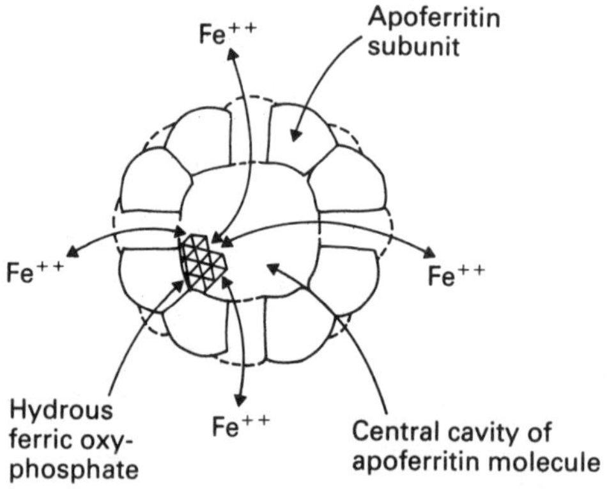

Fig. 3.1. *Schematic illustration of the route by which iron molecules enter or leave the ferritin molecule through pores in the spherical shell of apoferritin, a multimeric complex made up of 24 similar subunits. Iron is deposited as hydrous ferric oxide phosphate on the inner surface of the apoferritin shell, and can constitute up to 23 per cent of the dry weight of the ferritin molecule.*

Haemosiderin is the insoluble form of storage iron. It appears as golden yellow or brown granules in unstained tissues and in tissues stained with haematoxylin and eosin, or as blue granules when stained with potassium ferrocyanide. Haemosiderin contains more iron than ferritin (25–40 per cent). The exact chemical relationship between the two has not been precisely determined, but it is probable that as the ferritin molecule ages, there is partial denaturation of apoferritin and a corresponding increase in iron content, with haemosiderin being gradually formed. The haemosiderin then aggregates to produce microscopically visible granules. Inspection of the amount of haemosiderin in the bone marrow is an important method of assessing body iron stores.

Non-available tissue iron

Non-available iron is made up predominantly of the iron in muscle myoglobin, and to a lesser extent of iron in certain enzymes such as cytochromes, catalase and peroxidase. Its amount, estimated at about 500 mg, remains relatively constant, although it may be slightly reduced in severe iron deficiency anaemia.

PLASMA (TRANSPORT) IRON

Between 3 and 4 mg iron are present in the plasma, where it is bound to a specific protein, transferrin, a

β globulin of molecular weight 88 000, which is synthesized in the liver. Each molecule of transferrin binds one or two atoms of ferric iron.

The function of transferrin is the transport of iron. It is the means by which iron absorbed from the alimentary tract is transported to the tissue stores from tissue stores to bone marrow erythroblasts, and from one storage site to another. When transferrin reaches the storage sites or the bone marrow, it attaches to specific receptors on cells and liberates its ferric ions, which pass into the cell to be stored or utilized. Transferrin receptors have been demonstrated on reticulocytes and erythroblasts, and there is evidence that some of the bound transferrin is internalized within the cell prior to the release of iron. Plasma iron is continually being recycled with a turnover time of approximately three hours. The total amount of transferrin in the plasma is about 8 g, and a similar amount (binding 3–4 mg iron) is in the extracellular fluid, in equilibrium with plasma transferrin.

The level of *serum iron* in normal subjects averages about 20 μmol/l. Values are somewhat higher in men than in women, and show a diurnal variation, being higher in the morning than in the evening. Transferrin is present in the serum in a concentration which enables it to combine with 44–80 μmol of iron per litre. This value is known as the *total iron-binding capacity of the serum*. The percentage of the total iron-binding protein to which iron is attached is known as the *percentage saturation of the iron-binding protein*. This is calculated by dividing the serum iron value by the total iron-binding capacity, and expressing the result as a percentage. The average normal value is about 33 per cent saturation, i.e. the iron-binding protein is about one-third saturated. Many diagnostic laboratories now estimate the level of transferrin in the serum or plasma by techniques that utilize specific antibodies to transferrin and express the result as amount of protein per litre, the normal range being 2–3 g/l.

An immunoradiometric (labelled antibody) assay for measuring serum ferritin concentration was first established by Addison *et al.* (1972). The role of serum ferritin in iron transport is uncertain, but it is apparently derived from reticulo-endothelial cells and is cleared by hepatocytes. In normal subjects, the serum ferritin level is stable and shows little diurnal or day-to-day variation. Its concentration is related to body iron stores, and is age and sex dependent. Levels in children are high at birth, but rapidly fall and are low from 6 months to about 15 years of age. Serum ferritin concentrations in adults range between 15 and 300 μg/l, and the mean levels in men and women are 123 μg/l and 56 μg/l. In iron deficiency, concentrations are less than 12 μg/l. In iron overload, levels are very high, in some patients exceeding 10 000 μg/l (Jacobs & Worwood 1975).

Table 3.2. *Methods for assessing iron stores*

Quantitative phlebotomy
Liver biopsy (qualitative or quantitative)
Bone marrow aspiration and biopsy (qualitative or quantitative)
Urinary excretion of iron after infusion of chelating agent
Serum iron, total iron-binding capacity, and percentage saturation
Erythrocyte protoporphyrin
Serum and red cell ferritin
Dual energy computed tomography
Magnetic susceptibility

Serum ferritin concentrations generally correlate well with tissue iron stores, but in special situations, such as in infection and inflammation, some forms of malignancy (including acute leukaemia and active Hodgkin's disease) and liver disease, the serum level may be greater than 15 μg/l even when marrow iron is absent. However, a serum ferritin level of 12 μg/l or less is diagnostic of iron deficiency.

Methods employed in clinical practice for assessing iron stores are listed in Table 3.2, and their relative value in different situations is discussed by Brittenham *et al.* (1981) and Jacobs & Worwood (1984).

Absorption

The regulation of iron absorption is the primary mechanism by which the body controls its iron content, as capacity to excrete iron is extremely limited. The small intestine is highly sensitive to repletion or depletion of iron stores, and rapidly corrects imbalance by decreasing or increasing absorption. The daily intake of a normal adult on a mixed western-type diet contains 10–20 mg iron, of which 10 per cent or somewhat less (approximately 1–2 mg) is absorbed. Absorption is greater in women than in men, presumably because of the greater requirements due to menstrual loss and child-bearing. Iron is found in a wide variety of animal and plant foods, but in most in low concentrations. The chief dietary sources are meats, especially liver and kidney, egg yolk, green vegetables and fruit. Milk, particularly cow's milk, has a low iron content. Considerable amounts of iron may be added to food by cooking in iron utensils.

Most food iron in the gut enters two common pools (Hallberg 1981) that behave differently in terms of absorption. Absorption of non-haem iron present in vegetables, fruit and cereals is highly variable and is greatly influenced by other substances in the diet. Haem iron present in the haemoglobin and myoglobin of meat is well absorbed, and the overall composition of the diet is of less importance. The mechanism of absorption of haem iron also differs from that of other food iron. The diet of many people in the Third World consists almost entirely of cereals, and poor bio-availability of the limited amount of iron ingested is a major factor in the high prevalence of iron deficiency. To overcome this problem, iron fortification of flour has been adopted by some countries as a public health measure.

Non-haem iron is released from food as ferric or ferrous ions by the action of acid in the stomach. It is absorbed only in the ionic state, and almost exclusively as the ferrous form. Ferric ions are soluble at low pH, but tend to polymerize and become unavailable for absorption as the pH rises in the duodenum. Ferrous ions are more soluble under these conditions. The subequent fate of non-haem iron is determined largely by the influence of a variety of ligands in food, which complex with iron and act to facilitate or hinder absorption. Ascorbic acid is an important facilitatory substance which, in addition to reducing ferric to ferrous ions, forms low molecular weight iron chelates that remain soluble at the neutral pH of the gut lumen. Other facilitatory substances include meat, citric acid, amino acids and sugars. Tannin in tea is an important recently recognized inhibitory substance. A high phosphorus diet impairs absorption by forming insoluble ferric phosphate. Foods containing phosphates include bread, cereals and milk. Conversely, a low phosphorus diet may result in increased absorption. Phytic acid, which is present in most cereals, converts both ferrous and ferric salts into insoluble phytates, and may thus impair absorption (Charlton & Bothwell 1983).

Absorption of iron is most efficient in the duodenum and proximal jejunum. Non-haem iron attaches to surface glycoprotein receptors on the brush border of the mucosal absorptive cells. Following entry into the cell, depending on the body's requirement for iron, a proportion (possibly bound to a transferrin-like protein) is rapidly transferred across the cell and on to the portal circulation for distribution to tissue iron stores. Most of the remaining iron in the mucosal cell combines with apoferritin to form ferritin. The ferritin-containing cells are exfoliated from the mucosal surface at the end of their 2–3 day lifespan, and the iron is lost in the faeces (Conrad & Barton 1981). Haem enters the mucosal cell unchanged, and the iron is released within the cell by the action of the enzyme, haem oxygenase. Iron from this source then enters the common iron pool of the mucosal cell.

FACTORS MODULATING IRON ABSORPTION

Apart from the amount of available iron in the diet, the main factors influencing the amount of iron absorbed are: (a) the *size of the iron stores*; and (b) the *rate of erythropoiesis*.

Influence of iron stores

The state of the iron stores is a major determinant of the degree of iron absorption: depletion of iron stores causes increased absorption, and increased iron stores cause reduced absorption. Thus, in humans with iron deficiency, the amount of food iron absorbed is increased from the usual 5–10 per cent to 10–20 per cent.

Influence of erythropoietic activity

The effect of the rate of erythropoiesis on iron absorption has been shown by the fact that an increase in erythropoiesis due either to haemolysis or haemorrhage increases absorption, while depression of erythropoiesis by transfusion-induced erythrocytosis decreases absorption. The increase in absorption which occurs with erythroid hyperplasia in states of 'ineffective erythropoiesis' may be independent of the state of the iron stores.

The mechanism by which the body directs the small intestinal mucosa to increase or decrease iron absorption is not well understood. Current views on iron absorption and its control are discussed by Bothwell *et al.* (1979).

Excretion

The body is unable to regulate its iron content effectively by excretion, and normally cannot rid itself of any substantial amount of iron once it has been taken into the body beyond the stage of the intestinal mucosal cell. The amount of iron lost from the body per day is small—between 0.5 and 1.0 mg under physiological conditions. This figure does not take into account loss by menstruation in the female. The rate of loss is relatively constant and is independent of intake, occurring as a result of desquamation of epithelial cells, mainly from the alimentary tract, from excretion in the urine and sweat, and loss of hair and nails. Iron in the faeces consists almost entirely of unabsorbed iron and desquamated mucosal cells.

Iron balance

Under normal circumstances, iron absorption slightly exceeds iron excretion. As previously discussed, the diet normally contains 10–20 mg of iron, of which 10 per cent or less is absorbed, so that uptake varies from 1 to 2 mg per day. Basal losses range from 0.5 to 1.0 mg per day. Menstruation is an additional source of iron loss in females, the monthly loss being estimated at between 15 and 28 mg, i.e. between 0.5 and 1.0 mg per day for the whole 28-day menstrual cycle. Thus, the daily absorption necessary to compensate for daily loss is 0.5–1.0 mg in males, and about twice this amount, i.e. 1–2 mg, in females during the reproductive period of life (Table 3.3).

The daily iron requirement for haemoglobin synthesis is 20–25 mg. It has been pointed out that the body conserves its iron stores by re-utilizing the iron derived from the breakdown of the haemoglobin from aged red cells. In normal individuals, red cell destruction and formation take place at almost identical rates. Thus, in the absence of bleeding or increased demand, sufficient iron for haemoglobin synthesis is provided by the breakdown of haemoglobin during the destruction of aged red cells.

From a consideration of the above facts it is obvious that males are normally in a state of positive iron balance, i.e. the amount of iron liberated by the normal destruction of effete red cells together with the amount absorbed very slightly exceeds the amount required for haemoglobin synthesis and the amount lost by excretion.

Table 3.3. *Estimated iron requirements in mg per day**

	Urine, sweat, faeces	Menses	Pregnancy	Growth	Total
Men, post-menopausal women	0.5–1.0				0.5–1.0
Menstruating women	0.5–1.0	0.5–1.0			1.0–2.0
Pregnant women	0.5–1.0		1–2		1.5–2.5
Children	?0.5			0.6	1.0
Girls aged 12–15 years	0.5–1.0	0.5–1.0		0.6	1.0–2.5

*From Moore (1965).

However, in females of child-bearing age, the positive balance is only very slender, because of the additional loss by menstruation. Thus, a moderate increase in menstrual loss, especially if associated with impaired intake, can easily induce negative iron balance.

Iron deficiency anaemia

It has been estimated that 20 per cent of the world's population is iron deficient, and iron deficiency anaemia is the most common type of anaemia met with in clinical practice. It occurs at all ages, but is especially common in women of childbearing age, in whom it is an important cause of chronic fatigue and ill-health.

Iron deficiency anaemia is always secondary to an underlying disorder. In industralized communities, it is usually due to chronic, and often occult blood loss whereas in the Third World poor intake of iron or defective absorption are more frequent causes. Correction of the underlying cause is an essential part of treatment. It is important to remember that iron deficiency anaemia is sometimes the first manifestation of a serious disorder of the gastro-intestinal tract causing occult haemorrhage.

Pathogenesis

Iron deficiency anaemia develops when the supply of iron is insufficient for the requirements of haemoglobin synthesis. When iron balance becomes negative, the deficit is made good by iron mobilized from tissue stores, and an adequate supply of iron for haemoglobin formation is maintained. It is only when the tissue stores are exhausted that the supply of iron to the marrow for haemoglobin synthesis becomes inadequate, and hyprochromic anaemia develops.

Thus, iron deficiency may be regarded as developing in two stages: (a) the progressive depletion and ultimate exhaustion of available tissue iron stores; and (b) the development of anaemia (Fig. 3.2).

There are three major factors in the pathogenesis of iron deficiency anaemia:

an increased physiological demand for iron;
pathological blood loss; and
inadequate iron intake.

The relative importance of these three factors varies with the age and sex of the patient, but in general, blood loss is by far the most important. Frequently, more than one factor contributes to the anaemia.

INCREASED PHYSIOLOGICAL DEMAND FOR IRON

This increased demand occurs in *children during the period of growth* and in *women during their reproductive period of life*.

During the period of growth, there is a progressive increase in the number of red cells in the body and consequently in the total amount of haemoglobin. This results in an increased demand for iron by the marrow for haemoglobin synthesis. There is an additional, but much smaller, demand for the synthesis of myoglobin in the progressively increasing mass of other tissues. Growth is most rapid from the age of 6–24 months, the time of the greatest

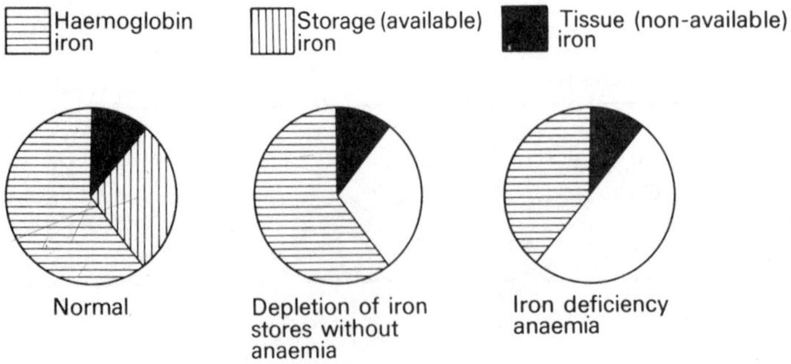

Fig. 3.2. *Stages in the development of iron deficiency.*

incidence of iron deficiency anaemia in young children.

During the reproductive life of the female, menstruation, pregnancy, parturition and lactation significantly increase the physiological requirements for iron. The average monthly loss from menstruation is 15–28 mg. Each pregnancy requires about 500–600 mg for the fetus and to cover blood loss at parturition, although this is partly compensated for by the absence of menstrual loss. Lactation causes further demands, even though the iron content of breast milk is relatively low.

PATHOLOGICAL BLOOD LOSS

Since 60–70 per cent of the total iron content of the body is contained in the haemoglobin of red cells, it is obvious that loss of blood to any extent causes lowering of the total body iron. The normal adult has tissue iron reserves sufficient to replace between one-third and one-half of the circulating haemoglobin (see Table 3.1). Once this reserve is exhausted, continued bleeding causes a state of iron deficiency. Blood loss from pathological lesions may cause iron deficiency anaemia at all ages and in both sexes, but the development of iron deficiency must be viewed especially seriously in adult males and in females after the menopause, in whom there is no physiological cause for the deficiency.

INADEQUATE INTAKE

Inadequate intake may result from either *nutritional deficiency* or *impaired absorption*. In western countries, inadequate intake is generally a contributing rather than a sole causative factor, except in the presence of increased physiological demand or haemorrhage.

Nutritional deficiency as a result of an inadequate diet is of major importance in infants and young children. It may also occur in adults due to poor economic circumstances, dietary fads or dislikes, and anorexia, especially in pregnancy. Poor bioavailability of dietary non-haem iron is an important factor in the Third World.

A long-standing impairment of absorption may result from gastrectomy or gastro-enterostomy, tropical sprue or coeliac disease in either children or adults.

Causes of iron deficency anaemia

FEMALES IN THE REPRODUCTIVE PERIOD OF LIFE

The highest incidence of iron deficiency anaemia is in women during the reproductive period of life, in whom it is a common cause of chronic fatigue and ill-health (Table 3.4). In a recent survey in Sweden, Rybo (1985) found that marrow iron stores were absent in 32 per cent of 38-year-old females. Iron deficiency anaemia is especially common in women with persistently heavy menstrual loss, and in women who have had many pregnancies in rapid succession. A mild degree of anaemia is not uncommon in young girls at the onset of menstruation. Significant blood loss may occur as a result of miscarriages, especially when these are repeated. It is important to remember that blood loss may occur from sites other than the uterus, e.g. the alimentary tract, and that when questioning does not suggest that the iron deficiency is due to uterine loss or pregnancies, further investigation is required.

Inadequate iron intake due to poor diet, anorexia (e.g. during pregnancy), diminished bio-availability, or impaired absorption, may act as a contributing factor. Thus iron deficiency anaemia is more common in women of lower economic status, probably due to the inadequate intake of foods rich

Table 3.4. *Major aetiological factors in iron deficiency anaemia*

Females in the reproductive period of life
Menstruation
Pregnancy
Pathological blood loss
Deficient diet
Adult males and post-menopausal females
Pathological blood loss
Infants and children
Deficient diet
Diminished iron stores at birth

in iron, such as meat, eggs and green vegetables, which are relatively expensive.

Pregnancy

Iron deficiency is the most common cause of anaemia in pregnancy. The majority of pregnant women with haemoglobin values of less than 10 g/dl are suffering from iron deficiency anaemia, although frequently there is definite iron deficiency in patients with haemoglobin values above this figure. The demands of previous pregnancies render women especially prone to iron deficiency, particularly when the interval between pregnancies is short. It is not uncommon for multiparous women or women with heavy menstrual loss to become pregnant with either pre-existing iron deficiency anaemia or no iron stores.

ADULT MALES AND POST-MENOPAUSAL FEMALES

It has been pointed out that the body carefully conserves its iron and that the iron derived from the normal breakdown of aged red cells is re-utilized for haemoglobin synthesis. The normal adult male has a tissue iron reserve of around 1–2 g, and furthermore, the average daily intake of iron in the food slightly exceeds average daily losses. As a consequence, blood loss is the only way in which iron deficiency can be induced in this group when there is normal dietary iron content and iron absorption.

Thus, in adult males, the vast majority of cases of iron deficiency are due to chronic haemorrhage, either present or past. The gastrointestinal tract is the usual source of the bleeding, but occasionally the bleeding is from the urinary tract, nose or lungs. Occasionally, iron deficiency anaemia occurs in young adult males in whom there is no obvious site of blood loss. It is probable that in such patients the requirements of growth during adolescence outstrip the intake. Rare cases of iron deficiency anaemia in this group are due to malabsorption of iron.

Careful investigation is often necessary to determine the cause of the bleeding, as clinical manifestations of the underlying disease may not be prominent. Gastrointestinal bleeding is not uncommonly intermittent, and thus the test for occult blood in the faeces may have to be repeated on several occasions before a positive result is obtained. The most frequent causes of gastrointestinal bleeding are listed in Table 3.5. Hookworm infestation should be considered as a possible cause of iron deficiency anaemia in persons from endemic areas who are visiting or who have migrated to non-endemic areas. The association of iron deficiency anaemia and eosinophilia suggests the possibility of hookworm or other parasitic intestinal infection. A search for the cause of the bleeding is particularly important in men in the age group where malignancy becomes common, as iron deficiency anaemia may be the first feature of an otherwise clinically 'silent' carcinoma of the stomach or colon. Omission to do this may result in failure to recognize an operable lesion.

Table 3.5. *Causes of iron deficiency anaemia due to chronic gastrointestinal blood loss*

Peptic ulcer
Haemorrhoids
Hiatus hernia
Carcinoma of the stomach
Carcinoma of the colon
Chronic aspirin ingestion
Oesophageal varices
Ulcerative colitis
Hookworm infestation

Haematuria, repeated epistaxis, and haemoptysis are uncommon causes of iron deficiency anaemia. The repeated epistaxes in hereditary haemorrhagic telangiectasia, however, commonly result in severe iron deficiency anaemia (p. 372).

In *post-menopausal women* the physiological demands for iron decrease, and iron deficiency anaemia is almost invariably due to chronic blood loss, either pathological uterine bleeding, bleeding from the alimentary tract, or from other sites, as in the adult male. Alimentary tract carcinoma and hiatus hernia, especially in obese women, are important causes of blood loss in this age group (Fig. 3.3). Post-menopausal uterine bleeding is often due to carcinoma of the uterus, and requires thorough investigation.

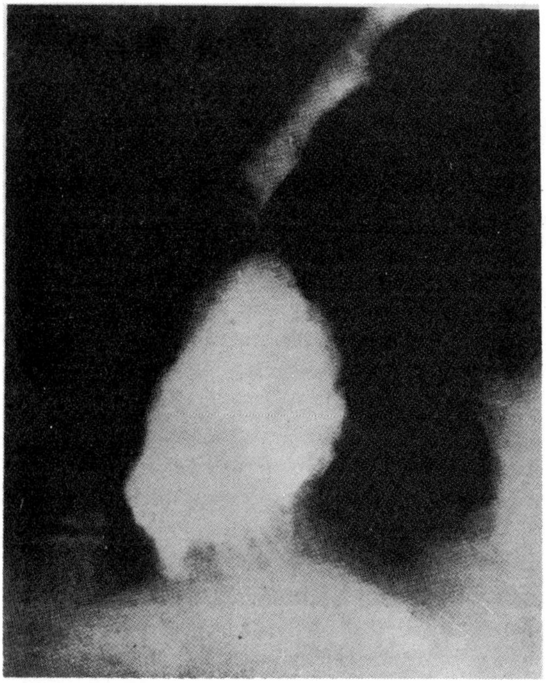

Fig. 3.3. *Hiatus hernia causing iron deficiency anaemia. Barium meal showing hiatus hernia. Mrs E.C., aged 61 years, presented with intermittent claudication and mild dyspnoea on exertion. On direct questioning, she admitted to mild dyspepsia. Blood—hypochromic microcytic anaemia (Hb 7.4 g/dl). Faecal occult blood test positive. Diagnosis—iron deficiency secondary to occult bleeding from hiatus hernia. Intermittent claudication disappeared following correction of the anaemia by treatment with intramuscular iron.*

INFANTS AND CHILDREN

Iron deficiency anaemia is the most common type of anaemia in infancy and childhood. The greatest incidence is between the ages of 6 and 24 months, but it is not uncommon up to the age of 5 years. It is relatively uncommon in children of school age.

The major aetiological factor is an inadequate intake of iron in the diet, which fails to meet the increased demands of growth. Inadequate antenatal stores may also contribute. Less common factors are blood loss, impaired absorption as in coeliac disease, and congenital abnormalities of the gastrointestinal tract.

The normal full-term infant has reserves of iron sufficient for about the first 4–6 months of life. These consist of iron present at birth and that released by breakdown of red cells during the neonatal period. As the iron stores derived from the mother are laid down mainly during the third trimester, the premature infant is born with diminished iron stores and is especially prone to develop anaemia. Other factors that may result in a baby being born with inadequate reserves are maternal iron deficiency and multiple pregnancy in which iron from the mother must be shared.

After the first 4–6 months of life, the infant is dependent on diet for supplies of iron. The majority of cases of iron deficiency in infants and young children are due to inadequate intake of iron. The usual problem is that supplemental feeding of iron-containing foods, e.g. vegetables, meat and eggs, is commenced too late. Faulty feeding may result from behaviour problems, and it is common under these conditions to find that the diet consists mainly of milk and carbohydrates, i.e. foods of low iron content. Such a diet may nonetheless have an adequate caloric content so that the infant is of normal or increased weight.

IRON DEFICIENCY ANAEMIA AFTER GASTROINTESTINAL SURGERY

Iron deficiency anaemia is common after gastrectomy and gastro-enterostomy. Anaemia may occur after both partial and total gastrectomy, but the incidence is greater the more extensive the gastrectomy. The anaemia is usually of mild to moderate degree, and it tends to be more marked in women of child-bearing age.

The major aetiological factors are chronic blood loss from inflamed mucosa about the anastomotic site and inability to increase absorption of food iron, possibly due to loss of gastric secretion. By-pass of the duodenum and excessively rapid passage of food through the small intestine may contribute. Depletion of iron stores due to bleeding before operation may also be a factor. Co-existent vitamin B_{12} or folate deficiency are not uncommon under these circumstances and may cause a dimorphic blood film, a modified marrow picture (p. 72), and an impaired response to administration of iron.

Clinical features

The clinical features result from the *anaemia* and the *effect of chronic iron deficiency on epithelial tissues.* Clinical features of the underlying disorder causing the anaemia are sometimes present.

ANAEMIA

The onset of iron deficiency anaemia is usually insidious. The symptoms are those common to all anaemias; the nature and severity vary with the degree of anaemia and the age of the patient. Lassitude, weakness, fatigue, dyspnoea on exertion, and palpitations are the most common symptoms. Angina and congestive cardiac failure may occur, especially in older patients. Menstrual disturbances are commonly associated with iron deficiency anaemia. Usually, menstrual loss is excessive, but decreased loss or even amenorrhoea commonly occurs after the development of severe anaemia. Excess menstrual loss is usually the cause rather than the result of the anaemia.

Pallor of the skin and mucous membranes is common. With more severe anaemia, the sclera is a pearly white, in contrast to the occasional slightly icteric tint of advanced pernicious anaemia.

EPITHELIAL TISSUE CHANGES

Changes in the epithelial tissues occur in a *small proportion* of patients with iron deficiency anaemia. They are most commonly seen in long-standing chronic iron deficiency states. Changes occur in the nails, tongue, mouth, oesophagus and hair. The finger nails become thin, lustreless, brittle, and show longitudinal ridging and flattening. In the most severe cases, the nails actually become concave or spoon-shaped—this is known as koilonychia. The characteristic change in the tongue is atrophy of the papillae, resulting in a pale, smooth, atrophic, shiny or glazed tongue, a feature which is not restricted to iron deficiency. Atrophy may be confined to the sides or may involve the whole tongue. Frequently this *atrophic glossitis* develops painlessly, but attacks of soreness and burning of the tongue are not uncommon, the tongue showing red inflamed areas denuded of papillae. The mucous membranes of the mouth and cheeks may also appear red. Rarely, *leukoplakia* of the tongue or mouth occurs. *Angular stomatitis* with redness, soreness and cracking at the angles of the mouth sometimes develops.

The *Plummer–Vinson (Paterson–Kelly) syndrome,* characterized by chronic iron deficiency anaemia and dysphagia, often with glossitis, is occasionally seen. It usually occurs in middle-aged or elderly women with severe chronic iron deficiency. The dysphagia appears to be due to constriction at the entrance of the oesophagus. Sometimes, a fine web or band, probably made up of desquamating epithelial cells, obstructs the oesophagus. This may be demonstrable radiologically as a 'post-cricoid web'. The patient localizes the obstruction at about the level of the larynx. Solid foodstuffs cannot be swallowed, and only fluids and soft foods can be taken in extreme cases. The dysphagia may be worse when the patient is tired. Iron therapy alone often improves the dysphagia, but in more severe cases the passage of a bougie may be necessary. This mucosal change is known to be associated with an increased incidence of post-cricoid carcinoma. The non-haematological effects of iron deficiency are reviewed by Jacobs (1982).

IRON DEFICIENCY ANAEMIA OF INFANCY AND CHILDHOOD

Pallor, irritability, listlessness and anorexia are the most prominent features in infants and young children. Cardiac enlargement is uncommon, although it may occur with severe anaemia. The changes in epithelial tissues seen in adults do not occur in infants, and are only rarely seen in older children.

Blood picture

The essential feature is a diminished concentration of haemoglobin in microcytic red cells. The degree of anaemia varies. It is usually of mild to moderate severity, but may be marked, especially in cases due to persistent, severe blood loss. The red cell count is reduced to a lesser degree than the haemoglobin level, and the count may be near normal even when the haemoglobin is reduced to 8–9 g/dl. The MCV and MCH are reduced, the degree of reduction depending on the severity of the anaemia. In severe cases, the MCV may be as low as 55 fl. The co-existence of vitamin B_{12} on folate deficiency occasionally results in the finding of a normal MCV and MCH in spite of depleted iron stores. The MCHC, if calculated directly from the haemoglobin level and centrifuged haematocrit (see Chapter 2, p. 24), is reduced in parallel with the MCV. The indirectly derived MCHC produced by modern automated cell counters is a less sensitive and reliable index of iron deficiency, and may be normal or only slightly reduced in severe iron deficiency.

In the blood film, the red cells are hypochromic, and there is anisocytosis and poikilocytosis. These changes are, in general, more marked in severe anaemia. The hypochromia varies in degree from a slight increase in the normal area of central pallor of the red cell to an extremely large area of central pallor surrounded by a small rim of haemoglobin concentrated at the periphery (Fig. 3.4). A small proportion of cells of normal haemoglobin content is usually present. Many cells, often the majority, are smaller than normal, and a few are tiny microcytes. A small number of slightly macrocytic cells, often polychromatic, are commonly present. Variation in shape is usual and is often marked. Elliptical forms are common, and elongated pencil-shaped cells may be seen. Target cells are commonly present in small numbers. The reticulocyte count is usually normal or reduced, but may be slightly raised, e.g. from 2 to 5 per cent, especially after haemorrhage. Normoblasts are uncommon, but occasionally appear in small numbers in severe anaemia or after haemorrhage.

The white cell count and differential are usually normal. The platelet count is usually normal, but may be slightly to moderately increased, especially in patients who are bleeding.

Bone marrow

The characteristic change in the marrow is erythroid hyperplasia; the increase is mainly in more mature forms. The predominant cells are polychromatic normoblasts which are commonly smaller than normal. Erythropoiesis is thus described as being micronormoblastic. The cytoplasm is decreased, and sometimes consists only of a small rim around the nucleus. It often stains irregularly, and sometimes has a ragged border. Cytoplasmic maturation

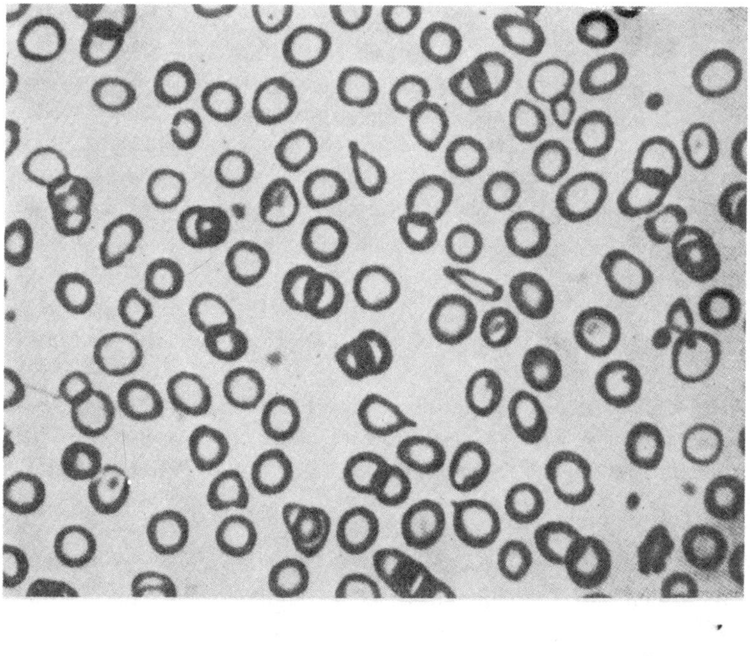

Fig. 3.4. *Photomicrograph of the blood film from a patient with hypochromic microcytic anaemia showing hypochromia, microcytosis, poikilocytosis and central pallor (× 710).*

appears to lag behind condensation of nuclear chromatin, so that the nucleus often appears almost pyknotic, despite the fact that the cytoplasm is still polychromatic. Granulopoietic cells and megakaryocytes are present in normal numbers and are of normal appearance. Examination of films of the aspirate and sections of trephine biopsies stained with potassium ferrocyanide shows that reticulo-endothelial iron is absent, and sideroblasts are greatly diminished.

Marrow examination is seldom necessary for diagnosis, unless there are unusual difficulties in the differentiation of iron deficiency anaemia from other causes of hypochromic anaemia (p. 50).

Biochemical findings

The level of serum iron is reduced to values usually ranging from 2.5 to 10 μmol/l. The total iron-binding capacity of the serum is increased, sometimes up to 100 μmol/l or even more, and the percentage saturation of the iron-binding protein is decreased to below 16 per cent. Serum ferritin is less than 12 μg/l in uncomplicated cases, but a level in the normal range does not necessarily exclude iron deficiency. In patients with chronic infection, inflammation, or malignancy, a serum ferritin level below 50 μg/l is often associated with reduced or absent iron stores.

Red cell protoporphyrin is increased to values ranging from 100 to 600 μg/dl (normal 20–40 μg/dl). The protoporphyrin accumulates in the red cells in the free form as there is insufficient iron to combine with it to produce haem. Estimation of red cell protoporphyrin has been used to diagnose iron deficiency before the development of overt hypochromic anaemia.

Diagnosis

There are two steps in diagnosis: to establish that the *anaemia is due to iron deficiency,* and to determine the *cause of the iron deficiency.*

TYPE OF ANAEMIA

The diagnosis of iron deficiency anaemia is often suggested by the clinical features, particularly the history, but it can be established with certainty only by blood examination. Satisfactory response to iron therapy confirms the diagnosis.

The history commonly reveals a known cause, particularly chronic haemorrhage. Koilonychia, when present, strongly suggests the diagnosis, as iron deficiency is its most common cause. Glossitis is of less diagnostic value as it occurs in pernicious anaemia and in certain other deficiency states.

Blood examination shows the typical hypochromic features, but differentiation from other causes of hypochromia such as thalassaemia is essential, and is considered later.

CAUSE OF THE IRON DEFICIENCY

The cause varies with the age and sex of the patient (Table 3.6). Careful consideration of the clinical features, especially of the history, will establish the cause in many cases, but further investigation is often necessary.

In *females of child-bearing age,* inquiry about menorrhagia, the number and frequency of pregnancies and miscarriages, and the nature of the diet usually indicates the probable causative factor or factors. If the history fails to suggest an adequate explanation for the anaemia, the possibility of occult gastrointestinal blood loss must be considered and appropriately investigated. Aspirin ingestion is a well recognized cause of gastritis resulting in occult blood loss. Thus a history of chronic aspirin ingestion should always be sought, especially when there is no obvious cause of gastrointestinal bleeding. It is important to realize that there is commonly no associated dyspepsia or abdominal discomfort. Aspirin ingestion as a cause of hypochromic anaemia should be especially considered in patients with chronic arthritis.

In *adult males,* most cases are due to gastrointestinal bleeding, the cause of which must be determined (see Table 3.5); this is also true for most *post-menopausal females.* In *infants and young children,* faulty diet is frequently established by the history.

Table 3.6 summarizes an approach to evaluation of the patient with iron deficiency anaemia. The special investigations are indicated by the provisional diagnosis made after consideration of the

Table 3.6. *Investigation of a patient with iron deficiency anaemia*

History

Females in the reproductive period of life

Menstrual history—especially menorrhagia
Pregnancies—number and frequency
Miscarriages
Diet
Alimentary blood loss as discussed in greater detail below
Haematuria, epistaxis, haemoptysis
Gastrointestinal surgery
Chronic aspirin ingestion

Males and post-menopausal females

Alimentary blood loss
(a) symptoms suggestive of gastrointestinal disorder—dyspepsia, weight loss, anorexia, abdominal pain, diarrhoea, constipation, alteration of bowel habits, dysphagia, acid regurgitation
(b) haemorrhoids
(c) haematemesis or melaena
Epistaxis, haematuria, haemoptysis
Gastrointestinal surgery
Diet
Chronic aspirin ingestion

Infants and children

Detailed dietary history, especially of supplemental feeding
Prematurity, multiple births or iron deficiency in mother
Gastrointestinal disturbance
Blood loss

Physical examination

Abdomen—abdominal mass, tenderness, features of liver disease
Rectal examination and proctoscopy
Pelvic examination
Telangiectasia of face and mouth

Relevant investigations*

Investigations commonly required

Examination of faeces for occult blood. Repeat several times if necessary
Upper gastrointestinal tract endoscopy or barium swallow, meal and follow-through (peptic ulcer, hiatus hernia, carcinoma of stomach, oesophageal varices, Meckel's diverticulum)
Colonoscopy or barium enema (carcinoma of colon and caecum, ulcerative colitis, diverticula, angiodysplasia)
Sigmoidoscopy (carcinoma of rectum, ulcerative colitis)
Microscopic examination of urine (haematuria)

Investigations occasionally required

Chest X-ray (haemoptysis)
Cystoscopy and/or pyelography (haematuria)
Examination of faeces for parasites (hookworm)
Liver function tests (cirrhosis of the liver)
Faecal fat, jejunal biopsy (malabsorption)
Laparotomy (persistent unexplained gastrointestinal bleeding)
Estimation of isotope-labelled red cell loss in stool (Meckel's diverticulum)
Selective mesenteric artery angiography (angiodysplasia)

*Disorders in which particular investigations are especially appropriate are bracketed with the investigation.

clinical features. They should always be performed in the order of maximum information yield and least inconvenience and expense to the patient.

Inspection of the stool and the test for occult blood in the faeces are of great importance in the detection of alimentary tract bleeding. Oral administration of iron causes the faeces to appear black and may simulate melaena, but does not in itself give a positive test for occult blood. Gastrointestinal bleeding is often intermittent, so that a single negative occult blood test does not exclude a lesion which can bleed, and the test may have to be repeated on several occasions before a positive result is obtained. The test is, however, very sensitive, and is rendered positive by loss of small amounts of blood at any site in the alimentary tract from oropharynx to anus.

Differential diagnosis of the hypochromic anaemias

The majority of cases of hypochromic anaemia are due to iron deficiency. Hypochromic anaemia is, however, commonly encountered in disorders in which the morphological abnormality is not due to unavailability of iron but to a block in iron utilization or globin synthesis in the red cell precursor. The establishment of an accurate diagnosis in the hypochromic anaemias is of great importance in ensuring correct treatment. The administration of iron to a patient with a hypochromic anaemia due to a cause other than iron deficiency is not only unhelpful, but leads to an undesirable increase in body iron stores. Diagnosis should be based on a carefully taken history, physical examination, and analysis of haematological and biochemical data. A scheme for the systematic laboratory investigation of hypochromic anaemias is illustrated in Table 3.7.

The hypochromic anaemias due to causes other than iron deficiency are thalassaemia, anaemia of chronic disease, and sideroblastic anaemia.

THALASSAEMIA

The homozygous form of beta thalassaemia is associated with red cell hypochromia, but the morphological changes are usually so bizarre that the condition is unlikely to be mistaken for iron deficiency. The heterozygous form, beta thalassaemia minor, is common in people of Mediterranean, African, Indian, and south-east Asian descent, and the blood film may be impossible to distinguish from that in iron deficiency. Similar considerations apply to heterozygous forms of alpha thalassaemia which are common in many of the regions where beta thalassaemia is found (p. 163).

Enquiry into the patient's ethnic origin and family history is an essential first step. The red cell count tends to be higher in thalassaemia than in iron

Table 3.7. *Systematic approach to laboratory investigation in the differential diagnosis of the hypochromic anaemias*

Hypochromic microcytic anaemia

↓

Iron studies

Ferritin	Reduced	Normal or increased	Normal	Normal or increased
Iron	Reduced	Reduced	Normal	Normal or increased
TIBC	Increased	Normal or reduced	Normal	Normal
Percentage saturation	Reduced	Reduced	Normal	Normal or increased
	↓	↓	↓	↓
	Iron deficiency	Anaemia of chronic disease	Haemoglobin studies	Bone marrow examination
			↓	↓
			Thalassaemia	Sideroblastic anaemia

deficiency, and target cells and basophilic stippling may be prominent on the blood film, but these changes are variable. More useful is the fact that the *degree of reduction of MCV and MCH in iron deficiency tends to parallel the severity of the anaemia, which contrasts with most cases of heterozygous thalassaemia in which the MCV and MCH are disproportionately low*. A number of discriminant functions derived by manipulation of red cell data produced by automated cell counters have been described as valuable in differential diagnosis, but none has been consistently accurate enough to be of clinical use. The red cell distribution width, an index of the heterogeneity of distribution of red cell size, i.e. anisocytosis, is generally normal in thalassaemia and increased in iron deficiency, but exceptions occur often enough to limit the diagnostic usefulness of the test (Bessman *et al.* 1983).

In uncomplicated cases of thalassaemia, iron studies exclude iron deficiency, and haemoglobin electrophoresis demonstrates the elevation of haemoglobin A_2 which characterizes beta thalassaemia minor, or less frequently the lone increase in haemoglobin F of the beta-delta form of thalassaemia minor. Haemoglobin electrophoresis is usually unrewarding in alpha thalassaemia minor, and haemoglobin H inclusions, diagnostic of alpha thalassaemia minor, should be sought in a brilliant cresyl blue-stained blood film. The combination of beta thalassaemia minor and iron deficiency is a common source of diagnostic confusion as the latter can cause the elevated haemoglobin A_2 to fall to a normal level. Thus, it is wise to re-check the haemoglobin A_2 in a patient whose MCV and MCH remain low following iron therapy in spite of recovery in haemoglobin level.

ANAEMIA OF CHRONIC DISORDERS (p. 102)

The anaemia and red cell morphological changes in chronic disease are usually only mild to moderate. Although the MCV is usually normal, it can occasionally be reduced and associated with hypochromia of mild degree on the blood film. History and physical examination may indicate the presence of chronic infection, malignant neoplasm, or inflammatory disorder such as rheumatoid arthritis. Athough the serum iron level is characteristically reduced, the overall pattern of normal or increased serum ferritin and decreased total iron-binding capacity is different from that of iron deficiency (Fig. 3.5). In occasional complicated cases with conflicting laboratory tests, examination of bone marrow aspirate for stainable iron is required for diagnosis.

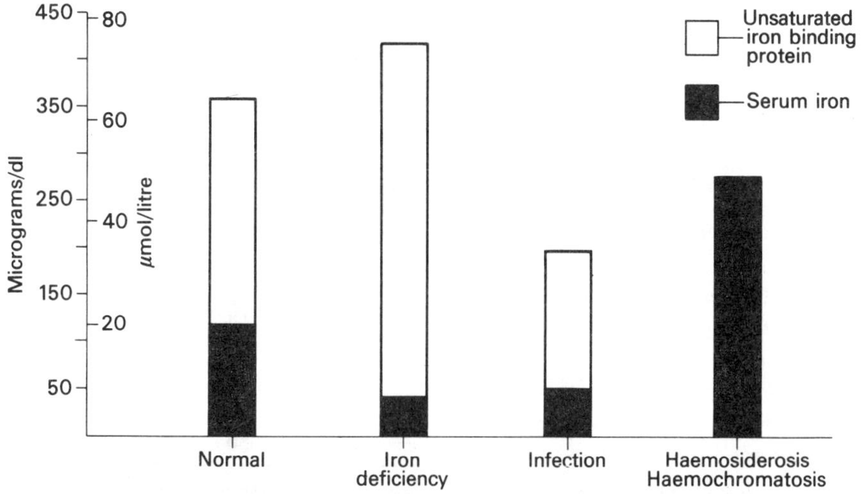

Fig. 3.5. *Serum iron and iron-binding capacity in different disorders affecting iron metabolism.*

SIDEROBLASTIC ANAEMIA (p. 56)

A dimorphic red cell picture on the blood film, with both normal and hypochromic red cells, is common in primary acquired sideroblastic anaemia, but the MCV is usually in the upper normal range. Iron studies exclude iron deficiency, and demonstration of ring sideroblasts in a Prussian blue-stained bone marrow aspirate confirms the diagnosis of sideroblastic anaemia.

Treatment

There are two essential principles in the management of iron deficiency anaemia: *correction of the disorder causing the anaemia* and *correction of iron deficiency*.

CORRECTION OF THE UNDERLYING DISORDER

Correction of the disorder causing the anaemia is of paramount importance. It varies from simple measures, such as cessation of aspirin ingestion or correction of dietary faults, to major surgical procedures to correct the cause of blood loss.

Appropriate medical or surgical procedures must be instituted to eliminate or alleviate blood loss. In women with persistently heavy menstrual loss for which there is no obvious organic cause, hormone therapy may be of help.

IRON ADMINISTRATION

General considerations in iron therapy

Objects of therapy. The objects of iron therapy are to restore the haemoglobin level to normal and to replenish the exhausted tissue iron stores. Both dosage and duration of therapy must be adequate to achieve these objects.

Route of administration. Iron may be administered by mouth or by parenteral injection, either intramuscular or intravenous.

Most patients respond satisfactorily to oral iron therapy; further, it is cheap and safe. Thus, oral therapy is the treatment of choice in most cases. Parenteral iron is expensive, and may be accompanied by undesirable side-effects, some of which are severe. However, parenteral treatment is useful in a small proportion of cases.

A response to iron therapy administered *without other haematinic agents* supplies important confirmatory evidence of the diagnosis of iron deficiency anaemia. For this reason, iron should be administered alone, and not with other haematinics, as this may confuse the interpretation of the response to treatment. Thus, oral preparations containing substances such as folic acid, vitamin B_{12} and other B vitamins should be avoided. There is no evidence that these supplements are of value in iron deficiency anaemia, and they considerably increase the cost of treatment.

Oral iron administration

A wide variety of oral iron preparations is available, and some are listed in Table 3.8. Ferrous salts are much more effectively absorbed than ferric salts, which must first be reduced to the ferrous form. Ferrous salts are unstable in solution, becoming oxidized to the ferric form, and are best given as coated (but not 'enteric-coated') tablets or capsules.

Sustained-release preparations are formulated to free the iron slowly as the tablet or capsule passes through the gastrointestinal tract, thus avoiding a high concentration of iron at any one site. They suffer the disadvantage of greater cost, and sometimes low release of iron from the formulation.

Table 3.8. *Oral iron preparations*

Preparation	Elemental iron content (mg)
Ferrous sulphate, 200 mg	60
Ferrous gluconate, 300 mg	35
Ferrous fumarate, 200 mg	65
Sustained-release preparation	
Ferrous sulphate, 350 mg	105

Several effective liquid preparations suitable for children are available.

CHOICE OF PREPARATION AND DOSE

The daily dosage should supply from 100 to 200 mg elemental iron. Ferrous sulphate is the preparation of choice, as it contains a high proportion of elemental iron, is efficiently absorbed, and is the cheapest of the ferrous salts. Most patients respond adequately to one tablet three times a day. Reasonable alternatives are ferrous gluconate or fumarate in a dose of one to two tablets three times a day.

Iron intolerance in the form of nausea, vomiting, abdominal discomfort or colicky pain, diarrhoea, and constipation sometimes occurs following the administration of conventional therapeutic doses. It is more common in pregnant women. Hallberg *et al.* (1966) observed intolerance after iron tablets in 25 per cent of patients but 14 per cent of those receiving *placebo* tablets also reported symptoms. *Symptoms are dose related and can usually be prevented or minimized by commencing with small doses which are then gradually increased, and taking the iron either with meals or immediately afterwards.* If symptoms are troublesome, the iron is discontinued for several days, then one tablet is taken with the main meal for one week, two daily the next week, and then three daily. If symptoms still occur, a sustained-release preparation should be tried. If these measures fail, the question of parenteral therapy should be considered.

RESPONSE

Adequate replacement of iron is followed by an increase in the reticulocyte count, which usually commences on the fourth day and lasts for about 12 days. The height of the response is inversely proportional to the haemoglobin level before treatment, and may reach around 16 per cent in severe anaemia. In general, the response is not as marked or as regular as the response of pernicious anaemia to vitamin B_{12}, and it is more practical to use the *rise in haemoglobin level as a measure of the effectiveness of treatment*. The haemoglobin level rises at an average rate of about 0.15 g/dl per day, usually commencing about one week after the institution of therapy. The rate of regeneration is more marked in the early stages, lessening as the haemoglobin value approaches normal.

Epithelial tissue changes, when present, are usually relieved, but response is often slow. The tongue papillae regenerate, and the tongue may ultimately appear normal. Soreness of the tongue and fissuring at the angle of the mouth disappear. The brittle flattened nails are replaced by nails of normal shape and texture. The dysphagia of the Plummer–Vinson syndrome is usually, but not always, relieved, and other measures, e.g. the passage of a bougie, are sometimes necessary, especially in long-established cases.

DURATION OF THERAPY

Iron is given in full doses until the haemoglobin level has been restored to normal. In uncomplicated cases this requires 4–10 weeks, depending on the severity of the anaemia. Smaller doses, e.g. one or two tablets of ferrous sulphate daily, are then given for a further 3–6 months, as this aids in replenishing the depleted iron tissue stores.

When the iron deficiency is due to chronic blood loss which cannot be controlled, a maintenance dose of iron is often necessary. The dosage varies with the degree of blood loss. Maintenance therapy is most often required in women with heavy menstrual loss; one common practice is to give such women oral iron in full doses for one week of each month. As an alternative to maintenance oral iron therapy, a course of parenteral iron may be given, and this may be the only effective approach when blood loss is severe and persistent.

FAILURE OF RESPONSE TO ORAL IRON

A proportion of patients respond incompletely to adequate doses of iron, or fail to respond at all.

Common causes of failure

The three common causes of failure to respond are wrong diagnosis, non-compliance, and persistent haemorrhage.

Wrong diagnosis. The clinical and haematological findings should be reviewed as the failure can be due to an incorrect assumption that the anaemia is due to iron deficiency.

Failure to take the tablets. It is not uncommon for patients to discontinue therapy or reduce dosage because of gastrointestinal disturbance. Careful questioning is often necessary to establish non-compliance.

Persistent haemorrhage. Persistent haemorrhage, if at all marked, causes partial or complete failure of response. When bleeding is severe, the haemoglobin level may actually fall, as the rate of the blood regeneration may not be able to keep pace with the rate of blood loss. The source of the bleeding, if not clinically obvious, is almost invariably the gastrointestinal tract.

Less common causes of failure

A complicating disorder that impairs bone marrow response. This may be:

chronic infection
chronic renal insufficiency
co-existing vitamin B_{12} or foliate deficiency.

These disorders may themselves be a cause of anaemia. When true iron deficiency due to haemorrhage or some other cause occurs at the same time as one of these disorders, response to iron therapy may be inadequate because of the inhibiting effect that these disorders exert on erythropoiesis.

Chronic infection as a cause of impaired response is especially important in children, but it also occurs in adults, in conditions such as chronic urinary tract infection. Chronic renal insufficiency is important as a cause of impaired response in older people in whom a degree of renal impairment is relatively common. The serum creatinine level should be determined in all patients with iron deficiency anaemia who inexplicably fail to respond to treatment.

Impairment of absorption due to alimentary tract disease. Absorption may be impaired following gastrectomy and gastro-enterostomy, and in sprue and coeliac disease.

Failure of absorption of unknown cause. Rarely, patients without overt gastrointestinal disease respond to parenteral, but not oral, iron. Many such cases are due to occult malabsorptive disease.

Parenteral iron administration

As stated above, most patients with iron deficiency anaemia respond adequately to oral iron therapy, which is the usual treatment of choice. However, parenteral therapy is indicated in a small proportion of cases. The pattern of response to parenteral therapy is similar to that with oral iron.

INDICATIONS FOR PARENTERAL IRON THERAPY

Intolerance to oral iron. Gastrointestinal symptoms can usually be relieved by modifying dosage or changing preparations, and only when these measures fail should parenteral iron be used.

Chronic blood loss. In cases of chronic blood loss in which the source of bleeding cannot be adequately controlled, orally administered iron may not satisfy the requirement of iron for replacement of lost blood. This type of chronic blood loss is most commonly seen with gastrointestinal lesions that do not respond to medical treatment and for which, for some reason, surgery is contra-indicated, e.g. certain subjects with peptic ulcer and hiatus hernia. Persistent menorrhagia and the repeated epistaxis of hereditary haemorrhagic telangiectasia are other causes of such blood loss.

Gastrointestinal disorders whose symptoms may be aggravated by oral iron. These disorders include peptic ulceration, ulcerative colitis, regional enteritis, and a functioning colostomy.

Impaired iron absorption. Impaired absorption may occur after gastrectomy and gastro-enterostomy, and in sprue and coeliac disease.

When rapid replenishment of iron stores is required. With marked anaemia discovered late in pregnancy, or in preparation for surgery, parenteral iron may be used as a preferable alternative to transfusion.

Parenteral iron preparations

Intravenous and intramuscular preparations are available, but are contra-indicated in patients with a history of allergy, especially asthma, and in those who have had a previous serious reaction to the preparation. Choice of route and preparation vary according to circumstances, e.g. whether the patient is in hospital, is able and willing to attend for repeated injections, or has suitable muscle mass for intramuscular injections. When the intramuscular route is chosen, iron–dextran or iron–sorbitol are suitable. When the patient is in hospital where adequate medical supervision is available, intravenous iron–dextran can be administered.

IRON-DEXTRAN

Iron–dextran (Imferon) is a colloid of ferric hydroxide with dextran, supplied in 2, 5, and 20 ml ampoules. Each millilitre contains the equivalent of 50 mg elemental iron. Thus the 2 ml ampoule contains 100 mg iron, the 5 ml ampoule 250 mg, and the 20 ml ampoule 1000 mg. It may be administered by either the intramuscular or the intravenous route, the former being preferred unless contra-indications are present.

After intramuscular injection, iron-dextran is slowly absorbed from the injection site via the lymphatics, and reaches peak concentration in plasma in 24–48 hours. It is taken up by reticulo-endothelial cells, mainly in the liver, from which the iron is transferred to erythroblasts.

The total dosage of iron is calculated by adding together the amount required to restore the haemoglobin value to normal and the amount required to replenish the tissue stores partially or completely. In patients whose blood loss has been arrested, partial replenishing of the stores with 500 mg iron is probably adequate, but in those with continuing blood loss, it is advisable to give 1000 mg.

The amount of iron in mg required to restore the haemoglobin to normal may be calculated as follows (Callender 1982):

Total dose = Haemoglobin deficit in g/dl ÷ 100
× ml blood vol. (65 ml × body wt in kg)
× 3.4 (mg iron per g haemoglobin)

INTRAMUSCULAR ADMINISTRATION

Iron–dextran is administered daily to weekly until the total amount required is given. Each dose should not exceed 2 ml. After filling the syringe from the ampoule, a new needle should be used, and the length of the needle should be such as to ensure a deep intramuscular injection. The injections are given into the upper, outer quadrant of the buttock, alternating the side on successive injections. The skin is moved aside at the site of injection and kept taut to prevent leakage back of the darkly stained fluid. The injection is given by a slow and steady pressure on the plunger, and the needle is quickly withdrawn ten seconds after the completion of the injection. The injection site is not massaged, but the patient is advised to move his/her legs for some minutes after injection. Local tenderness is common.

INTRAVENOUS ADMINISTRATION

Undiluted method

The total iron–dextran dose is given as a single bolus in a series of injections in a manner similar to intramuscular administration. A prior test dose of 0.5 ml iron-dextran diluted with 4–5 ml of the patient's blood should be injected slowly, and the patient then observed carefully for at least 30 minutes for side-effects. If the test dose is well tolerated, a therapeutic dose of up to 5 ml is given as a slow intravenous injection at a rate not exceeding 1 ml per minute. The patient should be under constant medical surveillance during the injections, and observation should be continued for at least one hour thereafter. The iron–dextran is irritating to the tissues, and the needle used for aspirating the ampoule contents should not be used for the intravenous injection. The injection must be ceased immediately if there is any suspicion that the needle is outside the vein. If extravasation occurs, the skin at the point of the needle becomes slate-grey in colour, and the patient complains of pain.

Total dose infusion method

The dose is diluted in a litre of isotonic saline or dextrose. In persons in whom circulatory overload is unlikely, saline is preferred as the incidence of phlebitis is thought to be less. Dextrose is employed in those in whom saline infusion is undesirable. The maximum concentration of iron used should not exceed 2.5 g (50 ml iron–dextran) per 1000 ml diluent.

For the first 20 minutes the infusion must be supervised closely and run slowly, e.g. at a rate of about 15 drops per minute. If no untoward reaction occurs in this time, the rate is increased to 45–60 drops per minute (1 litre over 4–5 hours) until the infusion is completed. Temperature, pulse rate and blood pressure are recorded every half hour in the first hour, and then hourly. The patient is watched for signs of side-effects and circulatory overload.

ADVERSE REACTIONS

The administration of iron–dextran is generally free from serious side-effects if the patient is truly iron deficient and the technique and dosage schedule are adhered to as described. It is also particularly important to confirm that the patient has no history of a previous reaction to iron–dextran. The intramuscular route is preferred unless there are compelling reasons for intravenous administration.

The most serious side-effect is an anaphylactic reaction, which most often occurs within the first few minutes of intravenous infusion. In addition to collapse, there may be fever, rigors, chest pain, dyspnoea, flushing, sweating, nausea and vomiting. Should this occur, the infusion must be immediately stopped and measures for treatment of anaphylactic shock instituted. Adrenalin, parenteral antihistamines, and hydrocortisone hemisuccinate should be available for immediate use.

Intramuscular or intravenous administration may be followed by delayed reactions. These include pyrexia, arthralgia, and myalgia, which often persist for up to four days, and rarely regional lymphadenopathy. Exacerbation of joint pain occasionally occurs in rheumatoid arthritis, and intravenous iron–dextran is best avoided in this disorder, except as a last resort.

IRON-SORBITOL-CITRATE

Iron–sorbitol–citrate (Jectofer) is suitable for intramuscular use only. It is rapidly cleared from the injection site because of its small molecular size, but up to 30 per cent of the dose is excreted in the urine in the first 24 hours. It is supplied in 2 ml ampoules, each ml containing 50 mg elemental iron. The total dose is calculated using the formula described for iron–dextran, and an additional amount is added to cover that lost in the urine.

Local reactions are minimal. Slight discomfort is occasionally experienced, and local staining of the skin is unusual. General reactions are similar to those of iron–dextran. Some patients notice an unpleasant taste or loss of taste. Patients with active urinary tract infections should not be treated with iron–sorbitol–citrate.

The sideroblastic anaemias

The sideroblastic anaemias (Table 3.9) are a group of disorders of varying aetiology in which the marrow shows marked dyserythropoiesis and an abnormal intramitochondrial accumulation of iron in erythroid precursors. Hypochromic as well as

Table 3.9. *Classification of the sideroblastic anaemias*

HEREDITARY
ACQUIRED
Primary
Secondary
Drugs and chemicals
Antituberculous (e.g. isoniazid, cycloserine)
Lead
Ethanol
Chloramphenicol
Haematological disorders
Myelofibrosis
Polycythaemia vera
Myeloma
Acute leukaemia
Hodgkin's disease
Haemolytic anaemia
Inflammatory disease
Rheumatoid arthritis
Systemic lupus erythematosus
Miscellaneous
Carcinoma
Myxoedema
Malabsorption

normochromic red cells are usually present in the peripheral blood, resulting in a dimorphic blood picture. Abnormalities in haem synthesis have been demonstrated in some patients.

Although relatively uncommon, the sideroblastic anaemias are being recognized with increasing frequency, especially as routine staining of bone marrow films for iron is now standard practice in most laboratories.

Siderocytes and sideroblasts

Siderocytes are red cells containing granules of non-haem iron which give a positive Prussian blue reaction. The granules also stain with Romanovsky dyes, appearing as basophilic granules referred to as *Pappenheimer bodies*. In health, siderocytes are not normally found in red cells in the peripheral blood, but small numbers are seen following splenectomy. Normal reticulocytes after release from the marrow are sequestered in the spleen where they complete haem synthesis and use the iron present in granular form in their *cytoplasm*. After splenectomy, this stage of reticulocyte maturation must occur in the peripheral blood, and cytoplasmic iron granules can be seen in some reticulocytes. The spleen also removes large siderotic granules present in disease states, and in the absence of the spleen these granules may persist for the lifespan of the red cell (Lewis 1983).

Sideroblasts are erythroblasts with Prussian blue positive iron granules in their cytoplasm. Three types (one normal and two abnormal) of sideroblast are defined on the basis of the number, size and distribution of the siderotic granules.

The *first type* is seen in normal bone marrow and represents iron that has not been utilized for haemoglobin synthesis. The granules are few in number, small, difficult to see, scattered through the cytoplasm, and not localized in the perinuclear zone. From 30 to 50 per cent of erythroblasts in normal marrow are sideroblasts of this type. They are not seen when iron deficiency is present.

The *second type* is abnormal and may be found in conditions in which the percentage saturation of transferrin is increased, e.g. with dyserythropoiesis (usually without a selective defect in haem or globin synthesis) or haemolysis. The siderotic granules are large and more numerous than normal, and are scattered diffusely through the cytoplasm. In this group of disorders the percentage of cells containing siderotic granules, and the number and size of these granules, is related to the percentage saturation of transferrin.

The *third type* is found in conditions in which haem synthesis is disturbed, e.g. the primary and secondary sideroblastic anaemias. No correlation exists between the percentage saturation of transferrin and the number and size of granules, or percentage of cells affected. The granules are more numerous and commonly large. They frequently form a complete or partial ring around the nucleus, when they are known as *ring sideroblasts*. The cause of the ring arrangement is clustering of abnormal iron-containing mitochondria around the nuclear border (Fresco 1981). Less commonly, the abnormal granules are diffusely scattered through the cytoplasm.

Hereditary sideroblastic anaemia

This rare disorder of sex-linked recessive inheritance has a presumed enzyme defect in haem synthesis. The affected males are anaemic. Carrier females may show no abnormality, or have mild red cell morphological changes with no anaemia. The condition is noted in childhood or young adult life. The anaemia is moderate to marked in degree. Hypochromic microcytic cells are prominent, although a minor population of normocytic cells is usually present, giving a dimorphic picture. The MCV and MCH are decreased. The serum iron is usually raised, with almost complete saturation of iron-binding capacity. Ring sideroblasts are present in the marrow in large numbers, and are typically mature erythroblasts. There is increased iron deposition in the tissues, and even haemochromatotic tissue damage may develop.

In general, treatment is unsatisfactory, although in some cases a partial response to high doses of pyridoxine occurs, although the typical red cell abnormalities remain. Secondary folate deficiency may develop which responds to folic acid.

Acquired sideroblastic anaemias

These acquired anaemias are classified as primary and secondary. They are uncommon but by no means rare, and are being recognized with increasing frequency.

PRIMARY

Primary acquired sideroblastic anaemia is generally regarded as a myelodysplastic disorder, and is referred to as *refractory anaemia with ring sideroblasts* (Type 2 in the French, American, British classification of Bennett *et al.* 1982).

This primary anaemia occurs in adults of both sexes, mainly in middle-aged and elderly subjects. It is characterized by insidious onset; symptoms may have been present for months or years. In some cases, the skin has a generalized dusky hue, especially on the arms and hands. The spleen is either not palpable or palpable just below the left costal margin. The liver may be either of normal size or moderately enlarged. The lymph nodes are not enlarged.

The anaemia is moderate to severe, but many patients have stable haemoglobin levels of 6–7 g/dl, or slightly higher. Some require repeated transfusion. The main feature of the blood film is the dimorphic red cell picture, and it is this feature that suggests the diagnosis.

Most of the red cells are normocytic or mildly macrocytic and normochromic, and there is a lesser population of microcytic hypochromic cells. A few target cells, stippled cells, siderocytes and sideroblasts are often present. The reticulocyte count is usually normal. The MCV is usually at the upper limit of normal or mildly elevated, and the MCH is normal or slightly reduced. The neutrophil count may be normal or decreased. Poorly granulated and Pelger–Hüet neutrophils are sometimes present. The platelet count is either normal, decreased or, less commonly, moderately increased. The neutrophil alkaline phosphatase score is subnormal in about 50 per cent of patients.

The bone marrow is hyperplastic, mainly due to erythroid hyperplasia. Erythropoiesis is usually normoblastic (commonly macronormoblastic) with a shift to the left, but varying degrees of megaloblastic change are not uncommon. There can be marked dyserythropoiesis with binucleate erythroblasts and cytoplasmic vacuolation in late normoblasts. Iron stain of the marrow aspirate shows that nearly all the erythroblasts have increased numbers of abnormal iron granules in their cytoplasm, many (both early and late forms) being ring sideroblasts. For a diagnosis of *refractory anaemia with ring sideroblasts* as defined by the French, American, British classification of myelodysplastic syndromes, at least 15 per cent of the erythroblasts must be ring sideroblasts. Dysmyelopoiesis and abnormal megakaryocytes may also be prominent (Singh *et al.* 1970). Chromosome abnormalities occur in 20–50 per cent of patients.

Ferrokinetic studies show that erythropoiesis is relatively ineffective. The serum iron and ferritin, and the red cell protoporphyrin, are usually moderately raised, and the percentage saturation of the iron-binding protein is increased. The serum bilirubin is normal or slightly increased.

Pathogenesis

Primary acquired sideroblastic anaemia is generally considered to be a clonal disorder of a haemopoietic progenitor cell in which the major manifestation is defective haem synthesis in erythroid precursors, due in most cases to a reduction in the activity of the enzyme ALA synthetase. The abnormalities in iron metabolism which are so prominent in the disorder are probably secondary to the impairment of haem synthesis. An alternative view is that the primary lesion is in the processing of erythroblast iron by abnormal mitochondria (Jacobs 1986).

Course and treatment

Most patients have a relatively benign course, and median survival is 5–10 years (Cheng *et al.* 1979). If symptoms of anaemia develop, 5–10 per cent of patients respond partially or nearly completely to large doses of pyridoxine, 200 mg daily. Secondary folate deficiency is common, and folic acid should be given if the serum folate level is low. Transfusion with red cells is given when symptoms require it, but should be kept to a minimum because of the possible development of toxicity due to iron overload. Iron-chelation therapy may be appropriate in patients with iron overload (p. 160). Neutropenia and thrombocytopenia are rarely severe enough to cause difficulties in management. In about ten per cent of patients the disorder evolves into acute leukaemia, almost always of the myeloid type.

SECONDARY

Drugs and chemicals

Of the *pyridoxine antagonists* used in the treatment of tuberculosis, isoniazid is the drug most commonly associated with the development of sideroblastic anaemia, which occurs after a few months of treatment. Other antituberculous drugs have been implicated in occasional cases.

Ring sideroblasts are sometimes seen in subjects with *lead poisoning* or receiving *chloramphenicol* therapy.

A dimorphic red cell picture with ring sideroblasts in the bone marrow is seen in up to 30 per cent of malnourished and usually folate deficient *alcoholic patients*, usually after a heavy drinking bout. The changes reverse rapidly on withdrawal of alcohol. In some such patients, abnormalities in the metabolism of pyridoxine, a co-enzyme in haem synthesis, have been found.

Association with haematological disorders

About ten per cent of patients with primary acquired sideroblastic anaemia develop acute myeloid leukaemia. Some patients with various malignant disorders who have been successfully treated with radiation and chemotherapy may also develop a sideroblastic anaemia which can evolve into acute leukaemia. Ring sideroblasts are also noted in some patients with acute leukaemia before and during cytotoxic chemotherapy, but they do not usually appear to have any effect on the basic behaviour of the disorder.

Radioactive iron studies

Radioactive iron (^{59}Fe) has been widely used as a probe to quantitate aspects of internal iron exchange in health and disease. Ferrokinetic studies once enjoyed considerable popularity in the investigation of the site, extent and effectiveness of erythropoiesis in haemolytic, aplastic and dyserythropoietic disorders, but appreciation of their theoretical and practical shortcomings has greatly reduced their use in recent years.

^{59}Fe is a γ-emitting nuclide with a half-life of 45 days, and is injected intravenously in the form of ferric citrate bound to transferrin. Blood samples are taken at intervals over the ensuing 1–2 hours, the plasma radioactivity measured, and a clearance curve plotted. The half-life of ^{59}Fe in plasma in health is 60–140 minutes. Additional blood samples are taken over the next two weeks, and the radioactivity in the red cells measured. In normal subjects, 70–80 per cent of the injected dose of ^{59}Fe appears in the circulating red cells by the seventh day. Uptake of the nuclide in the sacrum, liver and spleen is measured by external counters positioned over the three sites (Dacie & Lewis 1984).

The ferrokinetic study provides the following information:

plasma iron clearance;
plasma iron turnover (calculated from the plasma iron level and the clearance time);
efficiency of red cell iron utilization; and
surface counting patterns.

Plasma iron clearance and plasma iron turnover have been used as indicators of total marrow erythroid activity, and red cell iron utilization provides an estimate of the effectiveness of erythropoiesis, i.e. erythropoiesis that results in the production of red cells that survive for a significant time in the circulation. Surface counting patterns indicate the extent to which different organs take up the injected iron and have been used to estimate the degree of extramedullary erythropoiesis in the spleen in myelofibrosis (p. 334). The cyclotron-produced nuclide ^{52}Fe has a half-life of eight hours and is particularly suitable for the quantitation of splenic erythropoiesis (Pettit *et al.* 1976).

Iron kinetic studies fail to take into account reflux of iron into plasma following initial clearance, and their contribution to diagnosis and management of haematological problems has often been disappointing. More recent approaches are superior, but they are time-consuming and require computer analysis of data.

References and further reading

Iron metabolism and iron deficiency

Addison, G.M., Beamish, M.R., Hales, C.N. *et al.* (1972) An immunoradiometric assay for ferritin in the serum of normal subjects and patients with iron deficiency and iron overload. *J. Clin. Path.* **25**, 326.

Baird, McLean, A. & Sutton, D.R. (1972) Blood loss after partial gastrectomy. *Gut.* **13**, 634.

Bentley, D.P. (1982) Anaemia and chronic disease. *Clin. Haemat.* **11**, 465.

Bentley, D.P. & Williams, P. (1974) Serum ferritin concentration as an index of storage iron in rheumatoid arthritis. *J. Clin. Path.* **27**, 786.

Bessman, J.D., Gilmer, P.R. & Gardner, F.H. (1983) Improved classification of anemias by MCV and RDW. *Am. J. Clin. Path.* **80**, 322.

Beveridge, B.R., Bannerman, R.M., Evans J.M. *et al.* (1965) Hypochromic anaemia. A retrospective study and follow-up of 378 in-patients. *Quart. J. Med.* **34**, 145.

Bothwell, T.H., Charlton, R.W., Cook, J.D. *et al.* (1979) *Iron metabolism in man*, Blackwell Scientific Publications, Oxford.

Brittenham, G.M., Danish, E.H. & Harris, J.W. (1981) Assessment of bone marrow and body iron stores: old techniques and new technologies. *Semin. Hematol.* **18**, 194.

Burman, D. (1982) Iron deficiency in infancy and childhood. *Clin. Haemat.* **11**, 339.

Callender, S.T. (1982) Treatment of iron deficiency. *Clin. Haemat.* **11**, 327.

Cavill, I., Worwood, M. & Jacobs, A. (1975) Internal regulation of iron absorption. *Nature*, **256**, 328.

Cazzola, M. & Ascari, E. (1986) Red cell ferritin as a diagnostic tool. *Brit. J. Haemat.* **62**, 209.

Charlton, R.W. & Bothwell, T.H. (1983) Iron absorption. *Ann. Rev. Med.* **34**, 55.

Chisholm, M. (1973) Tissue changes associated with iron deficiency. *Clin. Haemat.* **2**, 303.

Chisholm, M., Ardran, G.M., Callender, S.T. & Wright, R. (1971) A follow-up study of patients with post-cricoid webs. *Quart. J. Med.* **40**, 409.

Conrad, M.E. & Barton, J.C. (1981) Factors affecting iron balance. *Am. J. Hemat.* **10**, 199.

Davidson, A., Van Der Weyden, M.B., Fong, H. *et al.* (1984) Red cell ferritin content: a re-evaluation of indices for iron deficiency in the anaemia of rheumatoid arthritis. *Brit. Med. J. 289*, 648.

Deiss, A. (1983) Iron metabolism in reticuloendothelial cells. *Semin. Hematol.* **20**, 81.

Drysdale, J.W., Adelman, I.G., Arosio, P. *et al.* (1977). Human isoferritins in normal and disease states. *Semin. Haemat.* **14**, 71.

Ellis, L.D., Jensen, W.N. & Westerman, M.P. (1964) Marrow iron. An evaluation of depleted stores in a series of 1,332 needle biopsies. *Ann. Int. Med.* **61**, **44**.

Finch, C.A., Deubelbeiss, K., Cook, J.D. *et al.* (1970) Ferrokinetics in man. *Medicine*. **49**, 17.

Finch, C.A. & Huebers, H. (1982) Perspectives in iron metabolism. *New Engl. J. Med.* **306**, 1520.

Hallberg, L. (9181) Bioavailability of dietary iron in man. *Ann. Rev. Nutr.* **1**, 123.

Hallberg, L., Hogdahl, A., Nilsson, L. *et al.* (1966) Menstrual blood loss and iron deficiency. *Acta Med. Scand.* **180**, 639.

Hallberg, L., Ryttinger, L. & Solvell, L. (1966) Side effects of oral iron therapy. *Acta Med. Scand.* (Supp.) **459**, 3.

Halliday, J.W. & Powell, L.W. (1982) Iron overload. *Semin. Hematol.* **19**, 42.

Hines, J.D., Hoffbrand, A.V. & Mollin, D.L. (1967) The hematologic complications following partial gastrectomy. *Am. J. Med.* **43**, 555.

Huebers, H.A. & Finch, C.A. (1987) The physiology of transferrin and transferrin receptors. *Physiol. Rev.* **67**, 520.

Huebers, H., Josephson, B., Huebers, E. *et al.* (1981) Uptake and release of iron from human transferrin. *Proc. Natl. Acad. Sci.* **781**, 2572.

Jacobs, A. (1969) Tissue changes in iron deficiency. *Brit. J. Haemat.* **16**, 1.

Jacobs, A. (1973) The mechanism of iron absorption. *Clin. Haemat.* **2**, 323.

Jacobs, A. (1982) Non-haematological effects of iron deficiency. *Clin. Haemat.* **11**, 353.

Jacobs, A., Miller, F., Worwood M. *et al.* (1972) Ferritin in the serum of normal subjects and patients with iron deficiency and iron overload. *Brit. Med. J.* **4**, 206.

Jacobs, A. & Worwood, M. (1975) Ferritin in serum. *New Engl. J. Med.* **292**, 951.

Jacobs, A. & Worwood, M. (Eds) (1981) *Iron in Biochemistry and Medicine, II*, Academic Press, London.

Jacobs, A. & Worwood, M. (1984) Assessment of iron stores. *Assoc. Clin. Pathol.* Broadsheet No. 111.

Layrisse, M., Cook, J.D., Martinez, C. *et al.* (1969) Food iron absorption: a comparison of vegetable and animal foods. *Blood*, **33**, 430.

Lee G.R. (1983) The anemia of chronic disease. *Semin. Hematol.* **20**, 61.

Moore, C.V. (1965) Iron nutrition and requirements. *Ser. Haemat.* **6**, 1.

Osterloh, K.R.S., Simpson, R.J. & Peters, T.J. (1987) The role of mucosal transferrin in intestinal iron absorption. *Brit. J. Haemat.* **65**, 1.

Pilon, V.A., Howantiz, P.J., Howanitz, J.R. *et al.* (1981) Day-to-day variation in serum ferritin concentration in healthy subjects. *Clin. Chem.* **27**, 78.

Powell, L.W., Alpert, E., Isselbacher, K.J. *et al.* (1975) Human isoferritins: organ specific iron and apoferritin distribution. *Brit. J. Haemat.* **30**, 47.

Rybo, E. (1985) Diagnosis of iron deficiency. *Scand. J. Haem.* Suppl.No.43, **34**, 1.

Walters, G.D., Miller, F.M. & Worwood, M. (1973) Serum ferritin concentration and iron stores in normal subjects. *J. Clin. Path.* **26**, 770.

Worwood, M. (1982) Ferritin in human tissues and serum. *Clin. Haemat.* **11**, 275.

Sideroblastic anaemias

Bennett, J.M., Catovsky, D., Daniel, M.T. *et al.* (1982) Proposals for the classification of the myelodysplastic syndromes. *Brit. J. Haemat.* **51**, 189.

Beris, P., Graf, J. & Miescher, P.A. (1983) Primary acquired sideroblastic and primary acquired refractory anaemia. *Semin. Hematol.* **20**, 101.

Bottomley, S.S. (1982) Sideroblastic anaemia. *Clin. Haemat.* **11**, 389.

Cartwright, G.E. & Deiss, A. (1975) Sideroblasts, siderocytes and sideroblastic anaemia. *New Engl. J. Med.* **292**, 185.

Cazzola, M., Barosi, G., Gobbi, P.G. *et al.* (1988) Natural history of idiopathic refractory sideroblastic anemia. *Blood* **71**, 305.

Cheng, D.S., Kushner, J.P. & Wintrobe, M.M. (1979) Idiopathic refractory sideroblastic anaemia: incidence and risk factors for leukaemic transformation. *Cancer,* **44**, 724.

Dacie, J.V. & Mollin, D.L. (1966) Siderocytes, sideroblasts and sideroblastic anaemia. *Acta Med. Scand.* Suppl. 445, **179**, 237.

Foucar, K., McKenna, R.W., Bloomfield, C.D. *et al.* (1979) Therapy-related leukemia: a panmyelosis. *Cancer,* **43**, 1285.

Fresco, R. (1981) Electron microscopy in the diagnosis of the bone marrow disorders of the erythroid series. *Semin. Hematol.* **18**, 279.

Hines, J.D. (1969) Reversible megaloblastic and sideroblastic marrow abnormalities in alcoholic patients. *Brit. J. Haemat.* **16**, 87.

Jacobs, A. (1986) Primary acquired sideroblastic anaemia. *Brit. J. Haemat.* **64**, 415.

Knapp, R.H., Dewald, G.W. & Pierre, R.V. (1985) Cytogenetic studies in 174 consecutive patients with preleukemic or myelodysplastic syndromes. *Mayo Clin. Proc.* **60**, 507.

Kushner, J.P., Lee, G.R., Wintrobe, M.M. *et al.* (1971) Idiopathic refractory sideroblastic anemia. Clinical and laboratory investigation of 17 patients and review of the literature. *Medicine,* **50**, 139.

Lewis, S.M. (1983) The spleen—mysteries solved and unresolved. *Clin. Haemat.* **12**, 363.

Lewy, R.I., Kansu, E. & Gabuzda, T. (1979) Leukemia in patients with acquired idiopathic sideroblastic anemia: an evaluation of prognostic indicators. *Am. J. Hematol.***6**, 323.

Losowsky, M.S. & Hall, R. (1965) Hereditary sideroblastic anaemia. *Brit. J. Haemat.* **11**, 70.

MacGibbon, B.H. & Mollin, D.L. (1965) Sideroblastic anaemia in man; Observations on seventy cases. *Brit. J. Haemat.* **11**, 59.

Singh, A.K., Shinton, N.K. & Williams, J.D.F. (1970) Ferrokinetic abnormalities and their significance in patients with sideroblastic anaemia. *Brit. J. Haemat.* **18**, 67.

Yunis, J.J., Rydell, R.E., Oken, M.M., *et al* (1986) Refined chromosome analysis as an independent indicator in de novo myelodysplastic syndromes. *Blood,* **67**, 1721.

Yunis, A.A. & Salem, Z. (1980) Drug-induced mitochrondrial damage and sideroblastic change. *Clin. Haemat.* **9**, 607.

Radioactive iron studies

Cavill, I. & Ricketts, C. (1981) Human iron kinetics. In: Jacobs, A. & Worwood, M. (Eds) *Iron in Biochemistry and Medicine II,* Academic Press, London.

Dacie, J.V. & Lewis, S.M. (1984) *Practical Haematology,* 6th Ed., Churchill Livingstone, London.

Finch, C.A., Deubelbeiss, K., Cook, J.D. *et al.* (1970) Ferrokinetics in man. *Medicine,* **49**, 17.

Pettit, J.E., Lewis, S.M., Williams, E.D. *et al.* (1976) Quantitative studies of splenic erythropoiesis in polycythaemia vera and myelofibrosis. *Brit. J. Haemat.* **34**, 465.

Chapter 4
The Megaloblastic Anaemias

The megaloblastic anaemias are characterized by distinctive cytological and functional abnormalities in peripheral blood and bone marrow cells due to impaired DNA synthesis. They usually result from a deficiency of one of the B group of vitamins, either vitamin B_{12} or folate. Much less commonly, they result from interference with DNA synthesis by other mechanisms, some of which involve congenital or acquired abnormalities of vitamin B_{12} or folate metabolism. Although less common than anaemias due to iron deficiency, the megaloblastic anaemias are a significant cause of ill-health in many parts of the world. Because of the generally excellent response to treatment, these anaemias are of great clinical importance.

In temperate zones, pernicious anaemia (vitamin B_{12} deficiency), nutritional folate deficiency, and folate deficiency due to malabsorption are the most common causes of megaloblastic anaemia. The folate deficiency may be absolute or conditioned, e.g. by the additional requirements of pregnancy. In tropical zones, folate deficiency due to a combination of inadequate intake and malabsorption is the cause of most cases, vitamin B_{12} deficiency being less prevalent.

Megaloblastic anaemia is so named because it is characterized by the appearance in the bone marrow of morphologically abnormal nucleated red cell precursors, which Ehrlich in 1880 called megaloblasts. Megaloblasts are abnormal in function as well as in appearance, with the result that the mature red cells formed from them are abnormal in size and shape, the most prominent abnormality being macrocytosis. The term *megaloblastic macrocytic anaemia* therefore describes the outstanding feature of both the bone marrow and the peripheral blood. However, although most megaloblastic anaemias have a macrocytic peripheral blood picture, the red cells are occasionally normocytic or even microcytic—usually when there is an associated deficiency of iron, e.g. in coeliac disease and pregnancy.

Differentiation from other macrocytic anaemias

In some disorders, macrocytic anaemia occurs in association with a normoblastic marrow. These normoblastic macrocytic anaemias are symptomatic anaemias, secondary to a number of well-defined disorders (Table 4.6, p. 95). With most of the disorders a macrocytic anaemia is unusual, a normocytic anaemia being the more common finding. The anaemia responds only to alleviation or cure of the underlying disease, and is uninfluenced by either vitamin B_{12} or folic acid therapy.

The causes of normoblastic macrocytic anaemia and their differentiation from megaloblastic anaemias are discussed on p. 95.

Vitamin B_{12} and folate metabolism

Vitamin B_{12} and folate are present in the normal diet of humans, and under physiological conditions are absorbed from the gastrointestinal tract in sufficient amount to supply the needs of the body. The general metabolism of these substances is discussed briefly below, as some knowledge is essential to an understanding of the mechanisms causing their deficiency (Table 4.1).

Table 4.1. *Vitamin B_{12} and folate metabolism*

	Vitamin B_{12}	Folate
Content in foods	Vegetables: poor Meat: rich	Vegetables: rich Meat: moderate
Effect of cooking	10–30% loss	60–90% loss
Adult daily requirements	2–4 μg	200 μg
Adult daily intake	5–30 μg	100–500 μg
Site of absorption	Ileum	Duodenum and jejunum
Body stores	2–5 mg	5–20 mg

Vitamin B_{12}

Vitamin B_{12} occurs naturally in foodstuffs. It plays an important role in general cell metabolism, acting as a co-enzyme in chemical reactions affecting the synthesis of DNA. In particular, it is essential for normal haemopoiesis and for maintenance of the integrity of the nervous system.

CHEMISTRY

Vitamin B_{12} was isolated in pure form in 1948 as cyanocobalamin, a red crystalline substance of molecular weight 1355, which belongs to the chemical family of cobalamins. The vitamin B_{12} molecule consists of two portions: a 'planar' group and a nucleotide lying at right angles to each other. The 'planar' group consists of a corrin nucleus of four pyrrole rings linked to a central cobalt atom; the nucleotide contains a 5,6-dimethylbenzimidazole base linked to ribose–phospate. *Cyanocobalamin*, which is found in only trace amounts in human tissue, has a –CN ligand attached to the cobalt atom. The physiologically active cobalamins in humans include *methylcobalamin* and *adenosylcobalamin*, which act as co-enzymes. *Hydroxocobalamin* is apparently a precursor of the other two forms, and is used therapeutically.

SOURCES

The vitamin B_{12} requirements of humans are obtained from foods, mainly those of animal protein origin; kidney, liver and heart are the richest sources, but lesser amounts occur in other foods including muscle meats, fish, shellfish, eggs, cheese and milk. Vegetables contain practically no vitamin B_{12}, in contrast to their high content of folate. The principal forms in the diet are adenosylcobalamin and hydroxocobalamin, which are bound to food protein.

Vitamin B_{12} is synthesized by micro-organisms, and the original source of all vitamin B_{12} in nature is bacterial synthesis. Many of these bacteria are normal inhabitants of the gastrointestinal tract, and the faeces normally contain the vitamin in large amounts. Vitamin B_{12} is synthesized only in the human large bowel. It is not absorbed from this site, and humans are thus entirely dependent on dietary sources.

ABSORPTION

Both active and passive mechanisms exist for the absorption of vitamin B_{12}. The active mechanism is mediated by gastric intrinsic factor and is responsible for the absorption of physiological amounts of vitamin B_{12} present in food. It is highly efficient: from 60 to 80 per cent of a 2 μg dose of vitamin B_{12} is absorbed through its operation. When food passes into the stomach, vitamin B_{12} is released from protein by the action of acid and proteolytic enzymes. *In vitro* studies by Allen *et al.* (1978) suggest that the B_{12} first combines with gastric 'R' protein, which is mainly derived from saliva and is immunologically identical to the major B_{12} transport protein, transcobalamin I (p. 64). As the complex proceeds down the small intestine, the 'R' protein is degraded by pancreatic enzymes, and the liberated vitamin B_{12} combines rapidly with intrinsic factor, a glycoprotein of molecular weight 44 000 secreted by parietal cells in the fundus and body of the stomach.

Normally, the amount of intrinsic factor secreted is far in excess of that needed for B_{12} absorption; only about 1–2 per cent of the total output is required under physiological conditions. One molecule of intrinsic factor binds one molecule of vitamin B_{12} and the attachment stabilizes the latter as it passes to the site of absorption in the distal small intestine. The intrinsic factor–vitamin B_{12} complex binds avidly to receptors on the brush border of ileal mucosal cells as long as calcium ions are present and the pH is above 6. Progress of the vitamin B_{12} across the mucosal cells is relatively slow; at least 8–12 hours elapses from ingestion to attainment of peak level in the circulation. It is not known whether intrinsic factor enters the mucosal cell or merely remains on the surface. Final release of vitamin B_{12} into the portal circulation appears to require the presence of a transport protein, transcobalamin II (TC II) with which the B_{12} binds for distribution to the tissues. The vitamin B_{12} in plasma is mostly methylcobalamin, with some adenosylcobalamin and hydroxocobalamin.

A second, less efficient, mechanism for absorption operates when the small intestine is presented with supraphysiological doses of vitamin B_{12}. No carrier molecule is involved, and passive absorption occurs equally in the jejunum and ileum. One per cent of a large oral dose of B_{12} is rapidly absorbed by this mechanism.

TRANSPORT

There are two major vitamin B_{12} binding proteins in plasma, transcobalamin I (TC I) and transcobalamin II (TC II). TC I is an α_1-globulin of molecular weight 60 000 which carries from 70–90 per cent of the circulating endogenous vitamin B_{12} (mainly methylcobalamin). It appears to function primarily as a storage protein and is not essential for vitamin B_{12} transport, as its absence does not lead to clinical signs of B_{12} deficiency. It is probably synthesized by granulocytes and is normally from 70–100 per cent saturated. A number of B_{12} binding proteins ('R' binders or cobalophilin) immunologically identical to TC I have been found in other body fluids (including gastric juice) and tissues.

TC II is a β-globulin of molecular weight 38 000, which is probably synthesized in the liver and is essential for the transport of vitamin B_{12} from one organ to the other and in and out of cells. It is largely unsaturated, binds newly absorbed or injected B_{12}, and readily releases the bound vitamin to tissues. Congenital deficiency of TC II leads to a severe megaloblastic anaemia (p. 92). A third plasma binding protein TC III, which is similar to TC I, binds only a small amount of circulating B_{12}.

Measurement of the unsaturated B_{12} binding capacity (UBBC), which in the normal subject reflects the amount of TC II and to a lesser extent TC I and TC III available in the serum for binding with added B_{12}, may be diagnostically useful in some disease states (Rachmilewitz *et al.* 1979). The normal range for serum UBBC is 500–1200 ng/l. The UBBC is usually elevated due to an increase in TC I in chronic myeloid leukaemia and acute promyelocytic leukaemia. It may be increased in other myeloproliferative disorders, but not to the same extent. In all these conditions, the vitamin B_{12} level is usually increased, but the UBBC correlates with extent of disease more closely than does the B_{12} level.

TISSUE STORES

The principal site for storage of vitamin B_{12} is the liver, which contains about 1500 μg. Kidneys, heart and brain each contain 20–30 μg. The total body content of vitamin B_{12} ranges from 2 to 5 mg. The storage form is largely adenosylcobalamin. Major routes of loss from the body are biliary excretion and desquamation of intestinal epithelial cells. A major fraction of the excreted vitamin is reabsorbed in the ileum by the intrinsic factor mechanism, resulting in an enterohepatic circulation.

FUNCTION

In spite of the profound clinical effects of vitamin B_{12} deprivation, its role in the normal metabolism of the human body seems deceptively limited. Only two biochemical reactions in humans are known with certainty to require vitamin B_{12} co-enzymes: the conversion of methylmalonyl–CoA to succinyl–CoA (adenosylcobalamin) and the synthesis of methionine from homocysteine (methylcobalamin). The homocysteine–methionine reaction is closely linked with the metabolism of folate, and deficiency of vitamin B_{12} is believed to lead to impaired conversion of methyltetrahydrofolate to tetrahydrofolate, which is then not available for DNA synthesis (see Fig. 4.2, p. 73). Thus, vitamin B_{12} deficiency, acting through derangement of folate metabolism, causes a clinical picture resembling in some respects that of folate deficiency itself. Folate metabolism and its interaction with vitamin B_{12} are discussed further on p. 66.

Folate

Folate, one of the water-soluble B vitamins, plays an essential role in cellular metabolism, and is required for a large number of reactions involving transfer of one-carbon units from one compound to another.

CHEMISTRY

Folic acid was synthesized in 1945 as a yellow crystalline powder of molecular weight 441 with the chemical name pteroylglutamic acid (PGA). The PGA molecule contains pteridine, one molecule of L-glutamic acid and one molecule of para-aminobenzoic acid. Folic acid does not exist as such in nature, but it is the parent compound of a large group of derivatives, referred to as folates, which play an important role as co-enzymes in cellular metabolism. Natural folates are polyglutamates (conjugated folates) in which further glutamic acid residues are attached to the basic glutamic acid moiety. Reduction to dihydro- and tetrahydrofolate derivatives is necessary for polyglutamate folate to participate in metabolic reactions, and a single carbon unit fragment (e.g. methyl or formyl group) is usually attached to the pteroyl part of the molecule.

Ninety per cent of food folates are polyglutamates (usually hexaglutamates), largely in the reduced formyl and methyl forms, and ten per cent are monoglutamates, also in the reduced form.

SOURCES

Folate is widely distributed in plant and animal tissues. The richest sources are liver, kidney, yeast and fresh green vegetables, especially leafy vegetables such as spinach and cabbage. Lesser amounts are present in other foodstuffs including muscle meat, some fruit, nuts and cereals. Milk has a moderately low folate content. Cooking in large quantities of water causes a loss of from 60 to 90 per cent of the folate content of food, and canning also causes significant loss. Although some folate is synthesized by bacteria in the large intestine, it is not available to the body as absorption takes place in the small intestine. The normal requirements of the body must therefore be totally supplied by the naturally occurring folate in food. The average daily diet contains between 100 and 500 μg 'total' folate, but there is considerable variation depending on economic status and dietary habits. The minimal daily requirement in adults for folate as PGA is 100–200 μg.

ABSORPTION

Folate is normally absorbed from the duodenum and upper jejunum, and to a lesser extent from the lower jejunum and ileum. Absorption of synthetic folic acid is a rapid active process: 80 per cent of a physiological dose is absorbed unchanged, with a peak serum level one hour after oral administration. Food folate monoglutamates are also readily absorbed, but the absorption of food polyglutamates is variable. Synthetic polyglutamates are absorbed almost as well as monoglutamates, but the presence of inhibitors reduces natural polyglutamate availability from some foodstuffs. Polyglutamates are cleaved to the monoglutamate form by the enzyme pteroylpolyglutamate (folate) conjugase within the mucosal cell. Most monoglutamates undergo further reduction and methylation in the mucosa, emerging into the circulation as methyltetrahydrofolate. Folate absorption is reviewed by Halsted (1980).

TRANSPORT

Folates circulate in plasma as methyltetrahydrofolate monoglutamate, either in the free form or weakly bound to a variety of proteins. A specific high-affinity folate binding protein may account for a small proportion of the binding capacity of plasma.

TISSUE STORES

Folates are mainly stored in the liver in the polyglutamate form. Liver and red cell folate is largely methyltetrahydrofolate polyglutamate. The total body content is 5–20 mg, and stores are exhausted in about four months if intake totally ceases. Normal loss occurs from sweat, saliva, urine and faeces.

FUNCTION

Folate co-enzymes are required for several biochemical reactions in the body involving transfer of one-carbon units from one compound to another. Two reactions that are important in the context of clinical folate deficiency are the *methylation of homocysteine to methionine* and the *synthesis of the pyrimidine nucleotide, thymidylate monophosphate* from deoxyuridylate monophosphate in the DNA synthesis pathway.

The importance of the vitamin B_{12}-dependent homocysteine–methionine reaction in the generation of tetrahydrofolate from methyltetrahydrofolate has already been discussed (p. 64). The synthesis of thymidylate from deoxyuridylate is a critical rate-limiting step in DNA synthesis and requires methylenetetrahydrofolate (see Fig. 4.2). The biochemical lesion of vitamin B_{12} and folate deficiency is further discussed on p. 73.

General considerations in vitamin B_{12} and folate deficiencies

Vitamin B_{12} deficiency

The human body contains between 2000 and 5000 μg vitamin B_{12} and has a daily requirement of about 2 μg. Thus, the body requirements of a person who develops a defect of vitamin B_{12} absorption can be supplied for a considerable period of time from the tissue stores. Clinical manifestations of deficiency develop only when the tissue stores are almost completely exhausted. This is well illustrated by the latent period of at least two years, and often much longer, before megaloblastic anaemia follows total gastrectomy (p. 83).

Causes (Table 4.2)

Vitamin B_{12} deficiency is practically always due to a disorder of the alimentary tract; very occasionally, it results from inadequate dietary intake. The mechanisms by which alimentary tract disorders produce the deficiency are: lack of intrinsic factor, impairment of the absorptive capacity of the intestinal mucosa, and interference with normal absorption by bacteria or parasites.

Clinical manifestations

There are three cardinal clinical manifestations of vitamin B_{12} deficiency of whatever cause:

- macrocytic megaloblastic anaemia
- glossitis
- peripheral neuropathy and subacute combined degeneration of the spinal cord.

These may occur either singly or, more usually, in combination, and in varying degrees of severity. It is especially important to realize that anaemia is sometimes minimal or absent in vitamin B_{12} deficiency. Neurological abnormalities appear to occur more frequently in pernicious anaemia than in other megaloblastic anaemias due to vitamin B_{12} deficiency.

Table 4.2. *Megaloblastic anaemias due to vitamin B_{12} deficiency*

Mechanism	Disorder
Decreased intake	Nutritional deficiency (p. 85)
Impaired absorption	
Gastric causes	Pernicious anaemia (p. 74)
	Gastrectomy (total or partial) (p. 83)
Intestinal causes	Lesions of small intestine (p. 84)
	Coeliac disease (p. 85)
	Tropical sprue (p. 87)
	Fish tapeworm infestation (p. 84)

Other causes of vitamin B_{12} deficiency include drugs (p. 85) and chronic pancreatic disease (p. 85). Vitamin B_{12} deficiency in infancy and childhood is discussed on p. 92.

Special tests in diagnosis

The main test for the detection of vitamin B_{12} deficiency is the serum vitamin B_{12} assay. To establish the cause of the deficiency, a radioactive vitamin B_{12} absorption test is performed.

SERUM VITAMIN B_{12} ASSAY

Two methods for measuring serum vitamin B_{12} concentration are available—a microbiological and a radio-isotope assay. In spite of a long-standing record of reliability as an indicator of B_{12} deficiency, the microbiological assay has been superseded in most laboratories by the radio-isotope assay, usually in the form of a commercially produced kit which is rapid, simple to perform and unaffected by the presence of antibiotics in the test serum. However, it occasionally gives results that do not correlate well with those obtained by microbiological assay and are at variance with the patient's vitamin B_{12} status as assessed by other clinical and laboratory criteria.

Microbiological assay

The principle of the test is that the serum to be assayed is added as a source of vitamin B_{12} to a medium containing all other essential growth factors for a B_{12}-dependent micro-organism. The medium is then inoculated with the micro-organism, and the amount of B_{12} in the serum is determined by comparing the growth as estimated turbimetrically with the growth produced by a standard amount of vitamin B_{12}. The two micro-organisms used for assay are *Euglena gracilis* and *Lactobacillus leichmanii*. The presence of antibiotics in the test serum interferes with the growth of *L. leichmanii*, and this assay yields false low results for such sera.

Using the Euglena assay, normal values range from 165 to 1000 ng/l (Anderson & Sourial 1983). Erythropoiesis usually becomes frankly megaloblastic in pernicious anaemia when the serum concentration falls below 100 ng/l. The *E. gracilis* assay is particularly satisfactory in providing a clear distinction between normal and pernicious anaemia sera.

Radio-isotope assay

The test involves isotope dilution of non-radioactive serum vitamin B_{12} by added ^{57}Co-labelled B_{12}. A carrier with B_{12} binding capacity is then used to adsorb a portion of the mixture of radioactive and non-radioactive vitamin B_{12}. The free and bound forms of the vitamin are separated, and the quantity of radioactive B_{12} adsorbed to the binding substance is measured. By comparison with measurements of a series of standards of known B_{12} content, the B_{12} level of the unknown serum is calculated. The original technique of Lau *et al.* (1965) employed intrinsic factor as the vitamin B_{12} binding substance, and separated the free and bound forms of the vitamin with protein-coated charcoal. Many variations have been described since.

Most radio-isotope assay methods yield higher vitamin B_{12} levels than microbiological assay on both normal and abnormal sera. Differences are particularly notable in sera from patients who have had a partial gastrectomy or are folate deficient. A more serious shortcoming of the radioisotope assay is the occasional finding of a normal vitamin B_{12} level in a patient in whom all other findings indicate unequivocally the presence of severe B_{12} deficiency. The factors responsible for discrepancies of this type have not been defined with certainty, although most evidence points either to faulty assay design or to the use of vitamin B_{12} binders other than pure intrinsic factor. Assay kits have been extensively modified in recent years in an effort to improve diagnostic performance, but some uncertainties remain (Cooper *et al.* 1986). An additional problem of interpretation arises when a low assay result is found in a patient in whom extensive investigation fails to reveal any other evidence of B_{12} deficiency or an underlying disorder capable of causing deficiency. Pregnancy or folate deficiency provide an explanation in some patients, but occasionally the cause for the low serum level is not apparent.

As with all laboratory tests, it is essential for the clinician interpreting the results to be aware of the type of assay used, its normal range, and possible limitations. It is equally important for each laboratory to exercise considerable care in the choice of assay method and to establish its own normal range rather than rely on results obtained by other laboratories or, in the case of commercial kits, those quoted by the manufacturer.

Reported normal ranges vary with the assay method employed. A commercial assay kit favourably assessed by Bain *et al.* (1982) gave a normal range of 165–684 ng/l. Vitamin-deficient patients had levels below 130 ng/l.

RADIOACTIVE VITAMIN B_{12} ABSORPTION TEST

The ability of the body to absorb vitamin B_{12} can be assessed by measuring the absorption of a small oral dose of ^{57}Co-labelled vitamin B_{12}. Further, the simultaneous administration of a source of intrinsic factor can be used to distinguish defective absorption due to lack of intrinsic factor and that due to other causes, e.g. impairment of the absorptive capacity of the intestinal mucosa. Most laboratories perform the test by measuring the amount of radioactivity in the urine (Schilling test). A recommended procedure has been published by the International Committee for Standardization in Hematology (1981).

The Schilling test

An oral dose of 1 μg radioactive vitamin B_{12} (cyanocobalamin) is administered to the fasting subject followed two hours later by a large parenteral injection of unlabelled B_{12} (1000 μg). The injection flushes out about one-third of the absorbed radioactive B_{12} into the urine in the next 24 hours. Normal subjects excrete ten per cent or more of the 1 μg dose in their urine. Patients with pernicious anaemia excrete less than five per cent, but occasionally up to seven per cent of the dose. Borderline results of up to ten per cent may occur in atrophic gastritis. If the patient absorbs normal amounts of vitamin B_{12}, no further testing is necessary. If absorption is subnormal, a second parenteral injection of unlabelled B_{12} is given 24 hours later, followed by a further test dose of radioactive B_{12} with intrinsic factor, and the B_{12} absorption is again estimated. If absorption returns to normal, a diagnosis of pernicious anaemia may be made. If absorption is again subnormal, a lesion of the small intestine is likely. Malabsorption due to abnormal bacterial flora in the small intestine may be corrected by a seven-day course of oral tetracycline.

Vitamin B_{12} deficiency itself may result in reversible malabsorption of vitamin B_{12} and other nutrients (Lindenbaum *et al.* 1974). Thus, in some patients with authentic pernicious anaemia, the impaired absorption of vitamin B_{12} in the Schilling test is not corrected by intrinsic factor. If, on other grounds, the diagnosis of pernicious anaemia seems likely, the test with intrinsic factor should be repeated after two months of vitamin B_{12} therapy.

The Schilling test is rapid and simple to perform. Important sources of error include incomplete urine collection, inactive intrinsic factor, and the presence of another diagnostic isotope in the urine which may be mistaken for radioactive vitamin B_{12}. Delayed excretion of the radioactive vitamin B_{12} in chronic renal disease also occasionally leads to erroneous results, and the patient's serum creatinine level should always be checked. Measurement of plasma radioactivity circumvents some of these problems and may be used as a supplement to the urinary excretion method. An inevitable consequence of the test is that the 'flushing' dose of non-radioactive B_{12} initiates therapy, and thus its timing in the sequence of investigations needs to be carefully considered. Clearly, blood samples for vitamin assays should be drawn before the parenteral injection is given.

A convenient variant of the Schilling test involves the simultaneous oral administration of free and intrinsic factor-bound radioactive vitamin B_{12}, the free form labelled with ^{58}Co and the bound form with ^{57}Co. The excretion of the two isotopes in a single 24-hour urine collection is analysed by differential counting, and an immediate estimate of the improvement in absorption caused by the addition of intrinsic factor is thus available. The test is presented in a kit form and is discussed by Domstad *et al.* (1981).

Response to treatment

Administration of either vitamin B_{12} or folic acid influences the manifestations of vitamin B_{12} deficiency. However, for reasons outlined below, *administration of folic acid is dangerous.*

VITAMIN B_{12}

In adequate doses, vitamin B_{12} administration results in: (a) reversion of erythropoiesis from megaloblastic to normoblastic, and return of the peripheral blood to normal; (b) healing of glossitis; and (c) cure of peripheral neuropathy and arrest, usually with some improvement, of subacute combined degeneration of the spinal cord.

FOLIC ACID

The results of folic acid administration are as follows:

1 Erythropoiesis reverts from megaloblastic to normoblastic. This is followed by improvement in the anaemia, but the haemoglobin does not always rise to normal values, and even when it does, some degree of relapse occurs after prolonged treatment.

2 Glossitis frequently, but not invariably, responds initially, but may relapse subsequently.

3 Nervous system manifestations are not relieved. Administration of folic acid has been said to accelerate the progress of neurological damage, and it is well documented that neurological lesions can progress even though the anaemia is undergoing significant improvement. For this reason, folic acid therapy is dangerous in megaloblastic anaemia due to vitamin B_{12} deficiency. When vitamin B_{12} and folate deficiencies co-exist, folic acid can be given together with vitamin B_{12} as the latter protects the spinal cord from damage.

Table 4.3. *Megaloblastic anaemias due to folate deficiency*

Mechanism	Disorder
Decreased intake	Nutritional deficiency (p. 88)
Impaired absorption	Coeliac disease (p. 85) Tropical sprue (p. 87)
Increased demand	Pregnancy, puerperium (p. 90) Haemolytic anaemia Myeloproliferative disorders Leukaemia and lymphoma Sideroblastic anaemia Carcinoma Inflammatory disorders Hyperthyroidism Skin disease
Drugs (p. 93)	

Folate deficiency in infancy and childhood is discussed on p. 92.

Folate deficiency: Causes (Table 4.3)

Deficiency of folate can result from:

1 *Inadequate intake.* Most cases of megaloblastic anaemia due to folate deficiency result from a subnormal intake. Inadequate dietary intake is a much more important factor than in B_{12} deficiency, partly because folate activity is more likely to be lost in cooking.

2 *Intestinal malabsorption.*

3 *Increased demand.* Marginal dietary deficiencies are more likely to become overt in the presence of increased demand, such as in pregnancy.

4 *Inability to utilize folate* due to the action of folate antagonists.

Clinical manifestations

There are two cardinal clinical manifestations of folate deficiency: *macrocytic megaloblastic anaemia,* and *glossitis.*

Deficiency of folate, in contrast to that of vitamin B_{12}, does not produce subacute combined degeneration of the spinal cord, but peripheral neuropathy is occasionally seen.

Special tests in diagnosis

In a classic paper, Herbert (1962) discussed the sequence of events in the development of folate deficiency in a healthy adult male during four-and-a-half months on a diet from which folate had been extracted. The first abnormality to develop was reduction in serum folate level (two weeks), followed by neutrophil hypersegmentation (seven weeks), reduction in red cell folate (18 weeks) and, finally, appearance of megaloblastic anaemia (20 weeks).

There are two main laboratory tests used to detect folate deficiency—the serum and red cell folate assays.

SERUM FOLATE ASSAY

Microbiological and radio-isotope methods are available for measuring serum folate concentration. The microbiological assay has several shortcomings, the most important being its extreme sensitivity to the presence of antibiotics and folate antagonists in the test serum. In most laboratories, it has been replaced by the radio-isotope assay, usually in the form of a commercial kit.

Microbiological assay

The folate activity of serum is due mainly to the presence of the folate co-enzyme, methyltetrahydrofolate; this compound is microbiologically active for *Lactobacillus casei* which is used for the assay. The principle of the test is similar to that of the microbiological vitamin B_{12} assay.

There is considerable variation in the normal range obtained in different laboratories. Levels below 3 μg/l suggest clinically significant folate deficiency. Levels in the range of 3–6 μg/l are less decisive and may not be associated with clinical or cytological features of folate deficiency. Low levels in serum probably represent the earliest subclinical stage of folate deficiency before the development of true tissue deficiency.

Radio-isotope assay

The assay is based on similar principles to that of the radio-isotope vitamin B_{12} assay, and uses labelled pteroylglutamic acid or methyltetrahydrofolate, and a folate-binding protein purified from cow's milk. Several commercial kits are available, and some permit concurrent assay of both folate and B_{12} (Raniolo *et al.* 1984).

Normal ranges for currently available commercial kits should be independently determined by each laboratory (Dawson *et al.* 1980).

RED CELL FOLATE ASSAY

Red cells contain 20–50 times as much folate as serum. The red cell folate level is usually a more reliable indicator of tissue folate stores than the serum folate, which fluctuates widely according to dietary intake. Microbiological or radio-isotope assay methods may be used. In general, correlation of results obtained with the two types of assay is less satisfactory than is the case with serum folate (Carmel 1983).

With the microbiological assay, normal values range from 160 to 640 μg/l, and Bain *et al.* (1984) have reported a range of 199–795 μg/l for a radio-isotope assay. Low red cell folate levels are found in patients with megaloblastic anaemia due to folate deficiency. However, in patients with pernicious anaemia, the red cell folate values are often subnormal, and thus the assay in isolation lacks specificity and is of limited value in the differential diagnosis of megaloblastic anaemia.

Response to treatment

Folate deficiency responds completely to folic acid administration. Vitamin B_{12} may cause partial remission of the anaemia.

Folic acid causes a reversion of erythropoiesis from megaloblastic to normoblastic with consequent return of the blood picture to normal, and prompt healing of glossitis. The serum folate level rises to normal or supranormal levels, and in those cases in which the serum vitamin B_{12} is subnormal, the B_{12} level rises to normal within days of commencement of folic acid therapy (p. 89).

Vitamin B_{12} in small physiological doses does not influence either the anaemia or the glossitis. On the other hand, therapeutic doses of B_{12} may result in relief of glossitis and a partial remission of the anaemia in some cases. However, the response is unpredictable and of varying degree, with wide variation in different patients.

Megaloblastic erythropoiesis

Megaloblasts are abnormal nucleated red cells which occur in the marrow of persons with either vitamin B_{12} or folate deficiency. Their abnormal appearance is due to disturbance of cell growth and maturation, resulting from interference with DNA synthesis, usually due to deficiency of vitamin B_{12} or folate. Megaloblastic erythropoiesis is accompanied by abnormalities in the granulocyte series and megakaryocytes.

Bone marrow morphology

ERYTHROPOIESIS

Megaloblastic changes occur at all stages of red cell development. Cells in the megaloblastic series are named as are their normoblastic counterparts (p. 4); the primitive cell is the promegaloblast, from which a series of maturing cells develop, namely basophilic, polychromatic and orthochromatic megaloblasts. Megaloblasts differ from their normoblastic counterparts in the following respects.

Cell size. Megaloblasts are larger than erythroblasts, with an increase in cytoplasm and nuclear size at every stage of development.

Nucleus. The chromatin network is more open, being arranged in a fine reticular fashion to give a stippled appearance (Fig. 4.1). As the cell matures the chromatin clumps, but the clumping is much less marked than in normoblasts at the same stage of development. Thus, the stippled appearance is commonly still well marked in polychromatic cells, and is sometimes seen in orthochromatic cells. The nucleus of the orthochromatic cell is commonly indented or lobulated, and one or more Howell–Jolly bodies may be present.

Dissociation of cytoplasmic and nuclear maturation. The maturation of the nucleus lags behind that of the cytoplasm: haemoglobinization of the cytoplasm proceeds at a faster rate than nuclear maturation.

Mitosis. Mitoses are more common, and are sometimes abnormal in appearance.

Maturation. Megaloblastic erythropoiesis is characterized by an increase in the proportion of more primitive cells ('maturation arrest'). In markedly megaloblastic marrows, promegaloblasts and basophil megaloblasts may constitute more than 50 per cent of the erythroblasts.

Prussian blue staining of the marrow shows an increase in the number and size of iron granules in erythroid precursors, although ring sideroblasts (p. 57) are rarely prominent. Iron in reticulum cells is increased.

LEUCOPOIESIS

Leucopoiesis is abnormal. The characteristic feature is the presence of large atypical granulocytes, which occur at all stages of development, but particularly at the metamyelocyte stage, resulting in 'giant stab'

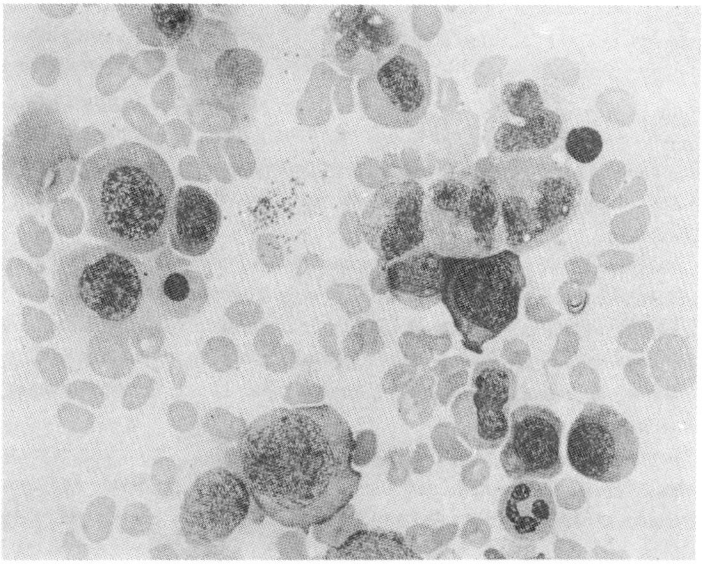

Fig. 4.1. *Megaloblastic erythropoiesis. Photomicrograph of a bone marrow film from a patient with pernicioius anaemia (× 550). Note stippling of the chromatin of megaloblastic erythroblasts.*

forms. The *giant stab cell* is up to 30 μm in diameter and has a large U-shaped nucleus, which may be somewhat irregular in outline and which sometimes stains poorly. These cells result from asynchronism between the development of nucleus and the cytoplasm. They probably die within the marrow, and the hypersegmented neutrophils of the peripheral blood do not appear to be derived from them. The absolute number of developing granulocytes in the marrow is actually increased, but their percentage is decreased because of the greater increase in nucleated red cells.

Megakaryocytes are usually present in normal or slightly increased numbers, but occasionally they are decreased; some are atypical and have a deeply basophilic agranular cytoplasm or hypersegmented nucleus.

RELATION OF MARROW CHANGE TO ANAEMIA

The marrow of patients with megaloblastic anaemia contains both megaloblasts and normoblasts, the relative proportion varying with the severity of the anaemia. Thus in marked anaemia megaloblasts predominate, while in mild anaemia megaloblastic changes are less prominent and many cells have characteristics intermediate between those of megaloblasts and normoblasts ('intermediate megaloblasts'). Maturation arrest is not prominent in intermediate megaloblastic marrows.

Peripheral blood picture

The classical blood picture of megaloblastic anaemia, irrespective of its cause, has the following features:

1 Anaemia with marked oval macrocytosis and an elevated MCV. The higher the MCV, the greater the incidence of megaloblastosis. MCV values above 125 fl are almost always associated with vitamin B_{12} or folate deficiency and a frankly megaloblastic bone marrow.

2 Neutropenia with hypersegmented neutrophils.

3 Mild, usually symptomless, thrombocytopenia.

The earliest change is the development of macrocytosis and an elevated MCV without anaemia. Anaemia then develops weeks, months or rarely years later, and as the level of haemoglobin falls, anisocytosis, macrocytosis and poikilocytosis become more prominent. Finally, neutropenia and thrombocytopenia develop.

Neutrophil hypersegmentation is present when more than five per cent of neutrophils have five lobes or the film shows at least one six-lobed cell (Lindenbaum & Nath 1980). Hypersegmentation is an early sign of vitamin B_{12} or folate deficiency, and is useful in the diagnosis of megaloblastosis with minimal or no anaemia. Other conditions in which hypersegmentation occurs are iron deficiency, myeloproliferative disorders, and chronic renal failure. In rare instances, the condition may be familial.

Effect of associated iron deficiency on the blood and marrow picture

In certain megaloblastic anaemias, notably those of coeliac disease, tropical sprue, partial gastrectomy, nutritional deficiency, pregnancy and infancy, iron deficiency is sometimes present at the same time as folate or B_{12} deficiency. Associated iron deficiency may partly mask the typical haematological features of the megaloblastic anaemia for the inexperienced observer. In some cases, the peripheral blood shows a double population of cells (dimorphic blood picture), some red cells being oval and well haemoglobinized, and others small and poorly haemoglobinized. In other cases, the masking takes the form of a lesser degree of macrocytosis, so that most cells are of normal size and the MCV is normal or even mildly reduced. However, careful scrutiny of the blood film usually shows a small number of oval macrocytes, and almost always neutrophil hypersegmentation. Other co-existing disorders that occasionally mask the typical haematological features of megaloblastic anaemia, and cause an inappropriately normal or low MCV, include thalassaemia, infection, chronic renal disease and rheumatoid arthritis (Spivak 1982).

The marrow findings in patients with associated iron deficiency are often not typical, with less marked megaloblastic changes than would be expected for the degree of anaemia: However, the features of intermediate megaloblasts can usually be detected, and giant stab forms are present.

Mechanism of anaemia

In megaloblastic anaemia, the anaemia results from failure of the megaloblastic bone marrow to compensate for a moderate reduction in red cell lifespan. Red cell survival studies have shown the presence of mild haemolysis, which is due to both intracorpuscular and extracorpuscular causes. Lack of vitamin B_{12} or folate causes slowing of DNA synthesis in developing erythroblasts with an accumulation of cells in the premitotic phase of the cell cycle. Some of these cells die within the marrow as shown by the ferrokinetic pattern of ineffective erythropoiesis. When raised serum bilirubin occurs, it is due both to haemolysis in the peripheral blood and to premature destruction of developing megaloblasts in the marrow. The neutropenia and thrombocytopenia also appear to result from ineffective production by abnormal precursor cells in the marrow.

The biochemical basis of megaloblastic anaemia

The key biochemical lesion common to both vitamin B_{12} and folate deficiency appears to be a block in DNA synthesis resulting from inability to methylate deoxyuridylate to thymidylate in the DNA synthesis pathway (Fig. 4.2). The methyl group for the deoxyuridylate–thymidylate step is supplied by the folate co-enzyme, methylenetetrahydrofolate. Deficiency of folate from any cause directly reduces the supply of methylenetetrahydrofolate, and thus interferes with the conversion of deoxyuridylate to thymidylate and the synthesis of DNA.

The mechanism by which vitamin B_{12} deficiency limits the availability of folate co-enzyme for DNA synthesis is not known with certainty. The *'methylfolate trap' hypothesis* proposes that the conversion of homocysteine to methionine is impaired by deficiency of vitamin B_{12} with resulting decreased formation of tetrahydrofolate and methylenetetrahydrofolate from methyltetrahydrofolate. Furthermore, the passage of methyltetrahydrofolate into cells is reduced as vitamin B_{12} is required for cell entry. The non-utilization of methyltetrahydrofolate, with reduction in available tetrahydrofolate for the synthesis of active polyglutamate co-enzyme forms of folate within the cell, constitutes the 'methylfolate trap'.

An alternative *'formate-starvation' hypothesis* to explain the impairment in folate co-enzyme supply in vitamin B_{12} deficiency has been proposed by Chanarin *et al.* (1980) on the basis of recent findings in animals exposed for long periods to the anaesthetic gas, nitrous oxide, which converts vitamin B_{12} from the active reduced form to an inactive oxidized

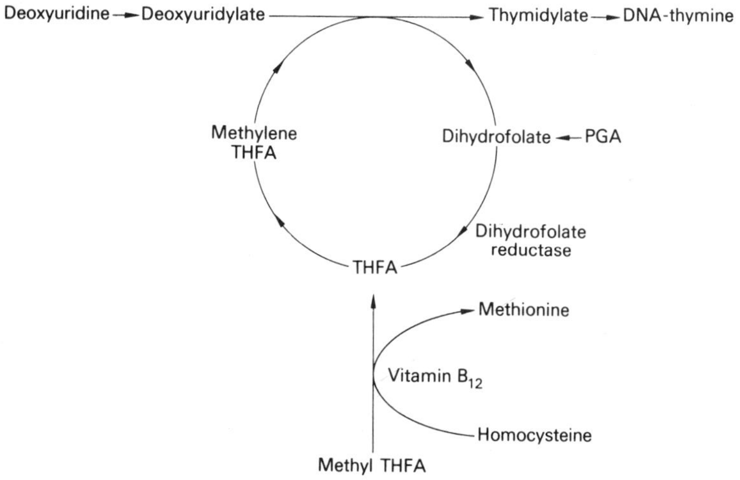

Fig. 4.2. *The metabolic interrelationship of vitamin B_{12} and folate, and their role in DNA synthesis. THFA: tetrahydrofolate; PGA: pteroylglutamic acid.*

form. They suggested that formyltetrahydrofolate is the optimal substrate for formation of folate polyglutamate, and that interference with methionine synthesis resulting from B_{12} deficiency directly impairs the supply of formate for generation of formyltetrahydrofolate from tetrahydrofolate. The metabolic interrelationships of B_{12} and folate in megaloblastic haemopoiesis are discussed by Das & Herbert (1976) and Chanarin *et al.* (1985).

dU suppression test. Short-term human *in vitro* bone marrow cultures can be used for investigation of the effects of vitamin B_{12} and folate deficiency on thymidylate and DNA synthesis. In normoblastic cultures, added deoxyuridine enters the DNA–thymine pathway and suppresses the incorportion of subsequently added tritiated thymidine into DNA. In vitamin B_{12} and folate deficiency, the added deoxyuridine causes less suppression, but the defect can be corrected by supplying the missing vitamin. The technique is referred to as the 'dU suppression test', and for laboratories with facilities for marrow culture it provides a rapid and convenient method for distinguishing between vitamin B_{12} and folate deficiency as the cause of megaloblastosis. However, the test has considerable limitations and can yield misleading findings, which are summarized by Wickramasinghe (1983).

Vitamin B_{12} deficiency: Pernicious anaemia

Pernicious anaemia was first described as a recognizable clinical entity by Addison in 1855. It is a chronic disorder of middle and old age, and the basic pathological lesion is gastric atrophy which results in vitamin B_{12} deficiency. The clinical features are those of vitamin B_{12} deficiency—macrocytic anaemia, glossitis and nervous system involvement—which occur either singly or, more usually, in combination, and in varying degrees of severity.

With adequate treatment the prognosis is excellent; the expectation of life in patients without marked nervous system involvement is approximately that of the general population of similar age.

Pathogenesis

The fundamental defect in pernicious anaemia is a failure of secretion of intrinsic factor (IF) by the stomach due to permanent atrophy of the gastric mucous membrane. In the absence of intrinsic factor, the vitamin B_{12} of food is not absorbed, resulting in vitamin B_{12} deficiency. Fig. 4.3 summarizes the main features of the pathogenesis.

The diffuse mucosal atrophy, which is referred to as *chronic atrophic gastritis,* is most marked in the body of the stomach; in 80–90 per cent of patients the antral mucosa is spared. The atrophic mucosa is heavily infiltrated by lymphocytes and plasma cells, and the atrophy is probably the end-result of degenerative changes that have been occurring progressively over many years. Histological examination reveals an almost complete absence of chief and parietal cells, frequently with a change to an intestinal type of epithelium. The atrophy not

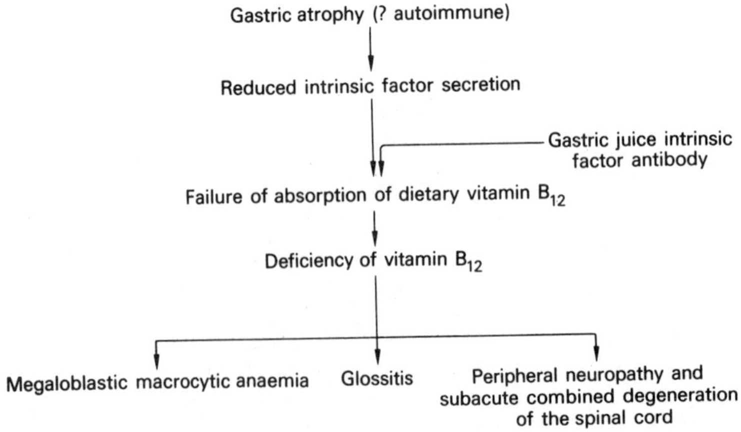

Fig. 4.3. *Pathogenesis of pernicious anaemia.*

only results in loss of intrinsic factor, but also affects the secretion of hydrochloric acid and pepsin. Thus a histamine or pentagastrin-unresponsive achlorhydria is almost invariable (p. 78), and the total volume of gastric secretion is reduced. The serum level of gastrin is elevated in about 80 per cent of patients, in whom the achlorhydria promotes release of the hormone from the antral mucosa. Radiological evidence of gastric atrophy is often seen on barium meal examination.

Chronic atrophic gastritis frequently occurs in the absence of pernicious anaemia. It may represent an early stage of a disorder which, given sufficient time, eventually evolves into overt pernicious anaemia. In a lesser number of cases, the chronic atrophic gastritis is probably a separate entity, unrelated to pernicious anaemia. Histologically, the gastric lesions are identical but, in terms of loss of intrinsic factor, the atrophy of pernicious anaemia is more severe.

The pathogenesis of the gastric atrophy of pernicious anaemia is uncertain. Current evidence suggests that it is the end-result of a complex interaction between genetic and auto-immune factors.

GENETIC FACTORS

There is evidence that genetic factors play a part, as in about ten per cent of patients more than one family member, of either the same or a different generation, is affected. The incidence of subnormal serum vitamin B_{12} levels, gastric auto-antibodies, and other auto-immune diseases is also increased in relatives. Blood group A is more common among patients and their relatives than in the general population. The disorder has a definite racial tendency; it occurs most frequently in people of northern European ancestry, and less frequently in people of southern European stock and in Asians. Certain physical characteristics, e.g. fair skin and blue eyes, are common in patients with pernicious anaemia.

AUTO-IMMUNE FACTORS

The concept of pernicious anaemia as an auto-immune disorder initially came from the finding that it occurred more frequently than expected in association with other auto-immune disorders, e.g. hyperthyroidism, hypothyroidism, and Hashimoto's thyroiditis. The discovery that gastric parietal cell auto-antibodies were frequently present in the serum and gastric juice added impetus to this hypothesis, and it has been presumed but not proven that these auto-antibodies were responsible for the atrophy of the gastric mucosa. The concept of pernicious anaemia as an auto-immune disease is discussed by Whittingham & Mackay (1985).

Antibodies against two distinct antigenic components of the gastric parietal cell have been found in the serum or gastric juice of most patients with pernicious anaemia.

Parietal cell antibodies

Serum antibodies to surface membrane and cytoplasmic antigens of gastric parietal cells are found in at least 85 per cent of patients with pernicious anaemia. They are also found in the sera of 35 per cent of patients' relatives, in 30–60 per cent of patients with chronic atrophic gastritis without pernicious anaemia, and in some normal people, particularly females over the age of 70 years. Antibodies also occur with increased frequency in the sera of patients with other auto-immune diseases, e.g. hyperthyroidism, hypothyroidism, adrenal insufficiency, and Hashimoto's thyroiditis. They are IgG antibodies, are usually demonstrated by immunofluorescent techniques, and may be found in gastric juice as well as serum. In general, they correlate with the presence of antral-sparing atrophic gastritis and hypergastrinaemia irrespective of the disease with which the gastritis is associated, and they are rarely, if ever, found in subjects who have a healthy gastric mucosa.

Intrinsic factor antibodies

Two types of intrinsic factor antibody are found in the sera of patients with pernicious anaemia. *Blocking antibodies* react with the vitamin B_{12}-combining site of intrinsic factor and inhibit subsequent binding of B_{12}. They are found in 50–70 per cent of patients. *Binding antibodies* attach to a site distant from the vitamin B_{12}-combining site and prevent linkage of the intrinsic factor–vitamin B_{12} complex to the ileal receptor. They occur less frequently than blocking antibodies, and are usually present only when the titre of blocking antibody is high. From about 20 to 30 per cent of patients have both antibodies. They are IgG antibodies which, apart from a small number of cases of hyperthyroidism, hypothyroidism, diabetes and adrenal insufficiency, occur only in pernicious anaemia. Unlike parietal cell antibodies, they do not occur in patients with chronic atrophic gastritis without pernicious anaemia. The antibodies may be measured by an assay system similar to the isotope vitamin B_{12} assay.

Intrinsic factor antibodies are also present in the gastric juice of 50–70 per cent of patients with pernicious anaemia. Gastric juice antibodies are usually of the blocking type, and are IgA immunoglobulins. There is no consistent correlation between the presence of serum and gastric juice antibodies. Overall, at least 70 per cent of patients have intrinsic factor antibody in either serum or gastric juice.

Cell-mediated immune reactions to intrinsic factor have also been demonstrated by several techniques in a large proportion of patients with pernicious anaemia and other auto-immune diseases.

SUMMARY

A totally satisfactory explanation of the pathogenesis of pernicious anaemia is not yet available. Immune mechanisms are believed by some to be responsible for the gradual destruction of gastric intrinsic factor-secreting mucosal cells. The demonstration of circulating humoral antibodies to intrinsic factor and parietal cells, and of cell-mediated immune reactions to intrinsic factor in the majority of patients, is supportive evidence for this hypothesis, but it has been difficult to obtain direct proof. The presence of intrinsic factor antibody in the gastric juice may determine the progression from chronic atrophic gastritis to pernicious anaemia by neutralizing the small amount of intrinsic factor still secreted by the atrophic mucosa.

A contrary view is that the gastric auto-antibodies of pernicious anaemia are merely epiphenomena resulting from the release of antigen from a gastric mucosa damaged by ill-defined acquired factors.

Clinical features

Pernicious anaemia is a disorder of the middle and older age groups, occurring with increasing frequency as age advances. Onset before the age of 40 years is uncommon, and under 30 years is rare. Any patient aged less than 40 years with a megalobastic macrocytic anaemia should be thoroughly investigated to exclude other causes, especially coeliac disease. Rare cases of pernicious anaemia in childhood have been reported (p. 92). Females are affected a little more commonly than males.

Onset. The onset is usually insidious; symptoms are often present for many months before the patient presents. The most common presentation is with symptoms of anaemia. Presenting manifestations are detailed in Table 4.4. *Occasionally, the condition is detected in apparently healthy non-anaemic subjects by the chance finding of an elevated MCV in a screening haematological examination.*

Anaemia. The symptoms common to all forms of anaemia are present in most cases, and are the most common presenting manifestations. Because of the insidious onset, the anaemia is usually moderately severe when the patient presents, but may be slight or absent. The skin is classically described as having a lemon tint, but this is usually seen only with marked anaemia, and is uncommon. However, slight scleral icterus may occur.

Glossitis. About 25 per cent of patients have glossitis, which occasionally antedates symptoms of anaemia by months or even years. It is frequently intermittent, so inquiry about attacks of soreness of the tongue during the previous several years should always be made in suspected cases. Occasionally the whole of the mouth and the throat are involved, and the patient may complain of burning pain on swallowing. The tongue is sometimes normal on examination despite the soreness, but in acute attacks, the tip, sides, and sometimes the whole tongue, are red and raw. The attacks cause loss of papillae, and the tongue becomes smooth and shiny. Some patients with the characteristic smooth tongue have no history of attacks of soreness. The sore tongue is rapidly relieved by vitamin B_{12} therapy.

Nervous system manifestations. These are common and may be the presenting feature. *There is no definite relationship between the degree of anaemia and the presence of neurological involvement.* Although anaemia is present in most cases with nervous system involvement, it is occasionally minimal or completely absent. The basic pathological lesions in the nervous system are axonal degeneration and demyelination of peripheral nerves and posterior and lateral columns of the spinal cord. The peripheral nerve lesion gives rise to a typical peripheral neuropathy in 40 per cent of patients, beginning in the periphery of the limb and progressing proximally. The cord lesion is of greater importance as it is more disabling and less amenable to therapy. The midthoracic region is usually involved first, the posterior column being affected before the lateral column.

The usual initial complaint is of *paraesthesia* in the feet. Paraesthesia is characteristically bilateral and symmetrical, and spreads gradually up the legs to the thighs. The hands may then be affected. Paraesthesia is followed by weakness in the legs and unsteadiness of gait due to loss of position sense. Fine movements of the fingers may be clumsy, and the patient may drop small objects.

When the patient's complaints are limited to paraesthesiae of the hands and feet, there are frequently no objective signs. With more extensive paraesthesiae, some impairment of sensation with absent or diminished reflexes and weakness of muscles may be present.

Definite evidence of *spinal cord involvement* occurs in about 15 per cent of cases. The most important clinical findings are loss of vibration sense due to posterior column involvement and the appearance of spasticity, hyperactive reflexes and extensor plantar responses due to lateral column involvement. The co-existence of peripheral nerve and cord lesions gives rise to paradoxical clinical findings, and the combination of flaccid weakness with extensor plantar responses may occur.

Retrobulbar neuritis is particularly prone to occur in males who are heavy smokers. Vitamin B_{12} deficiency may confer a special susceptibility to the neurotoxic effects of chronic cyanide exposure resulting from tobacco smoke.

Mild mental disturbances are common, and are occasionally the presenting manifestation. Patients who do not respond to vitamin B_{12} therapy probably have cerebral atherosclerosis rather than B_{12} deficiency. Delusions, confusion or hallucinations may occur, but vitamin B_{12} deficiency is an uncommon cause of dementia. The neuropsychiatry of vitamin B_{12} deficiency is reviewed by Shorvon *et al.* (1980).

Gastrointestinal manifestations. Diarrhoea occurs in about 50 per cent of cases, usually as mild recurrent attacks. Sometimes the pattern is of alternating constipation and diarrhoea. Anorexia and dyspepsia are common. Weight loss may occur, but most patients are well nourished. Marked weight loss always calls for investigation to exclude possible associated problems such as carcinoma of the stomach. Slight to moderate hepatomegaly is usual, and mild enlargement of the spleen is found in about ten per cent of cases.

Morphological and functional abnormalities of the *mucosa of the small intestine* are common. The abnormalities are consistent with the frequent presence of laboratory evidence of generalized malabsorption (Lindenbaum *et al.* 1974). The importance of malabsorption of vitamin B_{12} even in the presence of added intrinsic factor in assessing the results of the Schilling test is discussed on page 68.

Cardiovascular system. As pernicious anaemia occurs in the age group in which degenerative arterial disease is common, symptoms referable to the cardiovascular system are often prominent. Congestive cardiac failure may be precipitated either by anaemia or by blood transfusion.

Haemorrhagic manifestations are unusual except in the retina where haemorrhages are common, especially in severe anaemia. Occasionally, petechiae or small ecchymoses occur in the skin.

Mild pyrexia is common in untreated patients. *Amenorrhoea* may occur, and patients are usually infertile; fertility may be restored after vitamin B_{12} therapy. An occasional patient has vitiligo.

Blood picture

The blood film classically contains many oval macrocytes, as illustrated in Fig. 4.4. In general, the morphological abnormalities parallel the severity of the anaemia.

Haemoglobin levels range from the normal values for the sex of the patient to 3 g/dl or even less. The haemoglobin level is commonly 7–9 g/dl when the patient first seeks advice. The MCV is increased, commonly ranging from 110 to 140 fl, but both higher and lower values occur. The MCHC is normal but, because of the increased size of the cells, the MCH is increased, usually ranging from 33 to 38 pg. The MCV may be normal or reduced if a co-existing disorder associated with red cell microcytosis is present (p. 72). *Occasionally, the haemoglobin level is normal,* the only abnormality being macrocytosis with an elevated MCV.

In the blood film, the outstanding feature is the presence of macrocytic red cells, many of which are oval. Cells of normal size and microcytes are also present, and occasionally small fragmented and distorted cells are prominent. In the untreated patient, the reticulocyte count is seldom more than two per cent, but a few polychromatic and stippled cells are commonly present. A small number of nucleated red cells and cells containing Howell–Jolly bodies are often seen; the nucleated red cells may be typical megaloblasts, particularly when the anaemia is severe.

Table 4.4. *Presenting manifestations of pernicious anaemia*

Anaemia
Angina of effort
Congestive cardiac failure
Paraesthesiae
Glossitis
Recurrent diarrhoea
Anorexia, weight loss, abdominal pain
Mental disturbance
Visual disturbance

A moderate *leucopenia* ranging from 3 to 4 × 10^9/l is usual but not invariable; it is due to a reduction in neutrophils. Hypersegmented neutrophils are always present, and an occasional abnormally large polymorph with nucleus containing up to eight or nine lobes (macropolycyte) may be seen. A few myelocytes may appear in the peripheral blood.

A moderate *thrombocytopenia* is usual, with the platelet count ranging from 100 to 150 × 10^9 /l. Occasionally it may be lower, especially with severe anaemia, and cause haemorrhagic manifestations.

BIOCHEMICAL FINDINGS

The *serum bilirubin* is usually at the upper limit of normal, i.e. from about 14 to 17 μmol/l, but it may be slightly increased. Serum haptoglobin level is reduced. *Serum ferritin and iron* are elevated, but fall

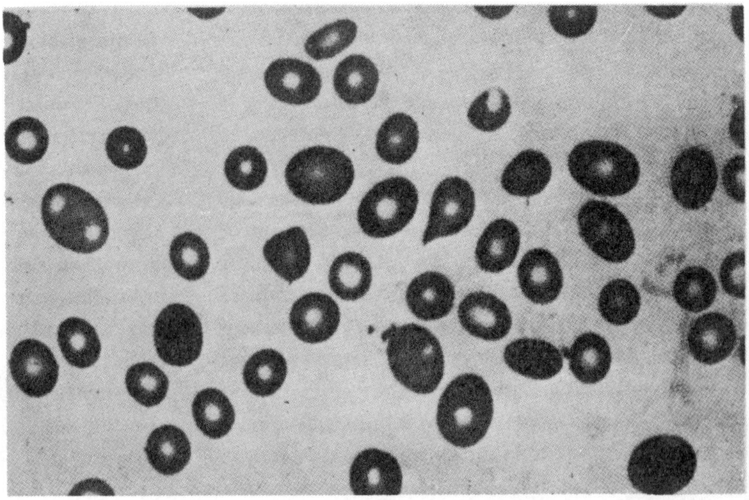

Fig. 4.4. *Pernicious anaemia. Photomicrograph of a blood film showing oval macrocytes, anisocytosis and poikilocytosis (× 520) Mr W.T., aged 71 years, presented with angina of effort, dyspnoea and weakness of three months' duration. No glossitis or paraesthesia was present. Hb: 6.5 g/dl. Vitamin B_{12} administration restored the blood picture to normal, with complete relief of angina and dyspnoea.*

within 48 hours of adequate treatment. *Plasma lactate dehydrogenase* is invariably increased, sometimes to very high levels. The direct Coombs' test is positive in up to ten per cent of patients due to complement-coating of the red cells.

The *serum folate* is usually normal, but it may be elevated or, rarely, reduced. The *red cell folate* is almost always reduced.

Bone marrow

Aspiration usually yields a large number of fragments. The fragments and cell trails are usually hypercellular. Erythropoiesis is intensely active and predominantly megaloblastic, and shows a 'shift to the left' with an increased proportion of more primitive cells. Granulopoiesis is active but the myeloid–erythroid ratio is reduced or even reversed. The morphological characteristics of the marrow have been described previously (p. 71). On rare occasions, erythropoiesis, although megaloblastic, is reduced in activity.

The marrow iron stain usually shows large amounts of iron in the fragments and in reticulum cells throughout the cell trails; abnormal sideroblasts are increased although 'ring' sideroblasts are usually *not* prominent. If the patient has iron deficiency, marrow iron stores are reduced or absent.

Chromosomal abnormalities are frequently observed on bone marrow culture, chromosome breakage being the outstanding finding. The abnormalities disappear after therapy.

Diagnosis

Diagnosis is based on the following features:

- clinical picture
- macrocytic blood picture
- megaloblastic bone marrow
- low serum vitamin B_{12}
- positive serum intrinsic factor antibody test
- characteristic radioactive vitamin B_{12} absorption test
- reticulocyte response to very small test doses of vitamin B_{12}
- elevated serum gastrin

Clinical picture. Occasional patients are not anaemic and have no symptoms or signs. More frequently, the diagnosis is suggested by a history of gradually increasing tiredness and lethargy, perhaps with some soreness of the tongue and/or symmetrical paraesthesiae of the extremities in a patient aged over 40 years with no abnormal physical findings apart from those due to anaemia. A family history is sometimes obtained. Signs of subacute combined degeneration of the spinal cord are strong presumptive evidence of pernicious anaemia, but are present in only about 15 per cent of patients.

Blood examination. This is essential, particularly the blood film. In anaemic patients the typical features of a megaloblastic macrocytic anaemia are present (p. 72), and are more marked the more severe the anaemia. It is important to emphasize that macrocytosis with an elevated MCV is often the first manifestation of vitamin B_{12} deficiency and may precede the development of anaemia by months or, rarely, years.

Bone marrow aspiration. This is generally not necessary in patients with a typical blood picture, but is essential in all doubtful cases. It should be performed before the administration of vitamin B_{12}, as this rapidly changes erythropoiesis from megaloblastic to normoblastic.

Serum vitamin B_{12} assay. The finding of a low serum vitamin B_{12} level is an essential prerequisite for the diagnosis of pernicious anaemia, and an assay should be performed in all suspected cases. Serum and red cell folate should also be assayed in case the patient's megaloblastic anaemia is due to folate rather than vitamin B_{12} deficiency, a *distinction that cannot be made with certainty from the clinical picture and haematological examination alone.*

Serum intrinsic factor antibody test. The presence of intrinsic factor antibodies is strong evidence in favour of a diagnosis of pernicious anaemia, although absence does not disqualify it. Parietal cell antibodies lack the positive diagnostic specificity of intrinsic factor antibodies, but their absence casts doubt on the diagnosis of pernicious anaemia. If both antibodies are present in the serum, the diagnosis is certain.

Radioactive vitamin B_{12} absorption test. This test is essential for the definitive diagnosis of pernicious anaemia in patients with a negative intrinsic factor antibody test. It provides direct evidence for the presence of vitamin B_{12} malabsorption; the second part of the test, with intrinsic factor, indicates whether lack of intrinsic factor is the cause of the malabsorption.

Serum gastrin level. A pentagastrin or histamine fast achlorhydria is almost invariable in pernicious anaemia, and 80% of patients have an elevated serum gastrin. The test is not specific for pernicious anaemia as increased levels may also occur in patients until atrophic gastritis and adequate vitamin B_{12} absorption.

PATIENTS WITH MINIMAL OR NO ANAEMIA

Diagnostic difficulty occasionally arises in untreated patients who present with nervous system involvement, and in treated patients in whom the diagnosis has never been adequately established.

Occasionally, patients with nervous system involvement are not anaemic, although they usually have at least some morphological abnormality, e.g. oval macrocytosis or marrow white cell changes. Once suspected, estimation of the serum vitamin B_{12} level, intrinsic factor antibody assay and, if necessary, a Schilling test will establish the diagnosis.

The patient who has been treated for 'pernicious anaemia' for many years without the application of modern diagnostic criteria for the disorder is a frequent clinical problem. Such a patient is haematologically normal with a high serum level of vitamin B_{12} resulting from regular vitamin B_{12} injections. Examination of serum for intrinsic gastric factor antibodies and, if necessary, a Schilling test usually clarify the diagnosis.

Prognosis

The prognosis depends largely on the degree of nervous system involvement at the time of diagnosis and its response to treatment. In patients with no involvement or with reversible changes, i.e. the majority of patients, prognosis with adequate treatment is excellent, and life-expectation is approximately that of normal people of similar age. However, a slightly increased and unpredictable risk exists of developing carcinoma of the stomach, especially in males (p. 82).

In patients with irreversible paraplegia, the prognosis is that of the paraplegia.

Treatment

Treatment will be considered under the following headings:

- administration of vitamin B_{12}
- symptomatic and supportive therapy
- follow-up and early detection of carcinoma of the stomach.

VITAMIN B_{12}

The essential feature of treatment is the administration *for life* of vitamin B_{12} in adequate doses. The reason for life-long therapy should be explained to the patient, together with the importance of attending regularly for injections and follow-up examinations.

The *objects* of vitamin B_{12} therapy are: (a) to correct the anaemia and to maintain a normal blood picture; (b) to arrest and reverse nervous system lesions when present, and to prevent them when absent; and (c) to replenish the depleted tissue stores. Adequate initial and maintenance doses are necessary to achieve these objects.

Vitamin B_{12} may be given as hydroxocobalamin or cyanocobalamin. Hydroxocobalamin offers some advantage as it is more available to cells and a greater proportion of the administered dose is retained by the body; the achieved serum vitamin B_{12} level falls more slowly than with cyanocobalamin (Hall *et al.* 1984). The B_{12} should be administered by deep subcutaneous or intramuscular injection.

Dose

Initial dosage. Several equally effective regimens have been recommended by different authorities. A practical regimen is to give 1000 μg hydroxocobalamin daily for one week. This will entirely restore the blood picture to normal and replenish vitamin B_{12} body-stores.

Maintenance dosage. When the above doses have

been given, the patient is maintained on 1000 μg hydroxocobalamin once every three months. There is no evidence that patients with neurological involvement benefit from larger doses. Maintenance therapy is given for life.

Toxic effects are uncommon, but local reactions or general allergic reactions occur rarely. They are probably due to impurities in the pharmacological preparation, rather than to the vitamin B_{12} itself.

The response to vitamin B_{12}

Symptoms. Subjective improvement commences from within 2–3 days with a sense of well-being and a return of appetite, even before there is any haematological response. The glossitis is rapidly relieved, and symptoms of anaemia improve as the haemoglobin rises. Symptoms of gout with accompanying hyperuricaemia occasionally occur around the seventh day.

Blood (Fig. 4.5). The first sign of response is in the reticulocyte count, which starts to increase on the second or third day, rises rapidly to a maximum on the sixth to eighth day, and falls gradually to normal on about the twentieth day. The height of the reticulocyte response is inversely proportional to the degree of anaemia, and may reach 40–50 per cent in patients with very severe anaemia. The increase in reticulocytes is followed shortly by an increase in the haemoglobin value which progressively rises, usually returning to normal in about 5–6 weeks, irrespective of the initial value. The MCV gradually falls, returning to normal in about ten weeks. The neutrophil count rises to normal, the response occurring a little later than the reticulocyte response. Occasionally, a temporary moderate neutrophilia occurs with some 'shift to the left'; a few myelocytes may appear. Hypersegmented neutrophils disappear after about two weeks. A mild thrombocytosis may occur before the platelet count returns to normal. The serum bilirubin, iron, lactate dehydrogenase and red cell folate return to normal.

Bone marrow. Erythropoiesis rapidly alters from megaloblastic to normoblastic. Changes are obvious within about six hours and, with adequate replacement, erythropoiesis is completely normoblastic after 3–4 days. Giant metamyelocytes persist for 12 days.

Hypokalaemia. This can occur soon after treatment is commenced, and is more likely to occur in

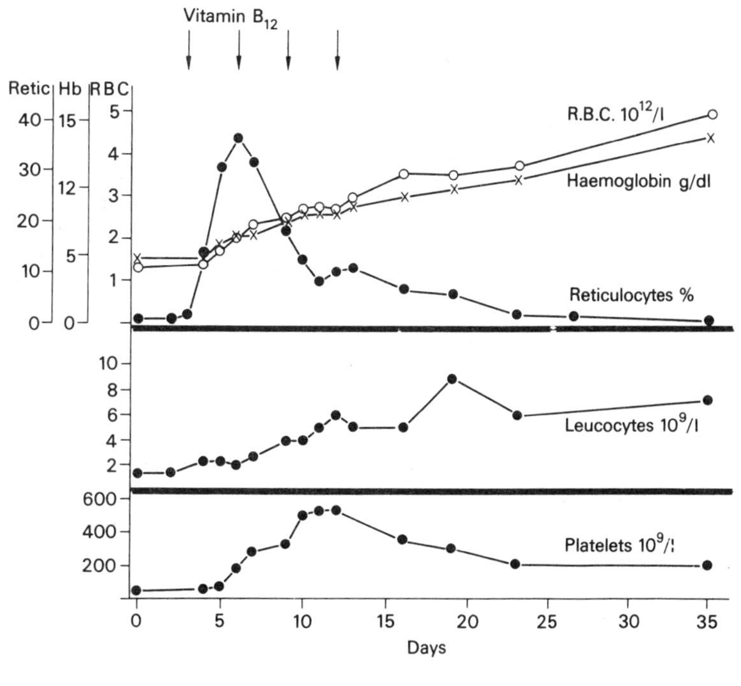

Fig. 4.5. *Pernicious anaemia: response to vitamin B_{12}. Four injections of vitamin B_{12}, each of 1000 μg were given over a period of two weeks. The reticulocytes started to rise on the 4th day after the first injection, increased sharply to reach a peak on the 6th day, and fell more slowly to normal values on about the 20th day. The red cell count and haemoglobin started to rise shortly after reticulocyte response, and rose progressively to normal values in about five weeks. The white cell and platelet response occurred slightly later than the reticulocyte response.*

subjects whose plasma potassium is already relatively low, and in those with more severe anaemia.

Nervous system manifestations. Vitamin B_{12} therapy is followed by reversal of the peripheral neuropathy and by arrest and slow improvement, to some degree, of the subacute combined degeneration of the cord. Recovery is maximum in the first six months of treatment, after which relatively little further improvement occurs.

Gastric abnormalities. The gastric mucosal atrophy and achlorhydria persist unchanged.

Supplements of iron are not required in most cases. However, occasionally bleeding, e.g. from haemorrhoids or alimentary tract malignancy, causes concomitant iron deficiency. Features of iron deficiency are often not obvious at the time of diagnosis, but develop during treatment when the haemoglobin has risen; full haematological remission does not occur until supplements of iron are given. Folic acid is dangerous in pernicious anaemia and should never be administered alone.

Failure of response to vitamin B_{12}

It is not uncommon for patients considered to have pernicious anaemia to fail to respond adequately to vitamin B_{12}. The usual explanation is *incorrect diagnosis.* The anaemia may be macrocytic but associated with a normoblastic marrow (see Table 4.6, p. 95). If the marrow is megaloblastic, it may be due to folate deficiency, sideroblastic anaemia (p. 58) or erythroleukaemia (p. 94). *Chronic infection* (particularly bedsores and urinary tract infection), *chronic renal failure, occult malignancy,* or concurrently administered *drugs,* e.g. chloramphenicol or alcohol, may impair the bone marrow response to vitamin B_{12} replacement. Ongoing *occult gastrointestinal bleeding* is another possible cause that should be excluded.

SYMPTOMATIC AND SUPPORTIVE THERAPY

The patient with pernicious anaemia is usually not critically ill, and the diagnosis should be fully established before specific therapy is undertaken. The average patient with only a moderate anaemia should be put to bed until the haemoglobin level reaches 9–10 g/dl. Congestive cardiac failure, if present, improves as the haemoglobin rises; the usual measures for its treatment should be instituted. *Physiotherapy* to improve muscular strength and co-ordination is important in patients with nervous system involvement. In paraplegic patients, every effort should be made to avoid urinary tract infections and bed sores.

In some cases, immediate measures may be necessary before the completion of diagnostic tests and commencement of appropriate specific replacement therapy. Although *blood transfusion* should be avoided if possible, it is indicated if the patient has significant problems due to anaemia. Packed red cells rather than whole blood should be given, and the transfusion should be slow and the venous pressure carefully monitored. Parenteral administration of diuretic before the transfusion may be indicated, especially in subjects with limited cardiac reserve.

If bleeding or infection is present, or the patient has other serious medical problems, e.g. chronic renal failure or severe liver disease, *emergency treatment* may be necessary. In most cases, a diagnosis of megaloblastic anaemia can be made from the blood and bone marrow appearances, but the precise causative factors may be in doubt. In this situation, full doses of both vitamin B_{12} and folic acid should be given by parenteral injection. It is essential to withdraw a sample of blood from the patient for appropriate serum assays before the injections are given. Failure to observe this rule will lead inevitably to diagnostic confusion.

Sudden death in patients with pernicious anaemia during treatment has been attributed to hypokalaemia resulting from entry of potassium from plasma into rapidly proliferating marrow erythroblasts. Estimation of serum potassium before and during initial therapy is advisable, with the administration of potassium supplements if hypokalaemia is likely to develop.

FOLLOW-UP AND EARLY DETECTION OF CARCINOMA OF THE STOMACH

Clinical and haematological examination should be made at six-monthly intervals after the haemoglobin level has returned to normal, for two main reasons: (1) to assess the adequacy of treatment; and (2) to detect the onset of carcinoma of the stomach. Inadequate vitamin B_{12} dosage or cessation of therapy is suggested by the recurrence or occurrence for the first time of glossitis or paraesthesiae, or by the reappearance of macrocytosis in the blood film (Savage & Lindenbaum 1983).

Carcinoma of the stomach develops three times more commonly in patients with pernicious anaemia (usually males) than in the general population of the same age. Thus, clinical and haematological changes that suggest the possibility of carcinoma of the stomach should be carefully monitored. Suggestive symptoms include loss of weight, anorexia, dyspepsia or abdominal pain, particularly if not previously present. Haematological changes include a fall in haemoglobin level and the development of hypochromia, both of which suggest occult bleeding. Barium meal examination and endoscopy should be carried out when any suspicion of carcinoma exists. Regular screening of well patients by endoscopy or exfoliative cytology is not warranted.

Megaloblastic anaemia following gastrectomy

The frequency of megaloblastic anaemia following gastrectomy depends on the extent of the gastrectomy, the nutritional state of the patient before and after operation, and the time since the operation.

Total gastrectomy

All patients who survive long enough following total gastrectomy, and who have not been given parenteral vitamin B_{12}, ultimately develop a megaloblastic macrocytic anaemia. Total gastrectomy results in complete loss of intrinsic factor and thus produces an abnormality similar to that of pernicious anaemia, i.e. failure of vitamin B_{12} absorption due to lack of intrinsic factor. However, the body has a considerable store of vitamin B_{12}, and the latent period between gastrectomy and the development of megaloblastic anaemia (which may be accompanied by glossitis and neurological involvement) is seldom less than 2 years and may be as long as 7–8 years. Many patients in whom total gastrectomy is performed for gastric carcinoma do not survive sufficiently long for vitamin B_{12} depletion to develop. Folate deficiency and iron deficiency may also develop as with partial gastrectomy (see below).

Treatment. It is advisable to give parenteral vitamin B_{12} prophylactically after total gastrectomy, in doses of 1000 μg hydroxocobalamin once every three months, for life. Alternatively, clinical and blood examinations can be performed at regular intervals, especially after two years have elapsed, to detect early signs of macrocytic anaemia or neurological involvement. When these disorders appear, treatment is as for pernicious anaemia.

Partial gastrectomy

Anaemia occurs in approximately 50 per cent of patients following partial gastrectomy (Hines *et al.* 1967). In the early post-operative years, iron deficiency is the main cause. Megaloblastic anaemia, usually due to vitamin B_{12} deficiency, and sometimes due to combined B_{12} and folate deficiency, is much less frequent and tends to develop later, often in association with iron deficiency. Subnormal serum vitamin B_{12} levels are found in up to 20 per cent of patients and may occur in the absence of overt megaloblastic anaemia. The B_{12} deficiency is due to loss of intrinsic factor-secreting mucosa by surgical resection and by atrophy or gastritis of the remaining gastric segment.

Defective absorption of vitamin B_{12} is demonstrable by the Schilling test in about 30 per cent of patients, the degree depending on the extent of gastric resection. Absorption is usually corrected by the addition of intrinsic factor. Improved absorption may also be achieved in some cases by administering the labelled vitamin B_{12} with food rather than in the fasting state. In patients in whom the conventional Schilling test is normal in spite of a reduced serum vitamin B_{12} level, a modified test using food-bound radioactive vitamin B_{12} may reveal an absorptive defect due to lack of release of vitamin B_{12} from food (Doscherholmen *et al.* 1983). Folate deficiency is mainly due to inadequate intake and increased demands, but malabsorption may contribute. Unfavourable haematological sequelae following vagotomy and pyloroplasty are rare.

Treatment. Yearly blood examinations are advisable after partial gastrectomy. If anaemia due to vitamin B_{12} deficiency develops, parenteral administration of B_{12} in the usual doses used for pernicious anaemia is indicated. Life-long B_{12} maintenance therapy and haematological follow-up are necessary.

Megaloblastic anaemia associated with lesions of the small intestine

Megaloblastic anaemia may occur as a complication of certain anatomical or inflammatory lesions of the small intestine; these include stricture, surgical anastomoses which produce a blind or by-passed loop of intestine, gastrojejunocolic and ileocolic fistulae, ileal resection, radiation damage, jejunal diverticulosis and regional ileitis. The majority of cases are due to vitamin B_{12} deficiency resulting from one of two mechanisms: (1) failure of absorption of vitamin B_{12} by the terminal ileum due either to removal by resection, bypassing by fistulae, or damage to the absorptive surface by inflammation or radiation; and (2) abnormal proliferation of organisms in the small intestine.

In cases of stricture or blind loops, depression of gut motility and stagnation of contents predispose to the abnormal bacterial proliferation, whilst with fistulae there is direct contamination by colonic content. The proliferating bacteria probably bind the intrinsic factor–vitamin B_{12} complex and thus compete with the host for the vitamin B_{12} in food or convert the B_{12} to physiologically inactive analogues (Brandt *et al.* 1977). The administration of broad-spectrum antibiotics may correct an abnormal Schilling test and cause temporary remission in patients with megaloblastic anaemia by sterilizing the gut contents and lessening competition for vitamin B_{12}. In cases associated with abnormal proliferation of bacteria, serum folate levels are often elevated, the organisms apparently synthesizing folate, which is then absorbed. In contrast, active regional enteritis is associated with decreased folate absorption, and serum folate levels are often low. The drug sulphasalazine also interferes with folate absorption and may be a contributory factor in some patients.

The clinical and haematological features are those of a megaloblastic anaemia due to vitamin B_{12} deficiency; neurological abnormalities occasionally develop. The anaemia usually responds to parenteral vitamin B_{12} in dosages as for pernicious anaemia, but folic acid administration is also necessary when folate deficiency is present. Surgical restoration of the normal continuity of the intestine with elimination of the blind or obstructed loop, or of the fistula, is also followed by relief of the anaemia, provided sufficient healthy terminal ileum remains.

Megaloblastic anaemia due to fish tapeworm

Megaloblastic anaemia due to vitamin B_{12} deficiency is occasionally seen as a complication of infestation with the fish tapeworm, *Diphyllobothrium latum*, in those countries where the worm is commonly encountered. These include the Scandinavian countries (particularly Finland), the USSR, and Japan. Although vitamin B_{12} malabsorption is common in individuals harbouring the worm, only a very small proportion develops a frank megaloblastic anaemia. In Finland, about 20 per cent of the population is infested, but only about 1 in 3000 persons become anaemic. In those with anaemia, the worm is always situated high in the small intestine and has probably been present for a long time. The living worm produces vitamin B_{12} deficiency by taking up the vitamin of the food, thus lowering the amount available to the host. The clinical picture resembles that of pernicious anaemia, and neurological signs may develop; however, the gastric juice always contains intrinsic factor. Parenteral administration of vitamin B_{12} results in cure; it can be discontinued when the worm has been expelled by antihelminthic therapy. Von Bonsdorff's monograph (1978) provides a comprehensive review of the subject.

Miscellaneous causes of B_{12} deficiency

Nutritional megaloblastic anaemia

Nutritional vitamin B_{12} deficiency occurs in people who for religious or other reasons do not eat meat or animal products. In most parts of the world, it is less common than nutritional folate deficiency (p. 88). The development of subnormal vitamin B_{12} levels and megaloblastic anaemia depends on the degree to which food of animal origin is excluded from the diet. Strict vegans eat no meat or animal products such as milk, milk products, and eggs. Some permit the taking of milk ('lactovegetarians'), but often the milk is boiled and much of the vitamin B_{12} destroyed. Severe megaloblastic anaemia due to vitamin B_{12} deficiency may occur in exclusively breast-fed infants born to vegetarian mothers.

In India, reduced serum levels of vitamin B_{12} are common in Hindu people, but a frank megaloblastic anaemia due to vitamin B_{12} deficiency alone is an unusual occurrence.

In cases where vitamin B_{12} deficiency is combined with folate and iron deficiency, some element of malabsorption is almost always present, and megaloblastic anaemia is frequent.

In temperate countries, most cases are found among vegetarians or migrant populations from tropical zones who retain their traditional eating habits and methods of food preparation. Serum folate levels are reduced if overall food consumption is poor, but in those who eat large amounts of vegetables, folate levels are often high. Many people tolerate moderately subnormal serum vitamin B_{12} levels for long periods without developing anaemia. The anaemia responds promptly to parenteral doses of vitamin B_{12} as given in pernicious anaemia. Subsequent daily administration of oral vitamin B_{12} in physiological doses of 5–10 μg should prevent recurrence in those patients who are not able or willing to increase their dietary intake of B_{12} (Chanarin *et al.* 1985).

Drugs

A number of drugs impair vitamin B_{12} absorption. They include phenformin, metformin, para-aminosalicyclic acid, cholestyramine, cimetidine, neomycin, colchicine and slow-release potassium chloride. Frank megaloblastic anaemia has only rarely been reported in spite of reduced serum vitamin B_{12} levels. Unusually prolonged exposure to the anaesthetic agent nitrous oxide may result in megaloblastic changes in peripheral blood and marrow (p. 73).

Chronic pancreatic disease

Malabsorption of vitamin B_{12} may occur in chronic exocrine pancreatic insufficiency (Schilling 1983). Allen *et al.* (1978) have suggested that the malabsorption is due to failure of degradation of the vitamin B_{12}-binding 'R' proteins in the small intestine, thus preventing subsequent transfer of B_{12} from the 'R' protein to intrinsic factor (p. 63). The abnormal Schilling test is not corrected by intrinsic factor, but improved absorption frequently follows oral administration of pancreatic extract. Absorption may be normal when the labelled B_{12} is administered with food, rather than in the fasting state. Although serum vitamin B_{12} levels may be reduced, megaloblastic anaemia is extremely rare.

Congenital disorders of vitamin B_{12}

Congenital disorders of vitamin B_{12} absorption, transport and metabolism are rare, although of great theoretical interest (p. 92). They include congenital intrinsic factor deficiency, familial selective vitamin B_{12} malabsorption (Imerslund–Grasbeck), inherited transcobalamin II deficiency and methylmalonic acidaemia (Rosenberg 1983).

Folate deficiency: Coeliac disease

Coeliac disease is the commonest cause of intestinal malabsorption in temperate zones, and is estimated to affect 0.03 per cent of the population. The condition is characterized by a lesion of the small intestinal mucosa which is related in an incompletely understood way to the ingestion of gluten, a protein present in some cereals. Withdrawal of gluten from the diet leads to healing of the small intestine and clinical improvement. The defect in absorption involves a wide range of substances including fat, protein, carbohydrate, vitamins and minerals, and the clinical picture varies depending on the nutrients most severely affected. The haematological aspects of coeliac disease are fully reviewed by Hoffbrand (1974).

Coeliac disease involves the jejunum predominantly, and thus folate and iron deficiency are the most common haematological complications. In untreated disease, absorption of both monoglutamate and polyglutamate folate is nearly always impaired, and serum and red cell folate values reduced. Iron absorption is also frequently impaired and serum iron levels reduced, particularly in children. Iron loss from the gut by exudation and cell exfoliation may contribute to the iron deficiency. Absorption of vitamin B_{12} is impaired in 50 per cent of patients, and the serum B_{12} level is subnormal in about 20 per cent. However, vitamin B_{12} deficiency is hardly ever severe enough to cause megaloblastic anaemia or neuropathy.

Clinical features

The disorder presents most frequently between the ages of 30 and 50 years. The sex incidence is equal. A history of symptoms suggestive of coeliac disease in childhood is given by approximately 25 per cent of patients.

The main *clinical manifestations* are weakness, intermittent diarrhoea, and loss of weight. Although diarrhoea occurs in most cases, it is not always a prominent symptom and is persistently absent in about 20 per cent of cases. The stools are characteristically fluid or semi-fluid, bulky, pale, frothy, offensive, and tend to float due to their high fat and gas content (steatorrhoea). Less typical presentations include megaloblastic anaemia, tetany, and spontaneous fracture due to osteomalacia or osteoporosis. Physical examination is usually normal, but advanced cases may show wasting, oedema, cheilosis and glossitis.

Patients with coeliac disease have an increased incidence of malignancy, either lymphoma of the small intestine or carcinoma of the gastrointestinal tract, especially of the oesophagus (Cooper *et al.* 1980).

Blood picture

Anaemia, usually of moderate but occasionally of marked degree, occurs in about 70 per cent of patients. In the majority, the blood film shows oval macrocytosis with an elevated MCV and all the typical features of a megaloblastic anaemia, but it may be microcytic hypochromic (particularly in children) or dimorphic with both macrocytosis and hypochromia. Target cells, Howell–Jolly bodies and thrombocytosis are occasionally noted on the blood film and indicate the occurrence of splenic atrophy (Marsh & Stewart 1970).

The *bone marrow* picture also varies. With severe anaemia, it is usually frankly megaloblastic, but with mild and moderate anaemia it is often predominantly normoblastic, although intermediate megaloblasts can usually be detected on careful examination, together with giant metamyelocytes. Marrow iron stores are partially or completely depleted.

Diagnosis

The diagnosis of coeliac disease is made from the clinical features and macroscopic inspection of stool, blood examination, demonstration of fat malabsorption, peroral jejunal biopsy, and a satisfactory clinical and histological response to withdrawal of gluten from the diet. The typical finding on jejunal biopsy is that of villous atrophy of the mucosa with loss of normal villi, giving rise to the appearance of a 'flat' mucosa.

Differential diagnosis. Diagnostic difficulty may occur in patients with coeliac disease who present with anaemia, especially when diarrhoea is not prominent or is absent. The anaemia is usually due to folate deficiency, and the finding of a low level of serum and red cell folate should prompt a search for clinical and laboratory evidence of coeliac disease. Less commonly the serum vitamin B_{12} level is reduced, and confusion with pernicious anaemia may result. A Schilling test and examination of serum for intrinsic factor antibodies usually clarify the diagnosis.

Treatment

At least 80 per cent of patients with a 'flat' jejunal mucosa respond clinically to a gluten-free diet, and most show healing of the mucosal lesion. Although the blood picture improves slowly to normal or near normal without administration of supplemental vitamins or iron, for practical purposes haematinics should always be given to the anaemic patient with laboratory evidence of vitamin or iron deficiency, as they significantly hasten haematological remission. In most cases the anaemia is due to folate deficiency, and folic acid should be given in a dose of 5 mg daily by mouth, until the blood picture and bone marrow have returned to normal and the patient has clearly achieved a satisfactory clinical response to the gluten-free diet. If iron deficiency is present, iron should be given, preferably by injection. Rebiopsy of the small intestine with demonstration of a favourable histological response to the gluten-free diet provides confirmation of the original diagnosis, and should be done in every case.

Folate deficiency: Tropical sprue

Small intestinal malabsorption occurs frequently among residents of, and visitors to, the tropics. In the majority of cases, no specific cause can be defined, and the syndrome is referred to as tropical sprue. The disorder is found in many parts of the tropics including India, Central America, China, the Middle East, South-East Asia, and the West Indies.

Absorption of polyglutamate folate is reduced, and if the illness is of sufficient duration, serum and red cell folate levels fall as stores are gradually depleted. When folate stores are completely exhausted, megaloblastic anaemia results. Vitamin B_{12} absorption, as measured by the Schilling test, is impaired in 50–95 per cent of patients, and the malabsorption is not corrected by intrinsic factor. In Caucasian subjects, vitamin B_{12} stores are sufficient to maintain supplies for at least three years, but in areas where the diet is largely vegetarian and vitamin B_{12} intake is low, subnormal serum levels and clinical manifestations of B_{12} deficiency may occur from after 2–3 months' deprivation. Serum vitamin B_{12} levels rarely reach the low levels seen in pernicious anaemia. In general, the nutritional reserves at the onset, and the severity and duration of the illness, are critical in determining the haematological manifestations and the rapidity with which they develop.

Pathology. Histological examination of intestinal mucosa obtained by peroral jejunal biopsy shows a wide spectrum of abnormality. In some severe cases, the mucosa is identical to that of coeliac disease, but more frequently the abnormalities are less florid. At the other extreme, morphological changes are minor and in no way different from those found in apparently healthy persons with little or no evidence of malabsorption living in the same area.

Clinical features. The onset is usually insidious, but the disorder occurs in an epidemic form with an acute onset in some areas. In the early stages of the illness, the main clinical features are intermittent or continuous diarrhoea, abdominal distension and pain, anorexia, nausea and vomiting. The stools are fluid or semi-fluid, and frequently contain mucus and blood. Later, the stools become pale, bulky and offensive, resembling the stools of coeliac disease, and the clinical picture is dominated by the manifestations of nutrient deficiency. Vitamin deficiency leads to glossitis, stomatitis, skin pigmentation and oedema. Wasting and weight loss occur. Although some patients completely recover in days or weeks, the usual course is characterized by remissions and relapses over a long period. Some patients have only relatively mild symptoms with little or no diarrhoea, and may present with anaemia rather than gastrointestinal symptoms. A late complication is the development of abdominal lymphoma as in coeliac disease.

Blood picture. Anaemia is common and is usually megaloblastic. In southern India, Baker & Mathan (1971) found that 64 per cent of patients had megaloblastic anaemia. Twenty-one per cent were due to vitamin B_{12} deficiency alone, 33 per cent were due to folate deficiency alone, and 44 per cent were due to a combined deficiency of both. Iron deficiency, and thus a dimorphic blood picture, is very common.

Diagnosis. The diagnosis of tropical sprue is made from the history of residence in the tropics, the clinical picture, macroscopic inspection of stool, blood examination, demonstration of the absorptive defect, and exclusion of other causes of malabsorption. Peroral jejunal biopsy is usually performed, although the histological changes of tropical sprue are seen in other conditions and are not specific for the disease.

Treatment. Bed rest, control of diarrhoea and vomiting, correction of fluid, mineral and nutritional deficiencies, and the administration of appropriate haematinics form the basis of treatment. Broad-spectrum antibiotics may result in a haematological response and lessen the diarrhoea in some cases. Long-term follow-up of patients is important to detect relapse or the development of lymphoma.

Nutritional megaloblastic anaemia due to folate deficiency

Megaloblastic anaemia resulting from nutritional causes is usually due to folate deficiency. Cases of combined folate and vitamin B_{12} deficiency may be seen, especially in the tropics. Nutritional anaemia due to vitamin B_{12} deficiency has been previously discussed (p. 85). The higher incidence of nutritional folate as compared to vitamin B_{12} deficiency is related to the smaller body-stores of folate and the greater liability of folate to destruction on cooking (see Table 4.1, p. 63). The folate content of food is low in relation to the minimum daily requirement of about 200 μg of folate, and if increased requirements, e.g. in pregnancy or infection, cannot be met from ingested folate, the limited amount of stored folate is rapidly depleted.

Causes. In *tropical zones,* the major causative factor is inadequate intake of folate due to poverty, or inappropriate cooking methods. Diets consisting of maize, rice or well-cooked beans result in a high incidence of folate deficiency. In contrast, areas in which green vegetables are consumed as a major part of the diet are relatively free from folate deficiency of purely dietary origin, provided the vegetables are cooked in a manner that preserves folate content. Tropical sprue (p. 87) is common in a number of tropical countries, and many cases of megaloblastic anaemia, apparently of nutritional origin alone, are probably the result of malabsorption associated with long-standing marginal dietary intake of folate and vitamin B_{12}.

In *temperate zones,* folate deficiency is usually caused by a deficient diet. There is considerable variation in prevalence, mainly depending on the age and socio-economic status of the population and the cooking methods employed. Several studies of elderly patients admitted to geriatric institutions have shown that 20–30 per cent have low serum folate levels. Reduction in red cell folate is less frequent, and most patients do not develop megaloblastic anaemia. Those who do are usually elderly, infirm people living alone, who are either too ill to prepare adequate meals or who have lost interest in eating due to deterioration of cerebral function. They are often women, perhaps edentulous, and they rarely admit to the paucity of their diet. Some, although purchasing adequate amounts of folate-rich food, may cook it for long periods in copious amounts of water, with resulting loss of folate.

Alcoholic patients whose appetite for solid food is suppressed by continual intake of alcohol, and who often have inadequate money to purchase folate-rich food, constitute another major group (p. 89).

Nutritional folate deficiency is also seen in ill patients who are anorexic or unable to increase their folate intake for other reasons. Thus, folate deficiency may occur after gastrectomy or in patients with chronic inflammatory bowel disease. Similarly, subnormal serum folate levels are frequently found in patients with chronic uraemia, but red cell folate levels are usually normal and megaloblastic anaemia is rare. Patients on long-term haemodialysis lose small amounts of folate through the dialysis membrane, but folate deficiency is unusual and dietary supplementation is generally not required (Sharman *et al.* 1982).

Finally, patients receiving intravenous fluid therapy or 'hyperalimentation' over long periods without added vitamins are at risk. An acute form of megaloblastic anaemia, often with pancytopenia, has been observed with increasing frequency in critically ill patients in intensive care units. In addition to folate deficiency, prior nitrous oxide anaesthesia (p. 73) may also be a factor in the development of megaloblastosis (Amos *et al.* 1982).

The *haematological* findings classically show the features of a megaloblastic macrocytic anaemia, and serum and red cell folate levels are low. The serum vitamin B_{12} level may also be reduced. In tropical zones, this is usually due to a true tissue deficiency of vitamin B_{12}. In temperate zones, the subnormal level frequently returns to normal within days of commencement of folic acid therapy even though vitamin B_{12} is not administered. Iron deficiency resulting from blood loss, e.g. hookworm infestation, and from a poor diet is commonly associated, and the blood picture may then have the features of a 'dimorphic' anaemia.

Diagnosis is based on exclusion of other causes of megaloblastic anaemia and a detailed dietary history. Inquiry concerning possible ingestion of drugs known to interfere with folate metabolism, e.g. anticonvulsants and trimethoprim, should be made.

Nutritional megaloblastic anaemia must be distinguished from megaloblastic anaemia due to malabsorption, especially from coeliac disease in which diarrhoea is not a prominent feature. In tropical countries, small intestinal disease is often present in addition to inadequate dietary intake, and tests for malabsorption should be undertaken.

Treatment consists of correction of the dietary defect when possible, and oral administration of folic acid in a dose to cover normal requirements; if serum iron and vitamin B_{12} levels are subnormal, these substances should also be administered. Treatment can be discontinued when the blood picture is normal and the patient is well, provided that an adequate diet is available. Folic acid fortification of food is under investigation in areas where dietary folate deficiency is prevalent.

Megaloblastic anaemia in alcoholic patients

The association of megaloblastic anaemia with excess alcohol ingestion is relatively common, and for this reason warrants separate consideration despite the fact that it is primarily nutritional in origin. Its prevalence varies widely depending on the general health, nutrition, social and economic status of the alcoholic population. The type of alcohol ingested is also important. Beer contains considerable amounts of folate, but whisky contains none and thus whisky drinkers are particularly prone to develop megaloblastic anaemia. Most studies, particularly from the United States, have been confined to so-called 'skid-row' alcoholics and have indicated an incidence of marrow megaloblastic change of 30–40 per cent. More recent work has suggested that major haematological abnormalities are unusual in alcoholics of higher socioeconomic status, the only stigma of excess alcohol ingestion being a mild macrocytosis without anaemia.

Most anaemic cases are clearly due to dietary folate deficiency and are associated with subnormal serum and red cell folate levels. Alcohol may also cause folate malabsorption or interfere with folate metabolism, and the fatty or cirrhotic liver of the chronic alcoholic may be unable to store and release adequate amounts of folate.

The evolution of anaemia in *actively drinking alcoholic patients* has been studied in detail by Eichner & Hillman (1971). The earliest abnormality observed in the marrow is nuclear and cytoplasmic vacuolation of erythroblasts and early myeloid precursors. This is apparently a direct toxic effect of alcohol, and the vacuoles disappear on withdrawal of alcohol. If alcohol ingestion continues and the diet is inadequate, the serum folate level falls sharply, the marrow becomes megaloblastic in 1–3 weeks, and finally 'ring' sideroblasts appear. If alcohol consumption is interrupted, the administration of a small physiological dose of oral folic acid reverts the megaloblastic marrow to normoblastic and cures the anaemia (Fig. 4.6). If alcohol intake continues, response to the folic acid is suboptimal, suggesting a direct inhibitory effect of alcohol on erythropoiesis.

The prevalence of subnormal serum and red cell folate levels in *chronic alcoholic patients* varies from 30 to 90 per cent depending on the social background and general nutritional status of the patients

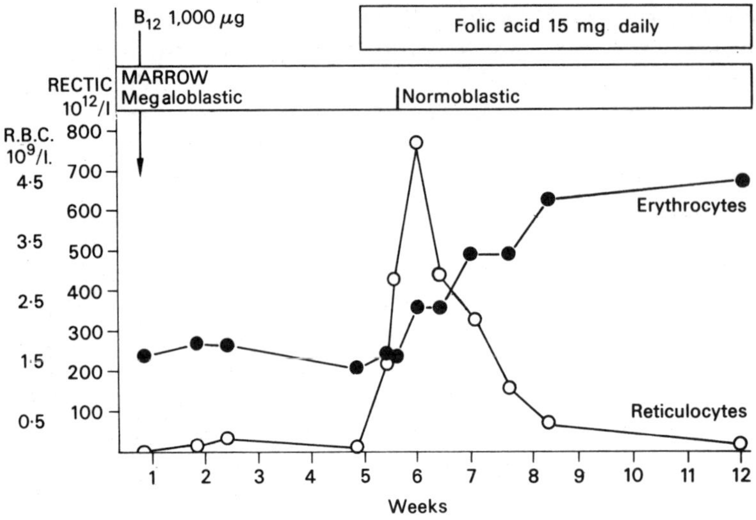

Fig. 4.6. *Mrs A.R., aged 50 years, presented with symptoms of anaemia and soreness of the mouth and throat of 4 months' duration, and a history of chronic alcoholism and poor diet. Blood—macrocytic anaemia. Bone marrow—megaloblastic erythropoiesis. No response to parenteral vitamin B_{12}. Clinical and haematological response to oral folic acid.*

studied. The serum folate level is often an unsatisfactory index of tissue folate status in alcoholic patients. It is occasionally normal in patients with frank megaloblastic anaemia, who subsequently respond to the administration of folic acid; in such cases, the red cell folate is usually reduced. Many patients with low serum and red cell folate levels are not anaemic, and marrow erythropoiesis may be normoblastic or only mildly megaloblastic. Progression to a frank megaloblastic anaemia is not inevitable.

Although folate deficiency is the usual cause of megaloblastic anaemia in alcoholic patients, alcohol can result in macrocytic and megaloblastic changes by a direct toxic effect on developing erythroblasts. Several surveys have shown that red cell macrocytosis is present in 80–90 per cent of chronic alcoholics who consume more than 80 g alcohol per day (Wu *et al.* 1974). In general, the patients are well nourished, and about 70 per cent have normal serum and red cell folate levels. The MCV is in the 100–110 fl range, there is no anemia, and the blood film shows round rather than oval macrocytosis and an absence of neutrophil hypersegmentation. Withdrawal of alcohol results in a gradual fall of the MCV to normal over three months. The marrows of such patients may be normoblastic or megaloblastic; megaloblastic changes revert to normal a few days after cessation of alcohol intake, but the marrow morphology and MCV are unaffected by folic acid therapy alone.

The serum folate level in actively drinking alcoholics needs to be interpreted with caution as alcohol itself may cause a rapid but reversible decline in serum folate levels as measured by microbiological and radio-isotope methods. The mechanism is uncertain. Haematological aspects of alcoholism are reviewed by Lindenbaum (1980) and Chanarin (1982).

Megaloblastic anaemia in hepatic cirrhosis

Frank megaloblastic anaemia due to folate deficiency is occasionally encountered in patients with cirrhosis arising from causes other than chronic excess alcohol ingestion. Inadequate dietary intake, increased folate requirements, and possible interference with folate metabolism are of aetiological importance.

Megaloblastic anaemia of pregnancy

Megaloblastic anaemia during pregnancy results from an inadequate intake of folate to meet the increased requirements of pregnancy. A small proportion of cases are due to latent coeliac disease first becoming manifest during pregnancy. Rare cases are due to the fortuitous association of pernicious anaemia, although this disorder is uncommon in the child-bearing age group.

The prevalence of megaloblastic anaemia of pregnancy varies in different populations, apparently depending on the nutritional status of the population. In well-nourished communities, florid forms are now rare, but mild cases occasionally occur in spite of the widespread use of prophylactic folic acid.

Pathogenesis. Folate is required by the fetus for normal development, and an adequate supply is assured at the expense of the mother. In normal pregnancy, the average folate requirement is increased three-fold. There is a progressive fall in serum folate values, subnormal levels occurring in about 50 per cent of patients in the last trimester. Reduction in the red cell folate level is less frequent. These changes are not necessarily accompanied by anaemia or abnormalities in the blood or bone marrow.

If pre-existing folate deficiency is present, or the dietary folate intake of the mother is inadequate to meet the increased demand, tissue deficiency of folate occurs and megaloblastic changes become evident in the bone marrow. Mild bone marrow changes, not necessarily associated with anaemia, are seen in 20–30 per cent of pregnant women in late pregnancy. In the occasional case, further progression to a frank megaloblastic anaemia occurs. Other factors, besides fetal demand, that may contribute to the development of anaemia include iron deficiency, co-existent haemolytic anaemia, urinary tract and other infections, anticonvulsant and trimethoprim therapy, and altered intestinal absorption of folate.

Clinical features. Megaloblastic anaemia of pregnancy tends to occur more frequently after multiple pregnancies than in first and second pregnancies. Onset is usually gradual in late pregnancy, but may be rapid, particularly when associated with the presence of infection. Anorexia, excessive vomiting, and moderate weight loss are common, and glossitis and diarrhoea are features in some cases. Breast milk contains folate and occasional cases occurring during prolonged lactation in a poorly nourished mother have been described. Spontaneous remission following delivery is usual, even in the absence of treatment. With early diagnosis and adequate treatment, the outlook for mother and child is good.

Blood picture. The degree of anaemia and abnormalities of red cell morphology vary. Frequently, the blood picture is similar to that of pernicious anaemia, with marked oval macrocytosis. However, in some cases these features are much less marked, and the anaemia may be normocytic rather than macrocytic and the MCV within normal range. Not uncommonly there is a concomitant iron deficiency, and the film is that of a 'dimorphic' anaemia (p. 72).

Bone marrow. When the anaemia is severe, erythropoiesis is frankly megaloblastic, but with lesser degrees of anaemia, careful scrutiny always reveals the presence of 'intermediate' megaloblasts, giant metamyelocytes, and hypersegmented neutrophils.

Diagnosis. Megaloblastic anaemia of pregnancy, although relatively uncommon, should be considered in any pregnant patient who is anaemic without obvious cause, especially in the third trimester or puerperium. Although there is a natural reluctance to perform bone marrow aspiration in late pregnancy, this examination is essential to establish a definitive diagnosis, as the levels of serum and red cell folate are often reduced at term in normal pregnancy and are not of great help. In some patients, the serum vitamin B_{12} is also subnormal, but the level usually returns to normal after folic acid therapy even though vitamin B_{12} is not given.

Prevention. Most authorities recommend the prophylactic administration of folic acid as well as iron during pregnancy. The daily supplement usually recommended is 300 μg. A number of proprietary tablets containing both iron and folic acid are available; combined preparations have the advantage that the patient need take only one tablet a day. Despite the prophylactic administration of these tablets, routine haematological examination in pregnancy is still an essential part of antenatal care. Megaloblastic anaemia of pregnancy is reviewed by Chanarin (1985).

Treatment. This is as for nutritional folate deficiency (p. 88).

Megaloblastic anaemia of infancy and childhood

Megaloblastic anaemia is rare in infancy and childhood. Nutritional megaloblastic anaemia and the megaloblastic anaemia associated with coeliac disease (p. 85) are usually due to folate deficiency. Megaloblastic anaemia in breast-fed infants of vegetarian mothers (p. 85), juvenile pernicious anaemia, congenital intrinsic factor deficiency, familial selective vitamin B_{12} malabsorption, and inherited transcobalamin II deficiency are associated with vitamin B_{12} deficiency.

Nutritional megaloblastic anaemia of infancy

Nutritional megaloblastic anaemia of infancy usually occurs between the ages of 5 and 12 months, and is uncommon after the first year. It is due to folate deficiency, caused primarily by dietary inadequacy; however, severe or prolonged infection and diarrhoea often act as aggravating factors. Premature babies are particularly at risk. They often become folate deficient and may develop megaloblastic anaemia at about 6–10 weeks. In the tropics, folate deficiency in infancy is usually part of the syndromes of kwashiorkor and protein-calorie malnutrition.

The *clinical features* are those common to all anaemias of infancy—pallor, irritability, listlessness and anorexia—often with associated infection of the respiratory or alimentary tracts. Failure to gain weight is usual, and fever is common. The anaemia is often severe. Marrow examination is essential for diagnosis. Death is common in untreated cases, infection frequently being the terminal event.

Treatment. The anaemia responds to the administration of folic acid by mouth, given in doses of 5 mg daily until the blood picture returns to normal and infection has been eliminated. Transfusion is sometimes needed in severely anaemic infants, but great care must be taken not to overload the circulation. Associated infections should be appropriately treated. Prophylactic folic acid is advisable in low birth-weight premature babies, and all neonates who have received an exchange transfusion or have had a prolonged infection.

Vitamin B_{12} deficiency in children

Four rare, but distinct, types of vitamin B_{12} deficiency in childhood and adolescence are recognized (Cooper 1976). *Juvenile pernicious anaemia* is similar to the adult form. A family history is usual, and most cases present after the age of ten years. The patients have gastric atrophy, achlorhydria and absent intrinsic factor secretion. Serum intrinsic factor antibodies are usually present, and an associated endocrinopathy may occur. *Congenital intrinsic factor deficiency* usually presents before the age of two years and is characterized by a selective failure of gastric intrinsic factor secretion, or possibly the secretion of structurally and functionally abnormal intrinsic factor. Gastric function and histology are otherwise normal. Serum parietal cell and intrinsic factor antibodies are absent. The condition is inherited as an autosomal recessive and has no genetic relationship to adult pernicious anaemia.

Familial selective vitamin B_{12} malabsorption (Imerslund–Gräsbeck) differs from the other types in that the basic abnormality is at the level of the small intestine rather than the stomach. Gastric histology and function (including intrinsic factor secretion) are normal, but vitamin B_{12} is not transported through the ileal mucosa into the circulation in spite of normal attachment of the intrinsic factor–vitamin B_{12} complex to the ileal receptors. The ileum is otherwise normal. Serum parietal cell and intrinsic factor antibodies are not present. The condition usually presents before the age of two years, and is inherited as an autosomal recessive. Proteinuria is a constant but unexplained accompanying manifestation.

Inherited transcobalamin II deficiency is an

extremely rare cause of neonatal megaloblastic anaemia in which the serum vitamin B_{12} level is paradoxically normal in spite of gross marrow megaloblastosis. Other inherited defects of vitamin B_{12} metabolism are reviewed by Matthews and Linnell (1982).

Congenital defects of folate metabolism

A number of congenital disorders of folate uptake, interconversion, and utilization are recognized. Some are associated with serious neurological impairment. Megaloblastosis is not a constant feature. They are reviewed by Rowe (1983).

Megaloblastic anaemia due to drugs

The administration of certain drugs may lead to the development of megaloblastic anaemia by interfering with the metabolism of folate. They fall into two broad groups: (1) drugs that only occasionally cause megaloblastic anaemia, the mechanism not being known with certainty. The anticonvulsant, phenytoin sodium, is the main drug in this group; and (2) drugs that inhibit the action of dihydrofolate reductase, a key enzyme in the metabolism of folate. If administered for a long enough period in sufficient doses, all drugs in the second group eventually cause megaloblastic anaemia. Patients receiving drugs in both groups are more likely to develop megaloblastic anaemia if additional factors leading to folate deficiency, e.g. poor diet, pregnancy, malignant disease, or malabsorption, are present. The drugs are listed in Table 4.5. Drug-induced megaloblastic anaemias are reviewed by Scott & Weir (1980).

Table 4.5. *Drugs causing megaloblastic anaemia*

Uncertain mechanism
Anticonvulsant drugs
Oral contraceptive agents
Dihydrofolate reductase inhibitors
Methotrexate
Trimethoprim
Triamterene
Pyrimethamine

Anticonvulsant drugs

Abnormalities of folate metabolism are seen in many patients receiving treatment for epilepsy with diphenylhydantoin (phenytoin) sodium and, to a lesser extent, with primidone. The patients are often also receiving phenobarbitone. Subnormal serum, red cell, and cerebrospinal fluid folate levels occur in about 50 per cent of patients receiving diphenylhydantoin. Mild haematological changes are also frequent; red cell macrocytosis and early marrow megaloblastic changes are seen in 30 per cent of patients. A low serum folate level is not necessarily followed by a fall in red cell folate even though administration of the drug is continued, and a low red cell folate may be present for long periods without the development of megaloblastic anaemia. The factors responsible for changing minor haematological abnormalities of no clinical significance into a frank megaloblastic anaemia in less than one per cent of patients on anticonvulsant therapy are not known with certainty, but superadded dietary folate deficiency may be important. The period between commencement of drug therapy and the onset of anaemia averages six years, but it may be as short as six months or as long as 20 years. The anaemia may be severe, and morphologically is identical to other megaloblastic anaemias due to folate deficiency.

The pathogenesis of the disordered folate metabolism is uncertain. The anaemia responds rapidly to the administration of folic acid in pharmacological dosage, and the anticonvulsant therapy may be continued. Long-term folic acid therapy is necessary when the patient needs to remain on anticonvulsants. Improvement has also been noted following withdrawal of the offending drug.

Oral contraceptive agents

Subnormal serum folate levels, and on rare occasions a frank megaloblastic anaemia, have been reported in patients taking oral contraceptives. At present the association must be regarded as tenuous, and other causes of folate deficiency, e.g. occult malabsorption, should be rigorously excluded before attributing a megaloblastic anaemia to oral contraceptives.

Dihydrofolate reductase inhibitors

The enzyme, dihydrofolate reductase, plays an important role in the metabolism of folate, and drugs that interfere with its action affect DNA synthesis to produce megaloblastic anaemia. Dihydrofolate reductase is necessary to regenerate metabolically active tetrahydrofolate from the dihydrofolate which is formed as a result of oxidation of methylenetetrahydrofolate in the deoxyuridylate–thymidylate step of DNA synthesis (p. 73, see Fig. 4.2). Several drugs inhibit dihydrofolate reductase and cause megaloblastic anaemia.

Methotrexate is a potent inhibitor of the enzyme and regularly causes marked megaloblastosis.

Trimethoprim, which is used as an antibacterial agent usually in combination with the sulphonamide, sulphamethoxazole, inhibits bacterial dihydrofolate reductase, but its effect on the human enzyme is relatively trivial. An occasional patient who has developed megaloblastic anaemia while receiving trimethoprim has been reported, but an alternative explanation for the development of megaloblastic anaemia has usually been available in the patients cited.

Pyrimethamine has caused megaloblastic anaemia in a number of cases, and long-term therapy should be monitored with regular blood examinations. *Triamterene* has also been reported to cause megaloblastic anaemia by a similar mechanism, but cases are rare.

Several drugs have been shown to interfere with vitamin B_{12} absorption without causing frank megaloblastic anaemia (p. 85). A number of other drugs, most of which are used primarily in the therapy of malignant disease, produce megaloblastosis by directly blocking DNA synthesis rather than by affecting vitamin B_{12} or folate metabolism. They include cytosine arabinoside, hydroxyurea, and 6-mercaptopurine. Renal transplant patients receiving azathioprine frequently develop macrocytosis and megaloblastic marrow changes. The drugs are listed by Scott & Weir (1980).

Megaloblastic erythropoiesis in other haematological disorders

Occasional cases of megaloblastic erythropoiesis occurring in patients with chronic haemolytic anaemia have been described. The megaloblastic change is due to a conditioned deficiency of folate resulting from increased requirements caused by the marrow hyperplasia; precipitating factors such as dietary deficiency or infection are usually present.

The possibility of superadded folate deficiency should be considered in any patient with chronic haemolytic anaemia in whom there is an unexplained fall in haemoglobin level and reticulocyte count from the usual 'steady state value, occurring either as an acute crisis or chronically over a period of months. If the marrow is megaloblastic and the serum folate level reduced, the administration of folic acid may result in a substantial improvement in the haemoglobin level. Very large doses of folic acid may be necessary in some cases. A similar conditioned deficiency may occur occasionally in myelofibrosis (p. 338), the leukaemias and lymphomas, myeloma, and sideroblastic anaemia (p. 58).

Other conditions in which folate requirements are increased and folate deficiency may occur include carcinoma, inflammatory disorders, widespread skin disease, and hyperthyroidism.

Megaloblastic anaemia unresponsive to vitamin B_{12} or folate therapy

A small number of rare disorders is characterized by megaloblastic marrow changes and normal serum levels of vitamin B_{12} and folate. Administration of the vitamins does not result in clinical or haematological improvement.

Orotic aciduria, an inherited disorder of pyrimidine metabolism, causes retardation of growth and development, and a megaloblastic anaemia. Orotic acid crystals are found in the urine, and the condition responds to the administration of uridine.

Erythroleukaemia may be associated with marrow

megaloblastosis. The abnormalities in the red cell precursors are often bizarre and are not necessarily accompanied by typical white cell changes.

The macrocytic anaemias

Macrocytic anaemia is defined as an anaemia in which the mean corpuscular volume (MCV) is increased. The reliability of the MCV estimation has been greatly improved by the advent of automated cell counters which directly measure the MCV. However, the MCV result is influenced by the method of instrument calibration, and there is as yet no universally accepted calibration method and thus no universally accepted normal range for the MCV. Most agree that an MCV in excess of 100 fl is abnormal and that such cells are macrocytic. When routine blood examination shows a raised MCV, the presence of macrocytosis must always be confirmed by careful examination of the blood film, which often gives important additional information about the type of macrocytic anaemia and its cause.

Classification

The macrocytic anaemias can be divided into two broad groups, based on the morphology of erythroid precursors in the bone marrow: (a) the megaloblastic macrocytic anaemias, associated with megaloblastic erythropoiesis; and (b) the normoblastic macrocytic anaemias, associated with normoblastic erythropoiesis. This distinction is of the utmost practical importance, as the two groups differ in aetiology, prognosis, and response to treatment.

The *megaloblastic macrocytic anaemias* are, in most cases, deficiency anaemias, resulting from deficiency of either vitamin B_{12} or folate; the mechanism producing the deficiency varies with the disorder. The anaemia responds well to the administration of the deficient substance.

The *normoblastic macrocytic anaemias* occur in association with a number of well-defined disorders (Table 4.6). With many of these disorders, a macrocytic picture is unusual, normocytic anaemia being the more common finding. The anaemias, despite the macrocytosis, are not influenced by either vitamin B_{12} or folic acid therapy, and respond only to alleviation or cure of the underlying causative disorder.

Table 4.6. *Conditions in which macrocytosis occurs in association with normoblastic erythroid precursors*

Macrocytosis common
Haemolytic anaemia
Post-haemorrhagic anaemia
Macrocytosis occasional
Alcoholism
Leukaemia, especially acute leukaemia
Liver disease
Aplastic anaemia
Sideroblastic anaemia
Myelodysplastic syndromes
Anaemia due to marrow infiltration or replacement (myelosclerosis, secondary carcinoma of bone, myeloma, malignant lymphoma)
Cytotoxic drug therapy
Hypothyroidism
Chronic obstructive airways disease
Scurvy

The macrocytosis is caused by the presence of reticulocytes or mature red cells of increased size, or both, in the peripheral blood.

Reticulocytes are slightly larger than normal mature red cells, and when present in increased numbers cause a mild to moderate degree of macrocytosis. In well-stained films they have a slight, diffuse basophilic tint. The macrocytosis of post-haemorrhagic anaemia and haemolytic anaemia is mainly due to reticulocytosis.

Mature red cells of increased size. The bone marrow in cases of normoblastic macrocytic anaemia commonly contains nucleated red cells which are macronormoblastic, i.e. cells that are larger than their normal counterparts of a similar stage of development, which they resemble in all other respects, including their nuclear structure. Mature erythrocytes derived from a macronormoblastic marrow are macrocytic. Macronormoblastic erythropoiesis may be due to: (a) an increase in the rate of erythropoiesis; this contributes to the macrocytosis of post-haemorrhagic anaemia and haemolytic anaemia; and (b) an abnormality of marrow function, as in aplastic anaemia, sideroblastic anaemia, leukaemia, and liver disease.

Table 4.7. *Summary of the investigation of a patient with megaloblastic macrocytic anaemia*

Clinical history
Age, race, family history
Duration of symptoms
Glossitis—present or past
Symptoms suggesting nervous system involvement—paraesthesiae, weakness of the legs, ataxia, precipitancy or hesitancy of micturition, urinary retention
Diarrhoea—present or past; characteristics of stool
Dietary history; alcohol intake
Pregnancy or recent delivery
Residence in tropics
Drug therapy
Abdominal operations or disease

Physical examination
General nutritional state
Scleral icterus
Tongue—evidence of acute or chronic glossitis
Abdomen—hepatomegaly, splenomegaly, operation scars
Evidence of peripheral neuropathy or subacute combined degeneration
Skin pigmentation
Evidence of specific nutritional deficiencies or other diseases.

Special investigations

INVESTIGATIONS TO ESTABLISH THAT THE ANAEMIA IS MEGALOBLASTIC:
Full blood examination
Bone marrow aspiration including marrow iron stain

INVESTIGATIONS TO ESTABLISH THE CAUSATIVE FACTORS:
Nature of deficiency
Serum vitamin B_{12} assay
Serum and red cell folate assay

Cause of deficiency
Radioactive vitamin B_{12} absorption test
Serum parietal cell and intrinsic factor antibodies
Tests of malabsorption
Pentagastrin or histamine gastric analysis
Radiological examination of stomach and small intestine
Jejunal biopsy

Response to treatment
Reticulocyte response and haemoglobin rise after therapy

The importance of the normoblastic macrocytic anaemias lies in the fact that they are often mistaken for megaloblastic anaemias, especially pernicious anaemia, and thus are treated with vitamin B_{12} or folic acid. *It should be noted that red cell macrocytosis and an elevated MCV may be seen in the absence of anaemia, marrow abnormalities, or deficiency of vitamin B_{12} or folate, particularly in alcoholic patients.* No cause may be apparent in some patients.

The macrocytosis of the megaloblastic macrocytic anaemias is usually much greater than that of the normoblastic macrocytic anaemias. In general, the higher the MCV, the greater the incidence of megaloblastosis, and MCV values above 125 fl are almost always associated with megaloblastic bone marrows. Also, the macrocytes are usually oval in the megaloblastic macrocytic anaemias, in contrast with the round macrocytes of normoblastic macrocytic anaemias. The clinical significance of macrocytosis is discussed by Davidson & Hamilton (1978).

The investigation of a patient with macrocytic anaemia

In the investigation of a patient with macrocytic anaemia, two questions must be answered:

1 Is the anaemia normoblastic or megaloblastic?

2 What is the cause of the anaemia?

IS THE ANAEMIA NORMOBLASTIC OR MEGALOBLASTIC?

Marrow examination is necessary to answer this question with absolute certainty.

In suspected megaloblastic anaemia, bone marrow examination is not absolutely essential when the peripheral blood picture is typical. If required, it should be performed before the administration of vitamin B_{12} or folic acid, as these rapidly cause reversion of megaloblastic erythropoiesis to normoblastic.

In suspected normoblastic anaemias, marrow aspiration may or may not be necessary, depending on whether the cause of the anaemia is obvious.

WHAT IS THE CAUSE OF THE ANAEMIA?

Normoblastic anaemias (Table 4.6) The cause of a normoblastic macrocytic anaemia is often suspected following consideration of the clinical and haematological features, and is then confirmed by appropriate investigations. In some disorders, marrow examination may be required for diagnosis.

Megaloblastic anaemias (Tables 4.2 and 4.3) Once it has been established by marrow examination that the anaemia is megaloblastic, two questions should be answered:

1 Is the anaemia due to deficiency of vitamin B_{12} or folate, or both?

2 What is the cause of the deficiency of vitamin B_{12} or folate?

Most disorders causing megaloblastic anaemia are associated with one main type of deficiency. For this reason, these two questions are complementary, as the answer to one usually helps to provide the answer to the other. Thus, in the patient whose clinical features suggest the underlying disorder, the nature of this disorder frequently gives a lead to the type of deficiency. Conversely, if the clinical features give little help about the causes of the disorder, a knowledge of the type of deficiency may give a clue.

The method of investigation of a patient with megaloblastic anaemia is summarized in Table 4.7.

References and further reading

Monographs, reviews

Chanarin, I. (1979) *The Megaloblastic Anaemias*, 2nd Ed., Blackwell Scientific Publications, Oxford.

Botez, M.I. & Reynolds, E.H. (Eds) (1979) *Folic Acid in Neurology, Psychiatry, and Internal Medicine*, Raven Press, New York.

Hall, C.A. (Ed.) (1983) *The Cobalamins. Methods in Hematology*, Vol. 10, Churchill Livingstone, Edinburgh.

Hillman, R.S. (1985) Vitamin B_{12}, folic acid, and the treatment of megaloblastic anemias. In: Gilman, A.G., Goodman, L.S., Rall, T.W. & Murad, F. (Eds) *The Pharmacological Basis of Therapeutics*, 7th Ed., MacMillan, New York.

Zagalak, B. & Friedrich, W. (Eds) (1979) *Vitamin B_{12}*, Walter de Gruyter, Berlin.

Metabolism of vitamin B_{12} and folate

Allen, R.H., Seetharam, B., Podell, E. *et al.* (1978) Effect of proteolytic enzymes on the binding of cobalamin to R protein and intrinsic factor. *J. Clin. Invest.* **61**, 47.

Chanarin, I. (1981) How vitamin B_{12} acts. *Brit. J. Haemat.* **47**, 487.

Chanarin, I., Lumb, M., Deacon, R. *et al.* (1980) Vitamin B_{12} regulates folate metabolism by the supply of formate. *Lancet*, **ii**, 505.

Chanarin, I., Deacon, R., Lumb, M. *et al.* (1985) Cobalamin–folate interrelations: a critical review. *Blood*, **66**, 479.

Colman, N. & Herbert, V. (1980) Folate-binding proteins. *Ann. Rev. Med.* **31**, 433.

Das, K.C. & Herbert, V. (1976) Vitamin B_{12}–folate interrelations. *Clin. Haemat.* **5**, 697.

Hall, C.A. (1979) The transport of vitamin B_{12} from food to use within the cells. *J. Lab. Clin. Med.* **94**, 811.

Halsted, C.H. (1980) Intestinal absorption and malabsorption of folate. *Ann. Rev. Med.* **31**, 79.

Herbert, V. (1962) Minimal daily adult folate requirement. *Arch. Int. Med.* **110**, 649.

Herbert, V. & Zalusky, R. (1962) Interrelations of vitamin B_{12} and folic acid metabolism: folic acid clearance studies. *J. Clin. Invest.* **41**, 1263.

Jacob, E., Baker, S.J. & Herbert, V. (1980) Vitamin B_{12}-binding proteins. *Physiol. Rev.* **60**, 918.

Kapadia, C.R. & Donaldson, R.M., Jr. (1985) Disorders of cobalamin (vitamin B_{12}) absorption and transport. *Ann. Rev. Med.* **36**, 93.

Marcoullis, G. & Nicolas, J-P. (1983) The interactions of cobalamin in the gastrointestinal tract. In: Glass, G.B. & Sherlock, P. (Eds) *Progress in Gastroenterology*, Vol. 4, Grune & Stratton, New York.

Noronha, J.M. & Silverman, M. (1962) On folic acid, vitamin B_{12}, methionine and formiminoglutamic acid metabolism. In: Heinrich, H.C. (Ed.) *Vitamin B_{12} and Intrinsic Factor, Second European Symposium, Hamburg 1961*, Enke Verlag, Stuttgart.

Rachmilewitz, B., Schlesinger, M., Rabinowitz, R. *et al.* (1979) The origin and clinical implications of vitamin B_{12} binders—the transcobalamins. In: Zagalak, B. & Friedrich, W. (Eds) *Vitamin B_{12}*, Walter de Gruyter, Berlin.

Schilling, R.F. (1983) The role of the pancreas in vitamin B_{12} absorption. *Am. J. Hematol.* **14**, 197.

Stenman, U-H. (1976) Intrinsic factor and the vitamin B_{12} binding proteins. *Clin. Haemat.* **5**, 473.

Diagnosis of vitamin B_{12} and folate deficiencies

GENERAL

Breedveld, F.C., Bieger, R. & Van Wermeskerken, R.K.A. (1981) The clinical significance of macrocytosis. *Acta Med. Scand.* **209**, 319.

Davidson, R.J.L. & Hamilton, P.J. (1978) High mean red cell volume: its incidence and significance in routine haematology. *J. Clin. Path.* **31**, 493.

Dawson, D.W., Fish, D.I., Frew., I.D.O. *et al.* (1987) Laboratory diagnosis of megaloblastic anaemia: current methods assessed by external quality assurance trials. *J. Clin. Path.* **40**, 393.

Hall, C.A. (1981) Vitamin B_{12} deficiency and early rise in mean corpuscular volume. *J. Am. Med. Ass.* **245**, 1144.

Herbert, V. (1962) Experimental nutritional folate deficiency in man. *Trans. Ass. Amer. Phys.* **75**, 307.

Herbert, V. (1987) Making sense of laboratory tests of folate status: folate requirements to sustain normality. *Am. J. Hematol.* **26**, 199.

Lindenbaum, J. & Nath, B.J. (1980) Megaloblastic anaemia and neutrophil hypersegmentation. *Brit. J. Haemat.* **44**, 511.

Lindenbaum, J. (1983) Status of laboratory testing in the diagnosis of megaloblastic anemia. *Blood*, **61**, 624.

Spivak, J.L. (1982) Masked megaloblastic anemia. *Arch. Int. Med.* **142**, 2111.

Wickramasinghe, S.N. (1983) The deoxyuridine suppression test. In: Hall, C.A. (Ed.) *The Cobalamins. Methods in Hematology*, Vol. 10, Churchill Livingstone, Edinburgh.

SERUM VITAMIN B_{12} *ASSAY*

Anderson, B.B. & Sourial, N.A. (1983) The assay of serum cobalamin by *Euglena gracilis*. In: Hall, C.A. (Ed.) *The Cobalamins. Methods in Hematology*, Vol. 10, Churchill Livingstone, Edinburgh.

Bain, B., Broom, G.N., Woodside, J. *et al.* (1982) Assessment of a radioisotopic assay for vitamin B_{12} using an intrinsic factor preparation with R proteins blocked by vitamin B_{12} analogues. *J. Clin. Path.* **35**, 110.

Beck, W.S. (1983) The assay of serum cobalamin by Lactobacillus leichmanii and the interpretation of serum cobalamin levels. In: Hall, C.A. (Ed.) *The Cobalamins. Methods in Hematology*, Vol. 10, Churchill Livingstone, Edinburgh.

Carmel, R. & Karnaze, D.S. (1986) Physician response to low serum cobalamin levels. *Arch. Int. Med.* **146**, 1161.

Cooper, B.A., Fehedy, V. & Blanshay, P. (1986) Recognition of deficiency of vitamin B_{12} using measurement of serum concentration. *J. Lab. Clin. Med.* **107**, 447.

England, J.M. & Linnell, J.C. (1980) Problems with the serum vitamin B_{12} assay. *Lancet*, **ii**, 1072.

Fish, D.I. & Dawson, D.W. (1983) Comparison of methods used in commercial kits for the assay of serum vitamin B_{12}. *Clin. Lab. Haemat.* **5**, 271.

Hutner, S.H., Bach, M.K. & Ross, G.I.M. (1956) A sugar-containing basal medium for vitamin B_{12} assay with Euglena; application to body fluids. *J. Protozool.* **3**, 101.

Kolhouse, J.F., Kondo, H., Allen, N.C. *et al.* (1978) Cobalamin analogues are present in human plasma and can mask cobalamin deficiency because current radioisotope dilution assays are not specific for true cobalamin. *New Engl. J. Med.* **299**, 785.

Lau, K.S., Gottlieb, C., Wasserman, L.R. *et al.* (1965) Measurement of serum B_{12} level using radioisotope dilution and coated charcoal. *Blood*, **26**, 202.

Mollin, D.L., Anderson, B.B. & Burman, J.F. (1976) The serum vitamin B_{12} level: Its assay and significance. *Clin. Haemat.* **5**, 521.

Zacharakis, R., Muir, M. & Chanarin, I. (1981) Comparison of serum vitamin B_{12} estimation by saturation analysis with intrinsic factor and with R-protein as binding agents. *J. Clin. Path.* **34**, 357.

SERUM AND RED CELL FOLATE ASSAYS,

Baril, L. & Carmel, R. (1978) Comparison of radioassay and microbiological assay for serum folate, with clinical assessment of discrepant results. *Clin. Chem.* **24**, 2192.

Bain, B.J., Wickramasinghe, S.N., Broom, G.N. *et al.* (1984) Assessment of the value of a competitive protein binding radioassay of folic acid in the detection of folic acid deficiency. *J. Clin. Path.* **37**, 888.

Carmel, R. (1983) Clinical and laboratory features of the diagnosis of megaloblastic anemia. In: Lindenbaum, J. (Ed.) *Nutrition in Hematology*, Churchill Livingstone, New York.

Dawson, D.W., Delamore, I.W., Fish, D.I. *et al.* (1980) An evaluation of commercial radioisotope methods for the determination of folate and vitamin B_{12}. *J. Clin. Path.* **33**, 234.

Hoffbrand, A.V., Newcombe, B.F.A & Mollin, D.L. (1966) Method of assay of red cell folate activity and the value of the assay as a test for folate deficiency. *J. Clin. Path.* **19**, 17.

Jones, P., Grace, C.S. & Rozenberg, M.C. (1979) Interpretation of serum and red cell folate results. A comparison of microbiological and radioisotopic methods. *Pathology*, **11**, 45.

Raniolo, E., Phillipou, G., Paltridge, G. *et al.* (1984) Evaluation of a commercial radioassay for the simultaneous estimation of vitamin B_{12} and folate with subsequent deviation of the normal reference range. *J. Clin. Path.* **37**, 1327.

Waxman, S. (1979) The value of measurement of folate levels by radioassay. In: Botez, M.I. & Reynolds, E.H. (Eds) *Folic Acid in Neurology, Psychiatry, and Internal Medicine*, Raven Press, New York.

ABSORPTION TESTS

Domstad, P.A., Choy, Y.C., Kim, E.E. *et al.* (1981) Reliability of the dual-isotope Schilling test for the diagnosis of pernicious anemia or malabsorption syndrome. *Am. J. Clin. Pathol.* **75**, 723.

Doscherholmen, A., Silvis, S. & McMahon, J. (1983) Dual isotope Schilling test for measuring absorption of food-bound and free vitamin B_{12} simultaneously. *Am. J. Clin. Pathol.* **80**, 490.

Grasbeck, R. & Kouvonen, I. (1983) The materials and processes of intestinal transport. In: Hall, C.A. (Ed.) *The Cobalamins. Methods in Hematology*, Vol. 10, Churchill Livingstone, Edinburgh.

International Committee for Standardization in Hematology (1981) Recommended methods for the measurement of vitamin B_{12} absorption. *J. Nucl. Med.* **22**, 1091.

Lindenbaum, J., Pezzimenti, J.F. & Shea, N. (1974) Small intestinal function in vitamin B_{12} deficiency. *Ann. Int. Med.* **80**, 326.

Pernicious anaemia

Ardeman, S. & Chanarin, I. (1963) A method for the assay of human gastric intrinsic factor for the detection and titration of antibodies against intrinsic factor. *Lancet*, **ii**, 1350.

Bessman, D. (1977) Erythropoiesis during recovery from macrocytic anemia: macrocytes, normocytes, and microcytes. *Blood*, **50**, 995.

Carmel, R. (1979) Macrocytosis, mild anemia and delay in the diagnosis of pernicious anemia. *Arch. Int. Med.* **139**, 47.

De Aizpurua, J.H., Cosgrove, L.J., Ungar, B. *et al.* (1983) Auto-antibodies cytotoxic to gastric parietal cells in serum of patients with pernicious anemia. *New Engl. J. Med.* **309**, 625.

Lawson, D.H. & Parker, J.L.W. (1976) Deaths from severe megaloblastic anaemia in hospitalised patients. *Scand. J. Haematol.* **17**, 347.

Lewin, K.J., Dowling, F., Wright, J.P. *et al.* (1976) Gastric morphology and serum gastrin levels in pernicious anaemia. *Gut*, **17**, 551.

Reynolds, E.H. (1979) The neurology of vitamin B_{12} deficiency. In: Zagalak, B. & Friedrich, W. (Eds) *Vitamin B_{12}*, Walter de Gruyter, Berlin.

Savage, D. & Lindenbaum, J. (1983) Relapses after interruption of cyanocobalamin therapy in patients with pernicious anemia. *Am. J. Med.* **74**, 765.

Shorvon, S.D., Carney, M.W.P., Chanarin, I. *et al.* (1980) The neuropsychiatry of megaloblastic anaemia. *Brit. Med. J.* **281**, 1036.

Stockbrugger, R.W., Menon, G.G., Beilby, J.O.W. *et al.* (1983) Gastroscopic screening in 80 patients with pernicious anaemia. *Gut*, **24**, 1141.

Whittingham, S. & Mackay, I.R. (1985) Pernicious anemia and gastric atrophy. In: Rose, N.R. & Mackay, I.R. (Eds) *The Auto-immune Diseases*, Academic Press, New York.

Megaloblastic anaemia following gastrectomy

Hines, J.D., Hoffbrand, A.V. & Mollin, D.L. (1967) The hematologic complications following partial gastrectomy. *Am. J. Med.* **43**, 555.

Mahmud, K., Kaplan, M.E., Ripley, D. *et al.* (1974) The importance of red cell B_{12} and folate levels after partial gastrectomy. *Am. J. Clin. Nutr.* **27**, 51.

Rygvold, O. (1974) Hypovitaminosis B_{12} following partial gastrectomy by the Billroth II method. *Scand. J. Gastroenterol.* (Supp.29), **9**, 57.

Megaloblastic anaemia associated with lesions of the small intestine

Brandt, L.J., Bernstein, L.H. & Wagle, A. (1977) Production of vitamin B_{12} analogues in patients with small-bowel bacterial overgrowth. *Ann. Int. Med.* **87**, 546.

Dyer, N.H., Child, J.A., Mollin, D.L. *et al.* (1972) Anaemia in Crohn's disease. *Quart. J. Med.* **41**, 419.

Hoffbrand, A.V., Tabaqchali, S., Booth, C.C. *et al.* (1971) Small intestinal bacterial flora and folate status in gastrointestinal disease. *Gut*, **12**, 27.

Schjonsby, H. (1970) Diverticulosis of the small intestine and megaloblastic anaemia. *Acta Med. Scand.* **187**, 3.

Swinson, C.M. Perry, J., Lumb, M. *et al.* (1981) Role of sulphasalazine in the aetiology of folate deficiency in ulcerative colitis. *Gut*, **22**, 456.

Megaloblastic anaemia due to fish tapeworm infestation and other miscellaneous causes of vitamin B_{12} deficiency

Allen, R.H., Seetharam, B., Allen, N.C. *et al.* (1978) Correction of cobalamin malabsorption in pancreatic insufficiency with a cobalamin analogue that binds with high affinity to R protein but not to intrinsic factor. *J. Clin. Invest.* **61**, 1628.

Chanarin, I., Malkowska, V., O'Hea, A. *et al.* (1985) Megaloblastic anaemia in a vegetarian Hindu community. *Lancet*, **ii**, 1168.

Matthews, J.H. & Wood, J.K. (1984) Megaloblastic anaemia in vegetarian Asians. *Clin. Lab. Haemat.* **6**, 1.

Rosenberg, L.E. (1983) Disorders of propionate and methylmalonate metabolism. In: Stanbury, J.B., Wyngaarden, J.B., Frederickson, D.S., Goldstein, L.J. & Brown, M.S. (Eds) *The Metabolic Basis of Inherited Disease*, 5th Ed., McGraw-Hill, New York.

Schilling, R.F. (1983) The role of the pancreas in vitamin B_{12} absorption. *Am. J. Hemat.* **14**, 197.

Von Bonsdorff, B. (1978) *Diphyllobothriasis in Man*, Academic Press, London.

Coeliac disease and tropical sprue

Baker, S.J. & Mathan, V.I. (1971) Tropical sprue in southern India. In Wellcome Trust Collaborative Study, *Tropical Sprue and Megaloblastic Anaemia*. Churchill, London.

Cooper, B.T., Holmes, G.K.T., Ferguson, R. *et al.* (1980) Celiac disease and malignancy. *Medicine*, **59**, 249.

Corazza, G.R. & Gasbarrini, G. (1983) Defective splenic function and its relation to bowel disease. *Clin. Gastroenterol.* **12**, 651.

Croese, J., Harris, O. & Bain, B. (1979) Coeliac disease; haematological features, and delay in diagnosis. *Med. J. Austr.* **2**, 335.

Halsted, C.H., Reisenauer, A.M., Romero, J.J. *et al.* (1977) Jejunal perfusion of simple and conjugated folates in celiac sprue. *J. Clin. Invest.* **59**, 933.

Hoffbrand, A.V. (1974) Anaemia in adult coeliac disease. *Clin. Gastroenterol.* **3**, 71.

Lindenbaum, J. (1979) Aspects of vitamin B_{12} and folate metabolism in malabsorption syndromes. *Am. J. Med.* **67**, 1037.

Marsh, G.W. & Stewart, J.S. (1970) Splenic function in adult coeliac disease. *Brit. J. Haematol.* **19**, 445.

Marsh & Stewart (1970) from p. 4–63.

Nutritional megaloblastic anaemia

Amos, R.J., Hinds, C.J., Amess, J.A.L. *et al.* (1982) Incidence and pathogenesis of actue megaloblastic bone marrow change in patients receiving intensive care. *Lancet*, **ii**, 835.

Baker, S.J. (1981) Nutritional anaemias; part 2, Tropical Asia. *Clin. Haemat.* **10**, 843.

Ballard, H.S. & Lindenbaum, J. (1974) Megaloblastic anemia complicating hyperalimentation therapy. *Am. J. Med.* **56**, 740.

Botez, M.I., Peyronnard, J-M., Bachevalier, J. *et al.* (1978) Polyneuropathy and folate deficiency. *Arch. Neurol.* **35**, 581.

Magnus, E.M., Bache-Wiig, J.E., Aanderson, T.R. *et al.* (1982) Folate and vitamin B_{12} (cobalamin) blood levels in elderly persons in geriatric homes. *Scand. J. Haemat.* **28**, 360.

Sharman, V.L., Cunningham, J., Goodwin, F.J. *et al.* (1982) Do patients receiving regular haemodialysis need folic acid supplements? *Brit. Med. J.* **285**, 96.

Wardrop, C.A.J., Heatley, R.V., Tennant, G.B. *et al.* (1975) Acute folate deficiency in surgical patients on amino-acid/ethanol intravenous nutrition. *Lancet*, **ii**, 640.

Megaloblastic anaemia in alcoholic patients

Chanarin, I. (1982) Haemopoiesis and alcohol. *Brit. Med. Bull.* **38**, 81.

Eichner, E.R. & Hillman, R.S. (1971) The evolution of anemia in alcoholic patients. *Am. J. Med.* **50**, 218.

Hillman, R.S. & Steinberg, S.E. (1982) The effects of alcohol on folate metabolism. *Ann. Rev. Med.* **33**, 345.

Lindenbaum, J. (1979) Aspects of vitamin B_{12} and folate metabolism in malabsorption syndromes. *Am. J. Med.* **67**, 1037.

Morgan, M.Y., Camilo, M.E., Luck W. *et al.* (1981) Macrocytosis in alcohol-related liver disease: its value for screening. *Clin. Lab. Haemat.* **3**, 35.

Wu, A., Chanarin, I. & Levi, A.J. (1974) Macrocytosis of chronic alcoholism. *Lancet*, **i**, 829.

Wu, A., Chanarin, I., Slavin, G. *et al.* (1975) Folate deficiency in the alcoholic—its relationship to clinical and haematological abnormalities, liver disease and folate stores. *Brit. J. Haemat.* **29**, 469.

Megaloblastic anaemia of pregnancy

Chanarin, I. (1985) Folate and cobalamin. *Clin. Haemat.* **14**, 629.

Cooper, B.A. (1973) Folate and vitamin B_{12} in pregnancy. *Clin. Haemat.* **2**, 461.

Giles, C. (1966) An account of 335 cases of megaloblastic anaemia of pregnancy and the puerperium. *J. Clin. Path.* **19**, 1.

Megaloblastic anaemia of infancy and childhood

Cooper, B.A. (1976) Megaloblastic anaemia and disorders affecting utilisation of vitamin B_{12} and folate in childhood. *Clin. Haemat.* **5**, 631.

Furuhjelm, U. & Nevanlinna, H.R. (1973) Inheritance of selective malabsorption of vitamin B_{12}. *Scand. J. Haemat.* **11**, 27.

Matthews, D.M. & Linnell, J.C. (1982) Cobalamin deficiency and related disorders in infancy and childhood. *Eur. J. Pediatr.* **138**, 6.

Rosenberg, L.E. (1983) Disorders of propionate and methylmalonate metabolism. In: Stanbury, J.B., Wyngaarden, J.B., Frederickson, D.S., Goldstein, L.J. & Brown, M.S. (Eds) *The Metabolic Basis of Inherited Disease*, 5th Ed., McGraw-Hill, New York.

Rowe, P.B. (1983) Inherited disorders of folate metabolism. In: Stanbury, J.B., Wyngaarden, J.B., Frederickson, D.S., Goldstein, L.J. & Brown, M.S. (Eds) *The Metabolic Basis of Inherited Disease*, 5th Ed., McGraw-Hill, New York.

Megaloblastic anaemia due to drugs

Blackwell, E.A., Hawson, G.A.T., Leer, J. *et al.* (1978) Acute pancytopenia due to megaloblastic arrest in association with co-trimoxazole. *Med. J. Austr.* **2**, 38.

Scott, J.M. & Weir, D.G. (1980) Drug-induced megaloblastic change. *Clin. Haemat.* **9**, 587.

Stebbins, R. & Bertino, J.R. (1976) Megaloblastic anaemia produced by drugs. *Clin. Haemat.* **5**, 619.

Wickramasinghe, S.N., Dodsworth, H., Rault, R.M.J. *et al.* (1974) Observations on the incidence and cause of macrocytosis in patients on azathioprine therapy following renal transplantation. *Transplant*, **18**, 443.

Megaloblastic anaemia unresponsive to vitamin B_{12} or folic acid therapy

O'Sullivan, W.J. (1973) Orotic acid. *Austr. N.Z. J. Med.* **3**, 417.

Chapter 5
Anaemia in Systemic Disorders; Diagnosis in Normochromic Normocytic Anaemias

Anaemia can develop as a secondary effect of disease processes that do not physically invade the bone marrow or markedly accelerate the destruction of erythrocytes. Diseases in which this effect is relatively common include chronic infectious or non-infectious inflammatory disorders, and certain types of malignancy. The erythrocytes are usually normochromic and normocytic, although minor degrees of hypochromia and microcytosis can develop, a change which is unrelated to iron deficiency. It is important to recognize that this type of anaemia is not caused primarily by a deficiency of haematinic agents, and that administration of haematinics does not correct the anaemia—the anaemia recovers only after alleviation of the primary disease process.

Anaemia that is normochromic and normocytic in type can develop in a wide variety of other states such as recent haemorrhage, renal failure, endocrine disorders, and in liver disease, although the latter can be macrocytic. These anaemias are, for convenience, considered in this chapter, and an approach to evaluation of the patient with normochromic normocytic anaemia is described at the end of the chapter.

Anaemia of infection

Minor degrees of anaemia are common in chronic infection, and occasionally in acute infection. This type of anaemia is particularly associated with infections accompanied by significant inflammatory features. In addition to causing anaemia in its own right, infection can also blunt the response of other types of anaemia to treatment, such as therapy with vitamin B_{12} in pernicious anaemia, or iron in iron deficiency anaemia.

The most common infections causing anaemia are those associated with chronic inflammation of female reproductive system, urinary tract, lung abscess, suppurative bronchiectasis, pneumonia, osteomyelitis, bacterial endocarditis, tuberculosis, typhoid, and abscesses at other sites.

The extent of anaemia associated with *tuberculosis* depends on the extent of the disease. When tuberculosis is localized mainly to one organ, e.g. the lung, the haemoglobin level is usually normal until the disease has made considerable progress, when a mild to moderate normochromic normocytic, or slightly hypochromic, anaemia may develop. Severe anaemia is rare in the absence of complications, e.g. tuberculous ulceration of the bowel, amyloidosis, or generalized dissemination.

With acute miliary tuberculosis, a moderate normochromic or slightly hypochromic anaemia is the rule. The bone marrow is usually involved in the miliary spread and thus contains tubercles. The amount of haemopoietic marrow is normal or increased. It is sometimes possible to obtain histological or bacteriological evidence of tuberculosis by marrow biopsy. Sections of aspirated marrow or the trephine biopsy occasionally contain tubercles, and the organism may be detected by culture of the aspirate. This method is thus sometimes useful in establishing the diagnosis in miliary disease.

The *clinical features* are predominantly those of the causative infection, as the anaemia is generally of moderate severity. Less commonly the anaemia is the presenting manifestation.

Blood picture. Haemoglobin levels are generally in

the range of 1–3 g/dl below the lower limit of normal for the age and the sex of the patient. Severe anaemia is rare, and its occurrence in a patient with infection should suggest the possibility of some other contributory factor, e.g. blood loss, haemolysis or renal failure. The degree of anaemia tends to be more marked the more severe and protracted the infection. The anaemia usually takes several weeks to develop after the onset of infection, then progresses slowly over several months until the haemoglobin level eventually stabilizes. The anaemia is generally normocytic and normochromic in type, but occasionally mild or moderate hypochromic (MCH 22–26 pg) and microcytic (MCV 70–80 fl) changes are present. Slight to moderate anisocytosis and poikilocytosis may be present. However, marked anisocytosis, poikilocytosis and hypochromia are rare in uncomplicated anaemia of infection. The reticulocyte count is not elevated.

The *bone marrow* aspirate reveals no diagnostic features. It is of normal or moderately increased cellularity. The myeloid : erythroid ratio may be increased, but it is difficult to establish whether this is due to increased granulopoiesis or decreased erythropoiesis, or both. In the absence of coincidental iron deficiency, the content of iron in reticulo-endothelial cells is generally increased.

Pathogenesis. This has been studied extensively (Cartwright & Lee 1971, Lee 1983). Anaemia with similar haematological features occurs in a number of chronic disorders, including carcinoma, lymphoma, rheumatoid arthritis, collagen vascular diseases and severe tissue injury, and thus the term *anaemia of chronic disorders* is perferable to the term *anaemia of chronic infection.* There is a mild haemolytic element, with a *modest* shortening of red cell lifespan, and the bone marrow is unable to increase production sufficiently to compensate for the mild degree of increased red cell destruction. The impaired marrow response appears to be due to at least two factors: (1) inappropriately decreased erythropoietin production for the degree of anaemia (Ward *et al.* 1971); and (2) impaired flow of iron from the reticulo-endothelial system to erythroblasts. Activated macrophages release substantial amounts of *interleukin-I,* which probably mediates many of the inhibitory effects on iron metabolism and erythropoiesis seen in the anaemia of chronic disorders (Lee 1983).

The impairment of iron transport is accompanied by characteristic biochemical changes. Levels of both serum iron and iron-binding capacity (transferrin) are reduced (Fig. 3.5, p. 51), and the percentage saturation of transferrin is reduced. *The pattern of hypoferraemia and decreased transferrin in the presence of normal or increased reticulo-endothelial iron is characteristic of this type of anaemia.* In contrast to the markedly reduced serum ferritin level in iron deficiency, the low serum iron level in the anaemia of chronic disorders is accompanied by a normal or elevated serum ferritin level.

Blood loss and *haemolysis* can contribute to anaemia in patients with infection, and should not be overlooked. Haemolysis can be produced by micro-angiopathy in sepsis, by release of haemolytic toxins by *Clostridium welchii* in gangrenous infections, and by auto-antibodies in certain types of mycoplasma infection.

Treatment. Eradication of the underlying infection is the only effective treatment. Administration of iron, vitamin B_{12} and folic acid is without effect in the uncomplicated situation. Blood transfusion raises the haemoglobin level but, especially when the anaemia is not marked, does not usually produce any significant clinical benefit, and in any case produces only a transient effect if the underlying illness is not eliminated.

Anaemia in collagen vascular diseases

Rheumatoid arthritis

Anaemia develops in many patients with active rheumatoid arthritis. It is usually of mild to moderate severity as in chronic infection, with haemoglobin levels of 9–11 g/dl in women, and somewhat higher values in men. Occasionally, especially in severe inflammatory disease, anaemia is more marked and the haemoglobin level falls to 7–8 g/dl, or even less.

Two main types of anaemia are seen in association with rheumatoid arthritis. The *most common* is a normocytic normochromic, or slightly to moderately hypochromic, anaemia in which the red cells show little variation in size and shape. The MCH is normal or slightly reduced. This anaemia is due to inflammatory effects of the rheumatoid arthritis *per se*, and its severity closely parallels the activity of the disease, as it is caused by the same mechanism as anaemia in chronic infection. It has the same characteristics as anaemia associated with chronic infection.

The *other* important form of anaemia is hypochromic microcytic anaemia due to iron deficiency, which in most instances is caused by occult gastrointestinal blood loss provoked by ingestion of non-steroidal anti-inflammatory drugs. Iron deficiency is particularly common in women of childbearing age and in juveniles. Nutritional deficiency may be a contributing factor to the development of anaemia in patients who prepare their own food, as their physical disability may cause them to neglect their diet. *Active rheumatoid disease may accentuate anaemia due to lack of haematinics, and may impair the response to treatment.*

Other causes of anaemia in rheumatoid arthritis include rare instances of folate deficiency and aplastic anaemia, the latter being a risk of therapy with agents such as gold, oxyphenbutazone, phenylbutazone, and penicillamine.

Treatment. The most effective measures in combating the anaemia are those that suppress the activity of the rheumatoid disease, as inflammatory activity is the major factor determining the severity of the anaemia. Reduction of disease activity is followed by a rise in haemoglobin level. In this type of normocytic or slightly microcytic anaemia, no improvement occurs following administration of iron—provided there is no associated iron deficiency, a factor that can be evaluated by estimation of the serum ferritin level. Obviously, iron replacement thereapy is indicated in subjects with a deficiency of iron. Response to blood transfusion in chronic active disease is transient, as in the case of anaemia associated with chronic infection.

Systemic lupus erythematosus (SLE)

Haematological abnormalities almost invariably develop at some stage in this disorder (Budman & Steinberg 1977). *Anaemia* occurs in more than half of patients with SLE. It is usually normocytic and normochromic, or slightly hypochromic, and of mild to moderate severity. Haemoglobin levels between 9 and 11 g/dl are most common, and the pathogenesis of this type of disorder is similar to that in anaemia in chronic infection. More severe anaemia can occur, especially in cases complicated by auto-immune haemolytic anaemia or renal insufficiency. Auto-immune acquired haemolytic anaemia with a positive direct Coombs' test develops in about five per cent of cases. However, a weakly positive Coombs' test is not uncommon in subjects without haemolysis, so that careful evaluation of indices of haemolysis is required in order to establish the type of mechanism responsible for any anaemia.

Other haematological abnormalities that can occur in association with anaemia involve both the leucocyte and platelet counts. The most common abnormality affecting the white cells is moderate leucopenia, with counts rarely less than 2×10^9/l. The differential count often shows a greater reduction in lymphocytes than in neutrophils, and a slight neutrophil shift to the left. Leucocytosis may occur in cases of acute onset, during exacerbations, as a result of bacterial infection, or during corticosteroid therapy. The absolute eosinophil count is usually within normal limits, but rarely is increased.

Moderate symptomless *thrombocytopenia* is relatively common. Occasionally, thrombocytopenia is severe and is almost always due to auto-antibody-mediated platelet destruction. Splenectomy is usually followed by an increase in platelet count as in idiopathic thrombocytopenia, but the tendency for unacceptably severe thrombocytopenia to recur at a later stage appears to be greater than in auto-immune thrombocytopenia in which there are no clinical or serological features of SLE. Occasionally, thrombocytopenic purpura or auto-immune haemolytic anaemia may precede other clinical features by months or years, so that the possibility of underlying SLE should be considered in all patients with apparent idiopathic thrombocytopenic purpura or auto-immune haemolytic anaemia.

The *clinical manifestations* that indicate the possible presence of SLE are protean and include arthralgia, polyarthritis, fever, malaise, weight loss, skin rash, albuminuria, renal insufficiency, hypertension, Raynaud's phenomenon, pneumonia, pleurisy, pericarditis, retinal changes, psychosis and convulsions. Slight to moderate enlargement of the lymph nodes and liver is present in about 25 per cent of cases, and enlargement of the spleen in 10–20 per cent. It is important to note that skin lesions are absent at both the onset and throughout the course of the disease in about 20 per cent of patients.

Confirmation of the diagnosis was formerly based on demonstration of the *LE cell* phenomenon in the laboratory (Dacie & Lewis 1984). Serum from subjects with SLE when incubated with leucocytes causes cell damage followed by ingestion of the resulting cellular debris by neutrophils, to produce a neutrophil distended by a large, homogeneous, round body which appears pale purple with Romanovsky staining. The responsible serum factor is an IgG auto-antibody but is, however, detected only in 80–90 per cent of cases with classical clinical features of SLE (Harvey *et al.* 1954). The 'LE cell' test is relatively tedious to perform and open to interpretative difficulties, to the extent that other serological and biochemical procedures for the detection of characteristic antinuclear or DNA-binding auto-antibodies have largely taken its place.

Antinuclear antibodies are detectable in most patients with active SLE, and are generally demonstrated by immunofluorescence methods. *Antibodies to double-stranded DNA* are very specific for SLE, and quantitation of these antibodies is of value both in diagnosis and in following the activity of the disease.

Polyarteritis nodosa

Normochromic normocytic anaemia of moderate severity is common in polyarteritis nodosa. Occasionally, anaemia is marked, especially in cases with renal insufficiency. Only very rarely does autoimmune acquired haemolytic anaemia develop. A moderate neutrophil leucocytosis is usual, with white counts ranging from 15 to 30 $\times$ 10^9/l, although this is not invariable. Eosinophilia occurs in about 25 per cent of cases, particularly in those with pulmonary involvement, in whom it may be marked. The erythrocyte sedimentation rate is almost invariably raised, often markedly. Bruising and purpura are not uncommon as a result of associated vasculitis, but the platelet count is commonly elevated, as it can be in most types of inflammatory state.

Dermatomyositis

Mild normocytic anaemia is common. The white cell count is usually normal, but sometimes moderately elevated. Moderate eosinophilia is occasionally present, but is much less common than in polyarteritis nodosa. The erythrocyte sedimentation rate is usually raised.

Scleroderma

Anaemia occurs in about 30 per cent of cases (Westerman *et al.* 1968) and most often appears to be related to the degree of activity of the disorder.

Cranial arteritis

Mild normochromic or hypochromic normocytic anaemia is common. A prominent feature is that the erythrocyte sedimentation rate is nearly always raised, and sometimes exceeds 100 mm/hour. The white cell count is normal or moderately increased, and mild eosinophilia is occasionally present.

Anaemia due to acute blood loss

The extent of the fall in the haemoglobin level following acute blood loss depends on the amount of blood lost and the interval that has elapsed from the time of bleeding, as illustrated in Fig. 5.1. Immediately after loss of blood from the circulatory compartment, there is a reduction in total blood volume, and the haemoglobin level in the residual blood is normal. The dominant clinical effects are those of circulatory volume depletion, with tachycardia and hypotension. Compensatory changes begin within hours, causing a progessive increase in plasma volume, until the total blood volume begins to approach the normal value after approximately 48 hours. This results in haemodilution of morphologically normal erythrocytes, the fall in the hae-

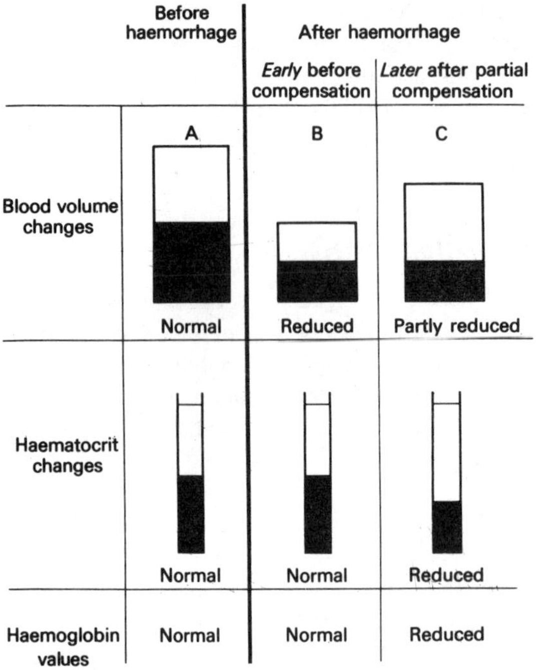

Fig. 5.1. *Changes in blood volume, plasma volume, total red cell volume, haemoglobin level, and haematocrit following acute haemorrhage (Walsh & Ward 1969).*

moglobin level commencing after several hours, and stabilizing after 2–5 days. *For this reason, estimation of the haemoglobin level within three hours of acute blood loss is not of value in assessing the degree of blood loss.*

After 24–48 hours, the first signs of red cell regeneration are usually indicated by an increase in polychromatic red cells, and a rise in the reticulcocyte count, which peaks after 5–7 days. The degree of increase depends on the severity of the anaemia, and seldom exceeds 15 per cent. The presence of the polychromatic cells, which are larger than mature cells, may cause a macrocytic picture. With severe haemorrhage, a few normoblasts may also appear in the blood, and these features sometimes lead to confusion with haemolysis as the cause of the anaemia.

Clinical features vary with the amount and rate of blood loss, and the capacity of the cardiovascular system to compensate. Early manifestations are mainly the effects of reduction of blood volume, with weakness, nausea, fainting, sweating, an ashen pallor, hypotension, and tachycardia. Restlessness, thirst, and air hunger are characteristic of severe circulatory failure with sudden blood loss. Later manifestations are those encountered in anaemia of any cause.

Treatment of acute blood loss aims to: (1) arrest the loss of blood; and (2) restore the blood volume to normal. When signs of circulatory failure are present, immediate infusion of a colloid solution of dextran or a plasma protein preparation is required to restore blood volume and cardiac output. Transport of oxygen by red cells is seldom a critical factor unless the patient was anaemic prior to the haemorrhage. Replacement of red cells by blood transfusion represents the second priority, once the circulation has been restored. As blood loss results in loss of iron, it is advisable to give oral iron for 1–2 months after severe blood loss to ensure a maximum rate of red cell regeneration.

Renal failure

Anaemia develops almost invariably in chronic renal failure with significantly impaired renal function; not uncommonly, patients with chronic renal failure first seek medical advice because of symptoms due to anaemia. In acute renal failure, the same mechanisms operate, but hypervolaemia due to plasma volume expansion may be an additional factor causing haemodilution, and *micro-angiopathy* is usually more common than in chronic renal failure.

Aetiology. The development of anaemia is not specifically related to the type of disease causing the renal failure, although the anaemia tends to be more severe in renal disease in which additional factors such as infection or blood loss are present. It occurs with primary diseases of the kidney or renal tract, e.g. chronic nephritis, chronic renal infection, cystic disease, or urinary tract obstruction, and with systemic diseases with renal involvement, e.g. SLE, polyarteritis, and amyloid disease. In some forms of progressive renal failure, the haematological picture of *micro-angiopathic haemolytic anaemia* develops when the causative disorder is associated with endothelial changes, or intravascular thrombosis or fibrin deposition.

Blood picture. The severity of the anaemia commonly shows a quantitative relation to the severity of the renal failure. Anaemia is unusual unless the blood urea is more than 9 mmol/l; however, mild to moderate anaemia occurs occasionally when active renal infection is associated with mild impairment of renal function, even though the blood urea is not raised. Anaemia is almost invariable with significant renal failure. Roscoe (1952) has shown that as the blood urea level increases from 8 to 40 mmol/l, the haemoglobin level falls progressively at an amount of about 2 g/dl for every rise of 8 mmol/l in the blood urea concentration, but when the blood urea level is about 40 mmol/l, further reduction in haemoglobin level does not occur. However, as individual variation is considerable, an accurate forecast of the haemoglobin level at any blood urea level cannot be made in a particular patient. Severe anaemia is more likely to occur when micro-angiopathic haemolysis is present.

The anaemia in uncomplicated cases is normochromic and normocytic. Moderate anisocytosis is common. Initially, poikilocytosis is not prominent, but in the later stages the development of 'burr' cells is common (Fig. 5.2). These are contracted cells which have one or more spiny projections on the surface. The appearance of fragmented, triangular, crescent-shaped, 'helmet' cells, and microspherocytes, in addition to burr cells, strongly suggests the development of *micro-angiopathic haemolytic anaemia* (p. 207). The reticulocyte count is usually normal, but a moderate increase (e.g. 5%), together with some polychromasia, may occur in patients with haemolysis.

Bone marrow aspiration yields a marrow of normal or moderately increased cellularity. Erythroblasts are usually normoblastic and are present in normal or increased proportions until severe uraemia develops, when erythroid hypoplasia may occur. Mild dyserythropoiesis sometimes occurs in severe renal failure. Leucopoiesis is usually normal, and megakaryocytes are present in normal numbers. The marrow iron content is normal.

Pathogenesis. Depression of erythropoiesis and increased red cell destruction both contribute to the anaemia of renal failure, but depression of erythropoiesis appears to be the more important factor. This is suggested by the impressive increase in haemoglobin level after administration of recombinant human erythropoietin in subjects with end-stage renal failure and severe anaemia (Winearls *et al*. 1986, Eschbach *et al*. 1987), an observation that indicates inadequate erythropoietin production is a very important factor under these circumstances.

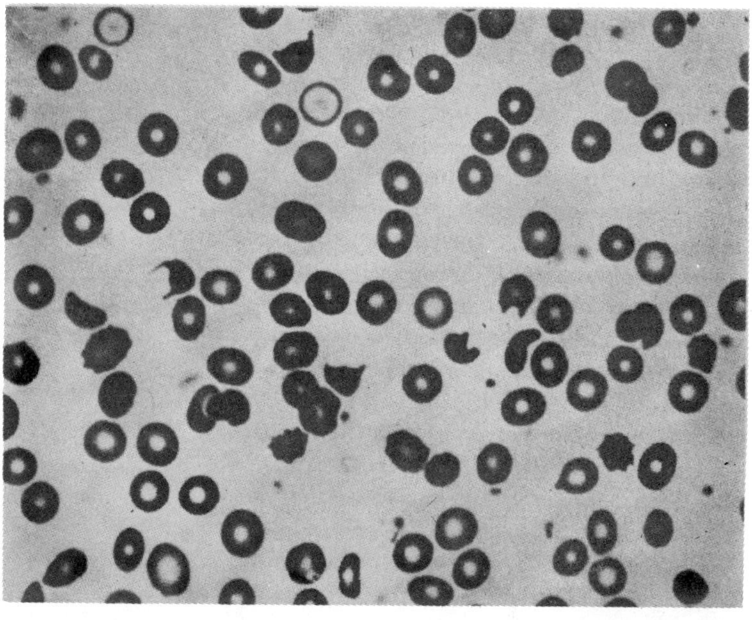

Fig. 5.2. *Photomicrograph illustrating poikilocytosis in a patient with renal failure. Some of the abnormal red cells have multiple projections characteristic of burr cells (× 570).*

Sometimes additional problems increase the severity of anaemia in renal failure, such as folate deficiency in subjects with a diet inadequate in folate, infection, haemolysis, and *blood loss*. The latter can be an ongoing problem in haemodialysis patients, in whom small amounts of blood are lost on a regular basis because of technical reasons (Eschbach *et al.* 1977), and also because *bleeding is enhanced by the inhibitory effects of uraemia on platelet function*.

Diagnosis. In many cases, the patient presents with other manifestations of renal failure and the anaemia is simply an incidental finding. Nevertheless, anaemia is occasionally the presenting manifestation of renal failure, especially when the other manifestations of renal insufficiency are not prominent. *Chronic renal failure should be considered as a possible cause of any normochromic normocytic anaemia in which the aetiology is not obvious.* Estimation of the plasma creatinine level should therefore be performed under these circumstances.

Treatment. In general, the anaemia of renal impairment in the absence of significant haemolysis is refractory to therapy, except for treatment that improves renal function and the production of erythropoietin, or the administration of erythropoietin.

One method by which renal production of erythropoietin can be promoted is by *renal transplantation*. A marked improvement in erythropoiesis is regularly observed 5–20 days after successful transplantation, as indicated by the onset of a reticulocytosis. The haemoglobin level rises to a plateau over the ensuing 8–10 weeks. Restoration of renal function after a phase of severe renal impairment is also followed after a lag period by recovery of erythropoiesis, but in subjects with unremitting severe renal failure, the anaemia had in the past been amenable to correction only by transfusion of red cell concentrates in the absence of any correctable factors.

Patients maintained on chronic haemodialysis often develop a relatively stable, moderately severe degree of anaemia with a haematocrit of the order of 0.2. Most patients adapt to this degree of anaemia, and as a general rule transfusions are administered only to those who do not. Iron deficiency can develop in patients on chronic haemodialysis; correction of the deficiency is an obvious step.

Preliminary indications are that substantial improvement in the anaemia can be produced by parenteral administration of *recombinant human erythropoietin* on a regular basis to compensate for the deficit in erythropoietin production in end-stage renal disease.

Anaemia in non-haematological malignancy

Anaemia is a common accompaniment of malignancy. In many patients, it is absent at the time of diagnosis but develops in the course of the illness. It is particularly common with malignancy of the alimentary tract, as a consequence of blood loss, and may be the presenting manifestation. A number of different factors can contribute, and it is common for several factors to operate in patients with malignancy.

The *type of anaemia* depends on the dominant underlying mechanism or mechanisms, and the most important are listed in Table 5.1. The anaemia is usually *normocytic*, but *hypochromic microcytic anaemia* due to iron deficiency occurs in patients with chronic bleeding. Occasionally a *leuco-erythroblastic anaemia* occurs when metastasis to bone has taken place.

Other blood changes that may occur in malignancy, especially with necrotic and infected tumours, are leucocytosis, an increase in the erythrocyte sedimentation rate, and the changes in

Table 5.1. *Factors that contribute to anaemia in patients with non-haematological malignancy*

Common factors
Blood loss
Infection
Chronic 'inflammatory-like' response
Less common factors
Bone marrow infiltration
Inadequate nutrition
Impaired renal function
Haemolysis
Myelosuppressive effects of treatment

iron metabolism common to anaemia of chronic disorders. Other occasional complications are disturbances of coagulation, e.g. from intravascular coagulation, or fibrinolysis.

Anaemia due to *blood loss* develops extremely commonly in carcinoma of the stomach and colon, and is particularly important as it may be the presenting manifestation which antedates symptoms referable to the alimentary tract. In most cases, the blood is altered and mixed with faeces so that it is not obvious to the patient. *The possibility of malignancy of the alimentary tract should always be considered in a patient of the appropriate age with an iron deficiency or normochromic anaemia without obvious cause. In the early stages, when bleeding is of minor degree, the oral administration of iron often results in a rise of the haemoglobin level, and the clinical improvement may distract attention from the possibility of a serious underlying cause.*

Infection may be an important contributing factor to anaemia in malignancy, such as in carcinoma of the bronchus or fungating lesions at any site. The mechanism by which the anaemia is produced is as previously considered under anaemia of chronic disorders, *a mechanism that can also operate in the absence of infection in subjects with advanced malignant disease.*

Metastasis to bone marrow occurs in about 20 per cent of all fatal cases of non-haematological malignancy. After the lungs and the liver, the bone marrow is the next most common site of 'blood-borne' metastases. Breast and prostate cancer are the *primary tumours* that most frequently metastasize to bone, but carcinoma of the lung, kidney, thyroid, and stomach, and malignant melanoma, also commonly metastasize there. Metastatic growth most frequently occurs in the sites normally occupied by red bone marrow, namely the vertebrae, ribs, sternum, pelvis, skull, and upper ends of the femur and humerus.

Anaemia is common in patients with secondary carcinoma of the bone marrow, but it can be absent even when widespread bone involvement is demonstrated by X-ray. Many factors in patients with advanced metastatic disease can contribute to the genesis of anaemia—malnutrition, infection, blood loss, micro-angiopathy, and effects of the type that produce the anaemia of chronic disorders—let alone replacement of haemopoietic tissue by tumour cells. The latter most frequently is not the major cause of the anaemia, in contrast to the situation in, for example, acute leukaemia.

In marrow metastasis, there may or may not be anaemia. When anaemia is present, it is usually normochromic and normocytic. A finding of diagnostic significance indicating the presence of marrow metastasis is a *leuco-erythroblastic* blood picture, in which nucleated red cells and granulocyte precursors are present (p. 274). Other features are anisocytosis, poikilocytosis, and occasional macrocytes and polychromatic cells. Sometimes a moderate leucocytosis is present, and sometimes a moderate degree of leucopenia, although the white cell count is rarely less than $2 \times 10^9/l$. With a leuco-erythroblastic picture there is usually a moderate proportion of metamyelocytes and myelocytes (usually less than 10 per cent), and even an occasional blast cell and promyelocyte.

Bone marrow. Tumour cells may be detected in the aspirated marrow, but trephine biopsy of the marrow yields a much higher proportion of positive results than does aspiration (Contreras *et al.* 1972). While they are most often seen in patients with X-ray evidence of bone involvement, tumour cells are also found in patients who do not have abnormal radiological features. A bone marrow trephine can establish the diagnosis of marrow metastasis not uncommonly in the absence of pain or abnormalities on X-ray or bone scan.

Tumour cells are, however, detected more frequently in biopsies performed at a site of bone tenderness or pain, or at an area shown by X-ray to be involved. Thus, before aspiration, the bones should be gently but systematically palpated and percussed to detect any areas of localized tenderness, and the X-rays should be studied. Aspiration may be difficult, and a 'dry' or small 'blood tap' is common, even when strong suction is used. A 'dry tap' may be due either to the fact that the needle has entered a solid mass of tumour tissue, or that the marrow cavity at the site of puncture is replaced by fibrous or bone tissue, as occurs in osteosclerotic secondaries. In cases of 'dry tap', a small amount of marrow may remain in the tip of the needle, from

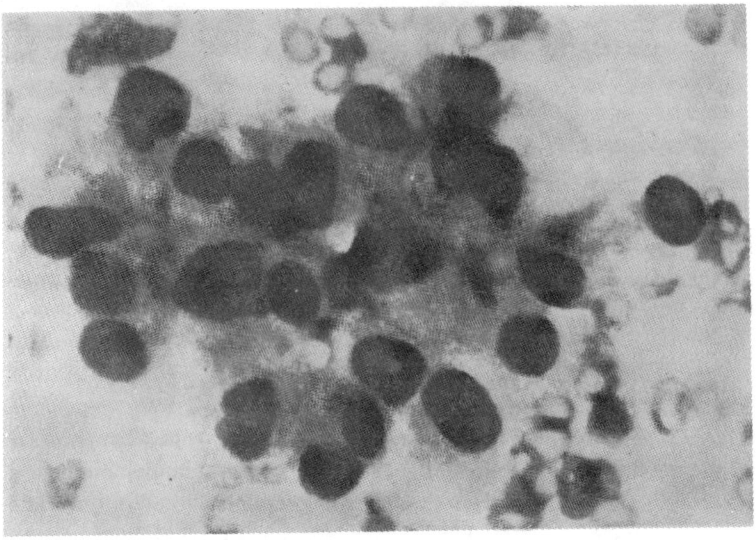

Fig. 5.3. *Photomicrograph of bone marrow aspirated from an elderly man with an enlarged, hard prostate, elevated plasma prostatic acid phosphatase, and leuco-erythroblastic anaemia. Note the clump of tumour cells in which carcinoma cells are tightly adherent to each other.*

which a satisfactory film may be made (Fig. 5.3). If aspiration at one site is technically unsatisfactory, or yields a non-diagnostic specimen, it should be repeated at another site. Trephine biopsy should be performed routinely. Negative biopsy findings do not, of course, exclude a diagnosis of metastatic involvement of bone marrow as the deposits are often discrete and separated by regions of non-involved haemopoietic tissue.

Prognosis. Leuco-erythroblastic anaemia commonly occurs late in the disease and is a poor prognostic sign, as death usually occurs in less than a year, often within 1–2 months. However, in patients with carcinoma of the breast or prostate, clinical remission that follows hormonal manipulation may be accompanied by an improvement in the blood picture, with a rise in haemoglobin level and platelet count, and disappearance or decrease in the proportion of immature cells in the blood film.

Interference with nutritional intake caused by anorexia, vomiting, dysphagia etc. can contribute to the production of anaemia by impairing intake or absorption of nutrients necessary for erythropoiesis, especially iron and folate, but it is rarely the sole cause of the anaemia. Megaloblastic macrocytic anaemia associated with carcinoma of the stomach is usually due to the development of carcinoma in a patient with gastric atrophy associated with pernicious anaemia (p. 83).

Haemolytic anaemia. Some shortening of red cell lifespan is common in disseminated malignancy, and is of importance since it may result in an unsatisfactory response to blood transfusion. A relatively uncommon, but definitely associated, form of severe haemolysis is *micro-angiopathic haemolytic anaemia,* which is seen particularly in metastatic mucin-secreting adenocarcinomas.

Liver disease

Anaemia is common in chronic liver disease, and occurs in about two-thirds of patients with cirrhosis. It is usually moderate in degree, but occasionally is severe. The number of quite different causes of anaemia in patients with liver disease is listed in Table 5.2, and the clinical and haematological picture depends on the dominant factor or factors responsible. Sometimes the cause of the anaemia is multifactorial.

Blood loss. In hepatic cirrhosis with portal hypertension, bleeding from oesophageal varices, peptic ulceration or haemorrhoids is common, and causes either normochromic anaemia when the haemorrhage is acute, or hypochromic anaemia with microcytosis when iron deficiency develops. Bleeding is often intermittent. Although bleeding from anatomically-defined lesions in the alimentary tract

Table 5.2. *Causes of anaemia in patients with liver disease*

Common	
Gastrointestinal bleeding	
Folate deficiency	
Hypersplenism	
Less common	
Haemolysis	
Bleeding due to haemorrhagic tendency	
'Anaemia of liver disease'	
Uncommon	
Viral hepatitis-related aplastic anaemia	
Auto-immune haemolysis	
Erythropoietic depression by high blood alcohol levels	

is the main cause of blood loss, the coagulation defects associated with severe liver disease are sometimes sufficiently marked to cause a generalized bleeding problem (p. 437). An additional cause of blood loss in patients with liver disease due to excessive ethanol intake is acute gastric erosions from which blood loss is promoted by concomitant effects of ethanol and aspirin.

Nutritional folate deficiency. Megaloblastic anaemia occasionally develops in association with hepatic cirrhosis, usually in alcoholics in whom the diet contains inadequate folate (p. 89).

Hypersplenism. When hepatic cirrhosis is complicated by portal hypertension, hypersplenism may develop, i.e. anaemia, leucopenia, and thrombocytopenia, either singly or in combination (p. 348). This condition rarely causes significant clinical problems in its own right, although it may worsen the extent of abnormalities produced by other disorders. It is frequently a cause of diagnostic confusion.

Haemolytic anaemia. Although red cell survival studies show that an extracorpuscular haemolytic element sometimes contributes to the anaemia due to liver disease *per se*, it is unusual for the typical clinical and haematological features of haemolysis to be present. *Acanthocytic red cells* (spur cells) may be present. These cells, which have an increase in membrane cholesterol, are more rigid than normal and may undergo splenic sequestration (Cooper *et al.* 1972). In extreme cases, acanthocytosis can be associated with haemolysis. Acute haemolysis can occur in alcoholics with fatty liver and extreme hyperlipidaemia, a situation described as *Zieve's syndrome* (Zieve 1966). Occasionally, auto-immune haemolytic anaemia, usually with a positive Coombs' test, occurs in patients with chronic active hepatitis (Sherlock 1985).

Anaemia of liver disease. The pathogenesis of the anaemia due to liver disease *per se* is not fully understood. Although it is related to impairment of liver function, it does not appear to parallel the degree of liver damage indicated by liver function tests, nor is it related to the duration of the disease. Both depression of erythropoiesis and accelerated red cell destruction contribute. The degree of anaemia is usually only moderate unless an exceptional degree of haemolysis is present. Most commonly, the morphologically abnormal red cells are macrocytes and target cells. The macrocytes tend to be round and not polychromatic, the presence of macrocytes usually causing an increase in the MCV of moderate degree, e.g. up to 110 fl. Even when the haemoglobin level is within the normal range, macrocytosis may be present. Variation in size and shape of the red cells is not prominent. Target cells are commonly present in moderate numbers, especially in jaundiced patients. A moderate reticulocytosis with values up to five per cent or more is common, together with moderate polychromasia and basophil stippling. The total white cell count is normal in the absence of complications, and the bone marrow contains either normal or increased proportions of normal erythroblasts, or macronormoblastic erythroblasts, which are larger than normal in size but lack megaloblastic features.

Hepatitis-related aplastic anaemia. Acute viral hepatitis is not specifically associated with anaemia, and the major haematological change during the acute phase is the presence of atypical lymphocytes (p. 223). However, aplastic anaemia develops rarely during the convalescent phase of what is usually typical infectious hepatitis A, and is often very severe (Camitta *et al.* 1974).

Treatment. The anaemia of liver disease *per se* is corrected only by improvement in liver function. Treatment is therefore directed towards the underlying disease of the liver, such as abstinence from alcohol in alcoholics. Iron should be given only when a diagnosis of iron deficiency has been clearly established, as iron overload is often present in chronic liver disease (Sherlock 1985).

Endocrine disorders

Myxoedema

Anaemia develops in about one-third to one-half of patients with hypothyroidism. Although anaemia tends to occur more frequently and to be more severe in patients with severe myxoedema, the anaemia does not necessarily parallel the severity of the other clinical features of the myxoedema. The degree of anaemia is seldom as marked as the degree of pallor suggests. It is usually mild or moderate, a haemoglobin level of 8–12 g/dl being usual, although lower levels occur. The MCV is usually in the normal range, but may be slightly raised (Horton *et al.* 1975). Microcytosis and hypochromia occur only when an associated iron deficiency is present. Overt macrocytosis in the blood film suggests the possibility of either pernicious anaemia, which has an increased incidence in this disorder, or folate deficiency. Moderate anisocytosis may occur, but poikilocytosis is slight. The total white cell count is usually normal, but mild leucopenia may occur in severe cases. The platelet count is normal. A moderate increase in the erythrocyte sedimentation rate is common.

The *bone marrow* is mildly to moderately hypoplastic, with marrow fragments containing an increased proportion of fat, and cell trails being less cellular than normal. The hypoplasia affects both red cell and white cell precursors, and thus the myeloid : erythroid ratio is normal.

Diagnosis. The diagnosis is usually suggested by the clinical features and thyroid function tests, and confirmed by recovery following thyroxine replacement. Frequently, there is no problem in diagnosis of the cause of the anaemia, as the patient presents with typical clinical features of myxoedema, and the anaemia is an incidental finding on blood examination. However, because of the pallor and lassitude, the patient is sometimes diagnosed as having 'anaemia', and the underlying myxoedema may be overlooked, particularly when the associated clinical features are not prominent. It is not uncommon for myxoedema to be thought on clinical grounds to be pernicious anaemia, as the two disorders tend to occur in the same age group and have overlapping clinical features.

Treatment with thyroxine is followed by a slow return of the haemoglobin level to normal over a period of months, sometimes 4–6 months. Iron, vitamin B_{12} or folic acid should be administered to those patients with hypothyroidism who also have proven deficiencies of these substances.

Hyperthyroidism

The haemoglobin level and red cell indices are usualy normal in hyperthyroidism. However, anaemia occurs occasionally, most often in patients in whom the disorder is of unusual severity or prolonged duration. The pathogenesis is uncertain, but it appears to be associated with impairment of iron utilization. An increased incidence of pernicious anaemia has been reported in patients with thyrotoxicosis.

Hypopituitarism

Mild to moderate anaemia develops in most cases of hypopituitarism. Haemoglobin levels usually range from 8 to 11 g/dl, although lower values may occur. The anaemia is normocytic or slightly macrocytic, and normochromic or slightly hypochromic. There is little variation in the size and shape of the red cells. The reticulocyte count and the serum bilirubin are normal. The total white count is normal or slightly reduced, and the differential count often shows a mild neutropenia with a relative lymphocytosis.

Because of the insidious onset and marked pallor, the anaemia may appear to be the most prominent clinical feature, and the underlying disorder may be overlooked. When macrocytosis is present, the condition may be confused with pernicious anaemia. The anaemia is refractory to haematinics, but appropriate hormonal replacement therapy results in a slow return of the blood picture to normal.

Addison's disease

The total red cell mass in the body is usually slightly reduced in Addison's disease, and mild normochromic normocytic anaemia is common. However, the decrease in plasma volume that can occur in untreated Addison's disease tends to mask the anaemia, with the result that the haemoglobin level is not infrequently in the low normal range. Institution of appropriate replacement therapy may thus be followed by an initial fall in haemoglobin level. The haemoglobin level is usually in the range of 10–12 g/dl, and seldom falls below 9 g/dl. Marked anaemia suggests a co-existing cause of anaemia, or the possibility that the adrenal insufficiency is secondary to pituitary hypofunction. Adequate replacement therapy results in a return of the blood count to normal in uncomplicated cases.

The total white cell and neutrophil counts are usually normal, but may be slightly reduced. The lymphocyte count is normal or slightly increased. During hypo-adrenal crises or infection there may be little increase in the white count, as the usual neutrophil leucocyte response is diminished. This is of practical importance as a crisis is often precipitated by infection, the presence of which cannot be excluded by a normal white cell count.

Protein malnutrition

An adequate dietary supply of protein containing essential amino acids is necessary for formation of haemoglobin in sufficient amounts to maintain a normal level of haemoglobin in the peripheral blood. Demands for the synthesis of haemoglobin have a high priority for the amino acid pool and take precedence over serum and tissue protein formation in states of protein malnutrition. This high priority of haemoglobin synthesis means that protein deficiency alone does not often act as a limiting factor in haemoglobin synthesis. Very considerable depletion of body stores of protein must occur before haemoglobin production is specifically impaired. Nevertheless, a diet adequate in good quality protein should be part of the routine treatment of all anaemic patients. Liver, beef, eggs, and milk products are good dietary sources of protein.

Anaemia due to protein deficiency occurs most frequently in the tropics, particularly in pregnant women and in children in association with kwashiorkor. The anaemia is usually mild to moderate in degree, and normocytic in type. The blood reticulocyte count is normal, and marrow erythropoiesis is normal or hypocellular. Episodes of transient marrow hypoplasia may occur. In the situations where protein malnutrition exists, there are often deficiencies of other nutrients, such as folic acid, vitamin B_{12}, riboflavin, vitamin A, and vitamin D. Patients respond to a high-protein diet, but features of iron or folate deficiency may develop during recovery, as subclinical iron or folate deficiency often co-exist, and are unmasked by the increase in haemoglobin production during the recovery phase. For this reason, supplements of iron and folate are recommended during treatment (Adams 1970).

Scurvy

Anaemia is common, but not invariable, in scurvy. In adults, the MCV is usually normal or slightly increased. In infants and children it is usually normochromic and normocytic, but occasionally hypochromic and microcytic due to associated iron deficiency. Megaloblastosis in ascorbate-deficient patients is usually due to deficiency of folate. This vitamin, like ascorbic acid, is heat labile and has a somewhat similar distribution in foods, so that deficiencies of the two frequently co-exist in infants, and in institutional or other settings where overcooking of food occurs. The degree of anaemia tends to be proportional to the severity of the scurvy, and is usually mild. The white cell count is normal or slightly decreased, and the platelet count is normal. The anaemia appears to be primarily due to impairment of erythropoiesis, but red cell survival studies have shown haemolysis in some cases. The administration of ascorbic acid completely corrects the anaemia, a prompt reticulocytosis usually occurring in 4–6 days in patients whose reticulocyte count is not already raised.

Pregnancy and anaemia

During the course of pregnancy, the haemoglobin level in most women falls, occasionally to below the lower limit of normal of 11.5 g/dl for non-pregnant adult females. This has been termed the 'physiological anaemia of pregnancy' and is a consequence of normally occurring increases in plasma volume. The fall in haemoglobin level commences about the 8th week and progresses steadily until the 32nd week, after which the level tends to stabilize, as illustrated in Fig. 5.4.

Individual variation in the degree to which the haemoglobin level falls is considerable. Some pregnant women show little change at all, whilst the level falls to 10.0 g/dl in others. After delivery, the haemoglobin level increases to normal by about the third month of the puerperium. The rise in haemoglobin level lags behind the rise in PCV when iron deficiency is present.

Red cells are normocytic, but a slight degree of anisocytosis is not uncommon, with an increased proportion of microcytes. The decrease in haemoglobin level reflects the *increase in plasma volume that occurs during pregnancy*. The mean increase is 43 per cent, although the individual range is extremely wide. The total volume of red cells rises by about 25 per cent, with less variation than the plasma volume (Low *et al.* 1965). This disproportionate increase in plasma volume results in haemodilution and a fall in haemoglobin level, the

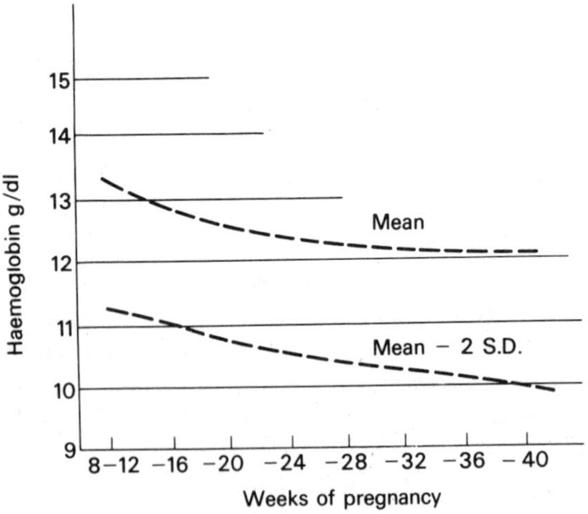

Fig. 5.4. *The mean level of haemoglobin and the lower limit of the normal range (two standard deviations below the mean) during the course of pregnancy in Australian women (Walsh & Ward 1969).*

maximum plasma volume occurring at 32–36 weeks of pregnancy, after which there is a slight decline until term. While the fall in haemoglobin level in healthy pregnant women is due primarily to hypervolaemia, it is often accentuated by the development of iron deficiency due to the drain on the maternal iron stores by the requirements of the fetus.

Treatment. Maintenance of the haemoglobin level at as high a level as possible is desirable because it enables the patient better to withstand complications such as haemorrhage, and increases well-being during the pregnancy and puerperium. Iron supplements should consequently be administered routinely to all pregnant women (p. 44).

Other physiological blood changes. The erythrocyte sedimentation rate is increased, especially in the third trimester, after which it rapidly returns to normal following delivery. A slight polymorph leucocytosis is common. The bone marrow may show moderate hyperplasia of all elements in the later stages of pregnancy.

General considerations of the causes of anaemia in pregnancy

Although the 'physiological' fall in haemoglobin level in pregnancy sometimes results in levels less than 11.5 g/dl, it very rarely reduces the level below 10 g/dl. The possibility of another cause for anaemia should be considered in all patients with levels lower than 11.5 g/dl, and certainly in all patients with levels less than 10 g/dl. *Further investigation to determine the cause of anaemia is essential and must include a full blood examination.*

Anaemia due to or aggravated by pregnancy. Iron deficiency anaemia is by far the most common cause of anaemia in pregnancy (p. 44). Megaloblastic anaemia due to folate deficiency is not uncommon in temperate zones, but is much more frequently seen in the tropics (p. 90). Protein malnutrition may cause anaemia in certain tropical regions (p. 113).

Anaemia unrelated to pregnancy. Anaemia occasionally represents the fortuitous association of pregnancy and an unrelated disorder. A common problem of diagnostic as well as therapeutic importance is anaemia in patients with thalassaemia minor or haemoglobinopathy, in whom low normal or marginally reduced haemoglobin levels are further reduced during pregnancy.

Puerperal anaemia. Anaemia first appearing in the puerperium is usually due to excess blood loss at parturition, but puerperal infection is another cause. Occasionally, megaloblastic anaemia due to pregnancy first becomes overt in the puerperium.

Investigation of normocytic anaemia

Normocytic anaemia is defined as an anaemia in which the MCV is within the normal range. In practice, the normocytic nature of an anaemia can usually be recognized by examination of the blood film. In most cases, all the red cells appear of normal size, but when anisocytosis is marked, microcytes or macrocytes, or both, may be present. Most normocytic anaemias are normochromic, i.e. the red cells appear normally haemoglobinized in the blood film, and the MCH is within the normal range. However, in some cases, a mild degree of hypochromia exists.

Normocytic anaemias form a significant proportion of anaemia seen in clinical practice. Table 5.3 lists the common causes of normocytic anaemia, and Table 5.4 summarizes an approach to the evaluation of the patient with normocytic anaemia. Although the anaemia associated with the disorders listed is usually normocytic, it is sometimes macrocytic, e.g. in aplastic anaemia or liver disease, and sometimes microcytic, e.g. in inflammatory states.

Table 5.3. *Classification of normocytic anaemias*

Disorders causing depression of erythropoiesis:
Infection*
Renal failure*
Disseminated malignancy*
Liver disease*
Collagen disease and other chronic inflammatory disorders*
Bone marrow infiltration*—leukaemia, lymphoma, multiple myeloma, myelofibrosis, metastatic myelofibrosis carcinoma
Aplastic anaemia
Endocrine disorders—myxoedema, hypopituitarism, Addison's disease
Protein malnutrition
Scurvy*
Blood loss with adequate iron stores
Haemolytic anaemia
Pregnancy

*Red cell survival studies have shown that shortened red cell survival also contributes to the anaemia, although the clinical and haematological features of florid haemolytic anaemia are absent.
Note that in some of these categories of anaemia there can be a minor to moderate degree of microcytosis (e.g. chronic inflammation) or macrocytosis (e.g. liver disease).

Assessment of the patient

The *clinical features* listed in Table 5.4 cover most of the points of diagnostic importance which require special emphasis in the assessment of a patient with normocytic anaemia.

BLOOD EXAMINATION

Red cell morphology. Marked anisocytosis and poikilocytosis are uncommon in the uncomplicated anaemia of haemorrhage, infection, renal insufficiency (except in the later stages), liver disease, aplastic anaemia, the collagen diseases, myxoedema, and hypopituitarism. Anisocytosis and poikilocytosis are often, but by no means invariably, prominent in disorders associated with bone marrow infiltration (leukaemia, lymphoma, multiple myeloma, myelofibrosis, and secondary carcinoma of bone). A dimorphic picture of normochromic and hypochromic red cells is common in refractory anaemia with ring sideroblasts.

White cell count and differential. A normal or slightly increased white cell count is usual with blood loss, infection, renal failure, and disseminated malignancy. The count is reduced in aplastic anaemia, commonly reduced in subleukaemic leukaemia and SLE, and may be normal or reduced in liver disease, lymphomas, and myxoedema. Nucleated red cells are seldom present in anaemia of infection, renal failure, liver disease, aplastic anaemia, myxoedema, or hypopituitarism. They are commonly, but by no means invariably, present in anaemia associated with bone marrow infiltration or myelofibrosis. Blast cells are usually present in acute leukaemia. Abnormal neutrophils with bilobed Pelger–Hüet nuclei or deficient granulation are suggestive of myelodysplastic disorders and myeloid leukaemia.

Reticulocyte count. The reticulocyte count is normal or reduced in infection, myxoedema, hypopituitarism, and aplastic anaemia. It is usually normal in renal failure, disseminated malignancy, liver disease, and disorders causing marrow infiltration, although a moderate increase (e.g. 4–10 per cent) occurs in some cases. A slight increase is common in chronic haemorrhage. Values over 10 per cent suggest either acute blood loss or haemolysis, and values over 15 per cent suggest haemolysis.

Table 5.4. *Summary of the investigation of a patient with normocytic anaemia*

History
Rate of onset
Blood loss
Alimentary symptoms
Bleeding tendency
Nocturnal polyuria
Bone pain
Symptoms suggestive of myxoedema or hypopituitarism
Alcoholism

Examination
Skin petechiae or ecchymoses
Conjunctivae—icterus, haemorrhage
Abdomen—hepatomegaly, splenomegaly, tenderness, mass, ascites
Signs associated with renal insufficiency—hypertension, retinal changes, proteinuria
Bone tenderness
Signs of myxoedema or hypopituitarism
Signs of infection
Pyrexia
Features of rheumatoid or other collagen disease

Blood examination
Red cell morphology
White cell count and differential
Reticulocyte count
Erythrocyte sedimentation rate

*Special investigations**
Bone marrow aspiration and trephine (aplastic anaemia, leukaemia, multiple myeloma, secondary carcinoma, lymphoma, myelofibrosis)
Faecal occult blood (gastrointestinal bleeding)
Barium meal, enema or endoscopy (gastrointestinal bleeding)
Microurine (urinary tract infection)
Blood urea and creatinine (renal insufficiency)
Skeletal X-ray (secondary carcinoma of bone, multiple myeloma, lymphoma)
Liver function tests (liver disease)
Blood culture (bacterial endocarditis)
Tests of thyroid function (myxoedema)
Tests for antibody to DNA (SLE etc.)
Tests for haemolysis (Table 8.2, p. 176)

*Disorders in which particular investigations are especially appropriate are bracketed with the investigation.

Erythrocyte sedimentation rate is normal, or only slightly raised, in blood loss due to benign disorders, and in myxoedema and hypopituitarism. It is almost invariably increased in anaemia due to infection, renal insufficiency, aplastic anaemia, the collagen diseases, and multiple myeloma. It is commonly increased in leukaemia, lymphoma (especially Hodgkin's disease), liver disease, and metastatic carcinoma in bone.

References and further reading

Infection and chronic disorders

Bentley, C.P. & Williams, P. (1974) Serum ferritin concentrations as an index of iron storage in rheumatoid arthritis. *J. Clin. Path.* **27**, 786.

Cartwright, G.E. & Lee, G.R. (1971) The anaemia of chronic disorders. *Brit. J. Haemat.* **21**, 147.

Dinant, H.J. & de Maat, C.E.M. (1978) Erythropoiesis and mean red cell life span in normal subjects and in patients with the anaemia of active rheumatoid arthritis. *Brit. J. Haemat.* **39**, 437.

Douglas, S.W. & Adamson J.W. (1975) The anaemia of chronic disorders: Studies of marrow regulation and iron metabolism. *Blood*, **45**, 55.

Lee, G.R. (1983) The anaemia of chronic disease. *Semin. Hematol.* **20**, 61

Ward, H.P., Kurnick, J.E. & Pisarczyk, M.J. (1971) Serum level of erythropoietin in anaemias associated with chronic infection, malignancy and primary haematopoietic disease. *J. Clin. Invest.* **50**, 332.

Tuberculosis

Corr, W.P., Kyle, R.A. & Boivie, E.J.W. (1964) Haematologic changes in tuberculosis. *Am. J. Med. Sci.* **248**, 709.

Fountain, J.R. (1954) Blood changes associated with disseminated tuberculosis. *Brit. Med. J.* **2**, 76.

Glasser, R.M. Walker, R.I. & Heron, J.C. (1970) The significance of haematologic abnormalities in patients with tuberculosis. *Arch. Int. Med.* **125**, 691.

Systemic lupus erythematosus, polyarteritis nodosa and dermatomyositis

Budman, D.R. & Steinberg, A.D. (1977) Hematologic aspects of systemic lupus erythematosus. *Ann. Int. Med.* **86**, 220.

Dacie, J.V. & Lewis, S.M. (1984) *Practical Haematology*, 6th Ed., Churchill Livingstone, London.

Harvey, A.M., Schulman, L.E., Tumulty, P.A. *et al.* (1954) Systemic lupus erythematosus: review of the literature and clinical analysis of 138 cases. *Medicine*, **33**, 291.

Miller, H.G. & Daley, R. (1946) Clinical aspects of polyarteritis nodosa. *Quart. J. Med.* **14**, 255.

Westerman, M.P., Martinez, R.C., Medsger, T.A. *et al.* (1968) Anemia and scleroderma. Frequency, causes and marrow findings. *Arch. Int. Med.* **122**, 39.

Acute haemorrhagic anaemia

Adamson, J. & Hillman, R.S. (1968) Blood volume and plasma protein replacement following acute blood loss in normal man. *J. Am. Med. Ass.* **205**, 609.

Finch, C.A. & Levant, C. (1972) Oxygen transport in man. *New Engl. J. Med.* **286**, 407.

Walsh, R.J. & Ward, H.K. (1969) *A Guide to Blood Transfusion*, 3rd Ed., Australian Medical Publishing Company, Sydney.

Renal failure

Caro, J., Brown, S., Miller, O. *et al.* (1979) Erythropoietin levels in uremic and anephric patients. *J. Lab. Clin. Med.* **93**, 449.

Carter, M.E., Hawkins, J.B. & Robinson, B.H.B. (1969) Iron metabolism in the anaemia of renal failure; effects of dialysis and of parenteral iron. *Brit. Med. J.* **3**, 206.

Eschbach, J.W., Cook, J.D., Schribner, B.H. *et al.* (1977) Iron balance in haemodialysis patients. *Ann. Int. Med.* **87**, 710.

Eschbach, J.W., Egrie, J.C., Downing, M.R. *et al.* (1987) Correction of the anemia of end-stage renal disease with recombinant human erythropoietin: Results of a combined phase I and II clinical trial. *New Engl. J. Med.* **316**, 73.

Mansell, M. & Grimes, A.J. (1979) Red cell and white cell abnormalities in chronic renal failure. *Brit. J. Haemat.* **42**, 169.

Nathan, D.G., Beck, I.H., Hampers, C.L. *et al.* (1968) Erythrocyte production and metabolism in anephric and uremic man. *Ann. N.Y. Acad. Sci.* **149**, 539.

Roscoe, M.H. (1952) Anaemia and nitrogen retention in patients with chronic renal failure. *Lancet*, **i**, 444.

Stewart, J.H. (1967) Haemolytic anaemia in acute and chronic renal failure. *Quart. J. Med.* **36**, 85.

Wallas, C.H. (1974) Metabolic studies on erythrocytes from patients with chronic renal disease on haemodialysis. *Brit. J. Haemat.* **27**, 145.

Winearls, C.G., Oliver, D.O., Pippard, M.J. *et al.* (1986) Effect of human erythropoietin derived from recombinant DNA on the anaemia of patients maintained by chronic haemodialysis. *Lancet*, **ii**, 1175.

Malignancy

Contreras, E., Ellis, L.D. & Lee, R.E. (1972) Value of the bone marrow biopsy in the diagnosis of metastatic carcinoma. *Cancer*, **29**, 778.

Delsol, G., Guiu-Godfrin, B., Guiu, M. *et al.* (1979) Leukoerythroblastosis and cancer. Frequency, prognosis, and pathophysiological significance. *Cancer,* **44,** 1009.

Garrett, T.J., Gee, T.S., Lieberman, P.H. *et al.* (1976) The role of bone marrow aspiration and biopsy in detecting marrow involvement by nonhematologic malignancies. *Cancer,* **38,** 2401.

Hansen, H.H., Muggia, F.M. & Selawry, O.S. (1971) Bone marrow examination in 100 consecutive patients with bronchogenic carcinoma. *Lancet,* **ii,** 443.

Liver disease

Camitta, B.M., Nathan, D.G., Forman, E.T. *et al.* (1974) Posthepatitic severe aplastic anaemia: an indication for early bone marrow transplantation. *Blood,* **43,** 473.

Cooper, R.A. , Diloy-Puray, M., Lando, P. *et al.* (1972) An analysis of lipoproteins, bile acids and red cell membranes associated with target cells and spur cells in patients with liver disease. *J. Clin. Invest.* **51,** 3182.

Douglass, C.C., McCall, M.S. & Frenkel, E.P. (1968) The acanthocyte in cirrhosis with hemolytic anemia. *Ann. Int. Med.* **68,** 390.

Douglass, C.C. & Twomen, J. (1970) Transient stomatocytosis with hemolysis: a previously unrecognized complication of alcoholism. *Ann. Int. Med.* **72,** 159.

Hines, J.D. (1969) Reversible megaloblastic and sideroblastic marrow abnormalities in alcoholic patients. *Brit. J. Haemat.* **16,** 87.

Klipstein, F.A. & Lindenbaum, J. (1965) Folate deficiency in chronic liver disease. *Blood,* **25,** 443.

Lieberman, F.L. & Reynolds, T.B. (1967) Plasma volume in cirrhosis of the liver: its relation to portal hypertension, ascites and renal failure. *J. Clin. Invest.* **45,** 1297.

Retief, F.P. & Huskisson, Y.J. (1969) Serum and urinary folate in liver disease. *Brit. Med. J.* **2,** 150.

Sherlock, S. (1985) *Diseases of the Liver and Biliary System,* 7th Ed., Blackwell Scientific Publications, Oxford.

Zieve, L. (1966) Hemolytic anemia in liver disease. *Medicine,* **45,** 497.

Endocrine disorders

Ardeman, S. Chanarin, I., Krafchik, B. *et al.* (1966) Addisonian pernicious anemia and intrinsic factor antibodies in thyroid disorders. *Quart. J. Med.* **35,** 421.

Baez-Villasenor, J., Rath, C.E. & Finch, C.A. (1948) The blood picture in Addison's disease. *Blood,* **3,** 769.

Horton, L., Coburn, R.J., England, J.M. *et al.* (1975) The haematology of hypothryoidism. *Quart. J. Med.* **45,** 101.

Jepson, J.H. & Lowenstein, L.* (1967) The effect of testosterone, adrenal steroids and prolactin on erythropoiesis. *Acta Haemat.* **38,** 292.

Nutritional deficiencies

Adams, E.G. (1970) Anaemia associated with protein deficiency. *Semin. Hemat.* **7,** 55.

Cox, E.V., Meynell, M.J., Northam, N.E. *et al.* (1967) The anaemia of scurvy. *Am. J. Med.* **42,** 220.

Goldberg, A. (1963) The anaemia of scurvy. *Quart. J. Med.* **32,** 51.

Pregnancy

Chanarin, I., Rothman, D. & Berry, V. (1965) Iron deficiency and its relation to folic acid status in prgnancy: results of a clinical trial. *Brit. Med. J.* **1,** 480.

de Leeuw, N.K.W., Lowenstein, L. & Yang-Shu Hsieh (1966) Iron deficiency and hydraemia in normal pregnancy. *Medicine.***45,** 291.

Hytten, F. (1985) Blood volume changes in pregnancy. *Clin. Haemat.* **14,** 601.

Low, J.A., Gottlieb. A.J., Delivoria-Papadopoulos, M. *et al.* (1965) Blood volume adjustments in the normal obstetric patient with particular reference to the third trimester. *Am. J. Obst. Gynaec.* **91,** 356.

Walsh, R.J. & Ward, H.K. (1969) *A Guide to Blood Transfusion.* 3rd Ed., Australasian Medical Publishing Company, Sydney.

Chapter 6
Pancytopenia; Aplastic Anaemia

Pancytopenia is the simultaneous presence of anaemia, leucopenia, and thrombocytopenia. Pancytopenia therefore exists in the adult when the haemoglobin level is less than 13.5 g/dl in males, or 11.5 g/dl in females; the leucocyte count is less than 4×10^9/l; and the platelet count is less than 150×10^9/l.

The presenting symptoms are usually attributable to the anaemia or the thrombocytopenia. Leucopenia is an uncommon cause of the initial presentation of the patient, but can become the most serious threat to life during the subsequent course of the disorder. Sometimes pancytopenia is detected as an incidental feature in a patient who has presented with symptoms of a disorder that is capable of depressing the levels of all cellular elements in the blood.

Table 6.1. *Causes of pancytopenia*

Aplastic anaemia
Subleukaemic acute leukaemia
Administration of cytotoxic agents and antimetabolites
Radiotherapy
Myelodysplastic disorders
Bone marrow infiltration or replacement:
Hodgkin's and non-Hodgkin's lymphoma, macroglobulinaemia
Multiple myeloma
Metastatic carcinoma in bone marrow
Myelofibrosis
Hypersplenism
Megaloblastosis—vitamin B_{12} and folate deficiency
Systemic lupus erythematosus
Paroxysmal nocturnal haemoglobinuria
Overwhelming infection
Miscellaneous

A wide variety of disorders can cause pancytopenia, as indicated in Table 6.1, although the frequency with which each condition is associated with pancytopenia differs considerably. However, pancytopenia is essentially always present at some stage in the course of aplastic anaemia, very common in subleukaemic leukaemia, relatively uncommon in lymphoma, and rare in metastatic carcinoma involving the bone marrow. The prognosis depends both on the severity of the pancytopenia and on the nature of the underlying condition.

Diagnosis in pancytopenia

Clinical features are those due to pancytopenia *per se*, and those of the causative disorder. Sometimes the clinical picture and examination of the blood readily indicate the nature of the causative disorder. The major diagnostic problems occur when there are no specific features in the blood to suggest the diagnosis, or when the clinical features are not sufficiently specific to point to the cause of an associated feature such as splenomegaly or lymphadenopathy.

Investigation of patients with pancytopenia

In most cases, the aetiology can be determined from consideration of the clinical features, blood examination, and examination of the bone marrow aspirate and trephine. When these data do not establish the diagnosis, further investigations are necessary. The nature and order of these investigations vary with the provisional diagnosis, and are appropriate for establishing the presence or absence of the disorders listed in Table 6.1. Certain biochemical investigations can, for instance, be helpful. Detection of an elevated serum lysozyme concentration, for example, in a patient with pancytopenia is indicative of an underlying myeloid neoplastic infiltrative process rather than aplasia of the bone marrow (Firkin 1972a). Occasionally, extensive investigation and/or prolonged observation are necessary before a definite diagnosis can be established.

The features of particular relevance to the investigation of a patient with pancytopenia are listed in Table 6.2. A careful examination of the blood film is often helpful in giving a lead to the diagnosis and, as marrow examination usually establishes the diagnosis, some of the more important points of these investigations are summarized below.

BLOOD EXAMINATION

Anisocytosis and poikilocytosis. Anisocytosis and poikilocytosis of moderate degree are common in

Table 6.2. *Outline of details required in the investigation of a patient with pancytopenia*

History
Age, sex, occupation, diet
Exposure to chemicals, drugs, or radiation
Bone pain
Fever, night sweats, malaise, weight loss, pruritus
Symptoms of disorders causing major splenic enlargement

Physical examination
Lymph node enlargement
Splenomegaly
Bone tenderness, deformity, or tumour
Hepatomegaly
Gum hypertrophy
Signs of disorders causing hypersplenism, especially portal hypertension
Evidence of primary malignancies often associated with metastasis to bone, especially breast, prostate and lung

Laboratory investigations
Essential investigations in all cases:
Peripheral blood examination. Especially note:
- anisocytosis and poikilocytosis
- white and red cell precursors
- abnormally increased or decreased granulation in neutrophils
- hypo- or hypersegmentation in neutrophils
- erythrocyte rouleaux formation
- erythrocyte sedimentation rate

Bone marrow aspiration and trephine

Further investigations where appropriate:*
Bone X-ray (multiple myeloma, metastatic carcinoma, lymphomas)
Chest X-ray (lymphomas, carcinoma of the lung, tuberculosis)
Serum alkaline and acid phosphatase level (metastatic carcinoma)
Serum protein electrophoresis (multiple myeloma, macroglobulinaemia)
DNA antibody, lupus erythematosus cell test (systemic lupus erythematosus)
Urinary Bence–Jones protein (multiple myeloma)
Needle biopsy of liver (hypersplenism, lymphomas, disseminated tuberculosis)

*Disorders in which a particular investigation has considerable diagnostic value are bracketed with that investigation.

acute leukaemia, but are by no means invariably present in this disorder. They are present, but less marked, in aplastic anaemia. Both changes may be quite conspicuous in metastatic bone carcinoma. They are usually less obvious in marrow infiltration by lymphomas or multiple myeloma. Poikilocytosis is often very marked in *myelofibrosis* (p. 334), pear- and tear-shaped poikilocytes being especially notable.

White and red cell precursors. These are almost invariably present in *myelofibrosis* as a relatively small proportion of the total nucleated cells in the blood. Such a *leuco-erythroblastic* picture is also common in *subleukaemic leukaemia* (p. 133) and *metastatic carcinoma* in bone (p. 109). It is less characteristic but can occur in multiple myeloma and marrow involvement by lymphoma. It is not typical of aplastic anaemia, so that its presence in pancytopenia suggests a diagnosis other than aplastic anaemia. In subleukaemic leukaemia and acute myelofibrosis, occasional typical or atypical 'blast' cells can be present and suggest the diagnosis. Immature lymphoid or plasmacytic cells can likewise occur occasionally in lymphoma (p. 284) and multiple myeloma (p. 304), respectively.

Abnormal granulation in neutrophils. Toxic granulation occasionally occurs in aplastic anaemia independently of infection, which is the usual cause of this abnormality.

Hyposegmentation or hypersegmentation in neutrophils. Hypogranular neutrophils are found in some myelodysplastic disorders (p. 258) and acute non-lymphoblastic leukaemias (p. 244). Pelger–Hüet-like cells (p. 244) are seen in myelodysplastic disorders and some leukaemias. An increased number of nuclear lobes is not specific for megaloblastosis, but this feature, coupled with macrocytic poikilocytic erythrocytes, strongly points to such a diagnosis.

Blood films. These may show rouleaux formation of slight to moderate degree in patients with a high sedimentation rate, but the marked rouleaux formation seen in cases of multiple myeloma (p. 303) and macroglobulinaemia (p. 310) is seldom seen in other causes of pancytopenia. Giant platelet forms may be seen in leukaemia and myelodysplastic syndromes, but platelet size is normal in aplastic anaemia.

Erythrocyte sedimentation rate. The sedimentation rate is commonly raised in many of the disorders causing pancytopenia. In aplastic anaemia, it is almost invariably raised. In multiple myeloma and macroglobulinaemia, values are commonly very high and may exceed 150 mm/hour; this is seldom seen in other disorders causing pancytopenia.

BONE MARROW ASPIRATION AND TREPHINE

A 'dry' or 'blood tap' is not uncommon in disorders causing pancytopenia, and repeated attempts may fail to obtain sufficient marrow particles for adequate examination. A marrow trephine biopsy should be routinely performed, as it not only provides information about the cellularity of haemopoietic elements, but also about the presence of reticulin and certain types of abnormal cells which are difficult or impossible to aspirate from the bony cavity. Sometimes the diagnosis can be established only when the procedure is performed at a site of focal bone involvement indicated by localized tenderness, deformity, or radiological abnormality.

Marrow aspiration is usually diagnostic in subleukaemic leukaemia, multiple myeloma, and aplastic anaemia. It is often diagnostic in marrow involvement by carcinoma and in myelodysplastic disorders. It can be helpful in non-Hodgkin's lymphoma and in macroglobulinaemia, but a trephine biopsy is necessary to establish the presence of myelofibrosis or involvement by Hodgkin's disease. The marrow in hypersplenism does not show any specific changes, but is usually hypercellular due to active erythropoiesis and leucopoiesis. When disseminated tuberculosis is suspected, a marrow film should be stained by the Ziehl–Nielsen method, and isolation of typical or atypical mycobacteria by culture should be attempted.

Aplastic anaemia

Aplastic anaemia is not the most common cause of pancytopenia, but it is a serious and usually chronic disorder which is described here in detail. The other conditions causing pancytopenia, as indicated in

Table 6.1, are discussed in detail in the relevant sections which deal with each particular disorder.

The term *aplastic anaemia* was introduced in 1888 by Ehrlich to describe a disorder of unknown aetiology characterized by anaemia, leucopenia, and thrombocytopenia resulting from aplasia of the bone marrow. The fundamental pathological feature is a reduction in the amount of haemopoietic tissue, causing an inability to produce normal numbers of mature cells for discharge into the bloodstream. Although there is a marked reduction in the total amount of haemopoietic tissue in the bone marrow, the marrow is not always uniformly hypocellular, and patchy areas of normal cellularity or even hypercellularity are sometimes interspersed between the areas of hypocellularity (Fig. 6.1).

Administration of cytotoxic agents and antimetabolites, or exposure to substantial amounts of ionizing radiation, also decrease the amount of haemopoietic tissue in the bone marrow, but the defect differs from that in aplastic anaemia in that it most commonly undergoes progressive recovery from the time that exposure to the offending agent is terminated. Ingestion of radioactive materials with a propensity to localize in bone can cause pancytopenia, which represents an industrial hazard formerly prevalent in the mining and handling of radioactive materials.

Classification

Aplastic anaemia is generally classified as follows:

1 *Idiopathic* when no cause, or any association with other conditions, is evident.

2 *Secondary* when the disorder is the result of exposure to certain drugs or chemicals, a sequel to certain viral infections, or related to certain other specific conditions. The most important relationships are with:

drug idiosyncrasy
chemical exposure
infectious hepatitis
pancreatic insufficiency
paroxysmal nocturnal haemoglobinuria
pure red cell aplasia

3 *Constitutional* when associated with inherited defects in DNA repair as seen in Fanconi's syndrome.

Selective aplasia of erythroid precursors is referred to as pure *red cell aplasia*, and the two main categories of this disorder exhibit different chemotherapeutic responses from aplastic anaemia. The

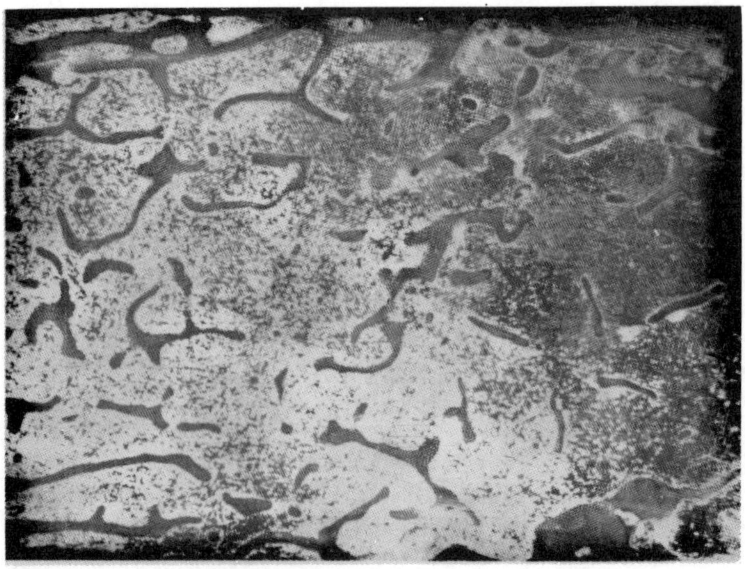

Fig. 6.1. *Bone marrow in aplastic anaemia. Histological section of bone marrow from a patient with idiopathic aplastic anaemia, showing an area of almost complete aplasia on the left, adjoining a smaller area of hyperplasia on the right. Marrow aspiration had previously yielded hypercellular marrow, evidently from a localized hypercellular region.*

major categories are classified as: *congenital* or Diamond–Blackfan anaemia, and *acquired* either with or without associated *thymoma*.

Aetiology of aplastic anaemia

In spite of the diversity of causative relationships, there are no fundamental differences in the course of the disorder, or the response to therapy. There is no unanimity of opinion as to the aetiology of aplastic anaemia, and it may represent a common end-result of different toxic mechanisms, which are abetted in some instances by an, as yet unexplained, increase in susceptibility to toxic processes in certain individuals.

A feature of the disorder, apart from in the relatively uncommon familial form, is that it often develops as a response to extrinsic factors—drugs and certain chemicals—which are normally tolerated by the majority of the population. Such *idiosyncratic* reactions to commonly employed therapeutic agents represent one of the most important causes of aplastic anaemia. It is, on the other hand, clear that the disorder can develop at least as frequently in absence of evident exposure to drugs or chemicals. Such instances are therefore due either to an idiosyncratic response to hitherto unrecognized extrinsic factors, or to a different type of pathological process. The response in aplastic anaemia patients who are recipients of transplanted genetically identical bone marrow from a healthy identical twin, indicates the existence in some cases of an ongoing toxic process which can injure haemopoietic tissue (Champlin *et al.* 1984). This toxic process can be suppressed by measures that involve potent cytotoxic and immunosuppressive capability, although the precise nature of the mechanism responsible for the injury to haemopoietic tissue remains unclear.

DRUG IDIOSYNCRASY

Idiosyncratic reactions are *qualitatively* abnormal reactions to a drug which cause hypoplasia of the bone marrow, and may occur when a drug is first given. The relationship to the daily or total ingested dose is very variable. Toxic effects sometimes appear only after large doses or prolonged courses, but have been reported to occur after small doses or short courses. The risk to any one individual in the population is small, but if the drug is widely used, the number of persons affected can become considerable.

Drugs that cause aplastic anaemia due to idiosyncrasy or hypersensitivity may be broadly subdivided into 'higher-risk' and 'lower-risk' drugs (Table 6.3). With 'higher-risk' drugs, the *per capita* incidence of individuals developing aplastic anaemia is relatively small, but nevertheless constitutes a fairly constant proportion of patients receiving the drug. With 'lower-risk' drugs, aplasia occurs only rarely, considerably less than in 1 in 10 000 patients treated. Oxyphenbutazone, chlorpromazine, phenylbutazone, gold salts, and chloramphenicol have, overall, been the drugs most commonly linked with aplastic anaemia.

Table 6.3. *Drugs associated with idiosyncratic aplastic anaemia*

Anticonvulsants	*Antirheumatic drugs*
methylhydantoin* (H)	oxyphenbutazone (H)
trimethadione* (H)	phenylbutazone (H)
paramethadione* (H)	indomethacin
aloxidone	gold salts* (H)
phenacemide*	diclofenac
methylphenylhydantoin	
methsuximide	
Antibacterial drugs	*Antidiabetic drugs*
chloramphenicol (H)	tolbutamide
sulphonamides*	chlorpropamide
isoniazid	carbutamide
arsenicals*	
Tranquillizers	*Miscellaneous*
meprobamate*	chlorothiazide*
pecazine	mepacrine
chlordiazepoxide	hydralazine
chlorpromazine* (H)	acetazolamide
promazine*	potassium perchlorate
thioridazine*	carbamazepine*
	tripelennamine

*Selective neutropenia or thrombocytopenia more common toxic effects; (H) relatively high-risk drug. Bithell & Wintrobe (1967) list references to original papers describing reactions to many of the drugs in this table.

Chloramphenicol produces two distinct patterns of haematological toxicity: dose-dependent *reversible haemopoietic depression* in all individuals, and *idiosyncratic aplastic anaemia* in a small proportion of individuals (Yunis & Bloomberg 1964).

The *reversible toxic effect* takes the form of an arrest of erythropoiesis and consequent depression of the reticulocyte count when serum levels of chloramphenicol are sustained at or above 15–20 μg/ml for at least several days. Production of platelets can also be depressed under these circumstances, leading to the development of thrombocytopenia (Scott *et al.* 1965). Examination of the bone marrow reveals decreased proportions of erythroid precursors which may also have vacuolated cytoplasm. These changes are normal pharmacological responses to relatively high blood levels of chloramphenicol, and occur in all individuals. Recovery of erythropoiesis and thrombopoiesis normally takes place in a matter of days when the administration of chloramphenicol is ceased.

Such an effect is not usually observed with conventional therapeutic doses, because the relatively high blood levels required to produce a significant degree of reversible toxicity are not achieved unless detoxification of the drug is impaired, either by hepatic disease or immaturity. This type of reaction is thus normally restricted to individuals receiving relatively high doses such as 50 mg/kg/day. As the response is readily reversible, it is not of serious clinical importance, unless it is not recognized and depression of all haemopoietic elements develops during protracted treatment.

Chloramphenicol causes this effect by depressing cellular proliferation as a result of its ability selectively to inhibit the synthesis of certain mitochondrial proteins normally produced by the protein synthesizing system in mitochondria. The affected proteins include cytochrome oxidase, an essential component of the major energy-generating system in the cell. The ensuing lack of energy availability leads to arrest of proliferation, which is evident first in rapidly dividing tissues such as erythroid precursors (Firkin 1972b).

Idiosyncratic aplastic anaemia, on the other hand, develops without a specific relationship to the daily or total ingested dosage of chloramphenicol. There may be a history of previous exposure to chloramphenicol, but this is far from inevitable. The majority of instances follow administration of chloramphenicol for several days or more at conventional dosages. Symptoms may not become evident for weeks or months, but the epidemiological evidence is overwhelming that this drug is a cause of aplastic anaemia (Best 1967).

Attempts to define the degree of risk in any individual taking a course of chloramphenicol suggest the incidence is approximately ten times greater than the background level of spontaneously occurring idiopathic aplastic anaemia (Wallerstein *et al.* 1969). It appears that somewhat fewer than 1 in 10 000 individuals develops aplastic anaemia when administered chloramphenicol, but such a degree of risk is unacceptable when alternative antibiotics with less serious side-effects are equally satisfactory in eradicating infection. Such widespread administration of chloramphenicol occurred at one point in time that it appeared responsible for an overall increase in the incidence of aplastic anaemia, and as a result the drug was withdrawn from general use in some countries. There is currently insufficient epidemiological data to establish whether the few reports of aplasia associated with the use of chloramphenicol eye-drops represent genuine idiosyncratic responses, or chance associations with a condition that can occur spontaneously.

Administration of a number of other therapeutic agents such as *gold salts* and *phenylbutazone* is associated with an increased incidence of aplastic anaemia (see Table 6.3). A large number of other drugs has been associated in a small number of instances with aplastic anaemia, but it is difficult to ascertain whether these represent chance relationships or otherwise. There is currently no evidence of a mechanism to account for the idiosyncratic response to any drug. Efforts to identify increased drug sensitivity in proliferating cultured myeloid progenitors from subjects who have had aplastic anaemia have in fact demonstrated the opposite finding of reduced susceptibility to the toxic action of the incriminated drug in the case of chloramphenicol (Howell *et al.* 1975), and phenylbutazone (Firkin & Moore 1978).

CHEMICAL EXPOSURE

The most important chemical associated with aplastic anaemia is *benzene*. This is a cyclic hydrocarbon and should not be confused with petroleum. Three factors influence the development of aplastic anaemia: susceptibility of the individual, duration of exposure, and concentration of vapour.

Aplastic anaemia is usually produced by inhalation of benzene vapour for considerable periods, as it has been mostly associated with prolonged confinement in poorly ventilated spaces in which benzene is employed as a solvent, often in glues. Other solvents, such as toluene and xylene, do not appear to have the same propensity for causing aplastic anaemia as benzene.

Benzene can also be found in products used in the home, and in hobbies. Paint removers, and adhesive and cleaning solutions, may contain benzene. The syphoning by mouth of petrol containing benzene has been followed by aplasia (McLean 1960). Aplasia has also been reported following exposure to the commercial solvent known as 'Stoddard's solvent', which is used as an all-purpose solvent, particularly as a dry-cleaning agent, paint thinner, and for cleaning machinery (Scott *et al.* 1959).

Aplastic anaemia has been attributed to inhalation of vaporized *lindane* (gamma benzene hexachloride) when used as an insecticide. The vaporizers that volatilize lindane have been widely used in homes, offices, public eating places and industrial workplaces. Lindane is also present in some spray insecticides used in the home and in agricultural work. Aplasia has also been reported following exposure to the insecticides *chlordane* and *chlorophenothane* (DDT), and to trinitrotoluene in explosives factories.

APLASTIC ANAEMIA AND INFECTIOUS HEPATITIS

Aplastic anaemia occurs as a rare, but recognized, sequel of infectious hepatitis, usually developing as an apparent idiosyncratic phenomenon after recovery from the hepatitis has taken place. It is most commonly associated with epidemic hepatitis infections (hepatitis A), and thus occurs more commonly in the younger age group affected by this type of hepatitis virus. Infections with a number of other viruses can cause marrow hypoplasia which is usually transient, although occasional instances of aplastic anaemia have been reported.

FANCONI'S ANAEMIA

Familial aplastic anaemia can occur, in which the onset is usually in the first decade of life. There *may* be associated abnormalities, such as patchy brown cutaneous pigmentation and neurological, renal, or skeletal malformations. Associated biological abnormalities are a diminished capacity for DNA repair and increased random chromosome breakage during mitosis. A resulting aberration involving DNA may serve as an initiating event in the development of aplastic anaemia, or of leukaemia which occurs more frequently in individuals with decreased DNA repair capability. Although an initial satisfactory response to anabolic agent therapy may occur, the disorder most commonly tends to pursue an inexorable course to fatal pancytopenia.

Clinical features

The behaviour of idiopathic aplastic anaemia is sufficiently similar to the secondary form for both to be considered together. Onset is often insidious, with symptoms of progressively worsening anaemia and an associated bruising or bleeding diathesis. Some have an apparently acute onset and present with bleeding or infection.

Symptoms of *anaemia* are as described for anaemia in general (p. 26), the most prominent being weakness, easy fatiguability, lassitude and dyspnoea on exertion. The *bleeding manifestations* are those common to thrombocytopenia in general (p. 376), and include haemorrhage into the skin, either as ecchymoses or petechiae, epistaxis, menorrhagia, and bleeding from the gums and alimentary tract. Cerebral haemorrhage is a not uncommon and often fatal complication. *Neutropenia* may result in infection, causing malaise, sore throat, ulceration of the mouth and pharynx, fever with chills and sweating, chronic skin infections, and recurrent chest infections. Pneumonia is a common complication, as is septicaemia, and both are frequent causes of death.

The outstanding feature on *physical examination* is the absence of objective findings apart from those resulting from anaemia, neutropenia, or thrombocytopenia. There is pallor, but no icterus. The spleen is rarely palpable, and the liver is palpable only as a complication of severe anaemia. Lymph nodes are not enlarged, although the regional nodes draining infected lesions may become palpable.

Blood picture

There is typically anaemia in which the red cells are normochromic and normocytic, although minor or moderate degrees of *macrocytosis* are surprisingly common. Other features commonly seen are *leucopenia*, particularly *neutropenia*, and *thrombocytopenia*. The absolute concentration of reticulocytes is usually depressed, red and white cell precursors are absent, and the erythrocyte sedimentation rate is usually elevated, sometimes to high values.

Haemoglobin levels are often as low as 7 g/dl, and may be considerably less. Red cell anisocytosis is common, and poikilocytosis can occur. Mean corpuscular volume can be elevated sufficiently to raise the possibility of megaloblastosis, but very large oval macrocytes as seen in the latter situation are uncommon. The percentage of reticulocytes can be subnormal, normal, or slightly increased, although the absolute count is usually not elevated, and is most commonly subnormal. A relatively high reticulocyte count is a good prognostic factor, although this is not an infallible guide to outcome. The leucocyte count may be normal at presentation, but tends to fall during the course of the disorder. There is typically a *relative* lymphocytosis. Red and white cell precursors are almost never present in the blood unless anaemia is extreme, and their presence suggests an alternative cause of pancytopenia such as leukaemia, myelofibrosis or bone marrow infiltration. The Ham's acid-serum test is occasionally positive in the absence of overt features of paroxysmal nocturnal haemoglobinuria (Lewis & Dacie 1967). Radioactive iron is cleared abnormally slowly from the blood, and surface counting demonstrates that the majority of the ^{59}Fe is taken up by the liver rather than the bone marrow. The serum iron level is usually elevated. Even the production of γ globulin is depressed in many patients, indicating that failure of the function of a wide range of haemopoietic elements can occur in this condition.

Bone marrow picture

Cellularity of haemopoietic elements can vary substantially at different sites in the bone marrow as illustrated in Fig. 6.1. In most cases, aspiration yields particles that are hypocellular. A 'dry' tap in which no material at all is obtained, or a 'blood' tap in which there is blood but no particles, can occur in this condition. It is therefore essential under such circumstances for a bone marrow trephine to be performed in order to assess the cellularity of the bone marrow.

In *aplastic and hypoplastic* particles, the proportion of fat cells increases, with a corresponding decrease in haemopoietic cells, varying from moderate reduction to complete absence (Fig. 6.2). All fragments should be examined, as some variation in cellularity may occur. Examination of an adequate number of fragments usually gives as much information about marrow cellularity as does a trephine biopsy, and is a most important part of the marrow examination in a suspected case of aplastic anaemia. Cell trails from hypoplastic fragments are either hypocellular or absent. The differential count of nucleated cells may reveal that erythropoiesis and leucopoiesis are equally reduced, or that one is relatively less affected. Plasma cells, reticulum cells and lymphocytes are *relatively* prominent, and in severely affected marrows comprise the majority of cells.

In *cellular* areas, the particles contain a reduced proportion of fat cells and an increased proportion of haemopoietic cells, and the trails are cellular. Haemopoietic tissue usually contains all cell series, but sometimes one cell type may predominate. Erythropoiesis is normoblastic but often *dyserythropoietic* features are present, particularly in the more

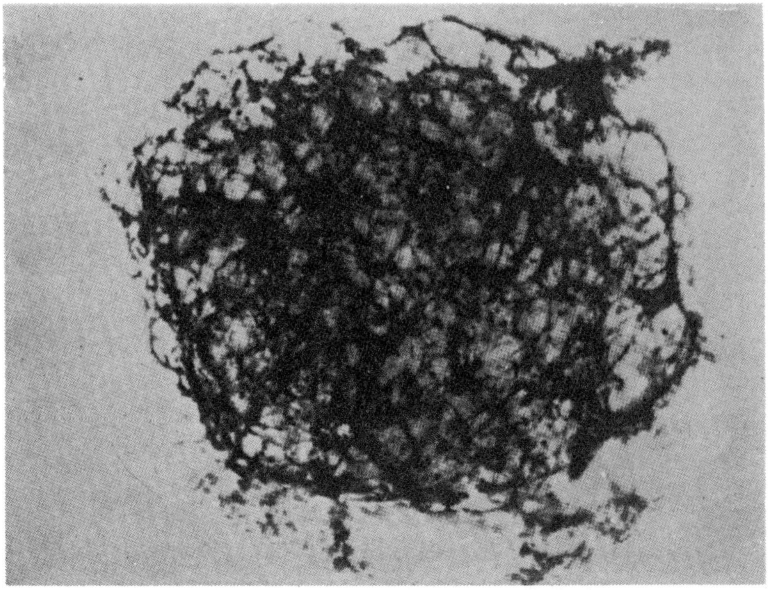

Fig. 6.2. *Particle of aspirated marrow in aplastic anaemia, consisting mainly of fat cells. Very few cells were present in the trail behind the fragment. Of the cells present, many were plasma and reticulum cells, both of which are relatively increased in the marrow in aplastic anaemia.*

mature erythroblasts. Megakaryocytes are commonly reduced in numbers even in cellular regions. The iron content is usually normal or increased.

Course and prognosis

Aplastic anaemia is a serious disorder which frequently terminates in death within six months. Mortality rates vary in different series from somewhat less than 50 per cent, to as high as 80 per cent in the first year after presentation. It is too early to be certain of the extent to which therapeutic modalities such as allogeneic bone marrow transplantation and administration of antithymocyte globulin will improve survival. Both forms of treatment are associated with some reduction in mortality, but transplantation is currently restricted to patients who have a histocompatible donor, and antithymocyte globulin administration is not always successful or sustained in its effect. It does, however, appear that one or other modality will enable a proportion of patients to survive who would otherwise die from the disorder.

Death is usually due to bleeding and/or infection, and most commonly occurs in the first six months from presentation. The longer the patient survives, the greater is the chance of improvement in haematological parameters, although partial remission can be followed by subsequent deterioration, and the risk of death remains greater than normal even in long-term survivors. It is not adequately appreciated that aplastic anaemia is generally a *chronic condition* in which the haemopoietic abnormality can persist for years in spite of the withdrawal of causative agents.

In many instances, haematological parameters have continued to deteriorate for a considerable period after exposure to an incriminated drug has ceased. Recovery to complete normality occurs in the minority of cases although the degree of abnormality in other survivors, as illustrated in Fig. 6.3, is frequently compatible with a clinically satisfactory state. Improvement, on rare occasions, can occur over a matter of weeks, but usually occurs slowly. The platelet count is particularly slow to rise, with thrombocytopenia often persisting after the haemoglobin level and leucocyte count have returned to normal (Vincent & de Gruchy 1967). Paroxysmal nocturnal haemoglobinuria sometimes develops during the course of the disorder (Lewis & Dacie 1967), and acute leukaemia in rare instances (Ellims *et al.* 1979).

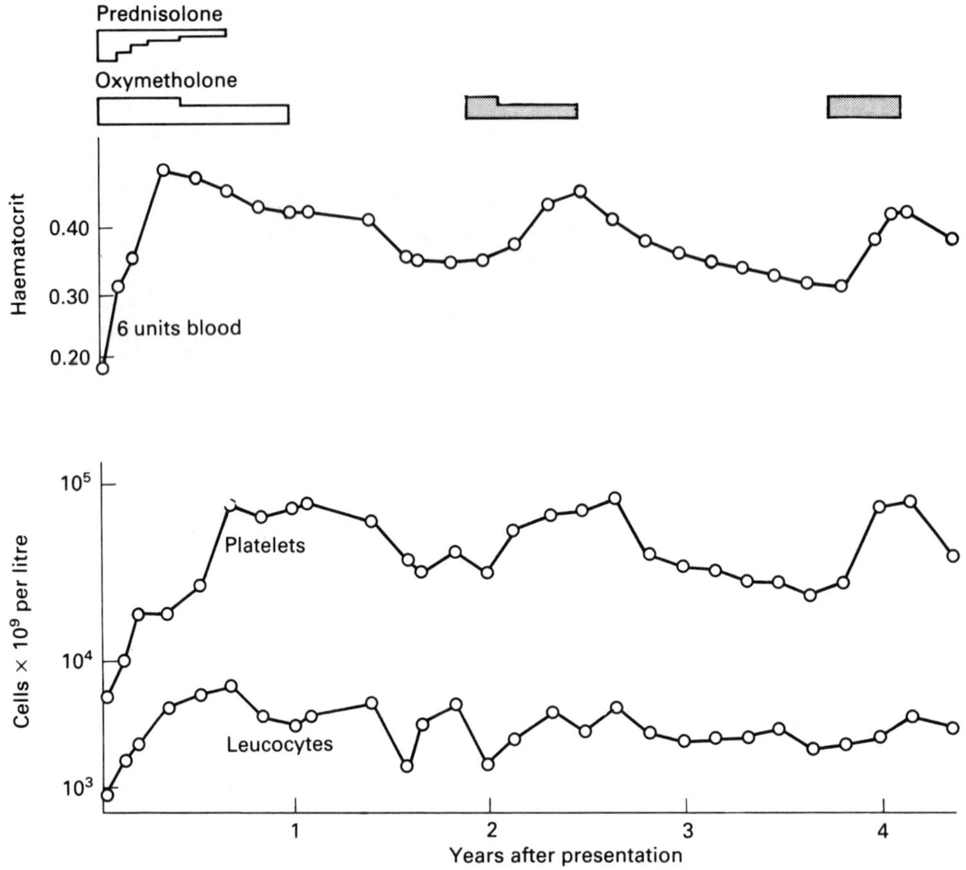

Fig. 6.3. *The course of the haematological indices in a subject with idiopathic aplastic anaemia, illustrating the chronic nature of the condition and the slow improvement that can occur in the haematocrit and platelet count in response to administration of oxymetholone.*

Outcome is difficult to predict in any one individual at presentation, and efforts have been made to identify factors associated with a good or bad prognosis. One analysis suggested that bleeding at presentation, male sex, abrupt onset, low absolute reticulocyte count, more severe thrombocytopenia, more severe neutropenia, and greater depression of haemopoietic cells in the marrow aspirate were associated with a worse prognosis (Lynch *et al.* 1975).

Prevention

Careful selection of therapeutic agents. Before prescribing a drug which is a potential cause of aplastic anaemia, the physician should weigh the risk of alternative measures for treating the disease against the risk associated with the drug. No potentially toxic drug should be used if an alternative, effective, non-toxic drug is available. Furthermore, no drug that carries a greater degree of risk than the disease should be used. Many reported cases of fatal aplastic anaemia result from administration of potentially toxic drugs to patients with relatively minor complaints which were either self-limiting, or for which an effective, safe, alternative therapy was available. A patient who has developed aplasia following exposure to a particular drug should never receive that drug again, and should be given a warning card to show to all future medical attendants.

Management

The course of the disorder is difficult to predict as it can progress rapidly to a fatal outcome, pursue a relatively indolent course, or recover in rare instances after several weeks. Such variability has made it difficult to establish with controlled trials the benefits of different management modalities. It is, however, clear that substantial improvement may occur after several months of severe pancytopenia, and a basic principle is *never to give up* attempts to achieve a satisfactory outcome. Management is considered under the following headings.

1 Identification and elimination of exposure to causative agent.
2 Supportive therapy:
  prevention and treatment of infection;
  prevention and treatment of haemorrhage;
  red cell transfusion for anaemia.
3 Measures to accelerate recovery from pancytopenia:
  bone marrow transplantation;
  antithymocyte globulin;
  anabolic agent administration;
  corticosteroid administration.

IDENTIFICATION AND ELIMINATION OF EXPOSURE TO CAUSATIVE AGENT

There is no doubt that aplastic anaemia is precipitated by ingestion or inhalation of certain drugs or chemicals. In such instances, it is logical to terminate the exposure as rapidly as possible in the hope this will lessen the ultimate severity of the disorder. One of the distressing features is that the condition can nonetheless inexorably progress over several months to a fatal outcome after only a brief period of exposure to certain drugs.

It may be difficult to establish the extent and identity of drugs or chemicals to which a patient with aplastic anaemia has been exposed in the relevant preceding period of about six months. Many patients simply do not reliably recall their medication history, and most do not know the extent to which they have been exposed to chemicals. Some insight into the nature of chemicals, such as benzene, with which individuals may have contact at work or in the home, is therefore valuable in the assessment of potential exposure to such agents. A more reliable drug history can usually be obtained from the patient's medical practitioner, but this will not reveal the ingestion of non-proprietary, so-called 'herbal' medications, which in some countries contain additives such as phenylbutazone.

SUPPORTIVE THERAPY

Prevention and treatment of infection

When the patient is *at risk* from infection because of neutropenia or because of glucocorticoid administration, several prophylactic measures are advisable. One is avoidance of areas of microbial contamination such as hospitals, where antibiotic-resistant organisms are common. Reduction of the load of nasal and oral bacteria in patients with severe neutropenia can be achieved with topical antiseptic preparations. Prophylactic antibiotic administration is not recommended, as it tends to alter the microbial flora to resistant organisms, and such a change is highly undesirable. Isolation of patients with extreme neutropenia in specialized low microbial environments imposes severe limitations on the patient. This may be tolerable during relatively limited phases of extreme neutropenia, such as in remission-induction therapy in acute leukaemia or in bone marrow transplantation, but impractical in a condition such as aplastic anaemia where little change may occur for prolonged periods. Development of *Candida albicans* infection occurs so commonly in association with administration of high dosages of corticosteroids that concurrent oral administration of a non-absorbable antifungal agent to suppress the load of such organisms in the mouth and gastrointestinal tract should be considered when corticosteroids are given.

Infection represents a serious threat to the severely neutropenic patient with aplastic anaemia. The absolute neutrophil count can fall when utilization of neutrophils due to infection exceeds the rate at which neutrophils are formed by bone marrow with diminished productive capacity. Such a development further reduces the defences against infection. Infection can also be associated with worsening of the degree of thrombocytopenia, and in already severely thrombocytopenic individuals can precipitate potentially fatal bleeding. Treatment of infection under such circumstances should be prompt and vigorous, employing the guidelines described for infection in neutropenia (p. 227). Oral antibiotics may be appropriate for minor episodes of infection in less severely neutropenic subjects, but intravenous broad-spectrum antibiotic therapy is indicated when the degree of neutropenia is severe, because of the tendency for the infection to progress rapidly to overwhelming sepsis.

Prevention and treatment of haemorrhage

Thromboctyopenia frequently results in bleeding in this condition. While prophylaxis against potentially fatal bleeding with random donor platelet transfusions has been shown to be of value in thrombocytopenic states of relatively limited duration, such as remission-induction therapy for acute leukaemia, it has not proved suitable for the more sustained period of thrombocytopenia in aplastic anaemia. A major factor is the development of iso-antibodies to allogeneic platelets which occurs in response to repeated platelet transfusions over weeks to months, ultimately rendering random donor platelet transfusions ineffective (Grumet & Yankee 1970). It has therefore been a common practice to reserve platelet transfusions for treatment of clinically significant bleeding, as 6–8 units of random donor platelets can markedly improve the haemostatic defect due to thrombocytopenia for up to several days. When random donor platelets are ineffective because of iso-antibodies, it is possible to obtain effective platelet support with platelets from donors with greater degrees of HLA compatibility, such as siblings, if sibling bone marrow transplantation is not contemplated (Grumet & Yankee 1970). Use of blood products from potential bone marrow donors is avoided in the hope of limiting the degree of rejection of subsequently transplanted bone marrow.

A simple but important preventive measure against bleeding is avoidance of the use of non-steroidal anti-inflammatory drugs. They have dual adverse effects: diminution of the functional capacity of platelets, and production of erosions in the upper gastrointestinal tract which tend to bleed. Menorrhagia can also be a serious problem, and the most practical approach to contain it is the uninterrupted administration of hormonal agents that prevent menstruation.

Red cell transfusion for anaemia

The object of transfusion is to raise the haemoglobin level to one at which anaemic symptoms are alleviated, and a comfortable life can be led for a reasonable period before transfusion is again required. Because of the better *in vivo* survival of red cells from recently taken blood, the use of blood taken within the previous few days is preferable. In the presence of bleeding, appropriately collected blood less than 24 hours old has the advantage of containing functionally effective platelets and coagulation factors; however, selective blood component therapy has generally replaced this practice.

Individual transfusion requirements vary from patient to patient, depending on the severity of the marrow depression and the extent of blood loss due to haemorrhage. Many patients require transfusion at regular intervals, but a few need only an occasional transfusion. It is not necessary to maintain the haemoglobin continually at normal levels. Many patients are comfortable for 6–8 weeks after the haemoglobin has been raised by transfusion to about 12–14 g/dl, provided that no bleeding occurs. Further transfusion is given when symptoms of anaemia again become prominent, usually when the haemoglobin level has fallen to around 7–9 g/dl. Transfusion requirements in women are often greater because of menorrhagia when menstrual activity is not suppressed by hormonal therapy.

In patients with marked bleeding, transfusion requirements are sometimes massive. Transfusions tend to become progressively less effective and are therefore required at increasingly shorter intervals, especially in patients who have received many transfusions. This is due to the addition of a haemolytic element to the anaemia. While this haemolysis sometimes results from the development of iso-antibodies, in many cases no such antibodies can be demonstrated. It appears that the spleen plays some role in the increased destruction of transfused red cells, as splenectomy may result in a lowering of transfusion requirements.

An important problem which may develop in patients receiving repeated transfusions is the occurrence of transfusion reactions, which may also lessen the efficacy of the transfusion. Sometimes these are due to the development of red cell iso-antibodies (p. 482) which can be detected by *careful cross-matching*. However, in many such patients, no red cell antibodies can be demonstrated, and it has been shown that the reactions may be due to development of antibodies to leucocytes or platelets. Such reactions can be reduced in severity or avoided by removing the leucocytes and platelets, by taking off the buffy coat when red cell concentrates are prepared by centrifugation, or by freezing the red cells. It is important also to avoid damage to veins which will prevent further transfusion, and thus the cut-down procedure should be avoided. Sometimes the amount of iron delivered by multiple transfusions is so great that clinical manifestations of haemochromatosis appear.

MEASURES TO ACCELERATE RECOVERY FROM PANCYTOPENIA

Bone marrow transplantation

Intravenous infusion of HLA-compatible bone marrow in order to engraft effective haemopoietic tissue in the patient's marrow cavity has achieved a considerable degree of success in the treatment of *younger* patients with *severe* aplastic anaemia (Storb *et al.* 1984). In the rare situation where the donor is an identical twin, the donor tissue is entirely histocompatible and does not give rise to immune-mediated attack on the tissues of the recipient, otherwise known as *graft-versus-host disease.* Bone marrow transplantation now tends to be restricted to patients under the age of 40 years, and is performed by infusion of marrow from an HLA-identical donor whose lymphocytes show little or no reactivity to recipient lymphocytes in the mixed lymphocyte reaction (p. 478). Greater degrees of HLA or mixed lymphocyte reaction incompatibility are associated with *rejection* of the bone marrow graft, or unacceptably severe graft-versus-host disease. The procedure as it is currently performed is one which is applicable to a minority of subjects with aplastic anaemia, as fewer than half have an HLA-compatible donor, and complications are of such severity in recipients over the age of 40 years that the procedure tends to be avoided in this age group.

The recipient is given such intense immunosuppressive treatment to prevent graft rejection that it causes extreme marrow suppression. Restoration of effective haemopoiesis by donor marrow infused at this time usually does not take place for 2–3 weeks, and thus specialized facilities and clinical expertise are required to support the patient during the intervening phase of life-threatening pancytopenia. For this reason, better results are obtained in specialized centres.

While most recipients survive the initial phase of pancytopenia, a distressing development is graft-versus-host disease in at least half of the survivors, despite attempted prophylaxis against the condition with immunosuppressive agents such as methotrexate or cyclosporin A (O'Reilly 1983). This is due to immunologically mediated attack by the immune system derived from donor marrow on host cells bearing minor antigenic differences, and it causes potentially fatal injury to tissues such as liver, bowel, and skin. There is commonly suppression of immune responses to pathogens, leading to infections such as pneumonia due to *cytomegalovirus, yeasts, fungi, Pneumocystis carinii* and other organisms. These infections are often fatal. The severity and frequency of such complications are currently sufficiently great for bone marrow transplantation to be restricted to subjects with very severe aplastic anaemia in whom alternative forms of management are associated with a very poor prognosis.

Antithymocyte globulin administration

Intravenous administration of immunoglobulin preparations containing antibody to human thymocytes for approximately one week is associated with improvement in haematological indices in about one-half of the treated subjects (Champlin *et al.*

1983). Improvement occurs relatively slowly, and uncommonly results in sustained normal values, although the degree of change confers considerable clinical benefit. Antithymocyte globulin thus provides potentially beneficial treatment for patients with aplastic anaemia in whom bone marrow transplantation cannot be performed because of advanced age or lack of a suitable donor. The antibody currently employed is mostly raised in the horse, and the patient must be carefully monitored during the infusion because of the low but real possibility of developing an anaphylatic response to horse serum components.

What is the best course of action when a histocompatible marrow donor has been identified? Results from allogeneic marrow transplantation are, generally speaking, superior to those obtained with antithymocyte globulin treatment in children and adolescents. A shift towards the reverse situation occurs as the age of the recipient increases further, and results are generally superior with antithymocyte globulin treatment in subjects over the age of 40 years, although allogeneic marrow transplantation still remains an option if the response to antithymocyte globulin is unsatisfactory.

Anabolic agent administration

Oxymetholone is currently the most commonly administered anabolic agent for the treatment of aplastic anaemia. A variety of androgens have been shown to produce a degree of improvement, and oxymetholone is one orally absorbable form associated with beneficial effects in some patients (Sanchez-Medal *et al.* 1964, Silink & Firkin 1968). Anabolic agents do not appear to decrease mortality in severe aplastic anaemia, but are of undoubted benefit in less severely affected cases because they can produce a delayed increase in the cellular elements of the blood (Fig. 6.3). The most dramatic effect is on the haemoglobin level, and may terminate dependence on transfusion. The dosage is usually 100 mg oxymetholone per day, or more, and in some responders, it can be withdrawn successfully after 6–12 months. In others, the haematological indices may deteriorate after oxymetholone withdrawal (Fig. 6.3), and further courses, or maintenance therapy, often effective at lower doses, may be required. Major side-effects include hepatic damage, a problem common to all orally absorbable androgens, and virilization in females.

Corticosteroid administration

Administration of corticosteroids in high dosages has occasionally been linked with improvement in aplastic anaemia. Therapy formerly often consisted of corticosteroids in combination with an anabolic agent, although it is uncertain whether the corticosteroids conferred any benefit. The lack of clearly established benefit in most patients is compounded by the undesirable side-effects of relatively high doses of corticosteroids, such as osteoporotic fractures, glucose intolerance, and increased susceptibility to infection.

Pure red cell aplasia

Congenital or Diamond–Blackfan anaemia

This form of anaemia characteristically develops in infancy, and differs from Fanconi's anaemia in that it is not accompanied by impaired production of leucocytes or platelets (Diamond & Blackfan 1938). It is a chronic disorder, caused by selective depletion of erythroid precursors. Although many explanations have been advanced to account for the lack of erythroblasts, there is currently no consensus as to the pathophysiology of the disorder. Anaemia may become extreme, and is not generally associated with other abnormalities, such as thymoma which can accompany acquired pure red cell aplasia. Diamond–Blackfan anaemia differs from acquired pure red cell aplasia and aplastic anaemia in that the majority of cases respond to glucocorticoid administration, and although maintenance therapy is usually required, the maintenance dosage that sustains effective remission is often surprisingly small. Spontaneous remission may occur during puberty.

Acquired pure red cell aplasia

The selective depletion of erythroblasts in this condition may involve only the more mature erythroblasts, although most commonly the entire erythroid series is affected. There is characteristically an acquired normochromic normocytic anaemia accompanied by a depressed absolute reticulocyte count in the chronic form of the disorder. While the leucocyte and platelet counts are usually normal, depression of leucocytes or platelets occasionally develops at some stage (Hirst & Robertson 1967).

Chronic acquired pure red cell aplasia differs from aplastic anaemia in that there is very good evidence of an auto-immune aetiology in the majority of cases. An association with thymoma is common, although in the minority, and the nature of the relationship with thymoma is poorly understood. A thymoma can be present many years before pure red cell aplasia develops, or alternatively, may have been excised apparently completely years beforehand. The association with many disorders of an established or presumed auto-immune nature, and the frequently beneficial response to immunosuppressive agents, suggests the condition is commonly due to immune-mediated injury to erythroid precursors.

Surgical excision of an associated thymoma has been reported to produce remissions, although such a result is far from inevitable (Hirst & Robertson 1967). Pure red cell aplasia unassociated with thymoma may occasionally respond well to glucocorticoid administration (Lee *et al.* 1978), but sustained benefit in terms of easily maintained or unmaintained remission is uncommon. Unmaintained remissions are achieved in about two-thirds of cases after courses of immunosuppressive agents, such as corticosteroids plus cyclophosphamide or azathioprine (Clark *et al.* 1984).

Differential diagnosis of pancytopenia

Aplastic anaemia is characterized by pancytopenia in which careful scrutiny of the blood film characteristically fails to reveal erythroid or leucocyte precursors. The erythrocyte sedimentation rate is often markedly elevated, and thus does not serve as a specific index of marrow depression due to infiltration by disorders associated with paraprotein production, such as multiple myeloma or macroglobulinaemia. Values in excess of 100 mm/hour are, however, sufficiently elevated to raise the possibility of the presence of the latter conditions.

Clinical examination usually reveals no positive findings other than those of anaemia, or of bleeding or infection resulting from thrombocytopenia or neutropenia, respectively. Lymph node enlargement is not characteristically part of the disorder, although regional nodes draining an infective focus may become moderately enlarged. The spleen and liver are usually impalpable.

Occurrence of one or more of the following signs in a patient with pancytopenia suggests a diagnosis other than aplastic anaemia: splenomegaly, hepatomegaly, lymph node enlargement, bone tenderness, immature white or red cells in the peripheral blood, normal erythrocyte sedimentation rate.

The diagnosis is usually established by examination of a *satisfactory* bone marrow aspirate containing at least a number of marrow particles, or of a bone marrow trephine. Uncommonly, the picture in the biopsied material is dominated by a focus of active marrow and may lead to an erroneous diagnosis of myelodysplastic syndrome.

Subleukaemic leukaemia is a more common cause of pancytopenia than aplastic anaemia. The leucocyte and platelet counts are depressed on presentation in an appreciable minority of subjects with acute leukaemia (p. 244), and the diagnostic problem arises in the subleukaemic group when there are very few or no blast cells evident in the blood film. Certain physical signs and, of course, examination of the bone marrow indicate the diagnosis. There may be lymphadenopathy, or enlargement of the liver or spleen, although these features can also be present in lymphoma and macroglobulinaemia. Features differentiating this condition from aplastic anaemia are summarized in Table 6.4.

Chemotherapy-related bone marrow depression is usually overtly linked to administration of cytotoxic agents or antimetabolites, and thus poses no diagnostic problem. The connection can, however,

Table 6.4 *Comparison of features of aplastic anaemia and subleukaemic leukaemia*

	Aplastic anaemia	Subleukaemic leukaemia
History	Relatively recent exposure to chemical agents or drugs in about one-half of cases	Occasionally exposure to radiation, alkylating agents or benzene in the past
Physical examination		
Sternal tenderness	Rare	Common
Splenomegaly	Uncommon. When present only slight	May be absent at onset, but can develop during course of illness
Lymph node enlargement	No generalized enlargement. Regional nodes draining infective lesions may be enlarged	Sometimes present and can develop during course of illness
Gum hypertrophy	Absent	Occasionally present
Blood examination		
Red cell morphology	Slight to moderate anisocytosis, often with some macrocytosis. Poikilocytosis of varying degree	Moderate anisocytosis and poikilocytosis usual
Neutrophils	Normal in morphology and granulation	Hypogranulation and Pelger–Hüet-like anomaly may be seen
Immature white and red cells	Usually absent	Absent or present only in small numbers at onset, but appear in the course of the illness. Blast cells predominate
Erythrocyte sedimentation rate	Almost invariably raised	Usually but not invariably raised
Bone marrow examination	Usually hypocellular. Occasionally normocellular or hypercellular. Examination at second site usually yields hypocellular specimen	Usually cellular or hypercellular leukaemic tissue. Chromosome abnormalities present in about one-half of cases

be obscure when pancytopenia due to bone marrow hypoplasia is caused by inappropriate administration of these agents, in the treatment of non-malignant conditions, and in situations where toxicity is enhanced by diminished drug elimination. Examples of diminished blood elimination include the retention of methotrexate in subjects with renal impairment, and diminished degradation of azathioprine or 6-mercaptopurine by concurrent administration of the xanthine oxidase inhibitor, allopurinol.

Myelodysplastic disorders can present with pancytopenia (p. 258). They are a heterogeneous group of haematological neoplastic conditions which do not fulfil the criteria of leukaemia, although the percentage of blast cells in some forms is above normal in the bone marrow, and blast cells may be present in the blood. Clinical examination can reveal enlargement of the liver or spleen, so that findings of this nature coupled with blasts in the blood film readily distinguish this condition from aplastic anaemia. Definition of the type of myelodysplastic syndrome is usually established by bone marrow examination, in which the usual cellular or hypercellular picture differentiates it from aplastic anaemia, and the constitution of the cell population usually, but not always, readily differentiates it from acute leukaemia (Bennett *et al.* 1982).

Bone marrow infiltration or replacement. Pancytopenia is occasionally present on presentation with *lymphoma*, either due to bone marrow infiltration in advanced stage disease, or to hypersplenism because of enlargement of the spleen. In most instances the biopsy of an enlarged, readily accessible lymph node establishes the nature of the disorder, although sometimes there is no palpable lymphadenopathy or detectable enlargement of the liver or spleen. The presence of lymphoma may be suggested by the presence of constitutional symptoms, such as fever, night sweats, malaise, and pruritus, or because of radiologically demonstrable mediastinal or hilar lymphadenopathy. It is often difficult to establish a diagnosis of Hodgkin's disease or non-Hodgkin's lymphoma of the nodular or large cell varieties by marrow *aspiration* when the bone marrow is infiltrated by these disorders. The *trephine biopsy* is more helpful, as it is far more likely to contain diagnostic material which is difficult to obtain by aspiration. *Waldenström's macroglobulinaemia* (p. 310) is relatively commonly associated with a clinical picture similar to that of advanced stage, well-differentiated non-Hodgkin's lymphoma, and may likewise be accompanied by pancytopenia due to bone marrow infiltration.

Multiple myeloma presents relatively frequently with pancytopenia, although the depression of the blood cell counts is usually only moderate in degree. Distinguishing features are a paraprotein on serum or urine protein electrophoresis, lytic lesions or osteoporosis in bone, and Bence Jones protein in urine. A histological diagnosis is usually established by examination of the bone marrow, which typically reveals an absolute increase in plasma cells, often with atypical morphological features (p. 304).

Infiltration of the bone marrow with *metastatic cancer* is a rare cause of pancytopenia, and is usually accompanied by a *leuco-erythroblastic* blood picture, where a relatively small proportion of the nucleated cells consist of erythroblasts and granulocyte precursors. Another infiltrative disorder of the bone marrow associated with pancytopenia and a *leuco-erythroblastic* blood film is *myelofibrosis* (p. 334). There is usually marked poikilocytosis with tear-shaped red cells and, almost inevitably, splenomegaly in myelofibrosis. The diagnosis in this condition, and in metastatic cancer of the bone, is best established by trephine biopsy of the bone marrow, as aspiration usually fails to obtain particles of bone marrow in myelofibrosis.

Hypersplenism usually causes relatively mild pancytopenia, and should be considered in any subject with splenomegaly (p. 348). In the absence of complicating factors, the bone marrow contains normal cellular elements which are usually increased in cellularity.

Megaloblastosis due to vitamin B_{12} or folic acid deficiency can, in the extreme case, cause potentially fatal pancytopenia. The blood film usually contains oval macrocytic red cells and hypersegmented neutrophils. Diagnosis is nearly always established by examination of the bone marrow, which is usually hypercellular and contains characteristic megaloblastic erythroid and granulocyte precursors, although on rare occasions the bone marrow is hypocellular.

Systemic lupus erythematosus is often accompanied by minor degrees of pancytopenia (Michael *et al.* 1951). Moderate anaemia is common and is usually of the type associated with chronic inflammation, although auto-antibody-mediated haemolytic anaemia is occasionally the cause. Mild leucopenia is also common, but the leucocyte count rarely falls below $2 \times 10^9/l$. Marked depression of the platelet count is more common than severe anaemia or leucopenia, and is usually mediated by autoimmune destruction of platelets. Examination of the bone marrow usually reveals relatively cellular tissue without abnormal cells, which excludes aplastic anaemia and infiltration by malignant processes. Arthralgia, skin rashes, and other clinical features of systemic lupus erythematosus may be present, and the diagnosis is confirmed by increased DNA-binding capacity or antinuclear antibody levels in the serum.

Paroxysmal nocturnal haemoglobinuria may present with pancytopenia in which haemolysis may be an inconspicuous feature. The diagnosis of this uncommon condition is indicated by increased susceptibility of red cells to lysis in isotonic sucrose or in the Ham's acid–serum test (p. 200).

Overwhelming infection can produce pancytopenia, and therefore is not immediately distinguishable on clinical grounds from aplastic anaemia in which sepsis has developed as a consequence of inadequate neutrophil production. Bone marrow examination is capable of differentiating between these conditions, as the cellularity is greater in the former situation, even though the more mature cells of the neutrophil series tend to be depleted. Disseminated tuberculosis is a less fulminant cause of pancytopenia of this type, and is readily overlooked unless bone marrow is subjected to Ziehl–Nielsen staining and culture for mycobacteria.

References and further reading

Alter, B.P., Potter, N.U. & Li, F.P. (1978) Classification and aetiology of the aplastic anemias. *Clin. Haematol.* **7**, 431.

Bennett, J.M., Catovsky, D., Daniel, M.T. *et al.* (1982) Proposals for the classification of the myelodysplastic syndromes. *Brit. J. Haemat.* **51**, 189.

Best, W. (1967) Chloramphenicol-associated blood dyscrasias, a review of cases submitted to the registry. *J. Am. Med. Ass.* **210**, 99.

Bithell, T.C. & Wintrobe, M.M. (1967) Drug-induced aplastic anaemia. *Semin. Haemat.* **4**, 194. (This article lists references to original papers describing toxic marrow reactions to many of the drugs listed in Table 6.3.)

Champlin, R., Ho, W. & Gale, R.P. (1983) Antithymocyte globulin treatment in patients with aplastic anaemia. *New Engl. J. Med.* **308**, 113.

Champlin, R., Feig, S., Sparkes, R. *et al.* (1984) Bone marrow transplantation from identical twins in the treatment of aplastic anaemia: implication for the pathogenesis of the disease. *Brit. J. Haemat.* **56**. 455.

Diamond, L.K. & Blackfan, K.E. (1938) Hypoplastic anaemia. *Am. J. Dis. Child.* **56**, 464.

Clark, D.A., Dessypris, E.N. & Krantz, S.B. (1984) Studies on pure red cell aplasia. XI. Results of immunosuppressive treatment of 37 patients. *Blood*, **63**, 277.

Ellims, P.H., van der Weyden, M.B., Brodie, G.N. *et al.* (1979) Erythroleukemia following drug induced hypoplastic anaemia. *Cancer*, **44**, 2140.

Firkin, F.C. (1972a) Serum lysozyme in haematological disorders: diagnostic value in neoplastic states. *Austr. N.Z. J. Med.* **1**, 28.

Firkin, F.C. (1972b) Mitochondrial lesions in reversible erythropoietic depression due to chloramphenicol. *J. Clin. Invest.* **51**, 2085.

Firkin, F.C. & Moore, M.A.S. (1978) Atypical phenylbutazone sensitivity of marrow colony forming units in phenylbutazone-induced aplastic anaemia. In: *Aplastic Anaemia*, University of Tokyo Press, Tokyo.

Grumet, F.C. & Yankee, R.A. (1970) Long-term platelet support of patients with aplastic anaemia. Effect of splenectomy and steroid therapy. *Ann. Int. Med.* **73**, 1.

Hirst, E. & Robertson, T.I. (1967) The syndrome of thymoma and erythroblastopenic anaemia. *Medicine*, **46**, 225.

Howell, A., Andrews, T. & Watts, R. (1975) Bone marrow cells resistant to chloramphenicol in chloramphenicol-induced aplastic anaemia. *Lancet*, **i**, 65.

Lee, C.H., Firkin, F.C., Grace, C.S. *et al.* (1978) Pure red cell aplasia: A report of three cases with studies on circulating toxic factors against erythroid precursors. *Austr. N.Z. J. Med.* **8**, 75.

Lewis, S.M. & Dacie, J.V. (1967) The aplastic anaemia-paroxysmal nocturnal haemoglobinuria syndrome. *Brit. J. Haemat.* **13**, 236.

Lynch, R.E., Williams, D.M., Reading, J.C. *et al.* (1975) The prognosis in aplastic anaemia. *Blood*, **45**, 517.

McLean, J.A. (1960) Blood dyscrasia after contact with petrol containing benzol. *Med. J. Austr.* **2**, 845.

Michael, S.R., Vural, I.L., Bassen, F.A. *et al.* (1951) The hematological aspects of disseminated (systemic) lupus erythematosus. *Blood*, **6**, 1059.

O'Reilly, R.J. (1983) Allogeneic bone marrow transplantation: current status and future directions. *Blood*, **62**, 941.

Sanchez-Medal, L., Pizzuto, J., Terre-Lorez, E. *et al.* (1964) Effect of oxymetholone in refractory anaemia. *Arch. Int. Med.* **113**, 721.

Scott, J.L., Cartwright, G.E. & Wintrobe, M.M. (1959) Acquired aplastic anaemia: an analysis of thirty-nine cases and review of the pertinent literature. *Medicine*, **39**, 119.

Scott, J.L., Finegold, S.M. Belkin, G.A. *et al.* (1965) A controlled doubled-blind study of the hematological toxicity of chloramphenicol. *New Engl. J. Med.* **27**, 1137.

Silink, S.J. & Firkin, B.G. (1968) An analysis of hypoplastic anaemia with special reference to the use of oxymetholone ('Adroyd') in its therapy. *Austr. Ann. Med.* **17**, 224.

Storb, R., Thomas, E.D., Buckner, C.D. *et al.* (1984) Marrow transplantation for aplastic anemia. *Semin. Hematol.* **21**, 27.

Vincent, P.C. & de Gruchy, G.C. (1967) Complications and treatment of acquired aplastic anaemia. *Brit. J. Haemat.* **13**, 977.

Wallerstein, R.D., Condit, P.K., Kasper, C.K. *et al.* (1969) Statewide study of chloramphenicol therapy and fatal aplastic anaemia. *J. Am. Med. Ass.* **208**, 2045.

Yunis, A.A. & Bloomberg, G.R. (1964) Chloramphenicol toxicity. *Prog. Hematol.* **4**, 138.

Chapter 7
Disorders of Haemoglobin Structure and Synthesis

The hereditary disorders of haemoglobin may be classified into two broad groups, the haemoglobinopathies and the thalassaemias. The *haemoglobinopathies* are characterized by the production of structurally defective haemoglobin due to abnormalities in the formation of the globin moiety of the molecule. The *thalassaemias* are characterized by a reduced rate of production of normal haemoglobin due to absent or decreased synthesis of one or more types of globin polypeptide chains.

The geographical distribution of the hereditary disorders of haemoglobin is shown in Fig. 7.1. It can be seen that the thalassaemias are widespread, with maximum prevalence around the Mediterranean littoral and in south-east Asia. The common abnormal haemoglobins, Hb-S and Hb-C are prevalent in tropical Africa and among Black populations in the New World. Hb-E is common in south-east Asia, and Hb-D Punjab in the Indian subcontinent. Hereditary disorders of haemoglobin are less common among people of northern European origin, but no ethnic group is totally spared.

In this chapter, the structure of haemoglobin is reviewed before the haemoglobinopathies and the thalassaemias are described.

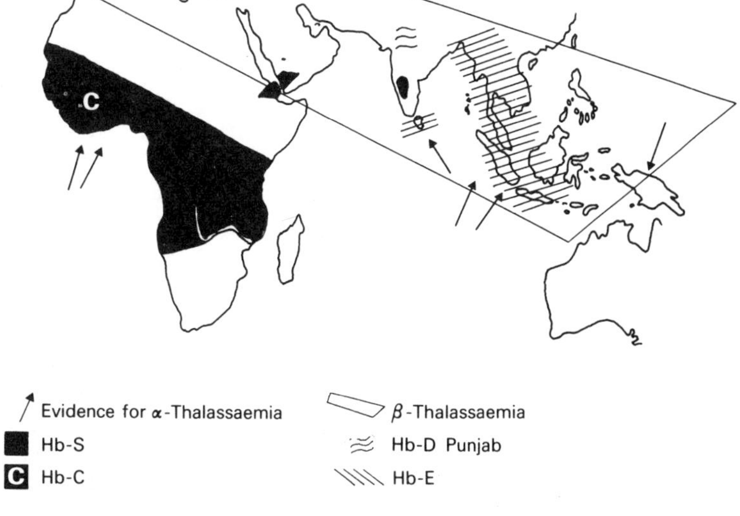

Fig. 7.1. *Geographical distribution of the clinically important haemoglobinopathies and the thalassaemias (prepared by Professor H. Lehmann; from Wintrobe et al. 1981).*

Normal haemoglobin

Haemoglobin is a conjugated protein of molecular weight 64 000, consisting of two pairs of polypeptide chains to each of which a haem is attached. Human haemoglobin exists in a number of types, which differ slightly in the structure of their globin moiety. However, the haem is identical in all types.

Haemoglobin types (Table 7.1)

Haemoglobin A (Hb-A) comprises about 97 per cent of the haemoglobin of adult red cells. It consists of two alpha (α) and two beta (β) chains with the structural formula $\alpha_2\beta_2$. The α chain contains 141 amino acids, and the β chain, 146. Small amounts of Hb-A are detected in the fetus as early as the eighth week of life. During the first few months of post-natal life, Hb-A almost completely replaces Hb-F, and the adult pattern is fully established by six months.

Haemoglobin A_2 (Hb-A_2) is the minor haemoglobin in the adult red cell. It has the structural formula of $\alpha_2\delta_2$, the delta (δ) chain containing 146 amino acids. The α chain is identical to that of Hb-A. Hb-A_2 is present in very small amounts at birth and reaches the adult level of 1.5–3.2 per cent during the first year of life. Elevation of Hb-A_2 is a feature of some types of thalassaemia and occasionally occurs in megaloblastic anaemia and unstable haemoglobin disease. Hb-A_2 may be reduced in iron deficiency.

Haemoglobin F (Hb-F) is the major respiratory pigment from early intra-uterine life up to term. It has the structural formula $\alpha_2\gamma_2$, each gamma (γ) chain consisting of 146 amino acids. The γ chains are designated $^G\gamma$ or $^A\gamma$ depending on whether they have glycine or alanine at position 136. At term, Hb-F accounts for 70–90 per cent of the total haemoglobin. It then falls rapidly to 25 per cent at 1 month, and 5 per cent at 6 months. The adult level of about one per cent is not reached in some children until puberty. Hb-F is elevated in some haemoglobinopathies and thalassaemia syndromes. It may be elevated in occasional cases of congenital and acquired aplastic anaemia, megaloblastic anaemia, paroxysmal nocturnal haemoglobinuria, sideroblastic anaemia, and in some forms of leukaemia. It is also occasionally raised in early pregnancy. The acid elution test (p. 141) indicates that Hb-F is unevenly distributed in the red cells in these conditions. Hb-F is measured by the alkali denaturation technique (p. 141). Weatherall *et al.* (1974) provide a more comprehensive list of hereditary and acquired conditions associated with raised Hb-F.

Hb-Gower 1 and *Hb-Gower 2* are confined to the embryonic stage of development. They contain epsilon (ε) and zeta (ζ) chains, Hb-Gower 1 being $\zeta_2\varepsilon_2$ and Hb-Gower 2, $\alpha_2\varepsilon_2$. *Hb-Portland* is found in trace amounts throughout intra-uterine life and in neonates. It has the structural formula $\zeta_2\gamma_2$. *Hb-Bart's* (p. 155) is also found in small amounts in cord blood if sensitive techniques are used. Both Hb-Portland and Hb-Bart's are increased in the cord blood of neonates with α-thalassaemia.

Table 7.1. *Normal human haemoglobins*

	Haemoglobin	Structural formula
Adult		
	Hb-A	$\alpha_2\beta_2$
	Hb-A_2	$\alpha_2\delta_2$
Fetal		
	Hb-F	$\alpha_2\gamma_2$
	Hb-Bart's	γ_4
Embryonic		
	Hb-Gower 1	$\zeta_2\epsilon_2$
	Hb-Gower 2	$\alpha_2\epsilon_2$
	Hb-Portland	$\zeta_2\gamma_2$

Haemoglobin structure

The structure of the haemoglobin molecule may be viewed at four levels of organizational complexity. The basic arrangement of linked amino acids forming four polypeptide chains, each attached to a haem molecule, is the primary structure. Each chain is arranged in a series of eight helical segments joined by short non-helical segments. Eighty per cent of the total length of each chain is in helical conformation, and this is referred to as the secondary structure.

The folding of each coiled chain into a specific

three-dimensional configuration is the tertiary structure. The four folded chains fit closely together to form a compact tetrameric molecule known as the quaternary structure. Each haem molecule is enclosed in a pocket by the folds of the chain. The integrity of the chains and their spatial relationships to each other and to the haem molecule are critical in the maintenance of stability of the molecule (p. 152) and its ability to transport oxygen (p. 153) (Perutz 1978).

Genetic regulation

Each individual receives one or more genes from each parent for each of the four major haemoglobin chains. β and δ chain synthesis are each under the control of single genes, but the gene loci of α and γ chains are duplicated.

Recent advances in molecular biology (Weatherall 1982) have greatly increased our knowledge of the fine structure of the human globin gene complex. The chromosomal organization of the α and β gene complexes is depicted in Fig. 7.2. The α gene complex is situated on the short arm of chromosome 16 and includes the duplicated α genes (α_1 and α_2), a non-functional pseudo-α gene ($\psi\alpha_1$) and two ζ genes, one of which is probably non-functional. The non-α gene complex is situated on the short arm of chromosome 11 and includes the β and δ genes, the duplicated γ genes ($^G\gamma$ and $^A\gamma$), the ε gene and a non-functional pseudo-β gene ($\psi\beta_1$). The DNA sequences of all the human globin genes have now been determined. Current concepts of globin gene structure are reviewed by Antonarakis *et al.* (1985).

Synthesis. The genetic information that directs the synthesis of individual globin chains in erythroblasts is encoded in the nucleotide base sequence of the corresponding gene DNA, each triplet codon of three nucleotide bases specifying a single amino acid. Each gene consists of regions (referred to as exons) that code for globin messenger RNA (mRNA) and other non-coding 'intervening sequences' (introns). Within the nucleus, the gene is transcribed into a large mRNA precursor from which the transcripts of the 'intervening sequences' are then removed by an enzymatic process called splicing. The modified mRNA moves to the cytoplasm where it combines with ribosomes and is translated into the globin chain.

Abnormal haemoglobins and the haemoglobinopathies

Many abnormal haemoglobins have been described. Each arises from a mutation affecting the gene directing the structure of a particular pair of polypeptide chains, and they are classified as α-, β-, γ- or δ-chain variants depending on the chains involved. The mutant gene is situated at the same

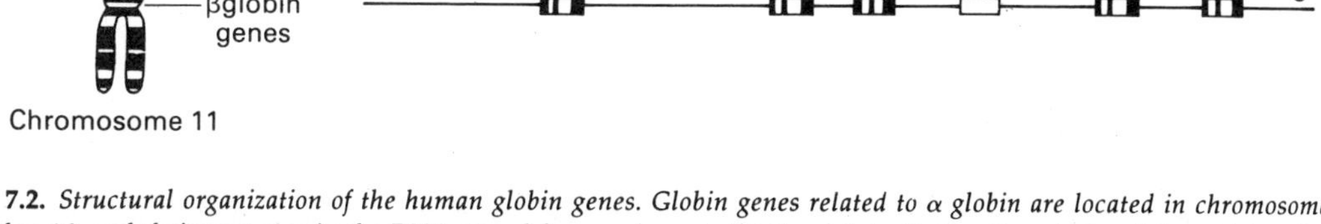

Fig. 7.2. *Structural organization of the human globin genes. Globin genes related to α globin are located in chromosomes number 16, and their sequence in the DNA strand from embryonic (ζ) through ineffective 'pseudo-gene' forms (ψ) to the two distinct adult (α) genes is illustrated. The corresponding sequence of the β-related globin genes on chromosomes number 11 from the embryonic ($\in$) through fetal (γ) and δ to adult β globin genes is also illustrated.*

chromosomal locus as (i.e. is an allele of) the normal gene controlling production of the corresponding normal chain.

When the possession of a haemoglobin variant gives rise to a clearly defined disease state, the affected person is said to have a haemoglobinopathy. It is important to appreciate, however, that the great majority of abnormal haemoglobins confer no harmful effect, and the individual remains asymptomatic and unaware of the abnormality within the red cell.

Types of structural abnormality (Table 7.2)

The majority of abnormal haemoglobins differ from the corresponding normal haemoglobin by the substitution of a single amino acid in one of their pairs of polypeptide chains. A small number have double amino-acid substitutions, and others have deletions of amino acids. At least eight abnormal haemoglobins have elongated chains, and the non-α chains of Hb-Lepore contain part of the δ- and part of the β-chain sequences. Finally, some haemoglobins have four identical polypeptide chains. A register of abnormal haemoglobins is kept by the International Hemoglobin Information Center and published regularly in the journal *Hemoglobin.*

Genetic regulation

Abnormal haemoglobins are inherited as autosomal co-dominants. Thus, subjects who inherit one normal and one abnormal gene are heterozygotes, and those who have two identical abnormal genes are homozygotes. Double heterozygotes are subjects who have inherited two different abnormal genes. The homozygous state is usually referred to as the 'disease' (e.g. the homozygous state for Hb-C is 'Hb-C disease'), and the heterozygous state as the 'trait' (e.g. 'Hb-C trait'). This rule has some exceptions, however. For example, unstable haemoglobin 'disease' is a reflection of a heterozygous state.

Each group of chain variants and the disorders associated with them have some common characteristics.

Beta-chain variant haemoglobins. Beta chains take part in the formation of Hb-A only, and thus β-chain variants are all variants of Hb-A. Heterozygous subjects synthesize both normal and abnormal β chains, and the abnormal haemoglobin is usually about 30–40 per cent of the total. Homozygous subjects synthesize the abnormal haemoglobin and the normal small amounts of Hb-A_2, but no normal β chains and thus no normal Hb-A. Heterozygotes for two β-chain variants have equal amounts of the two abnormal haemoglobins and a small amount of Hb-A_2 in their red cells. As β-chain synthesis commences in intra-uterine life, β-chain variants may be detected in the fetus. Clinical effects from the abnormal haemoglobin do not occur until after birth when γ-chain synthesis falls to a low level. The majority of abnormal haemoglobins are β-chain substitutions, and about 200 such variants have been described.

Alpha-chain variant haemoglobins. Alpha chains are involved in the formation of Hb-A, Hb-A_2, and Hb-F, and thus α-chain substitutions affect all these haemoglobins. Adult heterozygotes for α-chain variants produce both normal and abnormal Hb-A, Hb-F and Hb-A_2, the abnormal types having abnormal α chains in addition to the normal β, γ and δ chains. The major haemoglobin variant (the Hb-A variant) ranges from 15 to 45 per cent of the total haemoglobin in the red cell. About 100 α-chain variants have been described.

Table 7.2. *The common abnormal haemoglobins*

Haemoglobin	Structural formula
Hb-S	$\alpha_2\beta_2{}^{6\ \mathrm{glu} \rightarrow \mathrm{val}}$
Hb-C	$\alpha_2\beta_2{}^{6\ \mathrm{glu} \rightarrow \mathrm{lys}}$
Hb-E	$\alpha_2\beta_2{}^{26\ \mathrm{glu} \rightarrow \mathrm{lys}}$
Hb-D Punjab	$\alpha_2\beta_2{}^{121\ \mathrm{glu} \rightarrow \mathrm{gln}}$

Nomenclature

The abnormal haemoglobin of sickle-cell disease was first demonstrated in 1949. It was called Hb-S, but subsequent abnormal haemoglobins were allotted letters of the alphabet from C to Q. This system was seen to be inadequate, and it was decided that each new haemoglobin should be allotted a common name, usually the laboratory, hospital, town or district where the haemoglobin was found (e.g. Hb-Zurich, Hb-Kempsey), and a scientific name. The latter specifies the variant chain, the number of the abnormal amino acid, its helical position, and the nature of the substitution. Thus, Hb-S is $\beta^{6(A3)\ \mathrm{glu}\rightarrow\mathrm{val}}$.

In the event of a new haemoglobin having the same electrophoretic mobility as an already recognized variant, yet differing in amino-acid sequence, the new haemoglobin is identified by the letter of the older variant followed by the name of the abnormal chain and the place of discovery (e.g. Hb-Jα Oxford). Thus, there are several haemoglobins referred to as Hb-D and Hb-J. In practice, the name of the chain is often omitted (e.g. Hb-J Oxford) (Editorial Board, *Hemoglobin* 1979).

The haemoglobinopathies are often described in terms of phenotype, the haemoglobins being listed in order of decreasing concentration regardless of genetic considerations. Thus, sickle-cell trait is designated AS, and homozygous sickle-cell disease SS. The clinically important abnormal haemoglobins are listed in Table 7.2.

Laboratory diagnosis

Although definitive identification of an abnormal haemoglobin usually requires an array of sophisticated biochemical techniques, the initial investigation of the haemoglobinopathies is well within the scope of most routine clinical laboratories. The clinical findings, the patient's ethnic origin and family history, and preliminary haematological studies suggest the diagnosis, and haemoglobin electrophoresis demonstrates the presence of an abnormal haemoglobin. Other simple laboratory tests based on physicochemical properties of some abnormal haemoglobins, e.g. the sickle test, may permit a presumptive diagnosis at this point. Final definitive identification of the abnormal haemoglobin usually requires the assistance of a reference laboratory. The laboratory diagnosis of the haemoglobinopathies is discussed in detail by Huisman (1986).

Routine haematological and biochemical tests. Mandatory initial diagnostic tests are determination of the haemoglobin level, packed cell volume, red cell count and red cell indices, preferably by means of an electronic cell counter, together with a reticulocyte count and examination of a stained blood film by an experienced observer. Bilirubin estimation and other biochemical tests for the presence of haemolysis should also be performed.

Tests depending on physicochemical properties of abnormal haemoglobins. Tests of this type include the sickle test, the haemoglobin solubility test (Hb-S), the demonstration of intracellular haemoglobin crystals (Hb-C), Hb-H inclusions (α-thalassaemia) and Heinz bodies, the heat instability test and isopropanol precipitation test (the unstable haemoglobins), and oxygen dissociation studies (the high oxygen-affinity haemoglobins). These tests are described more fully under the relevant haemoglobinopathies.

Haemoglobin electrophoresis. Haemoglobin electrophoresis is the most useful method for the demonstration of abnormal haemoglobins. The haemoglobins are separated on a variety of supporting media on the basis of electric charge differences. Cellulose acetate electrophoresis at pH 8.6 is the method of choice in most clinical laboratories. Agar gel electrophoresis using a citrate buffer at pH 6.0 is useful in supplementing (but not replacing) the information gained from other methods, as the mobility of some abnormal haemoglobins on agar gel differs from that on other supporting media. The electrophoretic mobility of the commonly encountered normal and abnormal haemoglobins on cellulose acetate and agar gel is schematically depicted in Fig. 7.3. Further details of electrophoretic techniques may be obtained from Dacie & Lewis (1984).

Alkali denaturation. Hb-F is resistant to denaturation by alkali, and in clinical practice is estimated by the alkali denaturation technique. This test measures the percentage of alkali-resistant pigment remaining after exposure to alkali under standard conditions. Values over 2.5 per cent in adult subjects are regarded as elevated (Betke *et al.* 1959).

The acid elution test. Red cells containing Hb-F resist elution at an acid pH to a greater extent than do normal cells containing Hb-A. The acid elution or Kleihauer test (Kleihauer *et al.* 1957) makes use of

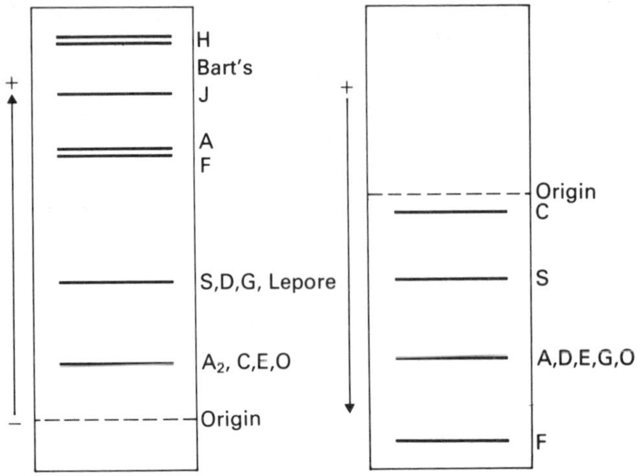

Fig 7.3. *Schematic representation of electrophoretic mobility of normal and some of the more common abnormal haemoglobins on cellulose acetate at pH 8.6 (left) and agar gel at pH 6.0 (right).*

this phenomenon to permit the cytochemical assessment of the Hb-F content of individual cells.

The sickle haemoglobinopathies

The sickle haemoglobinopathies are hereditary disorders in which the red cells contain Hb-S. They include the heterozygous (sickle-cell trait) and the homozygous (SS disease) states for Hb-S, and conditions in which Hb-S is combined with other haemoglobin structural variants or thalassaemia. In the deoxygenated state, the solubility of Hb-S is ten per cent of that of Hb-A. The conformational changes in Hb-S induced by deoxygenation cause the cells containing the abnormal haemoglobin to become rigid and deformed, assuming a sickle or crescent shape (Fig. 7.4).

The sickling of red cells in the circulating blood has two major pathological effects: (i) the distorted and rigid cells block small blood vessels, impairing flow and causing ischaemia and infarction; and (ii) repeated 'sickle–unsickle' cycles lead to loss of

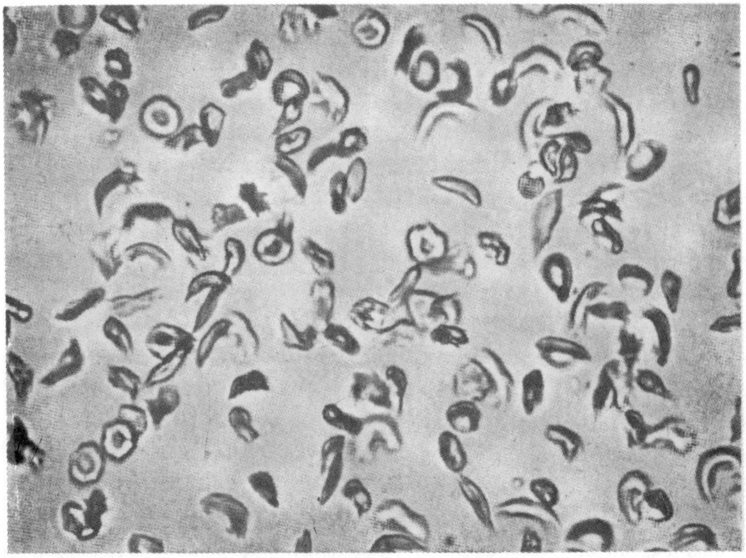

Fig. 7.4. *Sickle-cell preparation.*

fragments of red cell membrane, and the cells become spherocytic and fragile. They are removed prematurely by the reticulo-endothelial system, and to a lesser extent destroyed in the circulation resulting in both extravascular and intravascular haemolysis.

Hb-S differs from Hb-A in the substitution of valine for glutamic acid in the sixth position from the N-terminal end of the β chain. The precise mechanism by which this seemingly minor change in amino-acid sequence leads to such an important rearrangement of the molecule on deoxygenation is not known with certainty. Electron microscopy of sickle cells has shown bundles of long tubular fibres parallel to the long axis of the cell which are presumed to be of sufficient rigidity to distort the cell membrane. Each fibre consists of 14 or possibly 16 spirally-wound filaments, the filaments being composed of Hb-S molecules like beads on a string (Eaton & Hofrichter 1987).

Red cells containing large amounts of Hb-S begin to sickle at an oxygen tension of 50–60 mmHg. This tension is experienced by the cells in parts of the microcirculation, and thus sickling occurs *in vivo*. If the flow rate is rapid, sickling does not become fully established and the cells resume normal shape when they are swept back to areas of the circulation where the oxygen tension is higher. If the flow rate is slow, and the cells are delayed in areas where the oxygen tension is low, the cells sickle and there is further slowing of the circulation. Oxygen tension is further reduced, additional sickle cells accumulate, and finally complete blockage of the vessel occurs. Tissue ischaemia resulting from such vessel blockage is the basis of the painful crises that are a major clinical feature of the sickling disorders.

Several factors influence the degree of deoxygenation required to produce sickling of red cells containing Hb-S.

The amount of Hb-S in the red cell is clearly of importance as the cells of a patient with sickle-cell trait which contain less than 50 per cent Hb-S are less likely to sickle at a particular level of deoxygenation than the cells of a patient with homozygous sickle cell disease which contain nearly 100 per cent Hb-S.

The physical properties of the haemoglobin with which Hb-S is associated in the red cell may increase or decrease the liability of the Hb-S to sickle. Hb-C and Hb-D potentiate sickling, and patients heterozygous for these haemoglobins and Hb-S have moderately severe sickling disorder. Hb-F has the opposite effect and tends to diminish sickling (Noguchi *et al.* 1988).

Red cells of patients with homozygous sickle cell disease have a *reduced oxygen affinity*, and the oxygen dissociation curve of the blood is shifted to the right. Although this phenomenon assists the release of oxygen at the tissue level, it also results in the occurrence of sickling at a higher oxygen tension than would be the case if the dissociation curve was normal. Acidosis shifts the curve further to the right and similarly enhances the sickling process.

The packed cell volume and proportion of red cells containing Hb-S are also important in determining the increase in blood viscosity resulting from a fall in oxygen tension.

The sickle gene is the result of a point mutation in the codon for the sixth amino acid of the β globin chain, and is inherited as a Mendelian co-dominant. It occurs mainly in Blacks or persons with an admixture of Black blood, and is thus seen frequently in Africa and amongst Black populations in North and South America and the West Indies. It is also found in certain localities in Greece, southern Italy, Turkey, the Middle East, and India. The sickle gene is believed to confer some protection against *Plasmodium falciparum* malaria, and its geographical distribution is in accordance with this concept. The following sickle haemoglobinopathies are prevalent in communities where the sickle gene is found—sickle-cell trait, homozygous sickle-cell disease, sickle-cell thalassaemia, and sickle-cell Hb-C disease.

Laboratory diagnosis

SICKLE TEST

Red cells containing Hb-S take on a sickle shape when mixed with a freshly prepared solution of the reducing agent, sodium metabisulphite. The test is simple to perform, and detects both homozygotes and heterozygotes for the sickle gene.

HAEMOGLOBIN SOLUBILITY TESTS

The basis of these tests is the relative insolubility of reduced Hb-S in concentrated phosphate buffer. In practice, the haemoglobin is added to a solution of sodium dithionite, a reducing agent, in phosphate buffer. If Hb-S is present, the solution becomes turbid. Whole blood may be used, but the addition of saponin, a lysing agent, then becomes necessary. Several commercial kit tests are available, but many laboratories prepare their own reagents and the test may be automated. Homozygotes and heterozygotes for the sickle gene are detected. The simplified solubility tests using whole blood are marginally easier to perform than the sickle test, and are now widely used. The reagents must be freshly prepared, and a positive and negative control processed with the test sample.

HAEMOGLOBIN ELECTROPHORESIS

Although the sickle and haemoglobin solubility tests detect the presence of Hb-S, haemoglobin electrophoresis is mandatory for precise diagnosis of the sickle haemoglobinopathies. Hb-S may be demonstrated by electrophoresis on cellulose acetate at pH 8.6 in a position between Hb-A and Hb-A_2 (see Fig. 7.3). Although nearly 50 haemoglobin variants have a similar mobility to Hb-S, the only practical problem of any frequency caused by identical mobilities is the differentiation of homozygous sickle-cell disease from sickle-cell Hb-D disease. Red cells from patients with both conditions sickle, and as Hb-S and Hb-D migrate in the same position on cellulose acetate, the two diseases appear to be identical. The problem may be resolved by electrophoresis in agar gel at pH 6.0. On this medium, Hb-S and Hb-D separate widely. Thus, a two-band pattern on agar gel would confirm sickle-cell Hb-D disease, and a one-band pattern homozygous sickle-cell disease. The difficulty of differentiating the electrophoretic pattern of some cases of sickle-cell β thalassaemia from homozygous sickle-cell disease is discussed on page 150. The haemoglobin patterns of the haemoglobinopathies due to Hb-S are listed in Table 7.3.

Antenatal diagnosis of the sickle haemoglobinopathies is discussed on p. 161.

Sickle-cell trait

Sickle-cell trait, the asymptomatic carrier state for Hb-S, occurs in about eight per cent of American Blacks. In Africa, its prevalence rate in many populations is over 20 per cent, and reaches 50 per cent in some tribes. Sickle-cell trait is the *heterozygous state* for the Hb-S gene. Hb-S comprises

Table 7.3. *The Hb-S disorders: electrophoretic phenotypes*

	Haemoglobin (%)			
Disorder	A	A_2	F	S
Sickle-cell trait (AS)	55–70	2–4	N	38–45
Homozygous sickle-cell disease (SS)	0	2–5	1–20	75–95
Sickle-cell β thalassaemia				
S-β^+	10–30	4–8	2–10	60–85
S-β^0	0	4–8	5–30	70–90
S-HPFH	0	N	18–30	60–90
Sickle-cell Hb-C disease (SC)	0	35–50 $(C+A_2)$*	1–5	50–65
Sickle-cell Hb-D diesase (SD)	0	N	1–5	95(S+D)*
Sickle-cell trait α thalassaemia trait	65–75	N	N	20–30

*Hb-C cannot be separated from Hb-A_2, and Hb-D cannot be separated from Hb-S, on routine cellulose acetate electrophoresis. The electrophoretic phenotypes of the haemoglobinopathies associated with other abnormal haemoglobins follow the same general pattern as detailed for Hb-S. The above data are taken from papers quoted in the text and should be regarded as approximate only. N = normal; HPFH = hereditary persistence of fetal haemoglobin.

38–45 per cent of the total haemoglobin, the rest being Hb-A, Hb-A_2 and Hb-F (see Table 7.3). The cells do not contain sufficient Hb-S to undergo sickling at the lowest oxygen tension normally occurring in the body, and the red cell lifespan is normal. In the stained blood film, no sickle cells are present and the red cells appear normal. The MCV and MCH are also normal. However, sickling can readily be demonstrated by the sickle test, and the haemoglobin solubility test is positive. If the patient has concurrent α thalassaemia, the red cells are microcytic with a mild reduction in MCV and a Hb-S concentration of less than 38 per cent (Felice *et al.* 1981).

Sickle-cell trait does not cause anaemia, and in general is asymptomatic. If anaemia is present, other causes, e.g. iron deficiency, should be sought. A high proportion of affected subjects show defects in urine concentrating ability, and haematuria is an occasional complication. Rare episodes of splenic infarction during flight at high altitude in non-pressurized aircraft have been described, and severe hypoxia resulting from administration of anaesthetic agents and other respiratory depressants may in exceptional cases be associated with *in vivo* sickling and serious thrombo-embolic sequelae. There is some evidence that sickle-cell trait is a risk factor for sudden death during unaccustomed exercise (Kark *et al.* 1987), but most epidemiological studies suggest that no selective morbidity or mortality is attributable to the condition.

Homozygous sickle-cell disease

In the *homozygous state* for the Hb-S gene, the patient receives one Hb-S gene from each parent, both of whom show sickle-cell trait. The probabilities for each child of such a union to have normal haemoglobin only, sickle-cell trait, or homozygous disease are 25 per cent, 50 per cent, and 25 per cent. Homozygous sickle-cell disease occurs in 0.1–1.3 per cent of the American Black population.

In contrast to sickle-cell trait, the red cells contain sufficient Hb-S for sickling to be produced *in vivo* by the reduction of oxygen tension that occurs in the capillaries. The *in vivo* sickling is responsible for the clinical manifestations of the disease. These are chronic haemolytic anaemia, organ damage, and episodes of pain. The clinical picture is variable, with symptoms referred to a number of systems; in general, these symptoms cause more distress than those due to the anaemia.

CLINICAL FEATURES

The diagnosis is usually, but not invariably, made in *childhood*, often before the age of two years. Clinical manifestations are infrequent in the first six months of life, the high Hb-F levels protecting the red cells from sickling. Early childhood is a particularly dangerous period. Until recently, many children died in the first seven years, and even now in some tropical countries mortality is heavy. *Bacterial infection* is the most common cause of the early morbidity and mortality. Pneumococcal meningitis or pneumonia rapidly progressing to overwhelming septicaemia account for many deaths. The reasons for the greatly increased susceptibility to infection with *pneumococcus, meningococcus, E. coli* or *Haemophilus influenzae* are not known with certainty. Loss of splenic function (see below) and defective opsonization due to abnormalities in the alternate pathway of complement activation are probably important. Other complications in childhood include the hand–foot syndrome and the splenic sequestration syndrome. The *hand–foot syndrome* (dactylitis) is due to micro-infarction of the medulla of the carpal and tarsal bones. Overlying skin on the dorsa of the hands and feet is tender and swollen, and the child is febrile. The lesions, which are often symmetrical, heal without therapy, but leave permanent radiological sequelae and frequently recur. The *splenic sequestration syndrome* is caused by sudden pooling of blood within the spleen, often with acute hypovolaemia and shock. The spleen enlarges rapidly, and death may occur if the condition is not promptly recognized and a blood transfusion given. The syndrome tends to recur but is unusual after the age of six years.

Splenomegaly is usually evident by six months of age, and the spleen remains enlarged throughout early childhood. The presence of blood-film changes usually found in splenectomized patients (e.g. Howell–Jolly bodies and target cells) and failure of the spleen to accumulate radioactive sulphur colloid which is taken up avidly by the normal spleen, indicates that, even at this stage, a state of functional asplenia exists. Blood transfusion temporarily improves these abnormalities, but repeated episodes of infarction eventually lead to atrophy and 'autosplenectomy'; by eight years of age, the spleen is no longer palpable and its function is permanently impaired.

In the adult, clinical severity is highly variable. In many patients the disease is severe with frequent hospital admissions and inexorable deterioration. This is not always the case, however, and it has only recently been fully appreciated that a significant number of adults with homozygous sickle-cell disease are able to lead relatively normal lives, punctuated by only occasional episodes of illness. The emergence of this group of patients seems partly related to improvements in socio-economic conditions, particularly in tropical countries, with improved diet and better access to proper medical care. Recent studies have suggested that the co-existence of α thalassaemia exerts a favourable effect on some clinical and haematological manifestations (Higgs *et al.* 1982). The level of Hb-F within individual red cells also seems to be an important factor. Homozygous sickle-cell disease in parts of Saudi Arabia and India is associated with elevated Hb-F and is typically a very mild disorder. Apart from these well-defined subgroups, however, a clear correlation between Hb-F level and clinical course has been difficult to establish in the majority of cases of homozygous sickle-cell disease. Steinberg & Hebbel (1983) review factors that may be important in modifying the severity of the disease.

Although nearly all patients are anaemic to a greater or lesser degree, many adapt well to the anaemia. The oxygen dissociation curve of the blood is shifted considerably to the right, and the low oxygen affinity facilitates unloading of oxygen from the red cells to the tissues (p. 143).

Sickle-cell crises are a characteristic feature of the disease and are responsible for much morbidity. Sickle-cell crises may be vaso-occlusive, aplastic or, rarely, haemolytic. *Vaso-occlusive crises* consist of sudden attacks of bone pain, usually in the limbs, joints, back and chest, or of abdominal pain. Precipitating factors include infection (particularly malaria in tropical countries), physical and emotional stress, and extremes of ambient temperature, but in many adult cases no cause is obvious. The abdominal pain is commonly severe and may simulate a variety of acute abdominal emergencies. Affected patients are often febrile with nausea and vomiting, the abdomen is tender and rigid, and there is a marked neutrophilia. The pain may last for only a few hours or persist for several days. Bone pain varies in severity from mild to extremely severe and is usually accompanied by fever and constitutional symptoms. The pain is due to ischaemia and infarction and, although X-rays of painful bones often fail to show any changes, abnormalities are frequently demonstrated by radio-isotope techniques (Milner & Brown 1982). Marrow aspiration may reveal infarcted haemopoietic tissue. Fat embolism is a rare but potentially fatal complication of marrow infarction, and should be considered in sickle-cell crisis when there is deterioration in respiratory function. The frequency and severity of vaso-occlusive crises usually diminish with increasing age.

Aplastic crises occur when there is sudden cessation of marrow erythropoiesis related, in most cases, to infection with human parvovirus. Haemolysis continues and the red cell mass rapidly diminishes to life-threatening levels. The reticulocyte count falls and erythroid precursors are no longer evident in the marrow. Erythropoiesis recommences in 7–10 days with a surge of reticulocytes and nucleated red cells in the peripheral blood. Some so-called aplastic crises result from the development of megaloblastosis due to folate deficiency rather than true aplasia. Less frequently, the rate of haemolysis increases with an accelerated fall in the level of haemoglobin. The possibility of associated glucose-6-phosphate dehydrogenase (G6PD) deficiency and drug-induced haemolysis should be considered in these cases.

Although large population studies (Platt *et al.* 1984) have shown that, compared with controls, patients with homozygous sickle-cell disease are shorter, weigh less and show delayed sexual maturation, many individuals with the disorder are well developed and of normal height.

Conjunctival icterus is common, and the liver is often moderately enlarged and sometimes tender, probably due to micro-infarction. Cholelithiasis is common. The spleen is usually not palpable in adults. Signs of a hyperdynamic circulation are evident, with cardiac enlargement and systolic ejection murmurs and thrills. In occasional older patients, pulmonary hypertension and right ventricular hypertrophy and failure predominate. Obstruction of cerebral vessels, both large and small, may cause neurological manifestations which vary with the site and extent of obstruction; the most serious is hemiplegia which most commonly occurs in children under the age of 15 years.

Repeated attacks of acute febrile *pulmonary disease* with pleuritic pain and infiltrates on chest X-ray are common; they may be due to either infarction or infection, and differential diagnosis is often difficult. Causes of pulmonary vascular occlusion include *in situ* thrombosis, emboli from pelvic or leg veins, and marrow or fat emboli from infarcted bone. Pneumococcus is cultured from the sputum in some cases, but evidence of bacterial infection is often not obtained in adults. Progressive *loss of renal function* occurs in many patients, the usual early manifestation being a defect in renal concentrating ability due to distal tubular damage. Infarction of the renal medulla may cause papillary necrosis and haematuria. Female patients experience frequent urinary tract infections, and albuminuria is a common finding. Examination of the bulbar conjunctiva shows many small engorged comma-shaped vessels in the superficial vascular network, which disappear following transfusion. Occlusion of peripheral retinal arterioles is followed by arteriolar–venular anastomoses and neovascular proliferation. Infarction of the peripheral retina causes scarring and pigmentation. Severe cases show retinal detachment, vitreous haemorrhage, and glaucoma (Armaly 1974).

Chronic leg ulcers are common; they usually occur on the medial surface of the tibia just above the ankle, may be single or multiple, and are sometimes bilateral. Other clinical features include hearing loss, finger clubbing and priapism.

Skeletal X-ray often shows rarefaction and cortical thinning, and reflects gross expansion of the medullary space due to erythroid hyperplasia. Avascular necrosis of the femoral or humoral head is an occasional result of repeated bone infarction, and may cause severe arthritis. Some patients show an increased susceptibility to osteomyelitis, especially with *Salmonella* organisms.

Female patients may have reduced fertility, but pregnancy occurs and is associated with a high degree of maternal morbidity and fetal wastage. Sickle-cell crises and infective complications, particularly involving the urinary tract, are common.

BLOOD PICTURE

Haemoglobin values of 6–9 g/dl are usual, but they may be lower, and an occasional patient has a normal value. The anaemia is mainly due to a reduction in red cell lifespan, the $T_{50}Cr$ being about eight days. In some young patients with grossly enlarged spleens, hypersplenism is an important mechanism of red cell destruction. There is little ineffective erythropoiesis. Exacerbation of the haemolytic process may cause a sudden fall in haemoglobin; a similar fall results from an aplastic crisis. The anaemia is usually normochromic and normocytic, with a normal MCV and MCH. If the patient also has α thalassaemia (p. 163), there is some degree of microcytosis and reduction in MCV and MCH.

The stained film shows moderate anisocytosis and varying degrees of poikilocytosis. The poikilocytes may vary from elongated cells with either rounded or sharp ends to typical sickle cells, small numbers of which are usually, but not invariably, present. Sickle cells that retain their deformed shape after reoxygenation are referred to as 'irreversibly sickled cells' (ISC), and their number tends to remain constant for a particular patient. ISC are dense dehydrated cells with a high specific gravity, low MCV, high MCHC, an increased content of calcium, and very little Hb-F. They have probably been subjected to many 'sickle–unsickle' cycles, with gradually increasing membrane damage and loss which finally prevents them from resuming normal shape on reoxygenation. They have a lifespan of about two days. ISC are rarely seen in infants and young children, appearing after the age of six years at about the time of 'autosplenectomy'.

Oval cells are common, and occasional target cells and Howell–Jolly bodies are present. Reticulocytes are increased, with counts ranging from 10 to 20 per cent, and a few nucleated red cells may be present. The polychromatic cells in the stained films are usually of normal shape. Serum bilirubin is moderately increased, values between 17 and 34 μmol/l being usual. Neutrophil leucocytosis with a shift to the left is common, counts ranging up to 20–30 $\times$ 10^9/l. The platelet count is normal or moderately raised. The sedimentation rate is slow, even with marked anaemia, as the abnormal shape of the sickle cells prevents rouleaux formation. Subnormal serum folate levels are frequent, and the red cell folate may also be low. Serum haptoglobin and haemopexin are decreased, and methaemalbumin and free haemoglobin may be detected in some patients.

The sickle test and haemoglobin solubility test are positive, and heterogeneous distribution of Hb-F within the red cells may be demonstrated by the acid elution test. The haemoglobin consists mainly of Hb-S with a variable increase of Hb-F up to about 20 per cent, and normal Hb-A_2. There is no Hb-A (see Table 7.3).

DIAGNOSIS

Diagnosis is based on the demonstration of a positive sickle test or a positive haemoglobin solubility test in a patient of high-risk ethnic origin with a chronic haemolytic anaemia and a history of painful crises. The screening tests should always be confirmed by a comprehensive electrophoretic analysis to exclude the presence of modifying factors, e.g. unusually high levels of Hb-F, α or β thalassaemia, or other haemoglobin structural variants. Sickle-cell β thalassaemia, in particular, may present diagnostic problems; differences in the electrophoretic pattern of the two conditions are discussed on p. 149. The presence or absence of splenomegaly may be useful in differential diagnosis. The enlarged spleen of the sickle-cell β-thalassaemic patient persists into adulthood, whereas the homozygous sickle-cell patient's spleen atrophies and becomes impalpable.

PROGNOSIS

The prognosis is serious in childhood, the expected death rate in North American Black patients during the first decade of life being ten per cent. Principal causes of death are infection, acute chest syndromes, and the splenic sequestration syndrome. The prognosis for patients who survive the early years is more favourable, and the expected death rate during decades after the first is less than five per cent. Some American patients now live beyond the fifth or sixth decade (Steinberg & Hebbel 1983). The outlook for the Black patient in North America is discussed by Powars (1975), in Jamaica by Thomas *et al.* (1982), and in Ghana by Konotey-Ahulu (1974). Unusually mild forms of homozygous sickle-cell disease occur in certain ethnic groups in India and the Middle East.

TREATMENT

The reduction in mortality and morbidity that has occurred in patients with homozygous sickle-cell disease in recent years has been due mainly to improvements in living standards rather than spectacular medical advances. Nevertheless, regular medical care, preferably in the setting of a special clinic, has an important role to play in the maintenance of good health. Most serious acute complications occur during childhood, and should always receive prompt and intensive treatment. Parents should be made aware of the fulminant nature of pneumococcal infection, and prophylactic penicillin and pneumococcal vaccination during the years of greatest risk are advisable (Gaston *et al.* 1986). Adult patients are generally well between crises and adjust satisfactorily to their reduced haemoglobin level. Attempts to raise the haemoglobin by regular transfusion may result in increased blood viscosity and are usually not desirable unless the anaemia is causing serious symptoms or the patient is severely incapacitated by recurring crises. In the very occasional patient with hypersplenism, splenectomy may result in an improvement in the haemoglobin level. Splenectomy may also be indicated in selected young patients with recurrent episodes of acute splenic sequestration. Because of the risk of a conditioned folate deficiency (p. 94), a maintenance dose of folic acid should be given if the dietary intake is inadequate. Regular ophthalmic examination is desirable to detect early retinal lesions.

Factors that promote sickling and predispose to crises should be avoided. These include hypoxia, dehydration, and acidosis. Excess fatigue and exposure to cold and stress should also be avoided. Malaria prophylaxis in endemic areas should be maintained, and established infections diagnosed and treated promptly and vigorously with appropriate antibiotics. Trimethoprim should be avoided in patients not receiving folic acid supplements.

The principles of treatment of sickle-cell crisis are to keep the patient warm, to alleviate pain, to rehydrate, and to treat infection, hypoxia and acidosis. Analgesics should be chosen carefully, and drugs of addiction avoided if possible. Patients are often G6PD deficient, and additional haemolysis may be induced by analgesics. Partial exchange transfusion with fresh normal red cells is a useful technique to provide support over a period of crisis or to prepare a patient for a hazardous operation.

Close co-operation between physician, surgeon and anaesthetist is necessary if surgery is performed. Anaesthetic agents must be carefully administered, and adequate oxygenation maintained during and after the operation. Cardiac and pulmonary surgery are particularly hazardous.

Close supervision of pregnancy is essential. Prophylactic iron and folic acid should be given, and crises and infections promptly treated. Repeated transfusions with packed red cells or partial exchange transfusion may be necessary in some cases. Special care should be exercised during delivery and in the puerperium, and hypoxia strictly avoided. The management of sickle-cell disease in pregnancy is reviewed by Charache & Niebyl (1985).

There has been considerable recent interest in the possible prevention of sickling by chemical modification of the Hb-S molecule or by decreasing its concentration within the red cell. Several agents have received limited clinical trial, and others are currently under investigation (Serjeant 1985). Although there is considerable optimism that an ideal agent will eventually be developed, all so far tested have failed to demonstrate an acceptable combination of potent antisickling activity and lack of undesirable side-effects.

The management of homozygous sickle-cell disease in adults is reviewed by Charache (1981).

PREVENTION

Several centres in the United States and Great Britain provide screening for sickle-cell trait and genetic counselling (Scott & Castro 1979). Cord blood screening programmes for early detection of sickle-cell disease have also been established in several countries (Consensus Conference 1987). Prenatal diagnosis using techniques similar to those employed in the thalassaemias (p. 161) is available in a number of specialized clinics (Alter 1984).

Sickle-cell β thalassaemia

This disorder represents the double heterozygous state for the Hb-S and the β thalassaemia genes. It occurs mainly in persons of Greek and Italian descent, and in Blacks. The clinical and haematological manifestations are highly variable. In general, the condition resembles homozygous sickle-cell disease, but tends to be less severe. Much of the variability is ascribed to the existence of two types of sickle-cell β thalassaemia, one characterized by a complete absence of Hb-A due to the presence of a β^0 thalassaemia gene (see below) and the other Hb-A levels of 10–30 per cent due to a β^+ gene (p. 155).

In the *Mediterranean area*, sickle-cell β thalassaemia is usually a relatively severe disorder with little or no Hb-A in the red cells, an early onset, marked anaemia, and a high mortality rate in childhood. Painful crises, the hand–foot syndrome, and aseptic necrosis of bone all occur, and hepatosplenomegaly is usual. Some patients are less severely affected and reach adult life without major symptoms.

In *Blacks*, the condition is milder, and red cells contain 10–30 per cent Hb-A. Many patients have little disability and may be detected by a chance haematological screening examination. Some have occasional painful crises, but lead a normal life otherwise. A small proportion has a more serious illness, similar to that seen in Greek and Italian subjects. Splenomegaly is present in about 50 per cent of patients regardless of clinical severity. The disorder as seen in Jamaica is discussed in detail by Serjeant *et al.* (1979).

The *blood picture* in sickle-cell β thalassaemia is similar to that of β thalassaemia major (p. 158). The haemoglobin level in the β° type is 6–9 g/dl, and in the β^{+} type 10–11 g/dl. Microcytosis, marked hypochromia, and target cells are the main features of the blood film, and a small number of irreversibly sickled cells is often seen, particularly in the β° type. The MCV and MCH are greatly reduced, and the reticulocyte count mildly elevated.

The *haemoglobin pattern* of the β° type consists almost totally of Hb-S with a mild increase in Hb-F and Hb-A_2. There is no Hb-A. The β^{+} type consists of Hb-S, 10–30 per cent Hb-A, and a mild increase in Hb-F and Hb-A_2 (see Table 7.3). The electrophoretic pattern of the β^{+} type with Hb-S well in excess of clearly discernible Hb-A is characteristic and unlikely to be mistaken for any other sickle haemoglobinopathy. Cases with very small amounts of Hb-A may be diagnosed as homozygous sickle-cell disease, the Hb-A being visually lost in the increased Hb-F. Agar gel electrophoresis widely separates Hb-A and Hb-F, and facilitates identification of the small amount of Hb-A. The pattern of the β° type closely resembles that of homozygous disease, and the electrophoretic differential diagnosis usually depends on the demonstration of an increased Hb-A_2 level in the former condition. Examination of other family members for evidence of the thalassaemia gene should be undertaken in all putative cases of homozygous sickle-cell disease to avoid diagnostic error. Globin chain synthesis studies (p. 155) may be helpful in doubtful cases.

Sickle-cell Hb-C disease

Sickle-cell Hb-C disease results from the inheritance of the Hb-S gene from one parent and the Hb-C gene from the other. In general, although it resembles homozygous sickle-cell disease clinically, it is less severe. Growth, body habitus, and sexual development are normal. Most patients have painful crises and attacks of acute febrile pulmonary disease, but they are usually well between the crises, and the disease is compatible with longevity. Eye complications are often a prominent feature. Pregnancy occurs more frequently than in homozygous disease, but is almost as hazardous for mother and child as in the latter condition. Thromboembolic episodes and haematuria are particularly common. Jaundice is unusual, although about 60 per cent of adult patients have splenomegaly.

The patients are usually only mildly anaemic or may have a normal haemoglobin level. Numerous target cells are seen on the blood film, but irreversibly sickled cells are often not present. MCV and MCH are usually mildly reduced, and the reticulocyte count mildly elevated. The disorder as seen in Jamaica is discussed by Serjeant *et al.* (1973).

Sickle-cell Hb-D disease

Sickle-cell Hb-D disease is rare; it results from the inheritance of the Hb-S gene from one parent and the Hb-D gene from the other. It occurs mainly in Blacks, but Caucasians are occasionally affected. Clinically, it resembles homozygous sickle-cell disease, but is less severe and the patients are mildly anaemic. Most have a normal habitus and lead a relatively normal life with only very occasional painful crises. Numerous target cells are seen on the blood film. The electrophoretic pattern may be confused with that of homozygous sickle-cell disease (p. 144).

Other haemoglobinopathies

The haemoglobin-C haemoglobinopathies

Hb-C appears to have originated in West Africa where it affects 20 per cent of the population in some areas. The prevalence rate in the United States among Blacks is 2–3 per cent. It has occasionally been observed in Italians. Hb-C arises from the substitution of lysine for glutamic acid in the sixth position of the β chain. It is less soluble than Hb-A, and if present in sufficient amounts tends to form crystals within the red cell. The intracellular crystals may be seen in a wet preparation or after incubation of blood in three per cent sodium chloride solution at 37°C. Crystal formation occurs under these conditions in the red cells of patients with Hb-C disease and sickle-cell Hb-C disease, but is not observed in Hb-C trait (Ringelhann & Khorsandi 1972).

Hb-C is a slow-moving haemoglobin on cellulose acetate electrophoresis, migrating in the same position as Hb-E and Hb-A_2 (see Fig. 7.3).

Hb-C trait (heterozygous state) is generally asymptomatic; in the blood film the presence of numerous target cells is characteristic, but in occasional cases they may not be a marked feature. Red cell lifespan is normal.

Hb-C disease (homozygous state) is usually a benign illness characterized by compensated haemolysis with a normal haemoglobin level or a mild to moderate anaemia. It may be diagnosed as a result of a screening blood examination, but some patients have recurrent arthralgias or mild abdominal pain. Patients are of normal habitus, but splenomegaly is almost always present and there may be mild jaundice. Target cells are prominent in the blood film, ranging from 30 per cent to almost 100 per cent. The MCV and MCH may be mildly reduced, but are often normal. Occasional microspherocytes and nucleated red cells are usually present, and the reticulocyte count is often mildly elevated.

Sickle-cell Hb-C disease is not uncommon, and has been discussed earlier (p. 150).

Hb-C β thalassaemia has been described in American Blacks and more recently in Italians, Africans and Turkish people. In Blacks, it is usually asymptomatic and splenomegaly is uncommon. In other racial groups, it is more severe with a clinical picture of thalassaemia intermedia and frequent splenomegaly.

The haemoglobin-E haemoglobinopathies

Hb-E is found predominantly in south-east Asia, India, Burma, and Sri Lanka and amongst immigrant Indo–Chinese populations in western countries. Approximately 13 per cent of the population of Thailand, Cambodia and Laos is affected. Hb-E arises from the substitution of lysine for glutamic acid in the 26th position of the β chain. On cellulose acetate electrophoresis, Hb-E is slow moving and migrates in the same position as Hb-C and Hb-A_2. Agar gel electrophoresis permits differentiation, as Hb-E does not separate from Hb-A on this medium (see Fig. 7.3). The Hb-E disorders in Thailand are reviewed by Wasi (1981).

Hb-E trait (heterozygous state) is asymptomatic, and the haemoglobin level is normal. The red cell count may be elevated. The red cells are microcytic with a mildly reduced MCV and MCH.

Hb-E disease (homozygous state) may also be asymptomatic in some patients. It is characterized by compensated haemolysis with a normal haemoglobin level or a mild microcytic anaemia. There may be mild jaundice, and the liver and spleen are usually not enlarged. In the blood film, there is marked hypochromia, usually with many target cells. The MCV and MCH are reduced.

Hb-E β thalassaemia is relatively common in Thailand. It is a more severe condition than Hb-E disease. The clinical and haematological features resemble those of β thalassaemia major in most cases. Occasional patients are less severely affected. Death from infection in childhood is frequent, but some patients live until adult life.

Hb-E α thalassaemia is also common in Thailand. Several disorders of variable severity involving interactions between the α thalassaemia 1 and α thalassaemia 2 genes and Hb-E have been described.

The haemoglobin-D haemoglobinopathies

Hb-D occurs mainly in north-west India, Pakistan, and Iran, although it was first described in the United States. About three per cent of Sikhs living in the Punjab are affected. It is also found sporadically in Blacks and Europeans, the latter usually coming from countries that have had close associations with India in the past. The original Hb-D was called Hb-D Los Angeles, and it was later shown to be identical to Hb-D Punjab found in India and Pakistan. A number of other rarer abnormal haemoglobins, both α-chain and β-chain mutations, have similar electrophoretic mobilities and are also referred to as Hb-D. Hb-D Punjab arises from the substitution of glutamine for glutamic acid in the 121st position of the β chain.

The electrophoretic mobility of Hb-D on cellulose acetate is identical to that of Hb-S. On agar gel electrophoresis, Hb-D migrates with Hb-A, whereas Hb-S separates from Hb-A (see Fig. 7.3). Hb-D does not sickle. The Hb-D disorders are reviewed by Vella & Lehmann (1974).

The unstable haemoglobin haemoglobinopathies

The unstable haemoglobins are haemoglobin variants that undergo denaturation and precipitate in the red cell as Heinz bodies. Their presence results in a rare form of congenital non-spherocytic haemolytic anaemia.

The stability of the haemoglobin molecule depends on the maintenance of the normal configuration and internal contacts of the globin chains and on constant structural relationship between the haem groups and the surrounding haem pocket. The haem is held in position in the haem pocket by bonds between it and the amino acids of the surrounding chain. In the unstable haemoglobins, the firm binding of the haem group within the molecule is disturbed by replacement or deletion of one or more critical amino acids (Perutz 1978). Loss of the integrity of the haem pocket leads to the formation of methaemoglobin and precipitation of the globin. The precipitated globin adheres to the inner surface of the red cell membrane as Heinz bodies.

The spleen pits the Heinz bodies from the affected red cells as they circulate through it, and the resulting membrane damage leads to premature cell destruction. The structural abnormality of the haem pocket that causes haemoglobin instability leads in some cases to altered oxygen affinity of the molecule, which may influence the severity of symptoms.

Over 100 unstable haemoglobins have been described. They include Hb-Koln, Hb-Zurich, Hb-Hammersmith, and Hb-Sydney. Most arise from β-chain substitutions, and affected patients are heterozygous for the unstable haemoglobin and Hb-A. The condition is not limited to any particular racial group. Autosomal dominant inheritance has been noted in most families studied. In some cases, there is no family history. The disorder is fully reviewed by White (1976) who provides a list of the unstable haemoglobins.

LABORATORY DIAGNOSIS

Demonstration of Heinz bodies

Preformed Heinz bodies usually cannot be demonstrated by supravital staining in the red cells of patients with an unstable haemoglobin unless a splenectomy has been performed or haemolysis exacerbated by the administration of oxidant drugs. Sterile incubation of affected red cells at 37°C for 24 hours usually leads to their formation. Following splenectomy, Heinz bodies are present in at least 50 per cent of red cells.

Heat instability test

Haemoglobin instability may be directly demonstrated by this useful test which should always be used in the investigation of a patient with congenital non-spherocytic haemolytic anaemia. A fresh haemolysate is incubated with phosphate or tris buffer at 50°C for up to two hours. A precipitate rapidly forms if an unstable haemoglobin is present (Dacie & Lewis 1984).

Isopropanol precipitation test

This test is slightly more convenient than the heat instability test. A fresh haemolysate is incubated with an isopropanol–tris buffer at 37°C for up to 60 minutes. A precipitate rapidly forms if an unstable haemoglobin is present (Carrell 1986).

Haemoglobin electrophoresis

Demonstration of the unstable haemoglobin by electrophoresis is often less satisfactory than with stable haemoglobin variants. An abnormal band is present on cellulose acetate electrophoresis at pH 8.6 in about 75 per cent of the patients, but the band is often indistinct or slurred, especially if the haemolysate is not fresh. The electrophoretic mobility of Hb-Koln, the most common of the unstable haemoglobins, is similar to that of Hb-S. The proportion of unstable haemoglobin is highly variable. In most cases it is about 30 per cent, but it may be as low as 2 per cent or as high as 40 per cent. Hb-A_2 and Hb-F are elevated in occasional patients.

Clinical and laboratory findings

The clinical severity of the unstable haemoglobin haemolytic anaemias varies greatly. The anaemia may be so mild that the patient is unaware of any abnormality, and in an occasional case there may be no anaemia, the only sign of the disease being an elevated reticulocyte count. Alternatively, the anaemia may be severe and evident in the first year of life. Infection or the administration of oxidant drugs may cause an exacerbation of haemolysis.

Hb-Koln is the most commonly encountered unstable haemoglobin. It causes a well-compensated chronic haemolytic anaemia of mild to moderate severity with intermittent mild jaundice and splenomegaly. Cholelithiasis may occur, and the passage of dark urine is a feature in some patients.

The blood film shows only minor abnormalities, with minimal anisocytosis and poikilocytosis, variable hypochromia, punctate basophilia, and polychromasia. The reticulocyte count is always elevated, and the MCH is usually reduced. Red cell changes are more marked in splenectomized patients. Occasional patients have a mild thrombocytopenia. The mean red cell lifespan is 20–30 days (Bentley *et al.* 1974). Exacerbation of haemolysis by drugs has not been noted with Hb-Koln.

The approach to treatment varies with the severity of the haemolysis, but many patients manage satisfactorily with little medical attention and attain a normal lifespan. Blood transfusion is necessary for a sudden fall in haemoglobin level, and splenectomy has been useful in selected patients. Prompt therapy of infections and avoidance of oxidant drugs are important measures.

Haemoglobinopathies associated with polycythaemia

The movement of oxygen into and out of the haemoglobin molecule depends on changes in spatial relations between the α and β globin chains. Amino-acid substitutions that result in alterations of oxygen affinity are generally situated at critical areas of chain contact and interfere with the normal process of chain rearrangement associated with oxygenation and deoxygenation (Perutz 1978).

When the amino-acid substitution impairs ability to release oxygen at the tissue level, the abnormal haemoglobin is referred to as a high oxygen-affinity haemoglobin. The resulting anoxia stimulates compensatory erythropoietin production and hence erythrocytosis. The *in vitro* counterpart of the *in vivo* abnormality is the abnormal oxygen dissociation curve, which is 'shifted to the left' when whole blood from an affected patient is examined. The shift reflects the increased oxygen affinity, the fall in oxygen saturation for any given drop in partial pressure of oxygen being less than that found in normal adult blood.

At least 25 high oxygen-affinity haemoglobins with erythrocytosis have been described, the majority being β-chain substitutions, inherited as autosomal dominants. Affected patients are heterozygotes.

LABORATORY DIAGNOSIS

Haemoglobin electrophoresis. An abnormal electrophoretic band is demonstrable on cellulose acetate at pH 8.6 in about half of the patients. Separation of the abnormal haemoglobin on agar gel electrophoresis at pH 6.0 may be successful in some instances even in the absence of a cellulose acetate band, but in a significant number of cases no band can be demonstrated by conventional techniques. The abnormal haemoglobin constitutes 20–50 per cent of the total haemoglobin.

Oxygen dissociation studies. These are essential for definitive diagnosis, but are often not available outside specialist referral centres. Blood samples despatched by airmail may be satisfactory for analysis. The normal P_{50} value for whole blood is

25–30 mmHg. In patients with high affinity haemoglobins, levels range from 12 to 20 mmHg.

Clinical and laboratory findings. Affected patients have a haemoglobin level, packed cell volume, and red cell count at or above the upper limits of normal. White cell and platelet count are normal, and there is no splenomegaly. The patients are usually plethoric, but have no symptoms. Investigation of the plethora or a chance screening haemoglobin estimation may lead to detection. Blood gas analysis is normal. The absence of leucocytosis and thrombocytosis clearly distinguishes the disorder from polycythaemia rubra vera. More pertinent is the distinction from other forms of secondary erythrocytosis, familial or otherwise. If no obvious cause for the increased haemoglobin level is apparent, and especially if the subject is young and a family history with a dominant pattern of inheritance is obtained, the presence of an abnormal haemoglobin should be suspected. If an abnormal electrophoretic band cannot be demonstrated on cellulose acetate or agar gel electrophoresis, oxygen dissociation studies are necessary. Family members should be examined if available. The erythrocytosis of the high oxygen-affinity haemoglobins appears to be benign since the clinical syndrome has been found in apparently well subjects beyond middle age. Treatment is usually not necessary, but an occasional patient has benefited from phlebotomy. The high oxygen-affinity haemoglobins include Hb-Chesapeake, Hb-J Capetown, Hb-Kempsey, and Hb-Ypsilanti. They are listed and discussed in detail by Bellingham (1976).

The thalassaemias

The thalassaemias are a heterogeneous group of disorders with a genetically determined reduction in the rate of synthesis of one or more types of normal haemoglobin polypeptide chain. This results in a decrease in the amount of the haemoglobin involving the affected chain. In some forms of thalassaemia, the genetic mutation results in the synthesis of a structurally abnormal haemoglobin which is produced at a reduced rate.

Thalassaemia was originally described in Italians, Greeks, Spaniards and other peoples of Mediterranean origin. However, it is now realized that it is a common disorder with a widespread geographical distribution. It also occurs in the Middle East, India, south-east Asia, and in Blacks. Persons of Mediterranean origin in non-European countries may be affected. No population group is completely free from the condition, and it is now occasionally identified in persons of northern European origin.

Classification

The α and β chains of haemoglobin are synthesized independently under separate genetic control and, in the normal state, synthesis of the two chains is balanced. There are two main groups of thalassaemia, one affecting the synthesis of α chains, and the other affecting the synthesis of β chains; these are called α thalassaemia and β thalassaemia respectively. In β thalassaemia, the inadequate production of β chains leads to a reduction in the amount of Hb-A in the red cell, and a microcytic hypochromic anaemia results. The total haemoglobin is maintained in part by the production of γ and δ chains, and thus increased Hb-F or Hb-A_2 is usually found. The lack of β chains leads to accumulation of free uncombined α chains within the developing red cells. These chains aggregate and interfere with erythroid cell maturation and function, resulting in premature destruction of the cells in the marrow and consequent ineffective erythropoiesis (p. 159).

In α thalassaemia, the levels of Hb-A, Hb-F and Hb-A_2 are equally depressed since they all have α chains; there is usually a microcytic hypochromic anaemia. In the absence of sufficient α chains, excess β chains or γ chains aggregate to form Hb-H (β_4) or Hb-Bart's (γ_4). The inheritance of thalassaemia is co-dominant, and follows classic Mendelian principles. Alpha thalassaemia and β thalassaemia exist in both the homozygous and heterozygous states, and the genes for thalassaemia may interact with those of the haemoglobin structural variants.

Laboratory diagnosis

As in the structural haemoglobinopathies, the diagnosis of thalassaemia is initially suggested by the clinical findings, the patient's ethnic origin and family history, and the results of routine haematological tests. In the diagnosis of β thalassaemia, Hb-A_2 is quantitated by haemoglobin electrophoresis or microcolumn chromatography, and Hb-F by the alkali denaturation test. In α thalassaemia, red cell Hb-H inclusions are demonstrated by specific stains, and haemoglobin electrophoresis is used to detect Hb-H and Hb-Bart's. A definitive diagnosis may be made at this point in most cases. Globin chain synthesis rate and gene analysis studies, which require the assistance of a reference laboratory, are sometimes useful in difficult cases.

Routine haematological tests. The haemoglobin level, packed cell volume, red cell count, red cell indices, reticulocyte count, and examination of a stained blood film are essential initial tests. The MCV, which is measured electronically in many laboratories, is particularly useful. An MCV result of less than 80 fl alerts the clinician to the diagnosis of α or β thalassaemia, although iron deficiency and a number of chronic illnesses frequently seen in hospital practice also cause low levels. Serum iron, total iron binding capacity, ferritin, bilirubin, and other biochemical parameters of haemolysis should be measured.

Demonstration of Hb-H inclusions. When red cells containing Hb-H are incubated with a solution of a redox dye (e.g. brilliant cresyl blue), Hb-H, which is relatively unstable, precipitates and the red cells are pitted by numerous inclusions, an appearance likened to the surface of a golf ball. The inclusions must be distinguished from the reticulin of reticulocytes and from preformed Heinz body-like inclusions, which are numerous after splenectomy in patients with Hb-H disease.

Haemoglobin electrophoresis. Precise measurement of the Hb-A_2 level is required for the diagnosis of several types of β thalassaemia. Haemoglobin electrophoresis on cellulose acetate at pH 8.6 is widely used, the Hb-A_2 band being eluted from the strip and measured spectrophotometrically. A number of accurate microcolumn chromatographic methods are also available, some in pre-packaged kit form. They are quicker and more convenient to perform than electrophoretic methods and have replaced the latter in many laboratories (Brosious *et al.* 1978). If present in sufficient amounts, Hb-H and Hb-Bart's may be demonstrated by electrophoresis on cellulose acetate and starch gel at pH 8.6. They are referred to as 'fast' haemoglobins because they migrate in front of Hb-A towards the anode.

Globin chain synthesis rate studies. Studies of incorporation of radioactive amino acids into haemoglobin chains in immature red cells as a measure of relative rates of α- and β-chain synthesis have demonstrated unbalanced synthesis in α and β thalassaemia. Such studies are rarely necessary in the routine investigation of patients with thalassaemia but are important in antenatal diagnosis.

The *alkali denaturation test* for the measurement of Hb-F and the *acid elution test* are described on page 141. *Gene analysis studies* are described on page 162.

The β thalassaemias

The genetic mutation of β thalassaemia leads to a decreased rate of β-chain synthesis and consequently a reduction in the amount of normal Hb-A in the red cell. A microcytic hypochromic anaemia results. On the basis of the extent of reduction of β-chain synthesis, two main types of β thalassaemia are recognized. β^+ thalassaemia is characterized by incomplete suppression and β^o thalassaemia by complete absence of chain synthesis. Both β^o and β^+ types occur throughout the Mediterranean region. β^o thalassaemia predominates in south-east Asia, and β^+ is the usual type in Blacks. Although the two types cannot always be distinguished on clinical grounds in individual patients, the variable severity of β thalassaemia in some population groups is ascribed in part to the existence of these two thalassaemia genes.

Recent gene analysis studies have established that β thalassaemia may arise from any of between 40 and 50 different mutations of the β globin gene. The great majority are single base changes, and gene deletion is only rarely a cause. Most of the mutations affect the RNA splicing mechanism or block translation of mRNA into protein (Antonarakis *et al.* 1985).

At the clinical level, β thalassaemia occurs classically in two forms. Beta thalassaemia major, or Cooley's anaemia, is usually a severe illness characterized by major or total suppression of chain synthesis and is the homozygous form of the

Table 7.4. *The β thalassaemias and related syndromes: electrophoretic phenotypes*

	Haemoglobin (%)		
Disorder	A	A_2	F
β thalassaemia minor	90–95	3.5–7.0	1–5
δβ thalassaemia minor	80–95	1.0–3.5	5–20
β thalassaemia major			
β thal$^+$	10–90	1.5–4.0	10–90
β thal^O	0	1.5–4.0	98
HPFH (Black heterozygote)	60–85	1.0–2.0	15–35

HPFH = hereditary persistence of fetal haemoglobins.

disease. Beta thalassaemia minor, or trait, is a mild and sometimes asymptomatic condition and represents the heterozygous form. Suppression of β-chain synthesis is much less severe.

Some patients do not fit easily into these two clear-cut clinical categories. Patients may be clinically classified as thalassaemia intermedia if the severity of their disease lies between that of the major and minor forms. Thalassaemia intermedia encompasses a range of interactions between many different thalassaemia genes which result in milder defects of β-chain synthesis and globin-chain imbalance than occur in classical β thalassaemia major (Weatherall & Clegg 1981).

A classification of the commonly occurring types of β thalassaemia is outlined in Table 7.4.

Beta thalassaemia minor (trait)

This disorder is the *heterozygous state* for the β thalassaemia gene. It is characterized by a moderate reduction in β-chain synthesis as directed by a β thalassaemia gene inherited from one parent. The disorder is relatively common, e.g. it has been found in eight per cent of Greeks and five per cent of Italians in Australia. Clinically, it is usually a very mild disorder with little or no anaemia, no symptoms, and a normal life expectancy. The spleen may be palpable. The condition is commonly not diagnosed until adolescence or adult life, and may be detected in a routine haematological screening examination. It is often first diagnosed in pregnancy.

The haemoglobin level is usually normal or mildly reduced, but rarely less than 10 g/dl. The red cell count is often normal despite mild anaemia, and may be increased. The MCV and MCH are reduced, with values of 63–77 fl and 18–25 pg respectively. The MCHC is usually marginally reduced or normal. In occasional patients with concurrent α thalassaemia, the red cell indices are normal. Examination of the blood film show mild red cell anisocytosis, microcytosis, and hypochromia with variable numbers of target and stippled cells. The osmotic fragility test shows an increased resistance to haemolysis even when anaemia is absent. The serum bilirubin is normal or slightly raised.

In the great majority of cases, HbA_2 is increased. A small increase in Hb-F occurs in about 50 per cent; thus the absence of any increase in Hb-F does not exclude the diagnosis (see Table 7.4).

The main problem in diagnosis is the differentiation of β thalassaemia minor from iron deficiency in a person of Mediterranean origin. Clinical features are often not helpful. In the usual case of thalassaemia minor, red cell microcytosis, hypochromia, and reduction in MCV are relatively marked considering the mild or absent anaemia. This is not the case in iron deficiency in which there is closer correlation between the morphological abnormalities and the degree of anaemia. Red cell anisocytosis, as measured by the cell sizing facility on some modern electronic cell counters, is often more marked in iron deficiency (Bessman & Feinstein 1979).

Estimation of the serum iron, ferritin and transferrin, and of the red cell Hb-A_2 and Hb-F, usually provides a definitive diagnosis. When iron deficiency develops in a patient with thalassaemia minor, the elevated Hb-A_2 usually falls to normal but returns to a supranormal level when iron stores are replenished. If the Hb-A_2 and the Hb-F levels are normal, and the patient is not iron deficient, the possibility of α thalassaemia should be considered, and the test for Hb-H inclusions performed.

Treatment is generally not required in mild cases, and the benign nature of the disorder should be emphasized to the patient. Careful surveillance of the haemoglobin level during pregnancy is advisable, and prophylactic folic acid should be given. Although a patient with thalassaemia minor may become iron deficient, it is more usual for patients to receive oral or parenteral iron therapy for many years on the mistaken assumption that all hypochromic anaemias are due to iron deficiency. Thus, it is important to inform the patient of the diagnosis and the possible harmful effects of over-enthusiastic iron therapy.

Beta thalassaemia major

Beta thalassaemia major is the *homozygous state* for either the β° or β^{+} thalassaemia gene or, less commonly, the compound heterozygous state for the two genes. In its usual form in Italian or Greek patients, it is a severe disease which often results in death during childhood unless frequent blood transfusions are given. About one in every ten patients has a mild form which is compatible with survival into adult life with only occasional transfusions. This form of the disorder may be referred to as thalassaemia intermedia, although the haemoglobin constitution is usually identical to that seen in classical thalassaemia major. Extreme examples of the mild form, which sometimes occur in American Blacks, are completely symptomless or have only a mild anaemia. In some cases, the clinical heterogeneity appears to be due to the interaction of other genetic (for example, α thalassaemia or hereditary persistence of fetal haemoglobin) or environmental factors with the β thalassaemia gene.

CLINICAL FEATURES

The *newborn infant* with β thalassaemia major is not anaemic. The onset of anaemia is insidious, the initial manifestation being pallor, which is usually obvious within the first year of life and in severe cases within a few weeks of birth. Subsequent prognosis depends on whether the child is entered into a programme of regular blood transfusions (see below). If the disorder takes its natural course without active therapeutic intervention, growth and development in early childhood are retarded. The child fails to thrive, and anorexia, diarrhoea, loss of body fat, and recurrent fever occur. The severe anaemia usually results in cardiac dilatation. *Splenomegaly* is obvious by the age of three years, and the large spleen causes abdominal swelling and discomfort, and symptoms due to pressure on surrounding organs. Moderate to marked hepa-

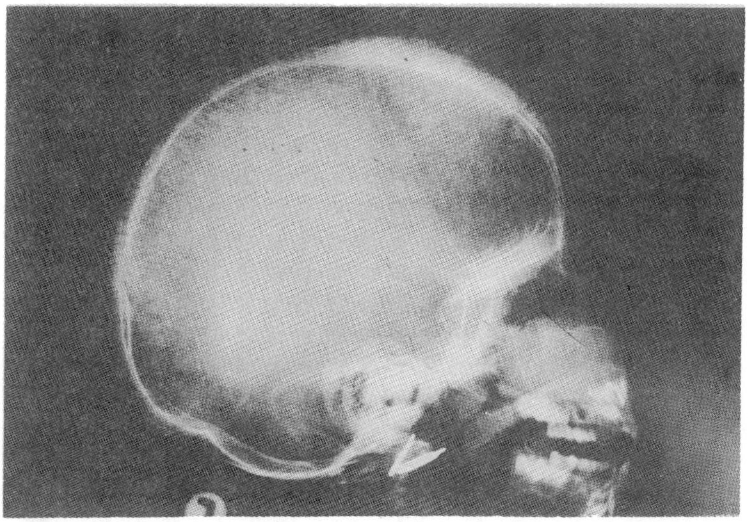

Fig. 7.5. *X-ray of skull in β thalassaemia major. From a girl of Italian descent, aged four years, with severe anaemia, jaundice, enlarged facial bones, and gross hepatosplenomegaly. The X-ray shows the typical 'hair-on-end' appearance of the cranial bone.*

tomegaly is also present. Clinical jaundice is uncommon, but is sometimes present to a mild degree. Changes in the *skeletal system* are constant; they result in a characteristic mongoloid facies due to expansion of the marrow in the malar bones, and in X-ray changes in the skull (Fig. 7.5), long bones, hands and feet (p. 179). Cortical thinning leads to pathological fractures, and bone pain may occur. Impairment of growth may result in small stature, the menarche is often delayed, and secondary sex characteristics undeveloped. Other occasional clinical features include epistaxis, skin pigmentation, leg ulcers and gall-stones. The children are susceptible to *severe infection* particularly if the spleen has been surgically removed, and septicaemia is an important cause of early mortality. *Pericarditis* occurs in about half of the patients. Streptococci are grown from the pericardial fluid in some cases, but the fluid is often sterile and the pericarditis may be related to iron deposition. *Extramedullary haemopoiesis* may occur, masses of haemopoietic tissue compressing the spinal cord. *Hypersplenism*, in addition to its complex role in the aetiology of the anaemia, often causes some reduction in platelet count, but rarely to a degree sufficient to result in haemorrhagic manifestations.

Children who receive regular transfusions grow and develop normally during the first decade and are spared most of the serious complications referred to above. However, in both treated and untreated patients, insidious deposition of iron in tissues during late childhood and early adolescence results in *organ dysfunction*. The increase in body iron is due to the combination of frequent transfusions and increased intestinal absorption resulting from ineffective erythropoiesis and chronic anaemia. Pancreatic haemosiderosis may cause diabetes, and cirrhosis results from iron deposition in the liver. Haemosiderosis of cardiac muscle leads to arrhythmias, heart block, and chronic congestive heart failure, and is the main cause of death after the first decade.

BLOOD PICTURE

In many respects, the blood picture resembles that of severe iron deficiency. The *anaemia* is usually severe, with a haemoglobin level of 3–9 g/dl. The erythrocytes show marked anisocytosis and poikilocytosis, which is often bizarre (Fig. 7.6); although microcytosis predominates, some cells are macrocytic and there are occasional spherocytes. Tear-drop cells are often seen but may be less frequent following splenectomy. Hypochromia is a striking

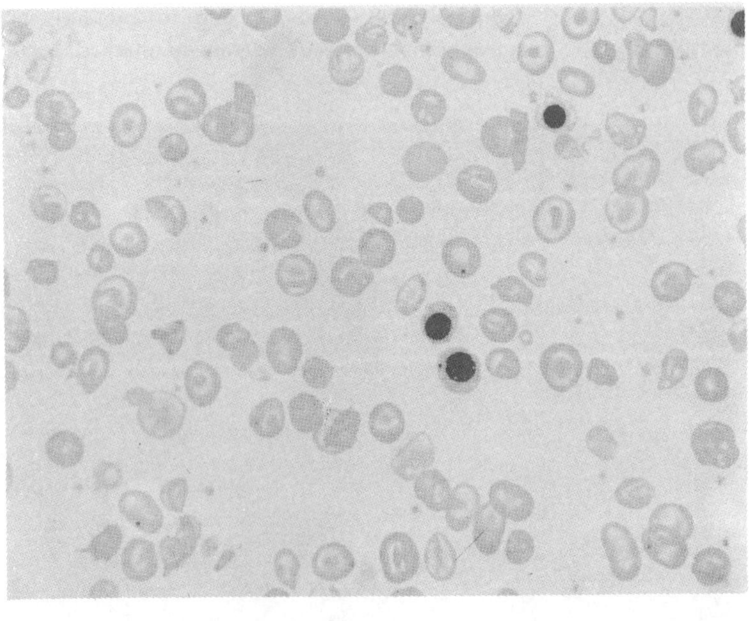

Fig. 7.6. *Thalassaemia major. Photomicrograph of a blood from a patient with β thalassaemia major. The pronounced poikilocytosis and target cell formation are well shown (× 385).*

feature; some cells appear as rings of haemoglobin with little or no central staining. Target cells are prominent. The MCV and MCH are significantly reduced; the MCHC is also reduced, but not to the extent suggested by the degree of hypochromia in the film. Normoblasts are almost invariably present, often in large numbers, especially post-splenectomy. Some of the normoblasts are primitive, but often they are small and mature with pyknotic nuclei. Granular cytoplasmic inclusion bodies, which represent aggregates of α chains, may be demonstrated by methyl violet staining in the cytoplasm of the normoblasts and reticulocytes of splenectomized subjects. Polychromasia and punctate basophilia are usually present to a moderate degree, and the reticulocyte count is raised to ten per cent or more. The reticulocyte count is usually higher in patients who have had a splenectomy.

The *white cell count* is usually raised, with values of 15–40 $\times$ 10^9/l or more. White cell counts obtained from electronic cell counters require correction for the presence of nucleated red cells. There is a shift to the left of the neutrophils, and some myelocytes are commonly present. The *platelet count* is usually normal, but may be reduced in patients with very large spleens.

The *osmotic fragility test* characteristically reveals an increased resistance to haemolysis. The serum bilirubin is usually slightly raised, and haptoglobin and haemopexin depleted. Methaemalbumin may be present in the plasma. Dark-brown urine is commonly observed, and this has been attributed to the presence of dipyrrole breakdown products of haemoglobin. The serum uric acid is frequently elevated, and clinical gout may occur. Haemosiderinuria is occasionally present. The serum iron and ferritin are invariably elevated, and transferrin completely saturated. Serum and red cell folate levels are often reduced. Plasma volume may be considerably elevated.

Bone marrow aspiration shows intensely hyperplastic erythropoiesis of a degree proportional to the anaemia. There is an increased proportion of basophilic and polychromatic normoblasts, which are frequently smaller than normal (micronormoblasts) due mainly to a decrease in cytoplasm. Methyl violet-positive inclusion bodies may be seen in some normoblasts and PAS-positive glycogen (p. 246) is also occasionally seen. Siderotic granules are commonly scattered throught the cytoplasm of the normoblasts. 'Ring' sideroblasts are occasionally seen, but are rarely a prominent feature. Fragment and reticulo-endothelial haemosiderin is normal or increased.

HAEMOGLOBIN PATTERN

The predominant haemoglobin is Hb-F which constitutes 10–98 per cent of the total (see Table 7.4). The percentage of Hb-F bears no relation to the degree of anaemia. Hb-A is present in small or moderate amounts in β^+ thalassaemia but is completely absent in β^o thalassaemia. Hb-A_2 is variable, being reduced, normal or occasionally increased. The acid elution test demonstrates a heterogeneous distribution of Hb-F in the red cells.

PATHOPHYSIOLOGY OF THE ANAEMIA

The anaemia of β thalassaemia major results from intramedullary red cell destruction, shortened red cell lifespan, and peripheral haemodilution due to an increase in plasma volume. It is currently believed that the principal lesion leading to intramedullary cell death and reduced lifespan is the formation of intracellular aggregates of α chains. Studies of haemoglobin synthesis have indicated that the deficiency of β-chain production leads to a large excess of α chains within the developing red cell. In some cells, γ chains are able to remove the excess α chains as Hb-F, but when γ-chain production is insufficient, the excess α chains rapidly precipitate. Depending on the amount of precipitation, the most severely affected cells are destroyed immediately in the marrow, and the less affected are released into the circulation. Erythrokinetic studies have confirmed the presence of severe ineffective erythropoiesis. The α-chain aggregates, which appear in the circulating cells as methyl violet-positive inclusion bodies, interfere with normal red cell membrane function and may contribute to reduced survival through this mechanism. More important, however, is the trauma inflicted as the aggregates are removed from the red cell by the process of pitting during passage through the spleen. Many cells are irreparably damaged, and are then destroyed in the circulation or phagocytosed by reticulo-endothelial cells in liver and spleen.

PROGNOSIS

Life expectancy in severe β thalassaemia major averages from 15 to 25 years. If untreated, death occurs from severe anaemia or infection before the age of five years. If regularly transfused, the patients die in the second or third decade from intractable congestive heart failure, cirrhosis, or diabetes. There are already indications that chelation therapy will result in a significant improvement in survival in future years. Occasional patients with the mild form of the disease survive into adult life with little disability and requiring few if any blood transfusions.

TREATMENT

Most patients with β thalassaemia major are severely anaemic, and many of the distressing symptoms of the condition are directly related to the anaemia. The compensatory mechanisms recruited by the body to improve the production of viable red cells may also cause symptoms, and in some patients are more troublesome than the anaemia itself. The expanding hyperplastic bone marrow leads to gross skeletal changes, particularly affecting the face; masses of extramedullary erythroid tissue compress vital structures; and increased iron absorption cause deposition of iron in parenchymal tissues. Thus, blood transfusion which alleviates the anaemia and suppresses the compensatory mechanisms is the basis of therapy.

The original aim of transfusion therapy was to maintain the haemoglobin at the lowest safe level. This usually involved blood transfusion at 5–10 weekly intervals. More frequent transfusions were considered unwise because of the iron content of the transfused blood (each unit of blood contains 250 mg iron) and the likelihood of accelerated development of haemosiderosis and organ failure.

More recently, it has been realized that an intensive transfusion policy offers considerable advantages for the patient, notwithstanding its additional contribution to body iron accumulation (Wolman 1969). Current hypertransfusion regimens are commenced in the first or second year of life and aim at maintaining a mean haemoglobin level of at least 10 g/dl by transfusion of concentrated red cells at 4–6 weekly intervals. Children treated in this way remain well with a normal pattern of growth and development until the early teens, when the effects of iron overload gradually appear. It is important to establish the patient's steady-state haemoglobin level before embarking on an intensive transfusion regimen. The patient should be phenotyped, and group-specific red cells (preferably rendered leucocyte-poor) should be used, if possible. To ensure prolonged *in vivo* survival, fresh blood is desirable, and a technique involving the transfusion of young red cells ('neocytes') obtained from donors by means of a cell separator is used in some clinics (Propper 1983).

In order to prevent the inevitable accumulation of iron, the iron-chelating agent desferrioxamine (DF) is used. DF is able to remove substantial amounts of storage iron via urine and stool, and, if commenced early in life, preferably at the same time as the regular transfusion regimen, will prevent (or at least delay) the occurrence of iron overload. In older patients with established iron overload, DF curtails further accumulation of hepatic iron and progression of fibrosis. In most cases, hepatic iron content decreases, liver function tests improve, and the level of serum ferritin falls. The drug is administered subcutaneously using a small portable infusion pump; the needle is inserted into the anterior abdominal wall and the dose infused over a 12-hour period daily for 5 days per week. Preliminary studies to establish a dose response curve are advisable to arrive at an optimal dosage regimen. The average daily dose for children is 50–60 mg/kg/day, and for adults approximately 2 g per day. The addition of vitamin C, 200 mg orally on each day of chelation, enhances iron excretion. In spite of its high cost, complexity of administration and potential for visual and auditory neurotoxicity (Olivieri *et al.* 1986), DF is now used widely in the treatment of children with thalassaemia major.

Massive splenomegaly is less of a problem since the advent of hypertransfusion regimens. Splenectomy has a definite place in the management of two groups of patients: in children with massive splenomegaly causing severe discomfort and symp toms due to pressure, and in patients with progressively increasing transfusion requirements. In hypertransfused patients, there is often a progressive shortening of the interval between transfusions, until ultimately transfusion is required very frequently. In most cases, immune allo-antibodies cannot be demonstrated, and the increased destruction appears to be due, at least in part, to a 'hypersplenic' mechanism, since splenectomy in such patients usually causes a significant fall in transfusion requirements. Red cell survival and sequestration studies using ^{51}Cr-labelled red cells are not helpful in assessing the likelihood of response to splenectomy.

Splenectomy should not be performed, if at all possible, until after the age of five or six years. There is a major risk of life-threatening infection in children who are splenectomized before this age. The reasons for the increased susceptibility to infection following removal of the spleen are not known with certainty, but are probably similar to those in sickle-cell disease (p. 145). *Pneumococcus, meningococcus* and *Haemophilus influenzae* are usually the organisms involved. Immunization with polyvalent pneumococcal vaccine is essential, and most authorities recommend prophylactic oral penicillin.

Prompt and aggressive antibiotic therapy should be commenced at the onset of the infection; provision of parenteral antibiotics to the parents of affected children for administration at the first sign of fever may be worthwhile.

Management of the various syndromes of organ failure that characterize the later course of the thalassaemic patient is often difficult. Iron deposition in cardiac muscle causes arrhythmias and chronic congestive cardiac failure which may be refractory to conventional therapy. The myocardium is very sensitive to digitalis, and consultation with an experienced cardiologist is advisable. Episodes of pericarditis are managed by bed rest, treatment of heart failure, and antibiotics if necessary. Spinal cord compression from masses of hyperactive erythroid tissue may require myelography and radiation therapy or laminectomy. Occasionally patients develop mild megaloblastic bone marrow changes, and a maintenance dose of folic acid may be warranted.

The place of *bone marrow transplantation* in the management of β thalassaemia major is currently under investigation. Lucarelli *et al.* (1987) have reported promising early results, but long-term data are not available and the procedure is associated with considerable morbidity from graft-versus-host disease and infection.

Ideally, children with thalassaemia should be treated in centres set up for their management. This permits establishment of the close relationship between patient, parents, and clinician which is essential for successful care of a serious chronic illness. The management of β thalassaemia major is reviewed in the comprehensive monograph of Modell & Berdoukas (1984).

PREVENTION

Screening programmes to detect asymptomatic, previously unknown, thalassaemic heterozygotes and to provide information and genetic counselling have been established in several countries in which the thalassaemia gene is prevalent throughout the whole population or in sectional ethnic groups (Silvestroni & Bianco 1983). The measurement of red cell MCV using an electronic cell counter has usually been used as the basic screening test (p. 155).

Antenatal diagnosis and selective termination in pregnancies at risk for homozygous β thalassaemia, Hb-Bart's hydrops fetalis (p. 165), and homozygous sickle-cell disease are now available in a limited number of specialized centres (Alter 1983).

Two methods are used:

Measurement of globin chain synthesis

A small sample of fetal blood is obtained at the 18th–20th week of gestation, either by placental needling under ultrasound guidance or by fetoscopic umbilical vein aspiration. Globin chain synthesis rates in fetal reticulocytes are measured (p. 155) and the $\beta:\gamma$ synthetic ratio is used to identify fetuses that are heterozygous or homozygous for the gene of interest. In a recent international survey conducted by Alter (1984), fetal mortality associated with the procedure was 5.4 per cent overall, and there was a 0.8 per cent diagnostic error rate.

Analysis of fetal DNA

Amniotic fluid is obtained by transabdominal amniocentesis during the 15th–18th week of gestation. Recently, first trimester diagnosis has been possible in some cases by using trophoblastic tissue obtained by transcervical aspiration (Old *et al.* 1986), and it is expected that this method will be increasingly favoured in the future.

Analysis of fetal DNA is performed by gene mapping techniques after extraction from fetal fibroblasts or chorion. The DNA is cut at specific sequences into small fragments with restriction enzymes obtained from bacteria. The resulting fragments are separated according to size by agarose gel electrophoresis and transferred onto nitrocellulose paper by a process called Southern blotting. The particular gene of interest is identified by hybridization with a specific radioactive probe, followed by autoradiography. The restriction fragments that are complementary to the probe hybridize with it and form a band on the X-ray film.

Using the above technique, several approaches have been used in the prenatal diagnosis of haemoglobin disorders (Weatherall 1985).

Direct identification of mutant genes. Those disorders in which the basic genetic abnormality is either a substantial gene deletion or a base substitution that alters a restriction enzyme cleavage site can be identified directly by gene mapping. These include Hb-Bart's hydrops fetalis in which there is deletion of the α gene, sickle haemoglobinopathies in which the base substitution alters a restriction site, and some types of β thalassaemia. The majority of β thalassaemias cannot be analysed in this way, but it is likely that a new technique using synthetically produced short DNA fragments (oligonucleotides) as probes will be increasingly used for these disorders in the future.

Restriction fragment length polymorphism (RFLP) analysis. RFLPs are normal variations (polymorphisms) in DNA structure between one individual and another that occur about once in every 100–200 nucleotide bases. They either remove a restriction enzyme cleavage site or introduce a new one, and may be analysed by gene-mapping techniques. They are inherited in a Mendelian fashion, and can be used as genetic markers to trace through families the mutant genes to which they are linked. RFLPs are common in the region of the β-globin gene complex, and the technique has been widely used in the prenatal diagnosis of thalassaemia.

Delta beta thalassaemia

A type of thalassaemia resulting from complete absence of both β- and δ-chain synthesis, in most cases due to extensive deletion of DNA in the β-globin gene complex, occurs in areas where the β thalassaemia gene is prevalent. The homozygous form of the condition is rare, and is characterized by a β thalassaemia major-like illness of moderate severity and 100 per cent Hb-F in the red cells. The heterozygous form is more common, and closely resembles β thalassaemia minor, both clinically and haematologically. Unlike β thalassaemia minor, however, the Hb-A_2 level is normal or reduced, and the only abnormality of haemoglobin constitution is an elevation of Hb-F which ranges from 5 to 20 per cent (see Table 7.4). The acid elution test demonstrates a heterogeneous distribution of Hb-F in the red cells.

The haemoglobin-Lepore syndromes

Occasional patients with apparent classical β thalassaemia minor or major have an abnormal haemoglobin, Hb-Lepore. Structural analysis has shown that Hb-Lepore is made up of normal α chains combined with chains that consist of parts of both δ and β chains. Three distinct types of Hb-Lepore have been described, namely Hb-Lepore Boston, Hb-Lepore Hollandia, and Hb-Lepore Baltimore. The abnormal chains are produced by $\delta\beta$ fusion genes which arise by unequal crossing over between parts of the δ and β globin genes during meiosis.

The Hb-Lepore syndromes are found in many population groups. They are particularly common in southern Italy and in parts of Greece and Yugoslavia. The disorder as seen in Italy is described by Marinucci *et al.* (1979). Hb-Lepore has a similar mobility to Hb-S on cellulose acetate electrophoresis. It does not separate from Hb-A on agar gel.

The *heterozygous state for Hb-Lepore* is a very mild disorder resembling β thalassaemia minor. Hb-Lepore constitutes about ten per cent of the total haemoglobin, Hb-F is slightly increased, and Hb-A and Hb-A_2 make up the remainder.

The *homozygous state for Hb-Lepore* is rare. Clinically and haematologically it resembles β thalassaemia major. Seventy-five per cent of the haemoglobin is Hb-F, and the remainder is Hb-Lepore. There is no Hb-A or Hb-A_2.

The *double heterozygous state for Hb-Lepore and β thalassaemia* is more common. It also resembles β thalassaemia major. About ten per cent of the total haemoglobin is Hb-Lepore, and Hb-A may be completely absent or comprise 20–40 per cent. The remainder of the haemoglobin is Hb-F and small amounts of Hb-A_2.

The Lepore haemoglobins have also been found in association with β-chain structural variants such as Hb-S and Hb-C.

Hereditary persistence of fetal haemoglobin (HPFH)

In most population groups, a small number of apparently healthy adult subjects with normal or near normal haematological findings have a raised Hb-F level. Two broad categories of this condition, which is referred to as 'hereditary persistence of fetal haemoglobin' (HPFH), have been described. In pancellular HPFH, the acid elution test (p. 141) shows a homogeneous distribution of Hb-F in the red cells, whereas in heterocellular HPFH, the Hb-F is heterogeneously distributed.

The commonest type of pancellular HPFH, the Black form, is due to deletion of part or all of the δ and β regions of the β-globin gene complex, and in most respects resembles $\delta\beta$ thalassaemia. In the homozygous state, there is a mild thalassaemia-like blood picture, and the haemoglobin consists entirely of Hb-F. Heterozygotes have a Hb-F level of about 25 per cent, and the only haematological abnormality is a slight reduction in MCH. Patients who are heterozygous for the HPFH and Hb-S genes have approximately 30 per cent Hb-F and 70 per cent Hb-S in their red cells. In the Greek form of pancellular HPFH, as yet observed only in heterozygotes, Hb-F is about 15 per cent. Heterocellular HPFH is less clearly defined, and the elevation in Hb-F is generally mild. In the Swiss form, Hb-F levels in heterozygotes are in the 2–5 per cent range.

The HPFH syndromes may cause diagnostic difficulty as they resemble some forms of β thalassaemia. In combination with the Hb-S gene, the disorder may be mistaken for homozygous sickle-cell disease or sickle-cell β thalassaemia with complete suppression of Hb-A. The absence of significant haematological abnormalities in the homozygous and heterozygous states, and the mild nature of the illness when combined with Hb-S in addition to the homogeneous distribution of Hb-F in the red cells as demonstrated by the acid elution test, permits differentiation of the HPFH syndromes. Wood *et al.* (1979) discuss the differential diagnosis.

The α thalassaemias

The α thalassaemias are disorders in which there is defective synthesis of α chains with resulting depression of production of the haemoglobins that contain α chains, i.e. Hb-A, Hb-A_2 and Hb-F. The deficiency of α chains leads to an excess of γ chains in the fetus, and of β chains in the adult. The γ chains form the tetramer Hb-Bart's (γ_4), and the unstable β chains precipitate and form Hb-H (β_4). The presence of Hb-Bart's and Hb-H in the red cell has serious consequences as both haemoglobins have a high oxygen affinity and thus are unable to deliver adequate oxygen to the tissues.

CLASSIFICATION

Clinical and haematological studies of α thalassaemia in the 1950s and 1960s identified four forms of the disorder (Table 7.5). Alpha thalassaemia 2 usually showed no abnormalities on routine haematological examination, and α thalassaemia 1 was a benign condition with a variable mild anaemia and red cell hypochromia. The clinical picture of Hb-H disease was intermediate between that of β thalassaemia minor and major, and infants with Hb-Bart's hydrops fetalis died *in utero* or shortly after birth.

Although this nomenclature is still widely used, advances in methods of gene analysis have greatly increased understanding of the genetic basis of α thalassaemia, and have provided a more rational basis for classification. Normal subjects have two linked α gene loci on the short arm of chromosome 16, and thus an α gene haplotype $\alpha\alpha/$ and genotype $\alpha\alpha/\alpha\alpha$ (see Fig. 7.2). The α thalassaemias are most commonly due to deletions of one or more of these genes. In most affected populations, two abnormal α gene haplotyes are found, namely α^+ ($-\alpha/$) which arises from deletion of one α gene and α^0 ($--/$) from deletion of both α genes. The majority of α-thalassaemia phenotypes result from the interaction of these two haplotypes, the clinical severity depending on the number of genes deleted up to the possible four. The α^+ ($-\alpha/$) haplotype usually involves the deletion of either 3.7 ($-\alpha^{3.7}$) or 4.2 ($-\alpha^{4.2}$) kilobases of DNA from the α globin gene complex. α^0 ($--/$) haplotypes are designated according to the geographical area in which they commonly occur, e.g. $--^{MED}/$, $--^{SEA}/$. A less common non-deletion form of α thalassaemia in which there is partial suppression of α-chain synthesis in the presence of an apparently normal complement of α globin genes ($\alpha\alpha^T/$ haplotype) has also been described in some population groups.

Alpha thalassaemia is common in South-East Asia, particularly in Thailand where 20 per cent of the population is affected. It also occurs in the Middle East, Greece, Italy, India, Africa, and the Pacific Islands. The prevalence rate among American Blacks is 25–30 per cent. The α^0 ($--/$) haplotype (and therefore Hb-H disease and Hb-Bart's hydrops fetalis) is restricted to south-east Asia and, to a lesser extent, the Mediterranean countries. The α thalassaemias are fully reviewed by Higgs & Weatherall (1983).

Alpha thalassaemia trait

Alpha thalassaemia trait is asymptomatic and is difficult to diagnose with certainty in adult life. It should be suspected in all patients of high-risk ethnic origin with a refractory microcytic hypochromic blood picture once iron deficiency and β thalassaemia minor have been excluded (Hegde *et al.* 1977). Two types are recognized, but in the individual case distinction is often not possible without globin-chain synthesis or gene-mapping studies.

Table 7.5. *Classification of the α thalassaemia syndromes*

Clinical	Genetic	Genotype	Number of genes
α thalassaemia 2	Heterozygous α^+ thalassaemia	$\alpha\alpha/-\alpha$	3
α thalassaemia 1	Homozygous α^+ thalassaemia	$-\alpha/-\alpha$	2
	Heterozygous α^0 thalassaemia	$\alpha\alpha/--$	2
Hb-H disease	Double heterozygote α^+/α^0 thalassaemia	$-\alpha/--$	1
Hb-Bart's hydrops fetalis	Homozygous α^0 thalassaemia	$--/--$	0

Alpha thalassaemia 2 (α^+ thalassaemia). This represents the heterozygous state for α^+ thalassaemia ($\alpha\alpha$/-α). In the newborn period, affected infants may have 1–2 per cent Hb-Bart's which they gradually lose over the ensuing months. In adult life, the haemoglobin pattern is normal, and Hb-H inclusions are not found at any stage. Haemoglobin level and blood film are normal, although the MCV and MCH may be mildly reduced.

Alpha thalassaemia 1 (α^0 thalassaemia). This represents the heterozygous state for α^0 (--/$\alpha\alpha$) or the homozygous state for α^+ thalassaemia (-α/-α). In the newborn period, 5–6 per cent Hb-Bart's is found, but the haemoglobin pattern is normal in later life. Hb-H inclusions are usually present in very small numbers, and a prolonged search may be necessary for their detection. The haemoglobin level is normal or only mildly reduced, but the red cells are usually mildly hypochromic and microcytic, and the MCV and MCH are reduced. Hb-A_2 is reduced in some patients.

Haemoglobin-H disease

Interaction of the α^+ (-α/) and the α^0 (--/) determinants gives rise to this form of α thalassaemia (-α/--) which is common in south-east Asia and is also seen in the Middle East and some Mediterranean countries. It is rare in Blacks.

Clinically, Hb-H disease is characterized by a moderate anaemia with a haemoglobin level of 8–9 g/dl, mild jaundice, and physical findings similar to, but generally less severe than, those of classical β thalassaemia major. The severity of the anaemia fluctuates, and it may fall to very low levels during pregnancy, intercurrent infection, or ingestion of oxidant drugs. Occasionally, the haemolysis is well compensated and the haemoglobin level normal. Splenomegaly is present in 85 per cent of patients, and cholelithiasis is common.

The *blood film* shows marked red cell morphological changes including severe hypochromia and microcytosis, target cell formation, and basophilic stippling. The MCV and MCH are low. Nucleated red cells are seen, and there is a mild reticulocytosis. Numerous *Hb-H inclusions* may be demonstrated with brilliant cresyl blue stain, and large Heinz body-like inclusions are also present if splenectomy has been performed.

The *haemoglobin pattern* consists of 2–40 per cent Hb-H, the remainder being Hb-A, Hb-A_2 (which is reduced) and Hb-F. A small amount of Hb-Bart's is present in some cases. In south-east Asia, 40 per cent of patients with Hb-H disease also have a small amount of an α-chain variant, Hb-Constant Spring. Neonates with Hb-H disease have about 25 per cent Hb-Bart's, and only very small amounts of Hb-H, but in most cases Hb-H gradually replaces Hb-Bart's over the first year of life.

Therapy is not required in most patients with Hb-H disease. Avoidance of oxidant drugs and prompt treatment of intercurrent infection is advisable. Blood transfusion may occasionally be necessary, and splenectomy has been successful in significantly elevating the haemoglobin in some carefully selected patients with consistently low levels. Folic acid administration is advisable, especially in pregnancy. Secondary haemochromatosis is rare, and administration of iron-chelating agents is not indicated.

Haemoglobin-Bart's hydrops fetalis

The most severe manifestation of the α thalassaemia gene is haemoglobin Bart's hydrops fetalis which is common in south-east Asia, but rare in other parts of the world where the α thalassaemia gene is found. Affected infants are homozygous for the α^0 determinant (--/--), both parents having heterozygous α^0 thalassaemia. There is almost total suppresion of α-chain synthesis with a gross excess of γ chains. The γ-chain tetramer, Hb-Bart's, has a high oxygen affinity, and severe tissue hypoxia results.

The *clinical picture* is similar to that of severe Rh haemolytic disease. Affected infants are either born dead or die within a few hours of birth. They are underweight, pale, mildly jaundiced, grossly oedematous, and have hepatosplenomegaly and ascites. The haemoglobin level is around 6 g/dl, and the blood film is grossly abnormal with anisopoikilocytosis, hypochromia, target cells, basophilic stippling, polychromasia, and large numbers of nucleated red cells. The reticulocyte count is high, and serum bilirubin elevated. The mother often has an associated toxaemia of pregnancy. Antenatal diagnosis of pregnancies at risk for homozygous α thalassaemia is now possible (p. 162).

The *haemoglobin pattern* consists of 80–90 per cent Hb-Bart's, with a small amount of Hb-H and a third 'fast' component, Hb-Portland. There is usually no Hb-A, Hb-A_2 or Hb-F.

Alpha thalassaemia and other haemoglobinopathies

Alpha thalassaemia is found in association with α-chain haemoglobin variants, e.g. Hb-Q and Hb-I; β-chain variants, e.g. Hb-E, Hb-S, and Hb-C; and with β thalassaemia.

Methaemoglobinaemia

Methaemoglobin (ferrihaemoglobin) is a derivative of normal haemoglobin (ferrohaemoglobin) in which the iron of the haem complex has been oxidized from the ferrous to the ferric form. It does not combine with oxygen and thus does not take part in oxygen transport. In normal red cells, methaemoglobin is continually being formed by the auto-oxidation of haemoglobin, but it is reduced as soon as it is formed; thus the concentration of methaemoglobin in the red cell under normal conditions is less than one per cent of the total haemoglobin. The reduction of methaemoglobin is accomplished by the enzyme NADH–methaemoglobin reductase (NADH–cytochrome b_5 reductase) in the presence of NADH. The NADH is generated by the Embden–Meyerhof pathway of glycolysis (Chapter 2, p. 19).

The term methaemoglobinaemia is used to describe the excess accumulation of methaemoglobin in the red cells. Methaemoglobin lacks the capacity to carry oxygen, and methaemoglobinaemia causes symptoms and signs of hypoxia. The great majority of cases of methaemoglobinaemia are due to the action of chemical agents that increase the rate of auto-oxidation of haemoglobin in the red cells. Rare cases are due to congenital metabolic defects of the red cell.

Toxic methaemoglobinaemia

The *causes* of toxic methaemoglobinaemia may be grouped as follows.

Drug causes. Drugs which may cause methaemoglobinaemia include phenacetin, acetanilide, sulphonamides, sulphones, prilocaine, primaquine and pamaquine, nitrates, nitrites and potassium chlorate.

Occupational causes. Methaemoglobinaemia in industry is most commonly due to absorption of nitro and amino aromatic derivatives, e.g. nitrobenzene, trinitrobenzene, and aniline. The substances are usually absorbed through the respiratory tract or skin, and the disorder is most often seen in workers in chemical factories and explosive plants.

Household causes. Chemicals capable of producing methaemoglobinaemia are present in a number of household substances; these include furniture and shoe polish (containing nitrobenzene), marking ink, shoe dyes and coloured crayons (containing aniline), perfumes, and flavouring essences. Acute methaemoglobinaemia is seen most often in children due to accidental ingestion of these substances. Methaemoglobinaemia has also been reported as a result of the use of aniline-containing inks to mark infants' napkins. Well-water sometimes contains high concentrations of nitrates, and in country areas the use of this water to prepare milk mixtures for infants has resulted in methaemoglobinaemia. Drug-induced methaemoglobinaemia is reviewed by Smith & Olsen (1973).

CLINICAL FEATURES

Cyanosis occurs when methaemoglobin constitutes about 15 per cent of the total pigment. In many cases, there are no clinical features other than cyanosis, but when the concentration of methaemoglobin reaches 30–45 per cent anoxic symptoms commonly develop. These include headache, dizziness, tachycardia, dyspnoea on exertion, muscular cramps, and weakness. In cases of acute poisoning, the concentration may exceed 60–70 per cent, and vomiting, lethargy, loss of consciousness, circulatory failure, and death may occur. In acute cases, the cyanosis develops within 1–2 hours of the ingestion of the toxic agent.

In chronic methaemoglobinaemia, a mild compensatory polycythaemia occasionally develops. Many of the substances that cause methaemoglobinaemia may also cause a haemolytic anaemia with Heinz-body formation.

DIAGNOSIS

Clinically, the diagnosis of methaemoglobinaemia is suggested by the presence of definite cyanosis with little or no dyspnoea. Methaemoglobin can be identified spectroscopically by its absorption band in the red part of the spectrum at 630 nm; this band disappears on the addition of yellow ammonium sulphide. When it is present in large amounts the blood has a chocolate-brown colour which does not disappear on oxygenation. Methaemoglobin does not appear in the plasma or urine except in the occasional case with associated haemolytic anaemia.

TREATMENT

Following removal of the causative agent, methaemoglobin is converted back to haemoglobin in a few days. Thus in chronic cases elimination of the causative drug or chemical results in disappearance of the cyanosis within several days.

In cases of acute methaemoglobinaemia due to poisoning, especially when symptoms are severe, more active treatment is necessary. Treatment consists of slow intravenous injection of methylene blue; the recommended dose is 2 mg/kg bodyweight for infants, 1.5 mg/kg bodyweight for older children, and 1 mg/kg bodyweight for adults, in a 1 per cent sterile aqueous solution.

Hereditary methaemoglobinaemia

Hereditary methaemoglobinaemia is rare. Two main types are recognized which differ in their fundamental effect and mode of inheritance.

Hereditary methaemoglobinaemia associated with NADH–methaemoglobin reductase deficiency. This disorder is transmitted as an autosomal recessive trait. Affected subjects are persistently cyanotic and usually have mild polycythaemia. Some have symptoms of anoxia. Mental retardation is an occasional association. Regular oral ascorbic acid therapy relieves the cyanosis and other symptoms when present. Deficiency of NADH–methaemoglobin reductase is reviewed by Schwartz *et al.* (1983).

Hereditary methaemoglobinaemia associated with haemoglobins-M. Several abnormal haemoglobins, referred to as haemoglobins-M, are associated with cyanosis. The disorder is transmitted as an autosomal dominant trait, and anoxic symptoms are usually absent. The cyanosis is not improved by the administration of methylene blue or ascorbic acid. The haemoglobins-M are reviewed by Nagel & Bookchin (1974).

Sulphaemoglobinaemia

Sulphaemoglobin is an abnormal sulphur-containing haemoglobin derivative allied to methaemoglobin. It does not act as an oxygen carrier and is not present in normal red cells. It is formed by the toxic action of the drugs and chemical agents that cause methaemoglobinaemia in persons who are either constipated or who are taking sulphur-containing medicines. A history of ingestion of sulphur-containing purgatives such as magnesium sulphate is not uncommon, and in occasional cases there is an associated anatomical abnormality of the bowel, e.g. stricture on diverticulosis. Methaemoglobinaemia and sulphaemoglobinaemia are often present together.

Sulphaemoglobin represents an irreversible change in the haemoglobin pigment; thus it does not disappear from the red cells once the causative agent is removed, but persists until the cells are destroyed at the end of their lifespan, progressively disappearing from the blood over a period of about three months. Furthermore, it is not converted to haemoglobin by either ascorbic acid or methylene blue.

Sulphaemoglobinaemia results in cyanosis, similar to that of methaemoglobinaemia. *Diagnosis* is established by spectroscopic examination and isoelectric focusing. Sulphaemoglobin occurs only in the red cells; it is not present in the plasma unless haemolysis occurs.

Treatment consists of removal of the causative agent and correction of constipation when present. Constipation is best treated by liquid paraffin or an enema; sulphur-containing laxatives such as magnesium sulphate should be avoided.

References and further reading

Monographs

Bunn, H.F. & Forget, B.G. (1986) *Hemoglobin: Molecular, Genetic and Clinical Aspects*, Saunders, Philadelphia.

Huisman, T.J.H. (Ed.) (1986) *The Hemoglobinopathies. Methods in Hematology*, Vol. 15, Churchill Livingstone, Edinburgh.

Modell, B. & Berdoukas, V. (1984) *The Clinical Approach to Thalassaemia*, Grune & Stratton, London.

Serjeant, G.R. (1985) *Sickle Cell Disease*, Oxford University Press, Oxford.

Weatherall, D.J. (1982) *The New Genetics and Clinical Medicine*, Nuffield Provincial Hospitals Trust, London.

Weatherall, D.J. (Ed.) (1983) *The Thalassemias. Methods in Hematology*, Vol. 6, Churchill Livingstone, Edinburgh.

Weatherall, D.J. & Clegg, J.B. (1981) *The Thalassaemia Syndromes*, 3rd Ed., Blackwell Scientific Publications, Oxford.

Wintrobe, M.M., Lee, G.R., Boggs, D.R. *et al.* (1981) *Clinical Hematology*, 8th Ed., Lea & Febiger, Philadelphia.

Normal haemoglobin: structure, synthesis and genetic regulation

Antonarakis, S.E. Kazazian, H.H. & Orkin, S.H. (1985) DNA polymorphism and molecular pathology of the human globin gene clusters. *Hum. Genet.* **69**, 1.

Jackson, I.J. & Williamson, R. (1980) Mapping of the human globin genes. *Brit. J. Haemat.* **46**, 341.

Nienhuis, A.W. & Benz, E.J. (1977) Regulation of hemoglobin synthesis during the development of the red cell. *New Engl. J. Med.* **297**, 1318.

Orkin, S.H., Antonarakis, S.E. & Kazazian, H.H.Jr. (1983) Polymorphism and molecular pathology of the human beta-globin gene. *Prog. Hemat.* **13**, 49.

Perutz, M.F. (1978) Hemoglobin structure and respiratory transport. *Sci. Am.* **239**, 68.

Weatherall, D.J., Pembrey, M.E. & Pritchard, J. (1974) Fetal haemoglobin. *Clin. Haemat.* **3**, 467.

Abnormal haemoglobins and the haemoglobinopathies

GENERAL

Alter, B. (1984) Advances in the prenatal diagnosis of hematologic diseases. *Blood*, **64**, 329.

Betke, K., Marti, H.R. & Schlicht, I. (1959) Estimation of small percentages of foetal haemoglobin. *Nature*, **184**, 1877.

Bradley, T.B. & Ranney, H.M. (1973) Acquired disorders of hemoglobin. *Prog. Hemat.* **8**, 77.

Dacie, J.V. & Lewis, S.M. (1984) *Practical Haematology*, 6th Ed., Churchill Livingstone, London.

Editorial Board, *Hemoglobin* (1979) Recommendations for nomenclature of hemoglobins. *Hemoglobin*, **3**, 1.

International Committee for Standardization in Hematology (1978) Recommendations of a system for identifying abnormal hemoglobin. *Blood*, **52**, 1065.

International Committee for Standardization in Haematology (1979) Recommendations for fetal haemoglobin reference preparations and fetal haemoglobin determination by the alkali denaturation method. *Brit. J. Haemat.* **42**, 133.

Kleihauer, E., Braun, H. & Betke, K. (1957) Demonstration von fetalem Hamoglobin in den Erythrocyten eines Blutausstrichs. *Klin. Wschr.* **35**, 637.

Livingstone, F.B. (1967) *Abnormal Hemoglobins in Human Populations*, Aldine Publishing Co., Chicago.

Milner, P.F. & Gooden, H.M. (1975) Rapid citrate-agar electrophoresis in routine screening for hemoglobinopathies using a simple hemolysate. *Am. J. Clin. Path.* **64**, 58.

Modell, B. (1983) Prevention of the haemoglobinopathies. *Brit. Med. Bull.* **39**, 386.

Old, J.M., Heath, C., Fitches, A. *et al.* (1986) First-trimester fetal diagnosis for haemoglobinopathies: report on 200 cases. *Lancet*, **ii**, 763.

Weatherall, D.J. (1985) Prenatal diagnosis of inherited blood diseases. *Clin. Haemat.* **14**, 747

THE SICKLING DISORDERS

Armaly, M.F. (1974) Ocular manifestations in sickle-cell disease. *Arch. Int. Med.* **133**, 670.

Ballas, S.K., Lewis, C.N., Noone, A.M. *et al.* (1982) Clinical, hematological, and biochemical features of Hb SC disease. *Am. J. Hematol.* **13**, 37.

Barrett-Connor, E. (1971) Bacterial infection and sickle-cell anemia. An analysis of 250 infections in 166 patients and a review of the literature. *Medicine*, **50**, 97.

Bertles, J.F. (1974) Hemoglobin interaction and molecular basis of sickling. *Arch. Int. Med.* **133**, 538.

Bookchin. R.M. & Lew, V.L. (1983) Red cell membrane abnormalities in sickle cell anemia. *Prog. Hemat.* **13**, 1.

Buckalow, V.M. & Someren, A. (1974) Renal manifestations of sickle-cell disease. *Arch. Int. Med.* **133**, 660.

Chang, H., Ewert, S.M., Bookchin, R.M. *et al.* (1983) Comparative evaluation of fifteen anti-sickling agents. *Blood*, **61**, 693.

Charache, S. (1981) Treatment of sickle cell anemia. *Ann. Rev. Med.* **32**, 195.

Charache, S., Scott, J.C. & Charache, P. (1970) 'Acute chest syndrome' in adults with sickle cell anemia: microbiology, treatment and prevention. *Arch. Int. Med.* **139**, 67.

Charache, S. & Niebyl, J.R. (1985) Pregnancy in sickle cell disease. *Clin. Haemat.* **14**, 729.

Consensus Conference (1987) Newborn screening for sickle cell disease and other hemoglobinopathies. *J. Am. Med. Ass.* **258**, 1205.

Dean, J. & Schechter, A.N. (1978) Sickle cell anemia: molecular and cellular bases of therapeutic approaches. *New Engl. J. Med.* **299**, 752.

Eaton, W.A. & Hofrichter, J. (1987) Hemoglobin S gelation and sickle cell disease, *Blood* **70**, 1245.

Embury, S.H. (1986) The clinical pathophysiology of sickle cell disease. *Ann. Rev. Med.* **37**, 361.

Felice, A.E., Altay, C.A., Milner, P.F. *et al.* (1981) The occurrence and identification of α-thalassemia-2 among hemoglobin S heterozygotes. *Am. J. Clin. Path.* **76**, 70.

Gaston, M.H., Verter, J.I., Woods, G. *et al.* (1986) Prophylaxis with oral penicillin in children with sickle cell anemia. A randomized trial. *New Engl. J. Med.* **314**, 1593.

Harkness, D.R. (1980) Hematological and clinical features of sickle cell disease: a review. *Hemoglobin*, **4**, 313.

Higgs, D.R., Aldridge, B.E., Lamb, J. *et al.* (1982) The interaction of alpha-thalassemia and homozygous sickle-cell disease. *New Engl. J. Med.* **306**, 1441.

Higgs, D.R., Pressley, L., Serjeant, G.R. *et al.* (1981) The genetics and molecular basis of alpha thalassaemia in association with Hb S in Jamaican negroes. *Brit. J. Haemat.* **47**, 43.

Horn, M.E.C., Dick, M.C., Frost, B. *et al.* (1986) Neonatal screening for sickle cell diseases in Camberwell: results and recommendations of a two year pilot study. *Brit. Med. J.* **292**, 737.

Horne, M.K. (1981) Sickle cell anemia as a rheologic disease. *Am. J. Med.* **70**, 288.

Kark, J.A., Posey, D.M., Schumacher, H.R. *et al.* (1987) Sickle-cell trait as a risk factor in physical training. *New Engl. J. Med.* **317**, 781.

Konotey-Ahulu, F. (1974) The sickle-cell diseases. Clinical manifestations including the 'sickle crisis'. *Arch. Int. Med.* **133**, 611.

Kramer, M.S., Rooks, Y. & Pearson, H.A. (1978) Growth and development in children with sickle-cell trait. *New Engl. J. Med.* **299**, 686.

McCurdy, P.R., Lorkin, P.A., Casey, R. *et al.* (1974) Hemoglobin S-G (S-D) syndrome. *Am. J. Med.* **57**, 665.

Milner, P.F. (1974) Oxygen transport in sickle-cell anemia. *Arch. Int. Med.* **133**, 565.

Milner, P.F. & Brown, M. (1982) Bone marrow infarction in sickle cell anemia: correlation with hematologic profiles. *Blood*, **60**, 1411.

Murray, N., Rerjeant, B.E. & Serjeant, G.R. (1988) Sickle cell-hereditary persistence of fetal haemoglobin and its differentiation from other sickle cell syndromes. *Brit. J. Haemat.* **69**, 89.

Noguchi, C.T., Rodgers, G.P., Serjeant, G. *et al.* (1988) Current concepts. Levels of fetal hemoglobin necessary for treatment of sickle cell disease. *New Engl. J. Med.* **318**, 96.

Pearson, H.A., Spencer, R.P. & Cornelius, E.A. (1969) Functional asplenia in sickle-cell anemia. *New Engl. J. Med.* **281**, 923.

Platt, O.S., Rosenstock, W. & Espeland, M.A. (1984) Influence of sickle hemoglobinopathies on growth and development. *New Engl. J. Med.* **311**, 7.

Powars, D.R. (1975) Natural history of sickle-cell disease—the first ten years. *Semin. Hematol.* **12**, 267.

Powars, D., Wilson, B., Imbus, C. *et al.* (1978) The natural history of stroke in sickle cell disease. *Am. J. Med.* **65**, 461.

Rucknagel, D.L. (1974) The genetics of sickle-cell anemia and related syndromes. *Arch. Int. Med.* **133**, 595.

Schmidt, R.M. & Wilson, S.M. (1973) Standardization in detection of abnormal hemoglobins. Solubility tests for hemoglobin S. *J. Am. Med. Ass.* **225**, 1225.

Scott, R.B. & Castro, O. (1979) Screening for sickle cell hemoglobinopathies. *J. Am. Med. Ass.* **241**, 1145.

Sears, D.A. (1978) The morbidity of sickle-cell trait. A review of the literature. *Am. J. Med.* **64**, 1021.

Serjeant, G.R. (1975) Fetal haemoglobin in homozygous sickle-cell disease. *Clin. Haemat.* **4**, 109.

Serjeant, G.R., Richards, R., Barbor, P.R.H. *et al.* (1968) Relatively benign sickle-cell anaemia in 60 patients aged over 30 in the West Indies. *Brit. Med. J.* **3**, 86.

Serjeant, G.R., Ashcroft, M.T. & Serjeant, B.E. (1973) The clinical features of haemoglobin SC disease in Jamaica. *Brit. J. Haemat.* **24**, 491.

Serjeant, G.R., Sommereux, A., Stevenson, M. *et al.* (1979) Comparison of sickle cell-β^0 thalassaemia with homozygous sickle cell disease. *Brit. J. Haemat.* **83**, 79.

Serjeant, G.R., Grandison, Y., Lowrie, Y. *et al.* (1981) The development of haematological changes in homozygous sickle cell disease: a cohort study from birth to 6 years. *Brit. J. Haemat.* **48**, 533.

Shurafa, M.S., Prasad, A.S., Rucknagel, D.L. *et al.* (1982) Long survival in sickle cell anemia. *Am. J. Hematol.* **12**, 357.

Steinberg, M.H. & Hebbel, R.P. (1983) Clinical diversity of sickle cell anemia: genetic and cellular modulation of disease severity. *Am. J. Hematol.* **14**, 405.

Stockman, J.A., Nigro, M.A., Mishkin, M.M. *et al.* (1972) Occlusion of large cerebral vessels in sickle-cell anemia. *New Engl. J. Med.* **287**, 846.

Thomas, A.N., Pattison, C. & Serjeant, G. (1982) Causes of death in sickle-cell disease in Jamaica. *Brit. Med. J.* **285**, 633.

Walker, B.K., Ballas, S.K. & Burka, G.R. (1979) The diagnosis of pulmonary thromboembolism in sickle cell disease. *Am. J. Hematol.* **7**, 219.

Warth, J.A. & Rucknagel, D.L. (1983) The increasing complexity of sickle cell anemia. *Prog. Hemat.* **13**, 25.

Wrightstone, R.N. & Huisman, T.J.H. (1974) On the levels of hemoglobins F and A2 in sickle-cell anemia and some related disorders. *Am. J. Clin. Path.* **61**, 375.

OTHER HAEMOGLOBINOPATHIES

Fairbanks, V.F., Gilchrist, G.S., Brimhall, B. *et al.* (1979) Hemoglobin E trait re-examined: a cause of microcytosis and erythrocytosis. *Blood*, **53**, 109.

Fairbanks, V.F., Oliveros, R., Brandabur, J.H. *et al.* (1980) Homozygous hemoglobin E mimics β-thalassemia minor without anemia or hemolysis: hematologic functional and biosynthetic studies of first North American cases. *Am. J. Hematol.* **8**, 109.

Lachant, N.A. (1987) Hemoglobin E: an emerging hemoglobinopathy in the United States. *Am. J. Hematol.* **25**, 449.

Ringelhann, B. & Khorsandi, M. (1972) Hemoglobin crystallization test to differentiate cells with Hb SC and CC genotype from SS cells without electrophoresis. *Am. J. Clin. Path.* **57**, 467.

Smith, E.W. & Krevans, J.R. (1959) Clinical manifestations of hemoglobin C disorders. *Bull. Johns Hopk. Hosp.* **104**, 17.

Vella, F. & Lehmann, H. (1974) Haemoglobin D Punjab (D Los Angeles). *J. Med. Gen.* **11**, 341.

Wasi, P. (1981) Haemoglobinopathies including thalassaemia. Part 1: Tropical Asia. *Clin. Haemat.* **10**, 707.

THE UNSTABLE HAEMOGLOBIN DISORDERS

Bentley, S.A., Lewis, S.M. & White, J.M. (1974) Red cell survival studies in patients with unstable haemoglobin disorders. *Brit. J. Haemat.* **26**, 85.

Carrell, R.W. (1986) Methods of determining hemoglobin instability (unstable homoglobins). In: Huisman, T.H.J. (Ed.) *The hemoglobinopathies. Methods in Hematology*, Vol. 15, Churchill Livingstone, Edinburgh.

Perutz, M.F. (1978) Hemoglobin structure and respiratory transport. *Sci. Am.* **239**, 68.

White, J.M. (1976) The unstable haemoglobins. *Brit. Med. Bull.* **32**, 219.

White, J.M. & Dacie, J.V. (1971) The unstable hemoglobins—molecular and clinical features. *Prog. Hemat.* **7**, 69.

HAEMOGLOBINOPATHIES ASSOCIATED WITH POLYCYTHAEMIA

Bellingham, A.J. (1976) Haemoglobins with altered oxygen affinity. *Brit. Med. Bull.* **32**, 234.

Jones, R.T. & Shih, T.-B. (1980) Hemoglobin variants with altered oxygen affinity. *Hemoglobin*, **4**, 234.

The thalassaemias

GENERAL

Bank, A. (1978) The thalassemia syndromes. *Blood*, **51**, 369.

Brosious, E.M., Wright, J.M., Baine, R.M. *et al.* (1978) Microchromatographic methods for hemoglobin A_2 quantitation compared. *Clin. Chem.* **24**, 2196.

Clegg, J.B. (1983) Hemoglobin synthesis. In: Weatherall, D.J. (Ed.) *The Thalassemias. Methods in Hematology*, Vol. 6, Churchill Livingstone, Edinburgh.

Clegg, J.B. & Weatherall, D.J. (1976) Molecular basis of thalassaemia. *Brit. Med. Bull.* **32**, 262.

Nienhuis, A.W., Anagnou, N.O. & Ley, T.J. (1984) Advances in thalassemia research. *Blood*, **63**, 738.

Old, J.M. & Higgs, D.R. (1983) Gene analysis. In: Weatherall, D.J. (Ed.) *The Thalassemias. Methods in Hematology*, Vol. 6, Churchill Livingstone, Edinburgh.

Steinberg, M.H. & Adams, J.G. (1982) Thalassemia: recent insights into molecular mechanism. *Am. J. Hematol.* **12**, 81.

Todd, D. (1984) Thalassemia. *Pathology*, **16**, 5.

BETA THALASSAEMIA

Alperin, J.B., Dow, P.A. & Petteway, M.B. (1977) Hemoglobin A_2 levels in health and various hematologic disorders. *Am. J. Clin. Path.* **67**, 219.

Alter, B.P. (1983) Antenatal diagnosis using fetal blood. In: Weatherall, D.J. (Ed.) *The Thalassemias. Methods in Hematology*, Vol. 6, Churchill Livingstone, Edinburgh.

Bessman, J.D. & Feinstein, D.I. (1979) Quantitative anisocytosis as a discriminant between iron deficiency and thalassemia minor. *Blood*, **53**, 288.

Efremov, G.D. (1978) Hemoglobins Lepore and anti-Lepore. *Hemoglobin*, **2**, 197.

Hamilton, S.R., Miller, M.E., Jessop, M. *et al.* (1979) Comparison of microchromatography and electrophoresis with elution for hemoglobin A_2 (Hb A_2) quantitation. *Am. J. Clin. Path.* **71**, 388.

Humphries, S.E. & Williamson, R. (1983) Application of recombinant DNA technology to prenatal detection of inherited defects. *Brit. Med. Bull.* **39**, 343.

Hoffbrand, A.V., Gorman, A., Laulicht, M. *et al.* (1979) Improvement in iron status and liver function in patients with transfusional iron overload with long-term subcutaneous desferrioxamine. *Lancet*, **i**, 947.

International Committee for Standardization in Haematology (1978) Recommendations for selected methods for quantitative estimation of Hb A_2 and for Hb A_2 reference preparation. *Brit. J. Haemat.* **38**, 573.

Kanavakis, E., Wainscoat, J.S., Wood, W.G. *et al.* (1982 The interaction of α thalassaemia with heterozygous β thalassaemia. *Brit. J. Haemat.* **52**, 465.

Lucarelli, G., Galimberti, M., Polchi, P. *et al.* (1987) Marrow transplantation in patients with advanced thalassemia. *New Engl. J. Med.* **316**, 1050.

Marinucci, M., Mavilio, F., Massa, A. *et al.* (1979) Haemoglobin Lepore trait: haematological and structural studies on the Italian population. *Brit. J. Haemat.* **42**, 557.

Mazza, U., Saglio, G., Cappio, F.C. *et al.* (1976) Clinical and haematological data in 254 cases of beta-thalassaemia trait in Italy. *Brit. J. Haemat.* **33**, 91.

Olivieri, N.F., Buncic, J.R., Chew, E. *et al.* (1986) Visual and auditory neurotoxicity in patients receiving subcutaneous deferoxamine infusions. *New Engl. J. Med.* **314**, 869.

Pippard, M.J. & Wainscoat, J.S. (1987) Erythrokinetics and iron status in heterozygous β thalassaemia, and the effect of interaction with α thalassaemia. *Brit. J. Haemat.* **66**, 123.

Pippard, M.J. (1983) Iron loading and chelation therapy. In: Weatherall, D.J. (Ed.) *The Thalassemias. Methods in Hematology*, Vol. 6, Churchill Livingstone, Edinburgh.

Pippard, M.J. & Callender, S.T. (1983) The management of iron chelation therapy. *Brit. J. Haemat.* **54**, 503.

Propper, R.D., Cooper, B., Rufo, R.R. *et al.* (1977) Continuous subcutaneous administration of deferoxamine in patients with iron overload. *New Engl. J. Med.* **297**, 418.

Propper, R.D. (1983) Transfusion management of thalassemia. In: Weatherall, D.J. (Ed.) *The Thalassemias. Methods in Hematology*, Vol. 6, Churchill Livingstone, Edinburgh.

Schwartz, E. (1969) The silent carrier of beta-thalassemia. *New Engl. J. Med.* **281**, 1327.

Silvestroni, E. & Bianco, I. (1983) A highly cost effective method of mass screening for thalassaemia. *Brit. Med. J.* **286**, 1007.

Weatherall, D.J., Pippard, M.J. & Callender, S.T. (1983) Iron loading in thalassemia—five years with the pump. *New Engl. J. Med.* **308**, 456.

Wolman, J.J. (1969) Health and growth of Cooley's anemia patients in relation to transfusion schedules. *Ann. N.Y. Acad. Sci.* **164**, 407.

Wood, W.G., Clegg, J.B. & Weatherall, D.J. (1979) Hereditary persistence of fetal haemoglobin (HPFH) and thalassaemia. *Brit. J. Haemat.* **43**, 509.

ALPHA THALASSAEMIA

Hegde, U.M., White, J.M., Hart, G.H. *et al.* (1977) Diagnosis of α-thalassaemia trait from Coulter Counter 'S' indices. *J. Clin. Path.* **30**, 884.

Higgs, D.R., Pressley, L., Clegg, J.B. *et al.* (1980) Detection of α thalassaemia in Negro infants. *Brit. J. Haemat.* **46**, 39.

Higgs, D.R. & Weatherall, D.J. (1983) Alpha-thalassemia. In: Piomelli, S. & Yachnin, S. (Eds) *Current Topics in Hematology*, Vol. 4, Alan Liss, New York.

Higgs, D.R., Wood, W.G., Barton, C. *et al.* (1983) Clinical features and molecular analysis of acquired hemoglobin H disease. *Am. J. Med.* **75**, 181.

Johnson, C.S., Tegos, C. & Beutler, E. (1982) α-Thalassemia. Prevalence and hematologic findings in American blacks. *Arch. Int. Med.* **142**, 1280.

O'Brien, R.T. (1973) The effect of iron deficiency on the expression of hemoglobin H. *Blood*, **41**, 853.

Steinberg, M.H. & Embury, S.H. (1986) α-Thalassemia in blacks: genetic and clinical aspects and interactions with the sickle hemoglobin gene. *Blood*, **68**, 985.

Wasi, P., Na-Nakorn, S. & Pootrakul, S. (1974) The α-thalassemias. *Clin. Haemat.* **3**, 383.

Wilkinson, T., Yakas, J., Knonenbeig, H. *et al.* (1986) α-Thalassemia British type ($\alpha\alpha$/--^{BRIT}) in an Australian family. *Pathology*, **18**, 193.

Methaemoglobinaemia and sulphae-moglobinaemia

Bodansky, O. (1951) Methemoglobinemia and methemoglobin-producing compounds. *Pharmacol. Rev.* **3**, 144.

Jaffe, E.R. & Hsieh, H.-S. (1971) DPNH-methemoglobin reductase deficiency and hereditary methemoglobinemia. *Semin. Hematol.* **8**, 417.

Nagel, R.L. & Bookchin, R.M. (1974) Human hemoglobin mutants with abnormal oxygen binding. *Semin. Hematol.* **11**, 385.

Park, C.M. & Nagel, R.L. (1984) Sulfhemoglobinemia. Clinical and molecular aspects. *New Engl. J. Med.* **310**, 1579.

Schwartz, J.M., Reiss, A.L. & Jaffe, E.R. (1983) Hereditary methemoglobinemia with deficiency of NADH cytochrome b5 reductase. In: Stanbury, J.B., Wyngaarden, J.B., Frederickson, D.S., Goldstein, L.J. & Brown, M.S. (Eds) *The Metabolic Basis of Inherited Disease*, 5th Ed., McGraw-Hill Book Co., New York.

Smith, R.P. & Olson M.V. (1973) Drug-induced methemoglobinemia. *Semin. Hematol.* **10**, 253.

Chapter 8
The Haemolytic Anaemias

Definition and classification

Haemolytic anaemias result from an increase in the rate of red cell destruction. The lifespan of the normal red cell is 100–120 days; in the haemolytic anaemias it is shortened by varying degrees, and in very severe cases may be only a few days.

The premature destruction of the red cell may result from two fundamental defects: (1) an *intracorpuscular* (intrinsic) abnormality of the red cells which renders them more susceptible to the normal mechanisms of cell destruction. The fault lies in the cells themselves. Normal compatible red cells transfused into a patient with an intrinsic red cell abnormality survive for a normal length of time, but the patient's cells when transfused into a normal recipient are prematurely destroyed; and (2) an *extracorpuscular* (extrinsic) abnormality due to the development of an abnormal haemolytic mechanism. Normal compatible red cells transfused into a patient with an extracorpuscular abnormality are prematurely destroyed, but the patient's cells transfused into a normal recipient survive for an approximately normal time.

The haemolytic anaemias may, therefore, be classified into two broad groups.

Haemolytic anaemias due to a corpuscular defect (intracorpuscular or intrinsic abnormality). These are mainly congenital. The basic defect may be in any of the three main components of the cell—the membrane, the haemoglobin molecule, and the enzymes concerned with cell metabolism.

Haemolytic anaemias due to an abnormal haemolytic mechanism (extracorpuscular or extrinsic abnormality). These disorders are acquired. The haemolysis may result from either an immune or a non-immune mechanism.

The various causes of haemolytic anaemia in these two groups are listed in Table 8.1. In a few disorders, both an intracorpuscular and extracorpuscular mechanism is present.

Compensated haemolytic disease. Shortening of the red cell lifespan does not necessarily result in anaemia, as compensatory bone marrow hyperplasia may increase red cell production six- to eightfold and maintain a normal haemoglobin level. Anaemia occurs only when the marrow hyperplasia is unable to compensate for the increased destruction. Thus anaemia is not invariable in the disorders listed in Table 8.1, and some authors prefer to describe them as the haemolytic disorders rather than the haemolytic anaemias. The term 'compensated haemolytic disease' is applied to haemolytic disorders in which anaemia is absent; they show reticulocytosis and erythroid hyperplasia of the bone marrow.

Haemolytic element in other anaemias. Red cell lifespan is often shortened in a number of anaemias that are not ordinarily classified as haemolytic anaemias. They include the anaemias associated with disseminated malignancy, leukaemia, malignant lymphomas, renal failure, liver disease, rheumatoid arthritis, and the megaloblastic anaemias. However, in these disorders the shortening of red cell lifespan is usually less than in the typical haemolytic anaemias and, in general, impairment of red cell production is the more important factor in the pathogenesis of the anaemia. The usual clinical features of a haemolytic anaemia are seldom present; jaundice is absent, the serum bilirubin is

Table 8.1. *Aetiological classification of the haemolytic anaemias*

Haemolytic anaemias due to intracopuscular (intrinsic) mechanisms

CONGENITAL

Membrane defects

Hereditary spherocytosis
Hereditary elliptocytosis
Hereditary xerocytosis and hydrocytosis

Haemoglobin defects

(a) Haemoglobinopathies:
  Sickle-cell anaemia
  Other homozygous disorders (Hb-C, Hb-E, Hb-D, etc.)
  Unstable haemoglobin disease
(b) Thalassaemia:
  β-thalassaemia major
  Hb-H disease
(c) Double heterozygous disorders:
  Sickle-cell β thalassaemia, etc.

Enzyme defects

(a) Non-spherocytic congenital haemolytic anaemia (Table 8.4, p. 189)
  (i) due to deficiency of pyruvate kinase or other enzymes of the Embden–Meyerhof pathway
  (ii) due to deficiency of glucose-6-phosphate dehydrogenase or other enzymes of the pentose phosphate pathway
(b) Drug-induced haemolytic anaemia and favism (p. 188)

ACQUIRED

Paroxysmal nocturnal haemoglobinuria

Haemolytic anaemias due to extracorpuscular (extrinsic) mechanisms

ACQUIRED

Immune mechanisms

Auto-immune acquired haemolytic anaemia (Table 8.5, p. 191)
(a) Warm antibody
(b) Cold antibody
Haemolytic disease of the newborn
Incompatible blood transfusion
Drug-induced haemolytic anaemia (p. 204)

Non-immune mechanisms

Mechanical haemolytic anaemia:
(a) Cardiac haemolytic anaemia
(b) Micro-angiopathic haemolytic anaemia (Table 8.10, p. 206)
(c) March haemoglobinuria

Miscellaneous

Haemolytic anaemia due to direct action of chemicals and drugs (p. 203)
Haemolytic anaemia due to infection
Haemolytic anaemia due to burns
Lead poisoning

within the normal range, and the reticulocyte count is normal or only slightly increased. Sometimes the haemolytic element is more marked than is usual; this may be suggested clinically by the fact that the haemoglobin rise after transfusion is poorly sustained.

Morphological characteristics. As judged by the red cell indices (p. 24), most haemolytic anaemias are either normocytic and normochromic, or macrocytic and normochromic. However, examination of the blood film frequently shows changes, particularly of shape, that are of diagnostic value. Abnormal cells which may be observed include spherocytes (p. 180), elliptocytes (p. 184), contracted cells, fragmented cells, stippled cells, acanthocytes, and stomatocytes.

Normal red cell destruction and haemoglobin breakdown

In normal subjects, the average lifespan of the red cell is 100–120 days. The normal mechanism of red cell destruction is not fully understood, but it seems probable that towards the end of the red cell's life, changes in the cell surface occur which make it more susceptible to phagocytosis by the reticulo-endothelial system in spleen, liver and bone marrow (Clark & Shohet 1985). Some intravascular destruction probably also takes place, but this mechanism seems to play only a minor role. The integrity of the red cell depends on its normal metabolic activities, which in turn are dependent on the effectiveness of its enzyme systems (p. 19). In particular, energy derived from the breakdown of glucose in the cell is important in maintaining cell integrity. As the cell ages, enzyme activity declines, and it is probable that ultimately the glycolytic system fails, resulting in an effete cell which is less deformable than normal and has acquired subtle surface membrane changes recognized by macrophages of the reticulo-endothelial system. Normal red cell metabolism is discussed in detail in Chapter 2, p. 17.

Haemoglobin breakdown

When senile red cells undergo phagocytosis, haemoglobin is released and broken down within the reticulo-endothelial cells. Globin is split from the haem and returns to the body's metabolic 'protein pool' where its amino acids are subsequently re-utilized. The porphyrin ring of haem is cleaved by the microsomal enzyme, haem oxygenase, yielding biliverdin and carbon monoxide. The biliverdin is further reduced to bilirubin by biliverdin reductase. Iron released from the haem during the initial cleavage reaction passes into the plasma where it combines with the iron-binding protein (p. 39), and is carried either to the marrow for re-utilization in haemoglobin synthesis, or to the body iron stores.

The bilirubin passes into the plasma, forms a firm complex with albumin, and is taken up by the liver. In the liver, bilirubin is conjugated with glucuronic acid to form bilirubin glucuronide, and is then excreted into the bile ducts (Fig. 8.1). Before its excretion by the liver, bilirubin is referred to as unconjugated, and after excretion as conjugated bilirubin. In normal subjects, the serum bilirubin is nearly all unconjugated. Conjugated bilirubin is more soluble in water than is unconjugated bilirubin. The glomerular membrane is permeable to the conjugated form which appears in the urine when its concentration in the serum is increased; unconjugated bilirubin is not found in the urine.

Following excretion by the liver the conjugated bilirubin passes via the bile ducts to the intestine, where it is reduced by the bacterial flora of the colon to a group of compounds, referred to generically as urobilinogen. From 10 to 20 per cent of the urobilinogen is absorbed from the bowel into the portal vein and is re-excreted by the liver into the bile, thus returning to the bowel. This is called the enterohepatic circulation of bile pigments. A small quantity of the absorbed urobilinogen is not excreted by the liver but passes into the systemic circulation and is excreted by the kidneys. Between 10 and 20 per cent of the total bilirubin excretion arises from sources other than normal red cell catabolism. These include premature destruction of immature red cell precursors in the bone marrow, breakdown of haem produced in excess of requirements for haemoglobin production, and turnover of non-haemoglobin haem within the liver. The formation and elimination of bilirubin are fully reviewed by Bissell (1975).

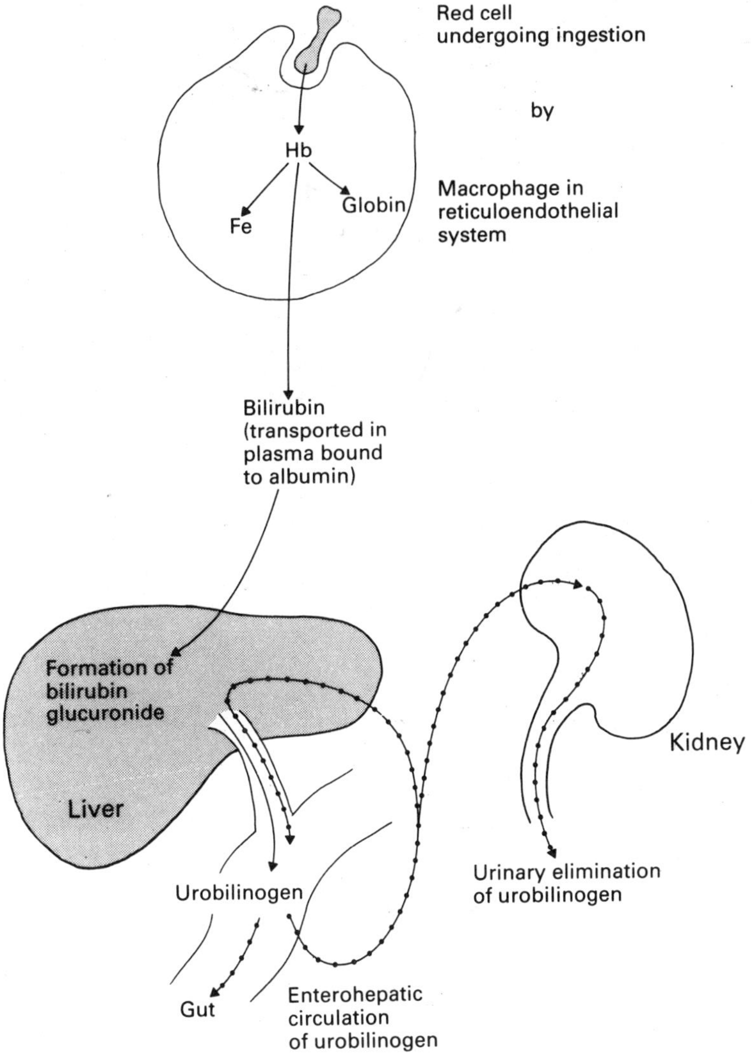

Fig. 8.1. *Haemoglobin breakdown and bilirubin metabolism.*

General considerations in the diagnosis of haemolytic anaemia

In the investigation of a patient with an anaemia suspected of being haemolytic, three questions must be answered:

1 Is the anaemia haemolytic?

2 If so, is the site of red cell destruction intravascular or extravascular?

3 What is the aetiology?

The *haemolytic nature* of the anaemia is determined from evidence of *increased haemoglobin breakdown* and of *bone marrow regeneration.* These features are common to all haemolytic anaemias, irrespective of their aetiology. In addition, evidence of *damage to the red cells,* when present, suggests that the anaemia is haemolytic. In doubtful cases, direct estimation of red cell lifespan can be made.

The *site* of red cell destruction is established by the presence or absence of free haemoglobin and haemoglobin breakdown products in the plasma and urine. *Intravascular haemolysis* is usually an acute process, the destruction of the red cells within the circulation releasing free haemoglobin. The haemolytic anaemias commonly associated with intravascular haemolysis are listed in Table 8.3 (p. 178). *Extravascular haemolysis* is essentially an exaggeration of the normal mechanism of removal of senescent red cells. The cells are recognized as abnormal by the reticulo-endothelial system, and phagocytosed prematurely. Haemoglobin is released and catabolized within the phagocytic cells, and although the serum bilirubin is elevated, no increase in free haemoglobin is detectable in the plasma.

The *aetiology* of the haemolytic anaemia is determined from a consideration of the clinical features and the results of special investigations. These are discussed in detail in the description of the individual haemolytic anaemias. Table 8.11 (p. 211) summarizes a method of investigation of a patient with suspected haemolytic anaemia.

General evidence of the haemolytic nature of an anaemia

Evidence of increased haemoglobin breakdown (Table 8.2)

HYPERBILIRUBINAEMIA AND JAUNDICE

A raised serum bilirubin and clinical jaundice are usual, but not invariable, in haemolytic anaemia. The serum bilirubin concentration usually ranges from 17 to 50 μmol/l, but higher values may occur, especially during a haemolytic crisis. The jaundice is of mild to moderate intensity, and is best seen in the sclerae. Clinical jaundice is not apparent until the serum bilirubin exceeds 40 μmol/l. The bilirubin level depends not only on the amount of haemoglobin broken down but also on the ability of the liver to excrete the increased amount of bilirubin presented to it. Thus the degree of hyperbilirubinaemia is not necessarily a reliable guide to the rate of haemolysis. Although usually present, *the absence of jaundice does not exclude the diagnosis of haemolytic anaemia.* The reason usually given to explain the absence of jaundice is that the normal reserve of the liver enables it to excrete the increased amounts of bilirubin. Haemolytic jaundice is not accompanied by pruritus or bradycardia.

Table 8.2. *General evidence of haemolysis*

Evidence of increased haemoglobin breakdown	
*Jaundice and hyperbilirubinaemia**	
Reduced plasma haptoglobin and haemopexin	
Increased plasma lactate dehydrogenase	
Haemoglobinaemia	Evidence of intravascular haemolysis
Haemoglobinuria	
Methaemalbuminaemia	
Haemosiderinuria	
Evidence of compensatory erythroid hyperplasia	
*Reticulocytosis**	
Macrocytosis and polychromasia	
Erythroid hyperplasia of the bone marrow	
Radiological changes in the skull and tubular bones (congenital anaemias only)	
Evidence of damage to the red cells	
Spherocytosis and increased red cell fragility	
Fragmentation of red cells	
Heinz bodies	
Demonstration of shortened red cell lifespan	

*Reticulocytosis and hyperbilirubinaemia (often but not invariably with jaundice) are the main criteria suggesting an overt haemolytic anaemia.

The bilirubin is unconjugated and does not appear in the urine. However, complications occasionally cause an increase in conjugated bilirubin, resulting in the appearance of bile pigments in the urine. The complications are biliary obstruction from gall-stones or pigment thrombus formation in the biliary canaliculi, and impairment of liver function due to associated liver disease, e.g. cirrhosis.

PLASMA HAPTOGLOBIN

Haptoglobins are α_2 glycoproteins which combine with haemoglobin and certain of its derivatives. They are formed in the liver and constitute about one per cent of the total plasma protein.

By combining with any haemoglobin present in the plasma, haptoglobin is responsible for the apparent renal threshold for haemoglobin. Haemoglobin molecules are small enough to pass through a normal glomerulus, but when combined with haptoglobin, the larger molecular size of the complex prevents passage. When haemoglobin is

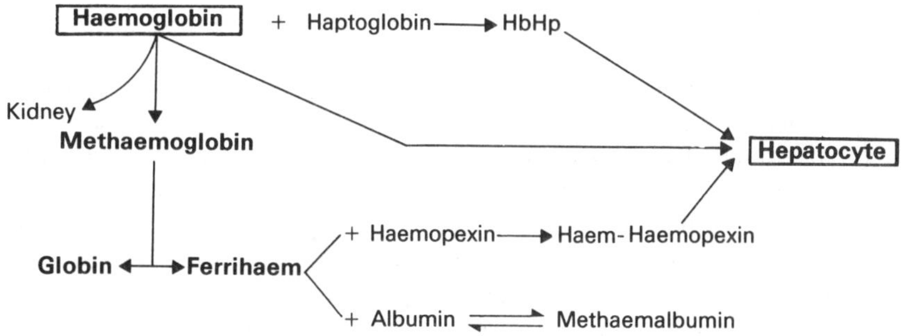

Fig. 8.2. *The fate of haemoglobin in the plasma. HbHp =haemoglobin–haptoglobin complex.*

released into the circulation in small amounts it combines with circulating haptoglobin and therefore none is excreted in the urine (Fig. 8.2).

The complex of haemoglobin and haptoglobin is rapidly removed from the circulation, mainly by the parenchymal cells of the liver. Following the transient release of haemoglobin into the circulation, the plasma haptoglobin level falls and returns to normal in 3–6 days. However, if there is continuous release of haemoglobin as in chronic haemolytic disease, the level remains depressed.

Plasma haptoglobin is normally expressed in terms of haemoglobin binding, and the normal level ranges from 0.3 to 2.0 g/l. The level is usually decreased in both extravascular and intravascular haemolytic disease. Haptoglobin is elevated due to increased hepatic synthesis in a number of acute and chronic systemic disorders, and thus normal or increased values do not necessarily exclude haemolysis.

PLASMA HAEMOPEXIN

Haemopexin is a plasma β glycoprotein which binds free haem in a 1:1 molar ratio. It does not bind haemoglobin. It is synthesized in the liver, and the normal plasma concentration ranges from 0.5 to 1.0 g/l.

When large amounts of haemoglobin are released into the plasma and the haptoglobin-binding capacity is exceeded, some of the resulting unbound haemoglobin is converted to methaemoglobin. The methaemoglobin dissociates into ferrihaem and globin, and the ferrihaem is bound by haemopexin thus preventing glomerular filtration of the small ferrihaem molecule. The ferrihaem–haemopexin complex is taken up by the liver, the parenchymal cells probably being the site of removal. In most cases of intravascular haemolysis, the plasma haemopexin falls to a low level.

PLASMA LACTATE DEHYDROGENASE

The plasma enzyme, lactate dehydrogenase, is moderately elevated in most cases of haemolytic anaemia, although the levels do not reach those encountered in the megaloblastic anaemias.

EVIDENCE OF INTRAVASCULAR LYSIS

When intravascular haemolysis occurs, haemoglobin from the destroyed red cells is liberated into the plasma. If the amount of haemoglobin released exceeds the haptoglobin-binding capacity, part of the unbound haemoglobin passes the renal glomerular membrane. It is re-absorbed in the proximal renal tubules, but appears in the urine if the absorptive capacity of the tubules is exceeded.

In the renal tubular cell, the globin is degraded to amino acids which are returned to the body stores, and the haem is catabolized to bilirubin. Haem iron enters a temporary storage depot in the cell. The gradual loss of the iron-laden tubular cells into the urine results in the appearance of urinary haemosiderin.

Some of the circulating unbound haemoglobin is converted to methaemoglobin, which dissociates into ferrihaem and globin. If the binding capacity of haemopexin is exceeded, the ferrihaem is bound by albumin in a 1:1 molar ratio with the formation of methaemalbumin. Methaemalbumin turnover is slow, and it is the last haem pigment to leave the plasma after an episode of intravascular haemolysis. The haem part of the methaemalbumin molecule is eventually taken up by the parenchymal cells of the liver. The appearance of methaemalbumin and depletion of haemopexin indicate severe intravascular haemolysis and are not seen unless plasma haptoglobin is also absent.

Some of the haemoglobin remains free in the circulation and is probably also taken up by the parenchymal cells of the liver. The fate of circulating haemoglobin is reviewed by Hershko (1975).

Haemoglobinaemia and haemoglobinuria. The level of free haemoglobin in the plasma of normal subjects is low, usually not exceeding 0.6 mg/dl. When intravascular haemolysis occurs and the haptoglobin binding capacity is exceeded, the plasma haemoglobin level rises to 100–200 mg/dl. When the plasma haemoglobin is markedly raised, the plasma has a pink or red colour, depending on the concentration of the haemoglobin. When the rise is moderate, e.g. 10–40 mg/dl, this colour may be lacking, not only because of the relatively low concentration but also because other pigments such as bilirubin, which gives a yellow colour, and methaemalbumin, which gives a brownish colour, may mask the pink tint.

When the renal threshold for haemoglobin reabsorption is exceeded, haemoglobinuria ensues (Table 8.3). The colour of the urine, which varies from pink to almost black, is due to the presence of two pigments—bright red oxyhaemoglobin and dark brown methaemoglobin which is produced by auto-oxidation of the haemoglobin in the urinary tract when the urine is acid. Haemoglobinuria must be carefully distinguished from haematuria.

Table 8.3. *Causes of haemoglobinuria*

Acute haemoglobinuria
Incompatible blood transfusion
Haemolytic anaemia due to drugs and chemicals
Favism
Paroxysmal cold haemoglobinuria
March haemoglobinuria
Haemolytic anaemia due to infections (mainly *Clostridium welchii*)
Blackwater fever
Haemolytic anaemia associated with eclampsia
Haemolytic–uraemic syndrome
Haemolytic anaemia due to burns
Snake and spider bites
Chronic haemoglobinuria
Paroxysmal nocturnal haemoglobinuria
Cardiac haemolytic anaemia
Cold haemagglutinin disease

Methaemalbuminaemia. The presence of methaemalbuminaemia is diagnostic of intravascular haemolysis, but its absence does not exclude it. Methaemalbumin may persist in small amounts for several days after an episode of acute intravascular haemolysis. Its presence imparts a golden to brown colour to the plasma, depending on its concentration. It is identified biochemically by Schumm's test.

Haemosiderinuria. Iron resulting from the breakdown of haemoglobin in the renal tubular cells (p. 177) is stored in the cells as haemosiderin and may be excreted in the urine as a result of cell desquamation. Haemosiderin can be demonstrated in the centrifuged sediment as Prussian blue-positive intracellular or extracellular granules. Haemosiderinuria is seen particularly in chronic intravascular haemolysis, and is especially typical of paroxysmal nocturnal haemoglobinuria in which haemosiderinuria persists even when haemoglobinuria is absent.

UROBILINOGEN EXCRETION

The main product of bilirubin breakdown is urobilinogen, which is excreted chiefly in the faeces and to a small extent in the urine. Measurement of its excretion can be used to detect increased haemoglobin breakdown, but difficulties in technique and interpretation limit the usefulness of the tests and they are now infrequently performed.

Evidence of compensatory erythroid hyperplasia

The increased red cell destruction in haemolytic anaemia is followed by erythropoietin-mediated hyperplasia of the erythroid tissue of the bone marrow. This hyperplasia results in reticulocytosis and the appearance of polychromatic macrocytes. The bone marrow shows normoblastic or macronormoblastic hyperplasia. In hereditary haemolytic anaemias, hyperplasia may result in radiological bone changes.

RETICULOCYTOSIS

The reticulocyte count is increased in the majority of patients with haemolytic disease. However, like the increase in serum bilirubin, the degree of reticulocytosis does not necessarily parallel the degree of anaemia, although in general the highest counts are usually found in the more anaemic patients. In normal subjects, the reticulocyte count varies from 0.2 to 2.0 per cent; in haemolytic anaemia it usually ranges from 5 to 20 per cent but occasionally rises to much higher values, e.g. 50–70 per cent or even more. In some patients with relatively mild compensated haemolytic disease, the reticulocyte count is at the upper limit of normal; nevertheless, repeated counts usually show mild transient rises, e.g. up to five per cent. The reticulocyte count may be used as an index of red cell production in haemolytic anaemia provided allowances are made for the reduction in total red cell count and the presence of 'shift reticulocytes' in the peripheral blood. Hillman & Finch (1985) discuss the application of correction factors to the reticulocyte count.

Nucleated red cells are commonly present in the peripheral blood in haemolytic anaemia. Their number is usually small, less than 1 per 100 leucocytes. In general, the higher the reticulocyte count and the more anaemic the patient, the more numerous are the normoblasts. With haemolytic disease in young children, particularly haemolytic disease of the newborn, normoblasts may be numerous. Normoblasts are also prominent in haemolytic disease that persists after splenectomy.

POLYCHROMATIC MACROCYTES

Erythropoietin causes premature delivery of reticulocytes from the bone marrow into the circulation. These less mature 'shift' reticulocytes are 30 per cent larger than mature reticulocytes and are easily recognized in Romanovsky-stained blood films by their size and polychromatic staining characteristics. Unlike the macrocytes of vitamin B_{12} or folate deficiency, they are round. Their presence is usually reflected in a moderate elevation of the MCV.

NORMOBLASTIC HYPERPLASIA OF THE MARROW

The aspirated marrow shows normoblastic hyperplasia. The marrow fragments are more cellular than normal and contain less fat, the cell trails are hypercellular, and the myeloid : erythroid ratio is reduced from the usual figure of about 3–4:1, sometimes to 1:1 or even less. The hyperplastic erythroid cells are commonly macronormoblastic.

SKELETAL RADIOLOGICAL ABNORMALITIES

In the hereditary haemolytic anaemias, the marrow hyperplasia is sometimes sufficiently marked to cause bony changes which can be seen on X-ray. The incidence, degree, and nature vary with the aetiological disorder. In general, the changes occur most frequently and are most marked in thalassaemia major, in which they are a constant feature. Changes are also common in sickle-cell anaemia but usually are less marked. In hereditary spherocytosis and the non-spherocytic congenital haemolytic anaemias, changes are uncommon.

In the *skull*, the hyperplasia results in broadening of the diploic space, with separation of the tables and thickening of the vault of the skull, especially of the frontal and parietal bones. The medulla is less dense, giving a ground-glass appearance, and the tables, especially the outer, are thinned. Bony trabeculae may develop at right angles to the tables giving rise to 'hair-on-end' or 'brush' appearance (see Fig. 7.5), which is common in thalassaemia major.

In the *tubular bones of the extremities*, marrow hyperplasia results in widening of the marrow cavity, thinning of the cortex, and decreased density of the medulla; the decreased medullary density contrasts with the trabecular pattern, which is often coarse and exaggerated. With marked changes, the bones may actually be increased in diameter. Changes are especially marked in the metacarpals, which before puberty are an excellent site for their demonstration. Similar changes may occur in the ribs. The vertebral bodies may be widened and shortened, giving a cupped appearance.

The above changes, when present, usually develop in the first few years of life. After puberty, the changes regress in the tubular bones of the extremities, while in the skull they persist and progress. In patients who survive to adult life, an irregular bony sclerosis may develop with resultant cortical thickening, narrowing of the marrow cavity, and periosteal reaction. These changes, which are most prominent in sickle-cell anaemia, are probably due to infarction following vascular thrombosis.

Evidence of red cell damage

In some haemolytic anaemias, changes in the red cells which result from damage by the extracorpuscular factor causing the haemolysis are present. The most important are spherocytosis, increased osmotic fragility, fragmentation, and Heinz-body formation; these changes, when present, strongly suggest that the anaemia is of haemolytic type.

SPHEROCYTOSIS

The normal erythrocyte is a biconcave disc. In haemolytic anaemia, cells which are less disc-like and more spheroidal are frequently found; they have a decreased diameter, and are known as spherocytes. The volume of the spherocyte is usually normal or only slightly reduced, but there is a reduction in surface area and consequently the surface area-to-volume ratio is reduced.

Spherocytes can be recognized by their appearance in the blood film, and their increased osmotic fragility in hypotonic saline solutions. In blood films, spherocytes appear as small, round, deeply staining cells in which the normal area of central pallor is lost (Fig. 8.3).

The spherocytes that occur in haemolytic anaemia are of two types: the *congenital spherocyte* of hereditary spherocytosis in which the spherocytosis is due to an intrinsic defect of the cell membrane (p. 182), and the *acquired spherocyte*, which is produced by the action of some abnormal extrinsic factor on a previously normal cell. Acquired spherocytosis may occur in auto-immune acquired haemolytic anaemia, haemolytic anaemia due to chemicals, infection, or burns, and in haemolytic disease of the newborn due to anti-A.

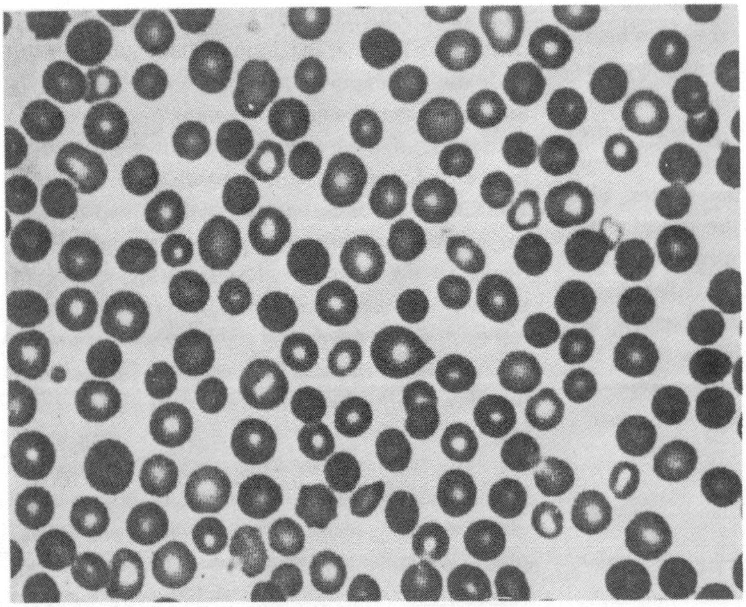

Fig. 8.3. *Hereditary spherocytosis. Photomicrograph of a blood film from a male aged 45 years, who presented with cholelithiasis due to pigment stones. The spherocytes appear as small, round, deeply staining cells (× 710).*

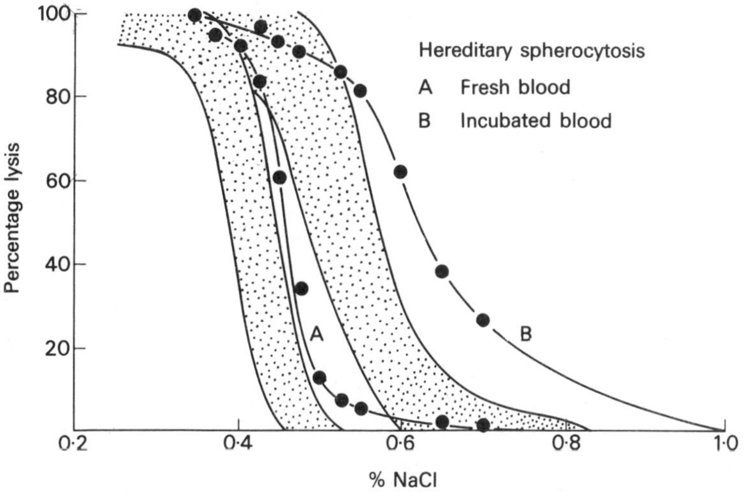

Fig. 8.4. *Red cell osmotic fragility curves in hereditary spherocytosis. The stippled area on the left represents the normal range for fresh blood, and on the right for sterile blood incubated at 37°C for 24 hours.*

Thus *spherocytosis occurs in a number of haemolytic anaemias of different aetiology and is not specifically diagnostic of any particular type of haemolytic anaemia.*

RED CELL OSMOTIC FRAGILITY

Spherocytes show an increased tendency to lysis in hypotonic saline solutions. In the osmotic fragility test, small quantities of blood are added to a series of saline solutions of increasing concentration, the percentage of haemolysis at each concentration is estimated, and the result plotted on graph paper. In normal subjects, an almost symmetrical sigmoid curve results. The mean corpuscular fragility (MCF) is the concentration of saline causing 50 per cent lysis; normal values range from 4.0 to 4.45 g/l NaCl (Fig. 8.4).

FRAGMENTATION

Fragmented red cells may be seen in certain haemolytic anaemias; the most important of these are chemical haemolytic anaemia (p. 203), cardiac haemolytic anaemia (p. 207) and the micro-angiopathic haemolytic anaemias (p. 207). Fragmented cells are seldom seen in normal blood, and in anaemia their presence in significant numbers suggests that the anaemia is haemolytic in type. Fragmented cells are irregularly contracted and sometimes stain deeply; crescent shaped and triangular cells are particularly characteristic (see Fig. 8.7, p. 208).

HEINZ BODIES

Heinz bodies are aggregates of denatured globin which may be demonstrated in the red cell by supravital staining as small round inclusions beneath the cell membrane. They occur in small numbers in normal red cells following splenectomy and in disorders in which the reducing power of the red cell is unable to counter excess oxidative stress. These include haemolytic anaemias due to direct toxic action of oxidant drugs or chemicals, hexose monophosphate pathway enzyme deficiencies, and the unstable haemoglobinopathies. Heinz body-like inclusions are also seen in α thalassaemia (p. 165) and β thalassaemia (p. 159). The spleen is able to pit the inclusions from the red cells, and thus they tend to be present in the circulation in greater numbers in splenectomized patients. Damage sustained in the pitting process is believed to hasten cell lysis.

Demonstration of shortened red cell lifespan

In most cases of haemolytic anaemia, the features described above establish the fact that the anaemia is haemolytic in nature. However, in doubtful cases, direct estimation of red cell lifespan by the use of radio-isotope-labelled red cells is necessary. The fundamental principle of the method is that red cells from a particular subject are labelled so that they can be identified in the blood of a recipient into whom they are injected. The presence and degree of increased red cell destruction is determined by following the rate of elimination of the labelled cells from the circulation.

Red cells may be labelled with radioactive chromium (^{51}Cr) or radioactive di-isopropyl phosphofluoridate ($DF^{32}P$ or ^{3}H–DFP). The radioactive chromium method is preferred in most laboratories as it permits surface body scanning, by which sites of red cell sequestration and destruction may be determined. The hexavalent chromium enters the red cells as chromate ion and, after conversion to the trivalent form, binds to the β chains of Hb-A. The International Committee for Standardization in Haematology has recommended methods for radio-isotope red cell survival studies (1980). The Committee suggested that the expression of results as $T_{50}Cr$, i.e the time taken for half the label to leave the circulation (25–34 days in healthy adults), should be replaced by the mean red cell lifespan (90–130 days).

In vivo ^{51}*Cr surface counting*. ^{51}Cr studies can be used to make an assessment of the primary site of red cell destruction by external *in vivo* measurements over the liver and spleen. Details are given by Dacie & Lewis (1984). The results are expressed as counts over the liver and spleen in excess of those expected. Although surface counting patterns are valuable in predicting response to splenectomy, the technique is not infallible and due regard must be taken of clinical features and other haematological data (Ahuja *et al.* 1972).

Hereditary haemolytic anaemias due to red cell membrane defects

Hereditary spherocytosis

Hereditary spherocytosis is a relatively common haemolytic disorder in which the fundamental abnormality is an intrinsic defect of the red cell membrane which results in the cell being of spherocytic shape. Spherocytes have a decreased surface area-to-volume ratio and are more rigid and less deformable than normal cells. Their rigidity prevents normal passage through the slit-like openings separating the splenic cords from the sinuses, and cells may be delayed in the splenic pulp for as long as ten hours before returning to the general circulation. This prolonged period of hypoxia and glucose deprivation compromises normal red cell metabolism, and there is loss of cell membrane, increased sphering, and rigidity. If the cell escapes from the hostile splenic environment, further conditioning on subsequent passage through the spleen leads to eventual phagocytosis by reticulo-endothelial cells in the spleen and other organs. Anaemia results when the rate of red cell destruction exceeds the rate of bone marrow regeneration.

Recent studies have suggested that the basic defect in hereditary spherocytosis lies in the red cell membrane skeleton, and qualitative and quantitative abnormalities of spectrin, the major protein of the membrane, have been demonstrated (Becker & Lux 1985). The most common finding is a simple reduction in the amount of spectrin (Agre *et al.* 1986); in some patients, the spectrin lacks the ability to attach to protein 4.1 (p. 17). The membrane abnormality is associated functionally with an increased permeability to sodium. An increased rate of passive movement of sodium into the cell is compensated for by an increased rate of active transport of sodium out of the cell by the cation pump mechanism (p. 19) which requires ATP derived from red cell glycolysis. The glycolytic rate of the cell is greatly increased as a compensatory mechanism to provide adequate ATP.

CLINICAL FEATURES

The disorder is inherited as an autosomal dominant trait, males and females being equally affected. Occasionally, there are no clinical features to suggest involvement of either parent but careful examination of the blood reveals an increased osmotic fragility in one parent. In approximately 25 per cent of patients, no abnormality can be demonstrated in the blood of either parent, and it is presumed that the condition has resulted from genetic mutation. Hereditary spherocytosis is not confined to any particular race, but it occurs most frequently in persons of British and northern European stock, in whom it is the most common form of hereditary haemolytic disease.

Onset. The majority of patients present with symptoms of anaemia or jaundice, or both. Less frequently, the patient presents with one of the complications of gall-stones or because of the accidental discovery of an enlarged spleen. The age at which diagnosis is established is determined largely by the severity of the disorder. Most patients present in the first ten years of life; occasionally the disorder is obvious shortly after birth. Mildly affected patients may not be diagnosed until adult life or even until old age; they may have no symptoms, and the disorder is discovered only when, on routine examination, they are found to have an enlarged spleen or mild anaemia, or when they are investigated after some other member of the family is found to be affected.

Jaundice, usually of moderate depth, occurs in most patients. However, it is seldom obvious in children in the first few years of life, and frequently does not appear until adolescence. Jaundice is sometimes intermittent. The serum bilirubin usually lies between 17 and 70 μmol/l. The urine contains no bile (and hence the condition was formerly known as familial acholuric jaundice) but may contain urobilinogen. Bile sometimes appears in the urine because of biliary obstruction caused by gall-stones, and, less frequently, because of liver damage.

The *spleen* is almost invariably enlarged. Enlargement is usually slight to moderate, but is occasionally marked. Typically the spleen is firm and non-tender, although it may become tender, especially during haemolytic crises.

Crises. The haemoglobin level of the individual patient tends to remain fairly constant. However, the course of the disease is characteristically punctuated by intermittent abrupt exacerbation of the anaemia, accompanied by constitutional symptoms. The crises vary in severity. They are often precipitated by infection (usually viral) but sometimes occur without obvious cause; they may occur in several members of the one family at about the same time. Minor crises appear to result from an increase in the rate of haemolysis (haemolytic crises), but major crises commonly result from a temporary marrow aplasia predominantly affecting erythropoiesis. Human parvovirus B19 has recently been recognized as a frequent aetiological agent in viral-induced aplastic crisis (Kelleher *et al.* 1983).

Constitutional symptoms may accompany the fall in haemoglobin. Haemolytic crises are commonly accompanied by an increase in the depth of jaundice, darkening of the urine, and an increase in the size of the spleen, which may become tender. In aplastic crises, the jaundice does not increase and may even decrease, the reticulocyte count falls, often almost to zero, and the erythroid cells of the marrow show either aplasia or maturation arrest. The reticulocyte count commonly increases again after 7–10 days, and is followed by a rise in haemoglobin. Occasionally, neutropenia and thrombocytopenia accompany the fall in haemoglobin. Folate deficiency may be an aetiological factor in some aplastic crises.

Pigment *gall-stones* develop in more than 50 per cent of cases; the incidence is higher with severe haemolysis, and increases with age. Pure pigment stones are not radio-opaque and can be demonstrated only by cholecystography or ultrasound examination. Mixed stones, containing calcium or cholesterol, may be visible in a plain X-ray of the gall-bladder area. Cholecystitis or obstruction of the common bile duct may result from the gall-stones, and sometimes they are the first clinical manifestation of the disease. The possibility of an underlying hereditary spherocytosis should be considered in any young patient with gall-stones.

BLOOD PICTURE

The blood picture typically shows anaemia with spherocytosis, an increased erythrocyte osmotic fragility, a raised reticulocyte count and serum bilirubin level, and a negative direct antiglobulin test.

The haemoglobin is usually 7–14 g/dl, but may fall below 7 g/dl during a crisis. In about 20 per cent of patients, the haemolysis is compensated and the haemoglobin level is normal. In the blood film, spherocytes are usually numerous and contrast sharply with the polychromatic macrocytes (see Fig. 8.3). In mildly affected patients, the number of spherocytes is small and they may be difficult to detect in the film. The MCV is usually normal but is occasionally slightly reduced. The MCH is normal but the MCHC is often increased, ranging from 34 to 40 per cent. Reticulocytes commonly range from 5 to 20 per cent; a small number of normoblasts may be present in patients with high reticulocyte counts. The red cell osmotic fragility of blood tested immediately on drawing is increased above the normal range in most patients. In mild cases, the increased fragility can sometimes be demonstrated only after incubation (see Fig. 8.4). The amount of spontaneous lysis which occurs on sterile incubation for 48 hours at 37°C (autohaemolysis) is increased. The increased autohaemolysis is substantially reduced, but usually not completely corrected, by the addition of glucose. A recent variation of the osmotic fragility test, the acidified glycerol lysis test is claimed to be particularly sensitive in the detection of minor degrees of spherocytosis (Zanella *et al.* 1980).

The survival in the patient's circulation of autologous red cells labelled with ^{51}Cr is shortened, and surface counting of radioactivity reveals excessive uptake over the spleen.

DIAGNOSIS

The diagnosis is based on the clinical and haematological features and the family history. Diagnostic difficulty may occur in mild cases detected for the first time in adult life. Occasionally, the disease in the relatives is very mild, and the blood, on routine examination, may appear normal. However, in affected relatives, the incubated osmotic fragility often shows an increase that is greater than normal.

Hereditary spherocytosis must be differentiated from other haemolytic disorders associated with spherocytosis (p. 180) and from other congenital haemolytic anaemias. Rare cases presenting in the neonatal period must be differentiated from other causes of neonatal anaemia or jaundice.

TREATMENT

Splenectomy is practically always followed by complete and sustained clinical remission, and is indicated in all patients except those who are symptom-free and well compensated. Even in these patients, splenectomy should be considered because of the risk of gall-stone formation and serious aplastic crisis. When diagnosis is made in childhood, splenectomy is probably better postponed until the age of about seven years, unless anaemia is severe and requires repeated transfusion, or growth is impaired. In very severe cases, splenectomy may be required in infancy. General health is not affected by splenectomy, although splenectomized young children are more susceptible to severe infection and should be immunized with polyvalent pneumococcal vaccine, preferably 1–2 months before splenectomy. Antibiotic prophylaxis during the first two years after splenectomy is also advisable. A cholecystogram or ultrasound examination should be performed prior to splenectomy and, if gallstones are present, cholecystectomy performed either at splenectomy or subsequently, at the discretion of the surgeon. Splenectomy is followed by a prompt cessation of haemolysis with a return of the haemoglobin to normal and disappearance of jaundice. Crises are unknown following splenectomy. Spherocytes still persist in the blood, but in the absence of the spleen they are no longer prematurely removed from the circulation, and their lifespan is normal or only slightly reduced.

A conditioned deficiency of folate resulting in megaloblastic erythropoiesis occasionally occurs, especially in pregnancy; it should be considered when there is an unexplained fall in haemoglobin. Treatment is with folic acid in standard doses.

Hereditary elliptocytosis (ovalocytosis)

Hereditary elliptocytosis is a common disorder, characterized by the occurrence of large numbers of elliptical cells in the peripheral blood. It is inherited as an autosomal dominant trait of variable expression, and is equally common in males and females. The gene determining the elliptocytosis is closely linked to the Rh locus on chromosome 1 in some, but not all, affected subjects.

The blood contains between 25 and 90 per cent oval cells, values over 50 per cent being usual. The abnormality is not apparent until the reticulocyte stage or later, and is not fully developed until after the first three months of life. The cells may be oval, elliptical, or rod-shaped, and there is no correlation between the degree of elliptocytosis, which often varies from one family member to another, and the severity of haemolysis The MCV is normal or slightly reduced, and the MCH is normal.

Clinically, several forms of the disorder may be recognized, but only two are encountered with any frequency: *mild elliptocytosis*, with no anaemia and minimal or no evidence of haemolysis, is the most common form; *mild elliptocytosis with haemolytic anaemia* occurs in about 15 per cent of affected subjects. The anaemia is mild or moderate with reticulocytosis ranging from 4 to 10 per cent, and a slightly increased serum bilirubin. The spleen is often palpable. Splenectomy usually results in clinical cure, although the elliptocytosis persists. Rare patients with severe haemolysis are homozygous for the gene, and may present with haemolytic anaemia in infancy.

Less common variants include spherocytic and stomatocytic forms and a more recently recognized entity, *hereditary pyropoikilocytosis*, in which the red cells show abnormal sensitivity to the effect of heat (Zarkowsky *et al.* 1975). The basic defect in hereditary elliptocytosis appears to be an intrinsic abnormality of the red cell membrane cytoskeleton due the presence of dysfunctional membrane proteins. Structural alterations in the spectrin molecule resulting in a disorderly arrangement of polypeptide chains, and diminished binding to other membrane proteins have been the most commonly encountered abnormalities. The disorder is fully reviewed by Palek (1985).

The disorder must be distinguished from *acquired ovalocytosis* which occurs in a number of disorders characterized by anisocytosis and poikilocytosis. These disorders include megaloblastic macrocytic anaemias, iron deficiency anaemia, thalassaemia, and myelosclerosis.

Hereditary xerocytosis and hydrocytosis

A hereditary haemolytic anaemia has been recognized in a small number of patients in which greatly increased red cell membrane permeability to the monovalent cations, sodium and potassium, leads to cellular dehydration or overhydration. The disorder is inherited as an autosomal dominant trait and has a wide spectrum of severity, from a compensated haemolytic state with normal haemoglobin level to severe anaemia presenting in early infancy. Splenomegaly is usually present.

Most cases may be classified into one of two groups—hereditary xerocytosis and hereditary hydrocytosis. In *hereditary xerocytosis* (or desiccytosis), the red cells are dehydrated and osmotically resistant, with reduced total cation content and elevated MCHC. Target cells and small, irregular microcytes predominate on the blood film. In *hereditary hydrocytosis* (or stomatocytosis), the red cells are overhydrated and osmotically fragile, with an increased total cation content and reduced MCHC. In the blood film, there are numerous stomatocytes, i.e. red cells with a linear, unstained area across the centre suggesting a mouth-like orifice. The disorder is reviewed by Wiley (1984).

Occasional stomatocytes are seen in blood films from apparently normal subjects. They occur in greater numbers in some alcoholic patients, and in Greek and Italian people resident in Australia. In the latter group, there may be mild haemolysis, but red cell electrolyte abnormalities are not present.

Hereditary haemolytic anaemias due to red cell enzyme deficiencies

Hereditary deficiencies of red cell enzymes are associated with two clinical syndromes: drug-induced haemolytic anaemia and non-spherocytic congenital haemolytic anaemia. *Drug-induced haemolytic anaemia* due to deficiency of the hexose monophosphate (HMP) pathway enzyme, glucose-6-phosphate dehydrogenase (G6PD), is of great clinical importance as the enzyme deficiency affects over 100 million people in many countries. Such people are not anaemic unless challenged by the administration of any of at least 20 therapeutic agents. Deficiencies of G6PD and other enzymes of the HMP and the Embden–Meyerhof pathway (p. 19) may be associated with life-long haemolytic anaemias, and these disorders are referred to as the *non-spherocytic congenital haemolytic anaemias.*

They are relatively rare. In this section, drug-induced haemolytic anaemia associated with G6PD deficiency is described first, followed by a brief account of the non-spherocytic congenital haemolytic anaemias.

Drug-induced haemolytic anaemia

Drug-induced haemolytic anaemia due to glucose-6-phosphate dehydrogenase deficiency has a high frequency in Mediterranean countries, in south-east Asia, and in Blacks. Population studies have shown a prevalence rate in American Blacks of 13 per cent, Nigerians 10 per cent, Sardinians 30 per cent, and Greeks 3 per cent. Other races affected include Indians, Chinese, Malays, Thais, Filipinos, and Melanesians. There is evidence to suggest that the defect confers some protection against falciparum malaria; thus it may lessen the severity of malarial infections in young children and infants.

The disorder is genetically transmitted by a sex-linked gene of intermediate dominance which is located on the end of the long arm of the X chromosome. Full expression of the trait occurs in hemizygous males, in whom the single X chromosome carries the mutant gene, and in homozygous females in whom both sex chromosomes (XX) carry a mutant gene. Intermediate expression is found in heterozygous females, in whom expression is variable. Female heterozygotes have been shown to have two populations of red cells, one with normal and one with markedly deficient enzyme activity; the relative proportion of the two populations results in G6PD activities that may vary from almost normal to those found for hemizygotes. Beutler (1978) provides a comprehensive review of all aspects of G6PD deficiency.

G6PD VARIANTS

More than 200 structural variants of G6PD have been identified (listed by Beutler & Yoshida 1988). Some are restricted to families or small ethnic groups. They are distinguished by a variety of biochemical techniques including electrophoresis, heat stability studies, and anlaysis of kinetic characteristics. Some of the variants are not associated with any clinical or haematological abnormality.

The G6PD of Caucasian subjects is called G6PD B+. Seventy per cent of Black males have G6PD B+, and 15 per cent have G6PD A+ which has a more rapid electrophoretic mobility. The 10–15 per cent of Blacks who develop haemolytic anaemia on drug administration have a variant called G6PD A− which, although having the same electrophoretic characteristics as G6PD A+, is unstable *in vivo* and is associated with low enzyme activity.

Drug-induced haemolytic anaemia in Greeks and Italians is usually due to the presence of G6PD Mediterranean. The deficiency of this enzyme is more severe than that of the Black A− type, and this is reflected in susceptibility to a wider range of drugs. Affected subjects may also develop neonatal jaundice and acute haemolysis on exposure to fava beans, both of which are rare in Blacks. The variant usually associated with drug-induced haemolysis in Chinese people is G6PD Canton. Cases of non-spherocytic congenital haemolytic anaemia (p. 188) have been described in association with many G6PD variants.

CLINCIAL FEATURES

The clinical features are those of an acute haemolytic anaemia. The severity of the haemolytic episode induced by a particular drug is, in general, related to its dose. The most detailed study of the clinical course has been in primaquine-sensitive Black volunteers, receiving 30 mg primaquine per day. This results in a self-limiting haemolysis, commencing in 2–3 days, and lasting for about 7 days, and followed by a return of the haemoglobin value to normal after 20–30 days despite continued drug administration. Clinically, some patients have only darkening of the urine, but the more severely affected complain of constitutional symptoms and are jaundiced. The self-limiting nature of the haemolysis is because red cell drug sensitivity is a function of cell age; older cells are destroyed, while younger cells are resistant. Haemolysis ceases and the haemoglobin level returns to normal when the older population of cells has been destroyed and only the younger cells remain. However, the resistance of younger cells is relative, as a second wave of haemolysis can be induced if the dose is suddenly greatly increased. In some non-Black subjects the haemolysis is not self-limiting; in such subjects withdrawal of the drug is of great importance.

Drugs that may cause haemolysis. Drugs and chemicals that have clearly been shown to cause clinically significant haemolysis in sensitive subjects are listed in Table 8.8, p. 202, which is based on Beutler's critical analysis of the literature (Beutler 1978).

Predisposing factors. Infections, both bacterial and viral, may cause haemolysis in sensitive subjects without the administration of drugs, or may accentuate drug-induced haemolysis; diabetic acidosis may act similarly. Persons with impaired renal function may have reduced drug elimination, leading to a higher blood concentration of a drug at a particular dosage and therefore to more severe haemolysis. This point is of particular importance in relation to drugs used in treating urinary tract infections.

Neonatal jaundice. In addition to the typical haemolytic state described above, G6PD deficiency has an association with neonatal jaundice and, rarely, kernicterus in Mediterranean, Chinese and, rarely, Black infants. The jaundice is sometimes accentuated by exposure to naphthalene or vitamin K derivatives. Affected infants are usually mildly anaemic.

HAEMATOLOGICAL FEATURES

The blood findings and red cell morphology in sensitive individuals are normal when not exposed to a drug causing haemolysis.

During the haemolytic phase, the red cells show polychromasia and basophilic stippling; spherocytosis may occur but marked poikilocytosis is unusual. The plasma haemoglobin rises, and haptoglobins are reduced; the presence of methaemalbumin in the plasma provides additional evidence of intravascular haemolysis. Heinz bodies appear in the red cells 1–2 days after the administration of the drug is begun; their number increases until the rate of haemolysis becomes rapid, and by the tenth day most or all of the cells containing Heinz bodies disappear. During the recovery phase only rare Heinz bodies are seen.

LABORATORY DETECTION

Screening tests

Several screening tests are available for the diagnosis of G6PD deficiency. Most demonstrate the presence or absence of G6PD by testing the ability of the red cells to generate NADPH from NADP, a reaction which directly depends on the availability of G6PD (p. 19).

Brilliant cresyl blue (BCB) dye test. NADPH reduces BCB to a colourless compound.

Methaemoglobin reduction test. Nitrite is used to oxidize haemoglobin to methaemoglobin. Methylene blue stimulates the hexose monophosphate pathway which, if intact, supplies NADPH, which in turn reduces brown methaemoglobin to red oxyhaemoglobin.

Fluorescent spot test. NADPH fluoresces when activated by long-wave ultraviolet light.

The screening tests satisfactorily detect hemizygous males and homozygous females. The proportion of female heterozygotes detected by the tests varies, but is up to 80 per cent with the methaemoglobin reduction test. The screening tests are described in detail by Dacie & Lewis (1984). Reagents for the BCB dye test and the fluorescent spot test are available commercially in kit form.

Enzyme assay

The enzyme assay method measures spectrophotometrically the rate of reduction of NADP to NADPH. Values in fully expressed hemizygous Black males range from 3 to 15 per cent, and in Mediterranean and south-east Asian subjects from 0 to 8 per cent. As mentioned, a wide variation of activity exists in heterozygote females.

DIAGNOSIS

The possibility of drug-induced haemolysis due to G6PD deficiency or favism (see below) should be considered in any patient with an unexplained acute haemolytic anaemia in which the antiglobulin test is negative, especially in persons of Black, Mediterranean or south-east Asian ancestry. When the diagnosis is suspected on clinical grounds, a screening test should be performed and, if possible, an enzyme assay. In fully expressed subjects, the timing of the assay is not important, but it may be in heterozygotes. Young cells have a higher G6PD activity than mature cells. The increase in young cells occurring during a haemolytic episode may therefore mask a G6PD deficiency in a heterozygote female. In fully expressed subjects with severe deficiency the rise in enzyme level, if it occurs at all, is not sufficient to obscure diagnosis. The assay should be repeated 2–4 months after the haemolytic episode in patients in whom the diagnosis of G6PD deficiency is definitely suspected, despite a normal G6PD activity on assay during or shortly after haemolysis.

Favism

Favism is a disorder characterized by acute haemolytic anaemia of sudden onset, often with haemoglobinuria and mild jaundice, which occurs in persons sensitive to the fava bean, *Vicia fava*, on ingestion of the uncooked or lightly cooked bean. Children aged between 2 and 5 years are characteristically affected; the condition is seen less frequently in adults. Some cases of haemolysis in breast-fed infants of mothers who have ingested fava beans have been described. Males are more frequently affected than females. Attacks occur most commonly in the spring when the beans are ripening. Inhalation of pollen from the fava bean plant may cause haemolysis in Sardinia, but this does not appear to occur in Greece. When due to pollen inhalation, haemolysis may be fulminating and begin within a few minutes, but with bean ingestion there is commonly a latent period of 24 hours to 9 days before onset of major clinical symptoms. The haemolysis varies in severity, but the anaemia is often severe; attacks usually last for 2–6 days, followed by spontaneous recovery, but death occurs occasionally. Irregularly contracted red cells in which the haemoglobin separates from the membrane ('blister cells') are particularly characteristic. Heinz bodies appear in most red cells early in the attack, but usually disappear by the third days.

Favism occurs mainly in Sardinia, Sicily, southern Italy, and Greece. However, cases are now being reported in persons of Mediterranean descent in the United States, Great Britain, Australia, and other countries; thus, it should be realized that the fava bean is the common European broad bean, which is widely grown and eaten in temperate climates. Although favism occurs typically in Mediterranean subjects carrying the severe Mediterranean type of G6PD deficiency, it may also occur in certain non-Mediterranean subjects with G6PD deficiency, including Chinese and Jews. It has been described in some English subjects in whom there was no apparent history of descent from races known to carry the disorder.

Persons susceptible to favism always have a deficiency of G6PD, but it appears that some other factor(s) (possibly genetic) are involved in the haemolytic attack that follows exposure to fava beans; thus some G6PD-deficient Mediterranean people can eat fava beans without haemolysis occurring. The disorder is reviewed by Belsey (1973).

The non-spherocytic congenital haemolytic anaemias

The non-spherocytic congenital haemolytic anaemias are a heterogeneous group of congenital anaemias occurring mainly, but not exclusively, in persons of northern European origin. They differ in severity and in haematological features, but as a group have in common the fact that spherocytes are not present on the blood film, the osmotic fragility of fresh blood is not usually increased, and splenectomy usually gives little or only moderate benefit. Most cases are due to an enzyme deficiency, although occasional cases are due to unstable haemoglobins (p. 152).

The deficiency may involve either the Embden–Meyerhof or the hexose monophosphate pathway, which were discussed in Chapter 2. Recently, deficiencies of non-glycolytic enzymes have also

Table 8.4. *Hereditary haemolytic anaemias due to enzyme abnormalities*

Associated with Embden–Meyerhof pathway deficiencies
Pyruvate kinase (over 300 cases reported)
Others (only small numbers of individual deficiencies reported):
Hexokinase
Glucose phosphate isomerase
Phosphofructokinase
Triose phosphate isomerase
Phosphoglycerate kinase
Aldolase
Associated with hexose monophosphate pathway deficiencies
Glucose-6-phosphate dehydrogenase (over 100 cases reported)
Others (only small numbers of individual deficiencies reported):
Glutathione reductase
γ-glutamyl cysteine synthetase
Gluthathione synthetase
Associated with abnormalities of nucleotide metabolism
Adenylate kinase deficiency
Pyrimidine 5′-nucleotidase deficiency
Hyperactivity of adenosine deaminase

been described (Table 8.4). The hereditary haemolytic anaemias due to enzyme deficiencies show continuous haemolysis.

EMBDEN-MEYERHOF PATHWAY

Enzyme deficiencies of the Embden–Meyerhof pathway are rare. By far the most common is pyruvate kinase (PK) deficiency, of which about 300 cases have been reported; it is described below. Other deficiencies (see Table 8.4) are reported in only small numbers. Most, but not all, have an autosomal recessive pattern of inheritance. In general, the haemolysis *in vivo* is considered to result from impairment of ATP production by the Embden–Meyerhof pathway, although the exact relationship of the metabolic lesion to premature red cell destruction is uncertain.

The deficiencies cause a non-spherocytic haemolytic anaemia, with considerable variation in severity; however, the anaemia is often severe. There are usually no clinical manifestations other than those of the haemolytic state. However, in triose phosphate isomerase deficiency, patients show neurological abnormalities and increased susceptibility to infection, probably due to enzyme deficiency of other tissues. Phosphofructokinase deficiency may be associated with muscular involvement, and phosphoglycerate kinase deficiency with mental changes.

For further details, the paper of Miwa & Fujii (1985) should be consulted; it gives a summary of each type and references to original case reports.

PYRUVATE KINASE (PK) DEFICIENCY HAEMOLYTIC ANAEMIA

Inheritance. The disorder is transmitted as an autosomal recessive trait; affected subjects are true homozygotes or inherit two different mutant genes, one from each parent (both of whom are clinically and haematologically normal). Most, but not all, reported cases have been in persons of northern European origin; both sexes are equally affected.

Clinical feature

The severity of the disorder shows considerable variation, and the clinical picture ranges from that of a severe haemolytic anaemia presenting in early infancy to a fairly well compensated haemolytic disorder of adults. However, in general, the defect is moderately severe and, in many reported cases, the clinical onset has been in infancy or early childhood. Less commonly the disorder presents in late childhood or early adult life. The common manifestations of a congenital haemolytic anaemia, namely jaundice and slight to moderate splenomegaly, are usual, but in less severely affected subjects presenting in the second or third decades clinical icterus may be absent. Hepatomegaly is common, especially in patients who have had numerous transfusions; cholelithiasis is also common. In general, the clinical and haematological features tend to remain fairly constant in the individual patient, but there may be variation in severity in the same family; intercurrent infection, pregnancy, or surgery may cause a temporary increase in anaemia.

Blood picture

Haemoglobin values show considerable variation, ranging from 5 to 12 g/dl. The increase in reticulocyte count also varies from patient to patient; before splenectomy it is usually slight to moderate, but after splenectomy high values, i.e. 50 per cent or more, are common. In most reported cases, the red cells have shown round macrocytosis of moderate to marked degree with a mildly elevated MCV and MCH. Polychromasia is usual, and a variable number of nucleated red cells may be present. A few cells with irregularly crenated margins, some of which are smaller than normal and stain deeply, are usually present. They are often more frequent after splenectomy. There is moderate to severe shortening of red cell lifespan as measured by the ^{51}Cr-labelling technique. The osmotic fragility of fresh blood is normal; after incubation, a population of cells showing increased resistance is apparent. The autohaemolysis test classically shows a marked increase of haemolysis uncorrected by glucose but corrected by ATP. The level of red cell 2,3-diphosphoglycerate is greatly increased, and ATP is usually reduced.

Diagnosis

The diagnosis should be considered in any case of non-spherocytic congenital haemolytic anaemia, especially when the clinical features suggest recessive inheritance. A fluorescent screening test for the diagnosis of PK deficiency is available. Assay of the red cell PK activity confirms the diagnosis; further evidence may be obtained by the demonstration of typical heterozygote values (about one-half of normal) in parents and other relatives. In double heterozygous subjects, values usually range from 5 to 25 per cent of normal but occasionally are higher. There is often poor correlation between the enzyme level and the severity of the haemolytic anaemia.

Treatment

The main form of treatment is blood transfusion as required for symptomatic comfort. Requirements vary significantly and may be heavy; nevertheless, some patients reach adult life without requiring transfusion. Splenectomy usually results in considerable improvement even though the haemolysis persists.

HEXOSE MONOPHOSPHATE PATHWAY

The most common, well-defined, non-spherocytic congenital haemolytic anaemia relating to this pathway is that associated with G6PD deficiency, of which over 100 cases have been reported. As previously described, deficiency of G6PD is much more commonly associated with haemolysis only after exposure to certain drugs (p. 186). Other hereditary deficiencies (see Table 8.4) are reported in only small numbers. The precise mechanism by which disorders of the hexose monophosphate pathway result in a shortened lifespan of the red cell is not known, but is probably related to failure to provide NADPH, which is necessary for the maintenance of an adequate level of reduced glutathione in the red cell and for prevention of oxidative denaturation of haemoglobin and cell membrane.

The chronic haemolytic disorders due to these deficiencies differ from those due to Embden–Meyerhof deficiencies in that: (a) they tend to be less severe; (b) the red cell ATP content is usually normal; (c) haemolysis may be exacerbated by drugs and fava beans; and (d) red cell morphological changes are slight or absent. In only relatively few reported cases has splenectomy been performed; it has either been without effect or has caused mild improvement.

Patients with *hereditary non-spherocytic haemolytic anaemia due to G6PD deficiency* have a chronic, mild to moderate anaemia present from birth; the anaemia may be exacerbated by the administration of drugs or by infection. Some cases present with neonatal jaundice. Patients are generally Caucasian males, mainly of northern European origin. Most cases are associated with G6PD enzyme variants (p. 186) with very low activity or marked instability. G6PD Mediterranean is probably the most common. Why this variant causes chronic haemolysis unrelated to drug ingestion in one ethnic group and drug-induced haemolytic anaemia in another is not known. Beutler (1978) lists G6PD variants associated with congenital non-spherocytic haemolytic anaemia and gives references to original case reports.

Nucleotide metabolism

Haemolytic anaemias associated with disorders of the purine and pyrimidine salvage pathways are reviewed by Paglia & Valentine (1981). The most common type, pyrimidine-5′-nucleotidase deficiency is characterized by a generally mild anaemia, marked basophilic stippling, and an increase in red cell pyrimidine-containing nucleotides.

Auto-immune acquired haemolytic anaemia

The term auto-immune acquired haemolytic anaemia (AIHA) is used to describe a group of haemolytic anaemias which result from the development of antibodies directed against antigens on the surface of the patient's own red cells, i.e. act as auto-antibodies. The antibodies are usually IgG or, less commonly, IgM or IgA and some bind complement. The *pathogenesis* of AIHA is uncertain. The formation of auto-antibodies may be due to a break-down in T-cell regulation of B cells with emergence of a hostile clone of immunocytes, or to a change in the structure of an antigen on the patient's red cells which is then recognized as 'non-self' by the immune system.

Table 8.5. *Classification of auto-immune acquired haemolytic anaemia*

Idiopathic (50 per cent)

Secondary (50 per cent)

DRUGS:
methyldopa, mefenamic acid, L-dopa, procainamide

UNDERLYING DISORDERS:
Infections—*Mycoplasma pneumoniae*, infectious mononucleosis, cytomegalovirus
Chronic lymphocytic leukaemia
Malignant lymphomas
Systemic lupus erythematosus
Other auto-immune disease—rheumatoid arthritis, chronic active hepatitis, myasthenia gravis, ulcerative colitis
Miscellaneous uncommon causes—carcinoma, sarcoidosis, ovarian teratoma

AIHA is an uncommon, but not rare, disorder. It occurs in every grade of severity, from a chronic mild asymptomatic state to an acute rapidly fatal disease.

Classification. AIHA is classified: (a) according to the temperature at which the antibody reacts with the red cells into warm antibody and cold antibody types; and (b) according to aetiology into idiopathic and secondary. A detailed aetiological classification is given in Table 8.5, and warm and cold antibodies are compared in Table 8.6.

Table 8.6. *The antibodies of warm and cold auto-immune acquired haemolytic anaemia*

		Cold AIHA	
	Warm AIHA	CHAD*	PCH†
Immunoglobulin class	IgG	IgM	IgG
Optimal reaction temperature	37°C	0–4°C	0–4°C
Antibody specificity	Often anti-Rh	Anti-I or anti-i	Anti-P
Immunochemical characteristics	Polyclonal	Monoclonal	Polyclonal
Serological behaviour *in vitro*	Incomplete	Agglutinin	Biphasic haemolysin
Protein on red cell surface	IgG 35% IgG + C 56% C 9%	C 100%	C 100%

*Cold haemagglutinin disease.
†Paroxysmal cold haemoglobinuria.

Warm antibody auto-immune acquired haemolytic anaemia

This type of haemolytic anaemia occurs at all ages, but adults are affected more frequently than children. The idopathic type affects females more commonly than males, and usually occurs after the age of 40 years. The secondary form may complicate a number of diseases (see Table 8.5), but chronic lymphocytic leukaemia, the malignant lymphomas, and systemic lupus erythematosus (SLE) account for most cases. The condition occurs as a complication of up to five per cent of cases of chronic lymphocytic leukaemia and SLE. Although methyldopa is now less frequently used in the treatment of hypertension, the administration of drugs remains an important cause of AIHA.

CLINICAL FEATURES

An insidious *onset* with symptoms of anaemia is usual. In most secondary cases the underlying disease is obvious when the haemolysis develops, although haemolytic anaemia is sometimes the first symptom, and the clinical manifestations of the underlying disease may not develop until months or even years later. Mild to moderate jaundice is usual, but is persistently absent in about 25 per cent of cases. The spleen is nearly always palpable, but rarely extends below the umbilicus. A very large spleen suggests the presence of chronic lymphocytic leukaemia or malignant lymphoma. Even when the spleen is impalpable, it is inevitably enlarged, a fact that may be demonstrated by radiography, radio-isotope scan, or at operation. Moderate hepatomegaly is usual. Lymph node enlargement does not occur in idiopathic cases, but is frequent in secondary cases. Haemoglobinuria is unusual, but occasionally occurs with an acute exacerbation of haemolysis. Haemosiderinuria is an occasional finding.

In young children, and in some adults, the onset may be sudden and follow a minor bacterial or viral infection. Anaemia develops rapidly, with jaundice and constitutional symptoms such as fever, headache, vomiting and pains in the abdomen and back. Intravascular haemolysis is evident, with haemoglobinaemia and haemoglobinuria; sometimes oliguria and even anuria develop. The spleen becomes palpable. Haemolysis usually ceases spontaneously after weeks or months and is followed by complete recovery. Rarely, death occurs from renal failure in severe cases. This form of transient acute warm antibody AIHA in children is usually idiopathic. In some instances it is associated with cytomegalovirus infection.

BLOOD PICTURE

The typical blood picture is of an anaemia with reticulocytosis, spherocytosis, and a positive direct antiglobulin test.

The haemoglobin level varies markedly. In compensated cases it is within normal limits, while in severely ill patients it may be 4 g/dl or less. A sudden drop to low values is the rule in acute cases. Spherocytosis is usually present in the active disease, but may be less obvious in the quiescent phase. Spherocytosis is accompanied by an increase in the osmotic fragility of fresh blood, but in general the increase on incubation is less consistent than in hereditary spherocytosis. When spherocytosis is mild it may not be obvious in the blood film and is revealed only by the osmotic fragility test. A mild increase in MCV is usual. Reticulocyte counts commonly range from 5 to 30 per cent, but may be higher, and small numbers of nucleated red cells are frequent. Rarely, the recticulocyte count is normal or even reduced due to an aplastic crisis (Liesveld *et al.* 1987) or folate deficiency. Polychromatic macrocytes are prominent in the film when the reticulocyte count is high and form a striking contrast to the microspherocytes. Erythrophagocytosis by monocytes may occasionally be observed.

The leucocyte count varies. In chronic cases of moderate severity, it is usually normal or, occasionally, moderately reduced. In acute cases or with severe haemolysis, leucocytosis is frequent, counts rising to 20–30 $\times 10^9$/l or even higher with a shift to the left. The platelet count is usually normal, but occasionally lowered, sometimes sufficiently to cause purpura. The serum bilirubin value usually ranges from 17 to 50 μmol/l, but is sometimes persistently normal despite continuing haemolysis.

The plasma haptoglobin level is reduced. The erythrocyte sedimentation rate is markedly increased in active states, but returns to normal during remissions. Immunoglobulin deficiency occurs in about 50 per cent of patients. IgA deficiency is most common, although some patients show deficiencies of IgG and/or IgM, or of all three immunoglobulins; occasionally there is an excess of an immunoglobulin. Serum and red cell folate levels may be reduced.

Blood drawn for routine examination often shows mild agglutination in the collection tube and on the blood film. This is not prevented by taking the blood into a warm syringe and keeping it at 37°, and represents agglutination of red cells heavily coated with incomplete antibody. It should not be mistaken for the usually more intense agglutination of cold haemagglutinin disease (p. 197).

IMMUNOLOGY

Auto-antibodies may be demonstrated *in vitro* in most cases of warm antibody AIHA. They are found on the red cell surface and in the serum.

Antibodies on the red cell surface

The presence of antibodies on the red cell surface is demonstrated by a positive direct antiglobulin test using a broad-spectrum antiglobulin reagent. More precise characterization of the coating immunoprotein is achieved with antiglobulin sera specific for immunoglobulin heavy chains and complement components. With these monospecific reagents, the red cells of 56 per cent of patients show coating with IgG and complement (C3), and 35 per cent with IgG alone. Nine per cent are coated with complement alone, and IgA or IgM coating is demonstrated on rare occasions. In SLE, the red cell coating is almost always IgG and complement, and in methyldopa-induced haemolytic anaemia, IgG alone (Issitt 1985).

Very small amounts of IgG can nearly always be demonstrated by sensitive techniques on the surface of red cells in which specific antiglobulin testing reveals coating by complement alone. Small amounts of IgG have also been demonstrated by similar methods on red cells from patients with 'Coombs' negative' warm antibody AIHA, in which the cells do not agglutinate with the usual broad-spectrum and specific antiglobulin sera. The amount of IgG on the red cell surface, as measured by the strength of agglutination in the conventional direct antiglobulin test, correlates poorly with the rate of red cell destruction in many cases. More sensitive techniques for measuring cell-bound IgG provide better correlation. Results of sequential quantitative antiglobulin tests on the red cells of individual patients, however, can often be related to fluctuations in severity of the haemolytic process.

It should be emphasized that there are a number of causes of a positive direct antiglobulin test besides AIHA (listed by Petz & Garratty 1980). Drugs are of particular importance, methyldopa (p. 205) being the most common cause of a positive direct antiglobulin test in the absence of haemolysis. Weakly positive tests due to complement coating are occasionally seen in ill patients, possibly as a result of immune complex absorption on the red cell surface with complement fixation.

Antibodies in the serum

The serum antibodies are usually incomplete antibodies, demonstrated by the indirect antiglobulin test or by the use of enzyme-treated red cells. They coat red cells optimally at 37°C but do not directly agglutinate, except in rare cases. Using the indirect antiglobulin test, serum antibody is detected in 60–80 per cent of patients. With more sensitive enzyme techniques, positive results are obtained in almost all affected patients. If serum antibodies cannot be demonstrated, a drug aetiology for the AIHA should be suspected. The antibodies are usually IgG, and frequently have blood group specificity within the Rh system. Thirty per cent of red cell eluates from affected subjects show Rh specificity if a panel of commonly occurring red cell types is used. If Rh null red cells are used, a further 35 per cent show some Rh specificity against a 'core' Rh antigen (Dacie 1975). The most commonly encountered Rh specificity is anti-e. Rh specificity is more frequently demonstrable in cases with IgG alone than with IgG plus complement red cell coating. Antibodies directed against other blood group antigens, e.g. U, LW, Kp^b, Wr^b, occur occasionally.

Studies on the subclass specificity of eluted IgG antibodies have shown that the majority are IgG_1. Most antibody molecules are polyclonal with mixed *K* and *λ* light chains.

SITE AND MECHANISM OF RED CELL DESTRUCTION

Red cell destruction in warm antibody AIHA is mainly extravascular by the macrophages of the spleen and to a much lesser extent the liver. Destruction within the circulation (intravascular haemolysis) may occur when the haemolytic process is particularly acute, and it is probable that even in chronic warm antibody AIHA there is always a minor element of intravascular red cell destruction. The exact mechanism of red cell destruction is not known with certainty, but the following sequence of events, reviewed by Frank (1985), seems likely.

Extravascular destruction (Fig. 8.5)

Red cells coated with IgG antibody are preferentially destroyed in the spleen. They attach to macrophages which have surface receptors for the Fc fragments of IgG subclasses IgG_1 and IgG_3, and are either completely phagocytosed or lose a small part of their membrane to the phagocytic cell and are rendered spherocytic. The spherocytic cells are released from the macrophages and destroved prematurely on subsequent recirculation through the spleen.

Red cells coated with complement at the C3b stage may also be phagocytosed by macrophages following adherence to a C3 receptor site on the macrophage surface. Only a small number of red cells are destroyed through this relatively ineffective mechanism. Most are released from the macrophages and resume circulation when the C3b is cleaved by factor I (C3b inactivator), leaving C3d on the red cell surface. Phagocytosis by this mechanism takes place throughout the reticulo-endothelial system (especially in the liver) and not preferentially in the spleen. The relationship between the amount of complement on the red cell surface and the degree of haemolysis is highly variable. Little or no haemolysis may occur in spite of the presence of large amounts of bound complement.

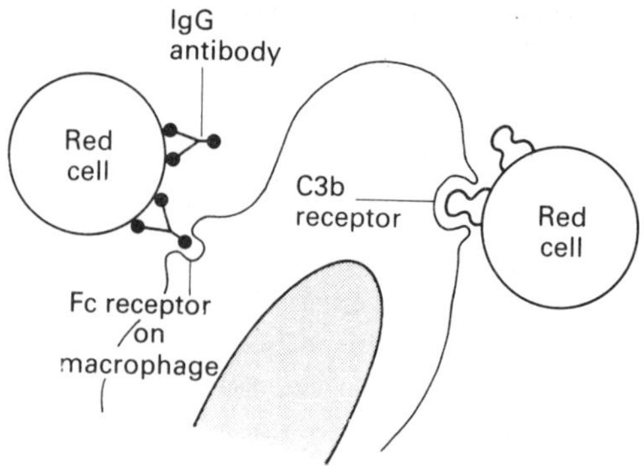

Fig. 8.5. *Schematic view of interactions between antibody or complement-coated red cells and specific receptors on the macrophage surface. Red cells coated with IgG_1 or IgG_3 attach via macrophage Fc receptors, and those coated with C3b via complement receptors. Most red cells attached by the latter mechanism are released following cleavage of surface C3b to C3d (for which there are no macrophage receptor sites) by factor I (C3b inactivator).*

Intravascular destruction

The rare finding of haemoglobinuria and haemosiderinuria in warm antibody AIHA indicates the presence of intravascular haemolysis. In these cases, complement fixed on the red cell surface by the IgG or IgM antibody is activated through the complete sequence to C9, which brings about cell lysis. Why the activation of the complement sequence terminates at the stage of C3 in most cases, and does not go on to completion, is not fully understood. The role of complement in immunohaematology is discussed by Petz & Garratty (1980).

DIAGNOSIS

Diagnosis is based on the demonstration of the typical findings of a haemolytic anaemia—jaundice, splenomegaly, anaemia, reticulocytosis, and a raised serum bilirubin—with a positive direct antiglobulin test. However, it must be realized that jaundice is absent in 25 per cent of patients.

Once the diagnosis is established, a search must be instituted for a cause. These are listed in Table 8.5. Bone marrow aspiration and trephine biopsy are indicated in most cases, and a careful search for evidence of leukaemia, malignant lymphoma, and megaloblastic red cell change should be made. Tests for the presence of SLE are important, and in acute cases in children and young adults, evidence of viral infection should be sought by appropriate cultures and serological studies.

COURSE AND PROGNOSIS

The course of the idiopathic form of disease is exceedingly variable and thus forecasting the outlook in a particular patient is difficult. Most patients respond, at least initially, to one or other form of treatment. In chronic cases, active haemolysis may continue for years, the degree of disability being proportionate to the anaemia. Spontaneous remissions occasionally occur; for this reason, the results of treatment are not always easy to assess. No patient can be said to be permanently cured if the antiglobulin test remains positive, even though the haemoglobin, reticulocyte count, and serum bilirubin values are normal. The possibility of relapse always remains, especially following infection.

Silverstein *et al.* (1972) reported a 91 per cent one-year and 73 per cent ten-year survival in all patients seen at the Mayo Clinic cover a ten-year period. They were unable to relate survival to age of patient at diagnosis, initial white cell, platelet or reticulocyte count, initial severity of anaemia, or presence of splenomegaly.

In secondary cases, the prognosis depends largely on the underlying disease, which in many cases is itself eventually fatal.

TREATMENT

Acute cases in children with moderate anaemia may recover without any treatment except for bed rest. In children with more severe disease, and in most adults corticosteroids, blood transfusion and splenectomy form the main basis of treatment. Immunosuppressive drugs may be used in certain cases.

Corticosteroids induce a prompt reduction in the rate of haemolysis in about 80 per cent of patients. Thus therapy with prednisone, either alone or combined with blood transfusion in more severe cases, is the initial treatment of choice. Response to corticosteroids cannot be correlated with any particular pattern of red cell immunoglobulin coating as shown by specific antiglobulin testing. There is considerable individual variation in the dosage required to induce and maintain remission. The initial dose of prednisone should be large, e.g. 60–80 mg daily. Parenteral hydrocortisone may be necessary in acutely ill patients. In general, the haemoglobin stabilizes within a week and then slowly rises to near normal or normal levels. The reticulocyte count falls as improvement occurs, but the fall is sometimes preceded by an initial transient rise. Treatment should be continued for at least three weeks before being considered ineffective. When remission occurs, dosage should be gradually reduced to the minimum necessary to maintain a haemoglobin level of at least 11 g/dl. The direct antiglobulin test usually remains positive for many months, although its titre may diminish. Serum antibody titres slowly fall over a period of 3–6 months. Some patients require no maintenance therapy; others require 5–15 mg prednisone, or more, daily. Second daily corticosteroid dosage may reduce the frequency of drug side-effects. In patients requiring large maintenance doses (in excess of 15 mg) over a long period of time, splenectomy should be considered (p. 196). When relapse occurs after remission, higher doses are reinstituted. Corticosteroids appear to reduce the degree of haemolysis in AIHA by decreasing antibody production and by inhibiting the clearance of antibody-coated red cells by the macrophages of the reticulo-endothelial system.

Blood transfusion is not required in patients with only moderate anaemia, but concentrated red cells should be used in severe cases whenever necessary to maintain a haemoglobin level and blood volume compatible with life. Transfusions should be kept to a minimum, especially when they appear to be ineffective. The transfused cells are often rapidly destroyed and the haemoglobin rise is transient, usually lasting only a matter of hours.

The auto-antibody on the patient's red cells and/or in the serum may cause difficulty both in blood grouping and cross-matching, and the tests should be performed by an experienced blood transfusion serologist. It is essential as a first step to exclude the presence of allo-antibodies in the serum, and an attempt should then be made to establish the specificity of the auto-antibody (Petz & Branch 1983). In some cases, limited specificity within the Rh system may be demonstrated, and it is possible to transfuse units negative for the relevant antigen. More frequently, the auto-antibodies are apparently non-specific, and all units of the correct ABO and Rh group cross-matched by the indirect antiglobulin and enzyme techniques show some incompatibility. When this occurs, the selection and slow administration of donor red cells showing the least incompatibility is usually advised. The patient's plasma haemoglobin should be monitored during the transfusion by performing a microhaematocrit at regular intervals and inspecting the plasma colour in the centrifuge tube. Masouredis & Chaplin (1985) present useful guidelines to the use ot blood transfusion in AIHA.

Splenectomy results in complete or near complete remission in about 60 per cent of patients. Splenectomy should be reserved for: (a) idiopathic cases which have not responded to adequate treatment with corticosteroids, and for secondary cases which have not responded to corticosteroids or to treatment of the underlying causative disorder; and (b) patients who have responded to corticosteroids, but in whom after some months there are still signs of activity, and who require large maintenance doses to sustain a reasonable haemoglobin level; even if a complete remission does not follow splenectomy, it is sometimes possible to control the anaemia with smaller corticosteroid doses than were required before splenectomy.

It is not possible to predict definitely from the clinical or haematological findings whether a particular patient will respond to splenectomy. Patients who respond well to corticosteroids are more likely to respond to splenectomy than those who do not. *In vivo* studies with ^{51}Cr-labelled red cells using surface counting techniques may be helpful (Ahuja *et al.* 1972). A good response to splenectomy can be anticipated in patients with excess counts over the spleen; however, even in patients in whom significant destruction is occurring in the liver, splenectomy may be beneficial in that it may be possible to maintain a symptomatically comfortable haemoglobin level with lower doses of steroid. The direct antiglobulin test often remains positive following splenectomy, irrespective of the clinical results. However, the serum antibody titre may fall when remission occurs. The patient who has a complete remission following splenectomy is not necessarily permanently cured as relapse may occur weeks, months, or even years later.

At operation the abdomen should be explored for enlarged lymph nodes and ovarian dermoid cysts. Accessory spleens should be searched for and removed. Histological examination of the spleen may give the first evidence of an underlying disorder, e.g. malignant lymphoma. Post-splenectomy thrombocytosis is frequently seen, particularly in patients who remain anaemic, and heparin therapy may be necessary when the platelet count rises to very high levels.

Immunosuppressive therapy with oral azathioprine in a dose of 2–2.25 mg/kg/day, or with cyclophosphamide, 1.5–2.0 mg/kg/day, has been used with some success. Careful monitoring of the neutrophil count is necessary. The occasional development of leukaemia and malignant lymphoma in patients receiving long-term azathioprine suggests that the drug should not be used unless absolutely necessary (Grunwald & Rosner 1979). It is generally reserved for those patients who fail to respond adequately to splenectomy and in whom further corticosteroid administration is without effect or is required in high dosage. *Oral folic acid*, 5 mg daily, should be given to all patients with continuing haemolysis.

Treatment of the causative disorder in secondary AIHA. In most secondary cases, the initial management is the same as for idiopathic cases, and the causative disorder is treated either concurrently or subsequently. The response to treatment varies; many patients respond despite persistence of the causative disease, although some do not. In patients with mild anaemia, treatment of the causative disease may be tried first; remission of the anaemia occasionally follows relief of the causative disorder. If AIHA develops in a patient with a previous history of malignant lymphoma or other neoplasm, a thorough check for recurrent disease should be made.

Cold antibody auto-immune acquired haemolytic anaemia

Auto-immune acquired haemolytic anaemia due to cold antibodies, i.e. auto-antibodies that react best with red cells at temperatures below 37°C, is less frequent than the warm antibody type. Two forms are recognized.

Cold haemagglutinin disease (CHAD) is characterized by a haemolytic anaemia of varying severity due to auto-antibodies that act as red cell agglutinins at low temperatures. *Paroxysmal cold haemoglobinuria (PCH)* is characterized by episodes of acute haemolysis due to auto-antibodies that act primarily as red cell lysins at low temperatures. Both CHAD and PCH may be idiopathic or secondary to an underlying illness.

COLD HAEMAGGLUTININ DISEASE (CHAD)

The idiopathic type of CHAD occurs in adults aged over 50 years, and is rare in children. Both sexes are equally affected, and most patients run a chronic course. The secondary form occurs as a rare complication of the malignant lymphomas, chronic lymphocytic leukaemia, Waldenström's macroglobulinaemia, or SLE, or as an acute transient haemolytic anaemia secondary to infectious mononucleosis or *Mycoplasma pneumoniae* infection (see Table 8.5). The disorder is reviewed by Crisp & Pruzanski (1982).

Clinical features

In idiopathic CHAD and CHAD associated with the malignant lymphomas, chronic lymphocytic leukaemia, or SLE, the onset is insidious with symptoms of anaemia. Two clinical patterns are recognized, depending on the thermal range of the antibody. Some patients experience episodes of acute intravascular haemolysis and haemoglobinuria in cold weather but maintain a normal haemoglobin level when the weather is warmer. Other patients have a well-compensated chronic haemolytic anaemia with a mild to moderate reduction in haemoglobin, perhaps slightly worse in the cold weather, but only rarely experience attacks of acute haemolysis. Agglutination of the patient's red cells as they traverse the cooler peripheral areas of the circulation results in varying degrees of obstruction of the microcirculation and symptoms and signs of cold sensitivity, e.g. Raynaud's phenomenon, acrocyanosis and, rarely, peripheral gangrene. These phenomena are more likely to occur in cold weather and are often absent in temperate climates.

Very occasional patients with idiopathic CHAD develop a malignant lymphoma as a terminal complication. More frequently, CHAD develops in a patient with a pre-existing lymphoma (Chaplin 1982).

Post-infectious CHAD, as seen in infectious mononucleosis and atypical pneumonia caused by *Mycoplasma pneumoniae*, typically has an acute onset in the second or third week of the infective illness. There is evidence of acute intravascular haemolysis with jaundice and splenomegaly. Cold sensitivity is usually not seen, and the haemolysis resolves in 2–3 weeks in most cases.

Blood picture

The typical blood picture is of an anaemia with red cell agglutination, reticulocytosis, and a positive direct antiglobulin test.

The red cell agglutination is the outstanding diagnostic feature. It is seen on blood films prepared from capillary specimens or from blood collected into an anticoagulant, and is often visible macroscopically in the collection tube. The agglutination may be avoided if the blood specimen is kept at 37°C before spreading and the slides are prewarmed. The haemoglobin level is reduced, but it rarely falls below 8 g/dl, and may be normal. It may fall to low values in acute exacerbations. Spherocytosis is usually present, but is less marked than in warm antibody AIHA. The reticulocyte count is mildly increased, and polychromatic macrocytes and occasional nucleated red cells are seen on the blood film. The white cell count and platelet count are usually normal. The serum bilirubin is mildly elevated and the plasma haemoglobin increased in active disease. Haemosiderin is often found in the urine in both active and quiescent phases. The red cell agglutination interferes with the function of automated cell counters, and spuriously high MCV results are obtained. Serum and red cell folate levels may be reduced.

Immunology

Most cases of CHAD are caused by an autoantibody referred to as anti-I. This antibody reacts with the I antigen which is found on the surface of nearly all adult human red cells but not on the surface of fetal red cells. The antibody is a complete antibody which agglutinates red cells with increasing strength as the temperature is lowered to 4°C, but is inactive at 37°C. Its lytic activity is much less marked than that of the Donath–Landsteiner antibody of paroxysmal cold haemoglobinuria (p. 199). Most patients with idiopathic CHAD or CHAD secondary to leukaemia, malignant lymphoma, or SLE have very high cold agglutinin titres, e.g. from 64 000 to 512 000. The agglutinin titres in CHAD secondary to *Mycoplasma pneumoniae* infection are usually not as high as in idiopathic CHAD. The agglutinating antibody in CHAD associated with infectious mononucleosis and some cases of malignant lymphoma is anti-i. This antibody strongly agglutinates umbilical cord red cells at low temperatures but is relatively inactive against adult red cells.

The anti-I antibodies of idiopathic CHAD and most types of secondary CHAD are IgM in type with κ light chains. An M-band is often evident on serum electrophoresis, and immuno-electrophoresis confirms that the abnormal band is a monoclonal IgM protein. The serum IgM level is elevated to about 6 g/l, but IgG and IgA are usually normal. The anti-I antibody of CHAD secondary to myco plasma infection is also IgM, but is usually polyclonal with mixed κ and λ light chains (see Table 8.6).

The direct antiglobulin test is positive if the blood specimen is drawn and kept at 37°C, and washed in warm saline before testing. The positive test is due to the presence of complement (C3d) on the red cell surface as demonstrated by specific antiglobulin sera. Serum complement is often depleted.

Site and mechanism of red cell destruction

As in warm antibody AIHA, red cell destruction in CHAD occurs both in the circulation and in the reticulo-endothelial system. The IgM antibody fixes complement to the patient's red cells in the cooler peripheral areas of the circulation. When the red cells return to areas of the body where higher temperatures prevail, the antibody dissociates from the red cell surface, leaving the complement still bound. Probably depending on the amount of complement and other factors, the complement sequence either terminates at the C3b stage or, less commonly, goes on to completion with intravascular lysis. The C3b-coated cells adhere to hepatic macrophages, and their subsequent fate is similar to that of the complement-coated cells in the warm antibody haemolytic anaemias (p. 194).

Prognosis and treatment

Progress of idiopathic CHAD is usually slow, and many patients remain relatively well, particularly if the upper thermal range of the antibody does not exceed 28°C. Protection from the cold weather, or a move to a more temperate climate, may be all that is needed. Corticosteroids and splenectomy are rarely of any benefit. Chlorambucil is of value in some patients, and usually leads to a reduction in the level of IgM in the serum. Occasional patients progress rapidly and require blood transfusion. Concentrated red cells are preferable, and the patient should be kept warm and the donor units warmed to body temperature before and during administration. Plasmapheresis has been used with success in some very severe cases. CHAD associated with infective illnesses is usually self-limiting.

PAROXYSMAL COLD HAEMOGLOBINURIA

Paroxysmal cold haemoglobinuria (PCH) is a rare disorder characterized by attacks of haemolysis with haemoglobinuria on exposure to cold, either local or general. It results from the development of a cold auto-antibody with strong lytic activity.

The disorder may be idiopathic or secondary to viral illnesses such as mumps, measles, or influenza. In children with viral illnesses, exposure to cold is not necessarily involved in precipitation of the haemolysis. In adults, the illness is usually chronic and takes the form of episodic haemolysis and haemoglobinuria precipitated by exposure to cold.

The degree of chilling required to cause haemoglobinuria varies; in some cases it is only slight, and may be limited to one part of the body, e.g. immersion of hands in cold water or taking a cold drink. After a period of minutes to several hours, the patient develops pain in the back and legs, sometimes with abdominal cramp and headache, and then a rigor with a sharp rise of temperature. The anaemia is usually severe (although short-lived), and red cell spherocytosis, erythrophagocytosis, and leucopenia are present on the blood film. The first specimen of urine passed after the rigor usually contains haemoglobin; haemoglobinuria disappears in several hours. The spleen may become palpable at the time of the attack, and transient jaundice is common on the day following the attack. Rarely, the degree of haemoglobinaemia is not sufficient to cause haemoglobinuria, and only constitutional symptoms occur.

The characteristic finding in the blood is a bithermic cold haemolysin which can be demonstrated by the Donath–Landsteiner test. The principle of the test is that the haemolysin in the patient's blood attaches to the red cells when the blood is chilled, and the sensitized cells are then haemolysed by complement when the blood is warmed to 37°C. The cold haemolysin is a complement-binding IgG antibody, and is usually found to have anti-P blood group specificity. The direct antiglobulin test is positive only during the episode of haemolysis. The positive result is due to the presence of complement on the red cell surface.

Paroxysmal nocturnal haemoglobinuria (PNH)

This uncommon disorder is characterized by chronic haemolytic anaemia with intermittent haemoglobinuria. The fundamental abnormality is an acquired defect of the red cell membrane—possibly a deficiency of *decay accelerating factor*, a complement regulatory protein—which renders it unusually sensitive to lysis by the complement of normal serum. Rosse *et al.* (1974) demonstrated three distinct red cell populations in PNH: two populations of intermediate and extreme sensitivity to complement lysis, and a third population that is resistant. *In vivo*, haemolysis of PNH cells appears to be due to activation of complement by the alternate rather than the classical complement pathway. Precise details of the mechanism that triggers the alternate pathway in PNH are still uncertain.

The surface of the red cells appears normal when examined microscopically on a stained blood film, but studies with transmission and scanning electron microscopy have demonstrated irregular cells with surface pits and protruberances.

Pathogenesis

The pathogenesis of PNH is unknown. It has a definite relationship to aplastic anaemia. In 25 per cent of patients, the disease commences as aplastic anaemia, the clinical and laboratory features of PNH appearing later. Evidence of PNH may be transient and confined to *in vitro* serological tests only, the disease continuing to behave as aplastic anaemia. Aplastic anaemia associated with PNH is usually idiopathic, but rare cases following congenital aplasia and aplasia secondary to drugs and chemicals have been described. Marrow aplasia may also occur during the course of classical haemolytic PNH. The PNH *in vitro* red cell defect is occasionally present in patients with myelosclerosis, although evidence of haemolysis is absent. Rare cases of acute leukaemia following PNH have been described. The most plausible view of the pathogenesis of the disorder is that it is due to the injury-induced development of an abnormal clone of stem cells giving rise to defective red cells, white cells, and platelets. The disorder is fully reviewed by Sirchia & Lewis (1975).

Clinical features

PNH usually appears first in adult life, most commonly in the third or fourth decade, and affects both sexes equally. It is not hereditary, and is unrelated to race. The onset is insidious, the patient presenting with symptoms of anaemia or haemoglbinuria, or both. *Haemoglobinuria* is the cardinal clinical feature, and is seen at some stage of the disease in nearly all patients; it is present at the onset in approximately 50 per cent. Its severity fluctuates, reflecting variations in the intensity of intravascular haemolysis and the level of plasma haemoglobin. It is related to sleep irrespective of whether sleep is taken by night or day. The reason for this phenomenon is not clear. Characteristically, only the urine passed during the night or in the morning on waking is red, but in severe cases all urine samples are coloured, although daytime samples are lighter. Bouts of haemoglobinuria alternate with periods of remission lasting weeks or months, during which haemoglobinuria is absent. Rarely, haemoglobinuria is absent for years or even for the whole course of the disease. Abdominal or lumbar pain and pyrexia occasionally accompany an attack of haemoglobinuria. Attacks of increased haemolysis and haemoglobinuria are sometimes precipitated by stress, infection, exercise, pregnancy, vaccination, menstruation, blood transfusion, surgery, and the administration of drugs, e.g. iron. Mild jaundice is usual. Slight enlargement of the spleen and liver is common.

Haemosiderinuria is a constant and characteristic finding; at autopsy, the renal tubules are heavily impregnated with haemosiderin. Some patients lose considerable amounts of iron as haemoglobin and haemosiderin, and may develop iron deficiency. No free red cells are present in the urine.

Unusual modes of presentation may cause diagnostic difficulty in patients with minimal haemolysis. Venous thrombosis is a frequent complication, and may cause severe headaches or attacks of abdominal pain and nausea. Progressive diffuse hepatic venous thrombosis (Budd–Chiari syndrome) causes abdominal pain, fever, increasing hepatomegaly, jaundice, and ascites, and usually terminates in hepatic failure and death.

Blood picture

The blood picture shows anaemia of varying severity with moderate macrocytosis, polychromasia, moderate leucopenia due to a reduction in neutrophils, and mild thrombocytopenia. Reticulocytes are increased, but generally to a lesser extent than expected for the degree of anaemia. In iron-deficient patients, hypochromia and microcytosis are present. In the active phase, haemoglobin is usually found in the serum which may also have a brownish tint due to the presence of methaemalbumin. Hb-F is occasionally elevated. The serum bilirubin is moderately increased. The neutrophil alkaline phosphatase score is decreased but may be normal in the aplastic phase. Coagulation studies have demonstrated a hypercoagulable state which increases during haemolytic crises. In occasional cases, the direct antiglobulin test is positive. The *bone marrow* is hypercellular during the haemolytic phase of the disorder, with normoblastic erythroid hyperplasia and some dyserythropoiesis. Iron stores are often reduced, and mild megaloblastic changes may be observed. In the aplastic phase, there is a reduction in all marrow elements and iron stores may be normal.

Diagnosis

Diagnosis is usually suggested by the characteristic intermittent haemoglobinuria and the demonstration of haemosiderin in the urine, and confirmed by positive *serological tests*. The disorder should be considered in any patient with a refractory anaemia, particularly if reticulocytosis, pancytopenia, or a history of transfusion reactions is present.

Ham's acid serum test. This serological test is the definitive diagnostic test for PNH. The principle is that the patient's cells undergo haemolysis in compatible acidified serum at 37°C. The serum may be the patient's own or from another normal subject. From 10 to 50 per cent lysis is usually observed in a positive test. Lysis of red cells in the acid serum test occurs through the alternate pathway of complement activation.

Sucrose haemolysis test. This test is a useful screening test for PNH. It is more sensitive than the acid serum test, but lacks the latter's specificity. PNH red cells lyse when suspended in isotonic solutions of low ionic strength, if serum is also present.

More than 10 per cent haemolysis is said to be diagnostic of PNH, values of 5–10 per cent being borderline. Red cell lysis in the sucrose haemolysis test is probably mediated through the classical pathway of complement activation.

Details of the tests and their interpretation are given by Jenkins (1972) and Sirchia & Lewis (1975).

Course and prognosis

The disorder is chronic; the severity varies from mild cases which cause relatively little discomfort, to severe cases in which anaemia is marked and haemoglobinuria persistent. Some patients survive at least 20 years with good medical care, but the median survival is 5–10 years. Death occurs from anaemia, post-operative complications, visceral thrombosis (especially of portal and cerebral vessels), haemorrhage, infection, or some unrelated disorder. Post-splenectomy thrombo-embolism is a major cause of death in several series of cases. Rarely, spontaneous cure of the disease occurs.

Treatment

No specific treatment is available, and management is largely supportive. Transfusion with concentrated red cells relieves the anaemia for a considerable time, as the transfused cells have a normal lifespan in the patient. In some patients, there is a reaction to transfusion with exacerbation of haemolysis. This is probably due to complement activation triggered by an immune reaction between leuco-agglutinins in the patient's plasma and leucocytes in the transfused blood. Reactions can be avoided by washing the donor cells with saline before transfusion or by the use of filtered or frozen blood, which is largely free of white cells (p. 481). Factors known to precipitate haemoglobinuria, especially drugs, should be avoided. The administration of androgens is of value in some cases. Response is usually not immediate, and Rosse (1982) recommends a trial of therapy with oxymetholone, 10–50 mg daily for at least two months. Prednisone causes a reduction in haemolysis in some patients. Because of the problems of long-term administration its use should be restricted to patients with a severe exacerbation of haemolysis or those with significant transfusion requirements who have not responded to other measures. Splenectomy is of no value, and in the past has had a high mortality. If there is unequivocal bone marrow evidence of iron deficiency, oral iron therapy may benefit the patient. Gross haemoglobinuria occasionally follows initiation of iron therapy, particularly if administered by the parenteral route, which should be avoided if possible. Long-term anticoagulant therapy may be required for thrombotic complications. The management of PNH is reviewed by Rosse (1982).

Haemolytic anaemia due to drugs and chemicals

A number of drugs and chemicals may cause haemolytic anaemia. They fall into three broad groups: (1) those that have a direct toxic action on the red cell; the haemolysis is dose-related and occurs in most normal subjects provided that sufficient dose of the drug is given; (2) those that cause haemolysis as a result of a hereditary metabolic abnormality of the red cell; and (3) those that cause haemolysis by immunological mechanisms (Table 8.7).

Table 8.7. *Drug-induced haemolytic anaemias*

Direct toxic action of drugs and chemicals
Red cell metabolic abnormality
Hereditary enzyme deficiencies
Unstable haemoglobins
Immune mechanisms
Immune haemolytic anaemia
Auto-immune haemolytic anaemia

Table 8.8. *Drugs and chemical agents that may cause haemolytic anaemia*

Drugs that regularly cause haemolytic anaemia in normal subjects by direct toxic action

Acetylphenylhydrazine	Phenylhydrazine
Arsine	Potassium chlorate
Chloramines	Resorcinol
Copper	Sodium chlorate
Formaldehyde	Sulphanilamide
Naphthalene	Sulphapyridine
Para-aminosalicylic acid	Sulphasalazine
Phenacetin	Sulphones
Phenazopyridine	

*Drugs that cause haemolytic anaemia in subjects with hereditary metabolic abnormalities of the red cell (principally G6PD deficiency)**

Analgesics	*Sulphones*
Acetanilide	Dapsone
	Thiazole sulphone
Antimalarials	
Pamaquin	*Miscellaneous*
Pentaquine	Acetylphenylhydrazine
Primaquine	Methylene blue
	Nalidixic acid
Nitrofurans	Naphthalene (mothballs)
Nitrofurantoin	Niridazole
	Phenylhydrazine
Sulphonamides	Toluidine blue
Sulphacetamide	Trinitrotoluene
Sulphamethoxazole	
Sulphanilamide	
Sulphapyridine	
Sulphasalazine	

Drugs that cause haemolytic anaemia by immune mechanisms

Immune	Quinine
Amidopyrine	Rifampicin
Antazoline	Sulphasalazine
Cephalosporins	Stibophen
Chlorpromazine	Sulphonamides
Chlorpropamide	Teniposide
Cisplatin	Tetracycline
Dipyrone	Thiazides
Erythromycin	Thiopentone
Insulin	Tolbutamide
Isoniazid	Triamterene
Nomifensine	
Para-aminosalicylic acid	*Auto-immune*
Paracetamol	L-dopa
Penicillin	Mefenamic acid
Phenacetin	Methyldopa
Quinidine	Procainamide

*In addition to these drugs, many of the agents that regularly cause haemolysis in large doses may cause haemolysis in G6PD-deficient subjects in smaller doses.

Table 8.8 lists drugs and chemicals that may cause haemolysis.

Haemolytic anaemia due to direct toxic action

Haemolysis may result from drug therapy, occupational poisoning, and household poisoning. The majority of the drugs and chemicals or their metabolites are powerful oxidants which injure the red cell membrane and interfere with the cell's normal metabolism. They lead to the formation of methaemoglobin and to the denaturation of globin, which precipitates in the red cells as Heinz bodies. Characteristically, the red cells are contracted, distorted, and often spherocytic, reflecting direct injury to the cell membrane by the drug and damage sustained during circulation through the spleen. Many of the drugs and chemicals that regularly cause haemolysis in large doses may cause haemolysis in patients with G6PD deficiency, or an unstable haemoglobin in smaller doses. Drug-induced oxidative haemolysis is discussed in detail by Gordon-Smith (1980).

Drug therapy. Commonly used drugs that have been reported to cause this type of haemolysis include the sulphones, which are used in the treatment of leprosy and dermatitis herpetiformis, some sulphonamides, and para-aminosalicylic acid.

Occupational poisoning. Haemolytic anaemia may follow exposure to arsine (arseniuretted hydrogen) in submarines (storage batteries), chemistry laboratories, and factories. Accidental ingestion of phenylhydrazine or acetylphenylhydrazine occasionally occurs in chemistry laboratories, with similar results.

Household poisoning. Cases of acute haemolytic anaemia have been reported in young children who have swallowed mothballs containing naphthalene, and in infants as a result of skin absorption from napkins impregnated with naphthalene; some of these have been associated with G6PD deficiency.

Contamination of haemodialysis systems. Several outbreaks of acute haemolytic anaemia in patients undergoing chronic maintenance haemodialysis have been caused by contamination of the dialysate by chloramines, which are bactericidal oxidant compounds used for purification of urban water supplies (Caterson *et al.* 1982). Contamination of dialysis fluid by the sterilizing agent, formaldehyde, also results in acute haemolysis.

BLOOD PICTURE

The degree of anaemia varies and is usually proportional to the dose. It is often accompanied by one or more of the following features which result from the action of the toxic agent on the red cell: (i) irregular contraction and 'blister' or 'bite' cell formation (p. 188); (ii) spherocytosis; (iii) Heinz bodies (Fig. 8.6); and (iv) methaemoglobinaemia and sulphaemoglobinaemia. Evidence of intravascular haemolysis (haemoglobinaemia, haemoglo-

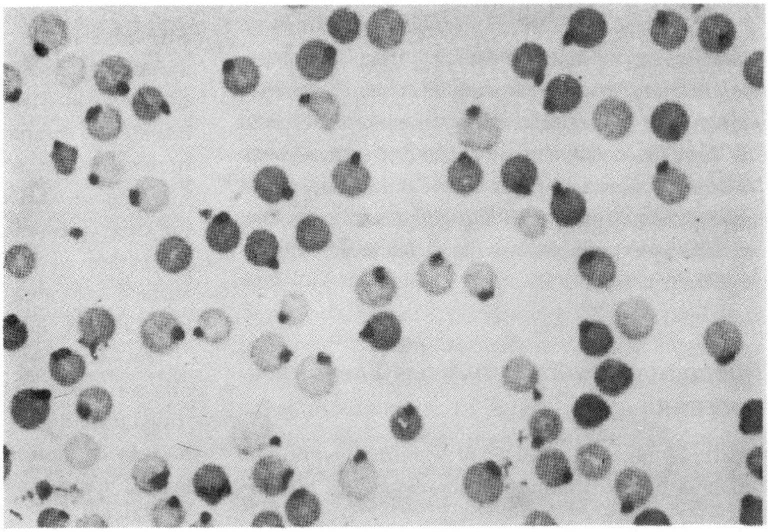

Fig. 8.6. *Heinz bodies. Photomicrograph of a blood film from a patient with nitrobenzene poisoning due to ingestion of furniture polish. There was marked methaemoglobinaemia and moderate haemolytic anaemia. Stained supravitally by brilliant cresyl blue (× 520).*

binuria, and methaemalbuminaemia) is also usually present.

The presence of the Heinz bodies, methaemoglobin, or sulphaemoglobin strongly suggests that the haemolysis is due to a chemical cause. However, their absence does not exclude such a cause, as some substances producing haemolysis do not result in their formation. Neutrophilia, sometimes with toxic granulation, is usual in acute chemical haemolytic anaemia, and a moderate platelet increase may also occur. A G6PD screening test and the heat-instability test for unstable haemoglobins should be performed. Analysis of urine for drug metabolites may help in cases in which the nature of the poison is uncertain.

Drug-induced haemolytic anaemia due to hereditary red cell enzyme deficiencies

Acute haemolytic anaemia due to certain drugs administered in standard doses may be associated with inherited red cell metabolic defects, of which by far the commonest is a deficiency of glucose-6-phosphate dehydrogenase (p. 186). With some other enzyme abnormalities, a pre-existing mild haemolytic anaemia may be aggravated by drug ingestion.

Drug-induced haemolytic anaemia due to unstable haemoglobins

Exacerbation of haemolysis by drugs has been demonstrated in some patients with haemoglobinopathies due to unstable haemoglobins. Hb-Zurich has been most extensively studied in this respect. The drugs involved have been similar to those causing haemolysis in G6PD-deficient subjects. The unstable haemoglobins are discussed more fully on page 152.

Immunological drug-induced haemolytic anaemia

Nearly 20 per cent of cases of acquired haemolytic anaemia due to immune mechanisms are attributable to the administration of drugs. Penicillin and methyldopa are most frequently incriminated, but a wide range of drugs (see Table 8.8) has the ability to initiate in the susceptible person immunological mechanisms that lead, directly or indirectly, to premature red cell destruction. Two forms of immunologically mediated drug-induced haemolytic anaemia are recognized.

Immune haemolytic anaemia in which antibodies are formed against the offending drug or its metabolites. Serum antibodies cannot be demonstrated *in vitro* with normal red cells unless the drug is also present in the test system.

Auto-immune haemolytic anaemia in which antibodies are formed against red cell antigens. Serum antibodies can be demonstrated *in vitro* with normal red cells in the presence or absence of the drug from the test system.

A number of cases has been reported in which there is evidence that cell destruction has been caused by both mechanisms acting simultaneously.

DRUG-INDUCED IMMUNE HAEMOLYTIC ANAEMIA

Two mechanisms appear to be involved in the pathogenesis of this type of drug-induced haemolytic anaemia. Some drugs, e.g. *penicillin* and *cephalothin,* have a strong affinity for the red cell membrane. When given to the patient in large doses they bind firmly to the membrane protein, and antibodies to the cell-bound drug are formed by the immune system. This is referred to as the *drug adsorption mechanism* (Petz & Garratty 1980). Other drugs, *e.g. quinidine, para-aminosalicylic acid* and *rifampicin,* do not bind firmly to the red cell membrane. Antibodies are formed directly against the drug (probably bound to a serum protein), and adsorption of the immune complex to the red cell surface activates complement, with ensuing cell lysis. This is called the *immune complex mechanism.*

The two types of drug-induced haemolytic anaemia are described in detail and a list of causative drugs provided by Petz & Garratty (1980) who also discuss laboratory diagnosis. Clinical and serological features are summarized in Table 8.9.

Table 8.9. *Immunological drug-induced haemolytic anaemias*

Clinical and haematological features	Immune (drug adsorption)	Immune (immune complex)	Auto-immune
Drug dose	Massive	Small	Prolonged administration
Onset	Rapid but not acute	Acute	Slow
Offset	Weeks	Days	Weeks
Site of haemolysis	Extravascular	Intravascular	Extravascular
Spherocytosis	Occasional	Usual	Usual
Renal failure	Rare	Frequent	Rare
Previous administration	Often	Often	Not usual
Direct antiglobulin test	Positive	Positive	Positive
Indirect antiglobulin test			
Without drug	Negative	Negative	Positive
With drug	Positive (cell-bound)	Positive	Positive
Antibody	IgG	IgM, C binding	IgG

The drug adsorption mechanism

Penicillin. More than 90 per cent of sera from adult subjects contains IgM antibodies which agglutinate normal red cells coated with penicillin *in vitro*. These antibodies are believed to result from the almost universal exposure of the normal population to penicillin in the environment. Penicillin can be detected on the red cell surface of all patients receiving high doses of penicillin, and three per cent of these patients develop a positive direct antiglobulin test without evidence of haemolysis (p. 193). A high concentration of IgG rather than IgM anti-penicillin antibody seems necessary for the development of haemolytic anaemia, and this occurs in rare patients who receive massive doses of penicillin intravenously over a long period.

The important serological finding in a patient with penicillin-induced haemolytic anaemia is a positive direct antiglobulin test due to red cell coating with IgG, in spite of negative tests for the presence of serum antibody. Serum antibody is, however, easily demonstrable if penicillin-coated red cells are used in the *in vitro* test system.

Cephalothin. Haemolytic anaemia due to cephalothin is rare. The mechanism of haemolysis seems similar to that of penicillin-induced haemolytic anaemia, but smaller drug doses are involved. Cephalothin and other cephalosporins may cause a positive direct antiglobulin test without haemolysis (p. 193).

The immune complex mechanism

This type of drug-induced haemolytic anaemia is rare. The serum anti-drug antibody is usually IgM in type, and the immune complex binds complement when adsorbed on the red cell surface. The positive direct antiglobulin test is due to complement, and immunoglobulins are not usually detectable. Serum antibodies are demonstrable only if the offending drug is included in the *in vitro* test system. In some patients, the antibody is directed against a drug metabolite rather than the drug itself, and it is necessary to use the metabolite in the test system to obtain a positive result. Salama and Mueller-Eckhardt (1985) have recently shown in studies on *nomifensine*-induced haemolytic anaemia that the serum or urine of a volunteer who has recently ingested a therapeutic dose of the drug is a convenient source of metabolite for serological testing.

DRUG-INDUCED AUTO-IMMUNE HAEMOLYTIC ANAEMIA

AIHA is a well-recognized complication of treatment with the anti-hypertensive agent *methyldopa*. About 15 per cent of patients on methyldopa develop a positive direct antiglobulin test without evidence of haemolysis when given the drug for a sufficient time (commonly from three months to one year) at sufficient dosage. The test gradually becomes negative once the drug is stopped; the time this takes depends on the initial strength of the antiglobulin test, and varies from one month to two years. The finding of a positive direct antiglobulin test in a patient receiving methyldopa is not an indication for cessation of the drug if valid clinical indications for its use are present. Regular clinical and haematological surveillance is desirable in such cases, however (Petz & Garratty 1980).

Between 0.01 and 0.1 per cent of patients treated with methyldopa develop overt haemolytic anaemia. The absence of haemolysis in the majority of patients taking the drug who have a positive direct antiglobulin test may be due to a methyldopa-induced defect in reticulo-endothelial function (Kelton 1985). The anaemia generally occurs within 18 months of commencing treatment, but has been diagnosed as early as 4 months and as late as 4 years. Onset of the anaemia is usually insidious, and the clinical, haematological, and serological features are similar to those of idiopathic warm antibody AIHA. The direct antiglobulin test is strongly positive due to IgG on the red cell surface, and serum antibodies can be demonstrated by the indirect antiglobulin test or by the use of enzyme-treated red cells. Addition of the drug to the test system is not necessary to obtain positive results. Antibody specificity within the Rh system is found in some cases. Following cessation of the drug, the clinical picture improves and the haemoglobin level rises; the haematological picture usually becomes normal fairly rapidly, but the antiglobulin test may take months to become negative.

Corticosteroids are effective and are used if symptoms are troublesome or if a rapid response is required.

About nine per cent of patients receiving *L-dopa* develop a positive antiglobulin test without evidence of haemolysis, and cases of haemolytic anaemia, similar to those occurring with methyldopa, have been described. *Procainamide* and the analgesic agent *mefenamic* acid have been cited as causes of auto-immune haemolytic anaemia in a small number of cases, and the drugs rarely give rise to a positive direct antiglobulin test without haemolysis. It should be stressed that the evidence for attributing a drug aetiology to a case of warm antibody AIHA is of necessity circumstantial as the auto-antibodies involved are identical to those found in idiopathic AIHA.

The mechanical haemolytic anaemias

Red cells may be injured by excess physical trauma as they circulate through the vascular system. Such direct injury takes the form of loss of areas of cell membrane, and may be followed by immediate cell lysis. Frequently, however, the injured membrane is resealed with the formation of grossly distorted, though still viable, red cells. The cells are recognized on the blood film as fragmented, contracted, triangular, and helmet-shaped forms, or microspherocytes. The abnormal cells circulate for a short period, but are destroyed prematurely in the circulation or by the reticulo-endothelial cells, and a frank haemolytic anaemia ensues. Evidence of both intravascular and extravascular haemolysis is usually present with variable degrees of haemoglobinaemia, haemoglobinuria, methaemalbuminaemia, haemosiderinuria, and hyperbilirubinaemia, depending on the severity of the process. Plasma haptoglobin is reduced or totally depleted, and lactate dehydrogenase is elevated. The main causes of the mechanical haemolytic anaemias are detailed in Table 8.10.

It should be remembered that distorted red cells may be caused by other mechanisms, such as chemical agents and physical agents, e.g. burns.

Table 8.10. *The mechanical haemolytic anaemias*

Cardiac haemolytic anaemia
Micro-angiopathic haemolytic anaemia
Haemolytic uraemic syndrome
Thrombotic thrombocytopenic purpura
Disseminated intravascular coagulation
Disseminated carcinoma
Malignant hypertension
Eclampsia
Immune disorders—SLE, scleroderma, polyarteritis nodosa, Wegener's granulomatosis, acute glomerulonephritis, renal transplant rejection
Haemangiomas (p. 442)
March haemoglobinuria

Cardiac haemolytic anaemia

Haemolytic anaemia is an occasional complication of open-heart surgical procedures, particularly those involving the use of valve prostheses (mainly aortic but also mitral) and the use of Teflon grafts for the repair of ostium primum and other defects. In cases associated with valve prostheses, malfunction of the prosthesis is almost always present. The haemolysis is considered to be due to direct mechanical trauma to the red cells, consequent on the development of turbulent blood flow in the vicinity of the prosthesis or Teflon graft. In mild cases, haemolysis is compensated and the haemoglobin level is normal. The reticulocyte count and serum bilirubin are slightly elevated; reduction of plasma haptoglobin and an elevated lactate dehydrogenase provide further evidence of subclinical haemolysis, and are useful screening tests.

In severe cases, there is marked anaemia with evidence of intravascular haemolysis. Haemosiderinuria is often a prominent feature. The blood film shows the presence of varying numbers of fragmented cells, similar to those seen in micro-angiopathic haemolytic anaemia. Occasionally, the iron loss from persistent haemosiderinuria results in red cell hypochromia; in such cases the administration of iron may in part relieve the anaemia. In patients with mild compensated haemolysis; iron and folic acid supplements and some restriction of physical activity may suffice.

If the haemolysis is persistently severe, re-operation to correct the functional defect is necessary. Minor degrees of compensated haemolysis may occur in unoperated patients with severe aortic valve disease.

Micro-angiopathic haemolytic anaemia

The micro-angiopathic haemolytic anaemias are mechanical haemolytic anaemias in which the red cell fragmentation is due to contact between red cells and the abnormal intima of partly thrombosed, narrowed, or necrotic small vessels. *In vitro* studies have established the mechanism by which red cells are traumatized as they are forced through a meshwork of fibrin clot. Although parts of the cell membrane are ruptured as the cells are folded around the fibrin strands, the membrane is resealed when the cells escape, and characteristic fragmented cells are formed. Further experimental evidence has correlated fibrin deposition within arterioles and capillaries (i.e. micro-angiopathy) with the appearance of fragmented red cells.

The main causes of micro-angiopathic haemolytic anaemia are detailed in Table 8.10.

THE HAEMOLYTIC URAEMIC SYNDROME

The triad of acute renal failure, thrombocytopenia, and haemolytic anaemia in infants and young children was first described by Gasser *et al.* (1955). A similar, if not identical, disorder occurs in adults, particularly post-partum females and patients undergoing therapy with cyclosporin and various chemotherapeutic agents. In children, its occurrence is usually sporadic, but some familial cases have been recorded. The pathogenesis is uncertain; the initiating event is thought to be damage to endothelial cells in the glomerular capillaries and renal arterioles, resulting in focal platelet clumping and microvascular coagulation and occlusion. The presence or absence of plasma factors that modify platelet behaviour have been demonstrated in some patients, and recent views on pathogenesis are discussed by Byrnes & Moake (1986).

Clinical features. Previously healthy infants and young children of both sexes are affected, particularly those between 5 and 12 months of age. Diarrhoea, vomiting, and pyrexia are the presenting features in most cases. Within 5–14 days, pallor and slight jaundice develop, and the child becomes oliguric. The urine is dark and contains protein, red cells, casts, and sometimes haemoglobin. Skin and mucous membrane bleeding may occur. The spleen is often palpable. Symptoms and signs of uraemia and cardiac failure develop, and in occasional cases there is evidence of nervous system involvement. Hypertension is present in about half the patients.

Blood picture. The anaemia is often severe and is accompanied by a neutropenia and thrombocytopenia of varying, and sometimes marked, degree. The blood film shows fragmented red cells and some microspherocytes. There is reticulocytosis, haemoglobinaemia, and moderate hyperbilirubinaemia, and the direct antiglobulin test is negative. Laboratory evidence of disseminated intravascular coagulation is present in some patients, but in others coagulation factors are normal or increased. The plasma urea level often reaches 50 mmol/l or more.

Treatment and prognosis. The outlook is serious, and mortality in adults is high. Death usually results from acute renal failure. More recently, results of treatment in children appear to be improving, and mortality rates of less than ten per cent have been reported. Renal failure and hypertension are treated by standard measures, and transfusions are given as symptomatically required. There is no consensus on the value of anticoagulants, fibrinolytic therapy, and antiplatelet agents. Encouraging results have been obtained recently with plasmapheresis and simple infusion of plasma (Misiani *et al.* 1982).

THROMBOTIC THROMBOCYTOPENIC PURPURA AND DISSEMINATED INTRAVASCULAR COAGULATION

Haemolytic anaemia with red cell fragmentation is a frequent feature of thrombotic thrombocytopenic purpura (Fig. 8.7). The anaemia is often severe with reticulocytosis, hyperbilirubinaemia, and normoblastaemia. Red cell fragmentation also occurs in some patients with disseminated intravascular coagulation (DIC). Jacobson & Jackson (1974) found fragmented cells in 43 per cent of patients with well-authenticated DIC, but the changes were severe in only three per cent. Haemolysis is usually mild.

DISSEMINATED CARCINOMA

Micro-angiopathic haemolytic anaemia is an occasional complication of metastatic carcinoma, and may be a presenting symptom. Mucin-secreting carcinomas of breast and stomach are the most common tumours involved, but the condition also occurs with carcinomas of pancreas, lung, and prostate. The anaemia, which is moderate to severe, usually has an abrupt onset, and there is often an associated thrombocytopenia. Fragmented red cells are present, and there is evidence of intravascular haemolysis. Nucleated red cells and immature granulocytes may also be noted. Clinical and laboratory evidence of disseminated intravascular coagulation is often present. The fragmentation is

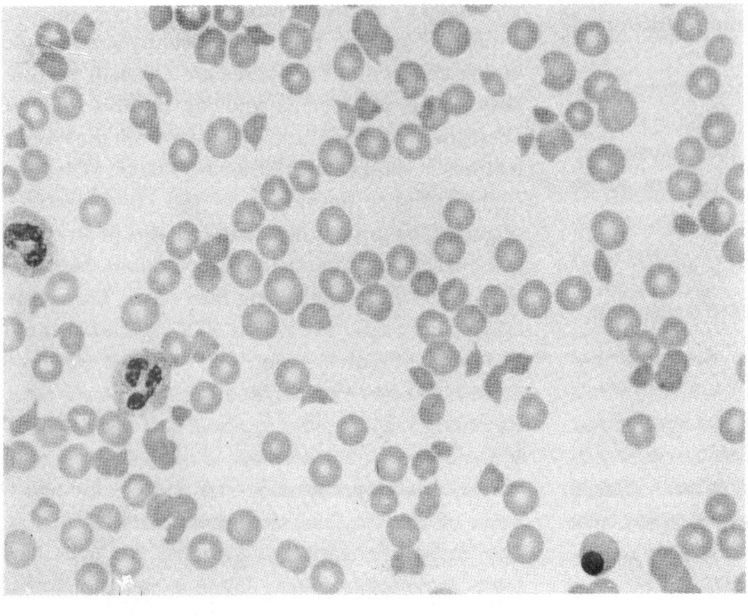

Fig. 8.7. *Micro-angiopathic haemolytic anaemia. Photomicrograph of a blood film from a patient with thrombotic thrombocytopenic purpura. The fragmented and irregularly contracted red cells are well seen (× 385).*

thought to be due to the forcible passage of red cells through small vessels containing embolic tumour cells or fibrin deposits. Treatment of the tumour may result in cessation of the haemolysis, and the use of heparin is justified in some cases to tide the patient over the period of tumour therapy. Details are given by Antman *et al.* (1979).

MALIGNANT HYPERTENSION AND ECLAMPSIA

Red cell fragmentation is a common finding in malignant hypertension, and may be associated with severe intravascular haemolysis and thrombocytopenia. The fragmentation is thought to be due to red cell damage resulting from arteriolar fibrinoid necrosis or intravascular coagulation, evidence of the latter being present in some patients. Severe micro-angiopathic haemolytic anaemia also occasionally occurs in eclampsia.

March (exertional) haemoglobinuria

March haemoglobinuria is a rare disorder in which haemoglobinaemia and haemoglobinuria follow exercise, classically in the upright position, notably on walking, marching, and running. The majority of patients are healthy, young, adult males, often soldiers or athletes who complain of the passing of red urine after marching or running, respectively. It may also occur in squash players. Haemoglobinuria usually lasts for several hours after the exertion, but in rare cases it persists for several days. It is often the only symptom but sometimes is accompanied by mild constitutional symptoms, e.g. nausea, abdominal cramps, aching in the back or legs, especially the thighs, or a burning feeling in the soles of the feet; these symptoms are usually relatively mild. The degree of haemolysis is seldom sufficient to cause anaemia.

The haemoglobinuria is due to traumatic intravascular haemolysis related to a mechanical effect on the blood within the vessels of the soles of the feet. The wearing of resilient insoles may be of value in prevention. A similar syndrome is seen in practitioners of karate who frequently strike hard surfaces with their hands. A recent view of haemolysis in runners is provided by Eichner (1985).

Haemolytic anaemia associated with bacterial infections and parasitic infestations

The anaemia of bacterial infection is predominantly due to bone marrow depression, but red cell survival studies have shown that a haemolytic factor contributes in some cases. However, infection with certain organisms, notably *Clostridium welchii*, results in frank haemolytic anaemia. Malaria is the classical example of haemolytic anaemia due to parasitic infestation.

Clostridium welchii infection

C. welchii infection regularly causes haemolytic anaemia, probably due to the direct action of toxin on the red cells. Most infections are due to post-abortal or puerperal infections. The severity of the haemolysis varies, but in cases of *C. welchii* septicaemia it is usually marked. With severe infections, the clinical picture is of an acutely ill patient with features of toxaemia and intravascular haemolysis. The anaemia is rapidly progressive and severe, with extreme spherocytosis, an increased osmotic fragility, and leucocytosis; the reticulocyte count may not be markedly increased.

Malaria

Anaemia is usual in malaria; it is often only mild or moderate but is occasionally severe, especially with falciparum infections. Its pathogenesis is complex and probably differs at different stages of the illness (Abdalla *et al.* 1980). Although the degree of anaemia often correlates poorly with the extent of red cell parasitization, destruction of parasitized cells in the circulation or spleen is an obvious factor, and a fall in haemoglobin often follows a chill. Depression of marrow erythropoiesis, dyserythropoiesis, hypersplenism, and immunological damage may also be involved in some patients. A mild leucopenia is usual, although leucocytosis may occur in association with fever and chills. The serum bilirubin may be raised. Diagnosis is established by demonstration of the parasites in the peripheral blood; they appear greatest in number at the time of the chill and in the following six hours. Failure to demonstrate the parasite does not exclude the diagnosis, especially in subsiding or chronic cases, and repeated examinations of thick blood films may be necessary. The blood picture returns to normal after cure of the infection. In cases of 'chronic' malaria, persistent anaemia and splenomegaly are usual.

Blackwater fever is a rare but serious complication of severe *Plasmodium falciparum* infection, characterized by an acute haemolytic anaemia with marked haemoglobinuria. Blackwater fever occurs chiefly in tropical and subtropical regions where malaria is endemic. There is no racial immunity, but Europeans, usually persons who have had repeated malaria attacks, are commonly affected. It frequently seems to be precipitated by the taking of antimalarial drugs, usually quinine, especially when the latter is taken irregularly for suppression or treatment.

Haematological aspects of malaria are reviewed by Perrin *et al.* (1982).

Lead poisoning

Changes in the blood, particularly basophil stippling of the red cells, are commonly present in persons exposed to lead. Stippling is now generally considered to be an unreliable criterion of lead intoxication, since the number of stippled cells does not correlate well with the intensity of exposure; occasionally, stippling is absent in patients with lead poisoning. Further, stippled cells can be found in increased numbers in a variety of haematological disorders, e.g. various haemolytic anaemias, leukaemia, and after exposure to other industrial toxins. Most cases of lead poisoning occur in persons working in lead industries. However, a certain number of non-occupational cases occur, most commonly in children, usually from the chewing of lead toys, furniture, or other articles painted with lead paint.

Anaemia is common in lead poisoning. It is usually of mild to moderate severity, haemoglobin values only rarely falling below 9 g/dl. The red cells are characteristically normocytic and normochromic, or microcytic and hypochromic, and may show mild polychromasia. A slight increase in reticulocytes is common.

The bone marrow shows erythroid hyperplasia with 'ring' sideroblasts and thus the anaemia of lead poisoning may be classified as a secondary sideroblastic anaemia (p. 58).

The *pathogenesis* of the anaemia of lead poisoning is not fully understood; it appears that the main factor is an interference with marrow haemopoiesis, but that there is also some haemolytic element, probably due to direct red cell membrane damage. There is evidence of inhibition of enzymes involved in haem synthesis; this is reflected in the increased free erythrocyte protoporphyrin and increased excretion of coproporphyrin and delta-aminolaevulinic acid (ALA) in the urine. Globin synthesis is also impaired.

Burns

Haemoglobinuria frequently occurs in severely burnt patients. It has been shown that heating of red cells to a temperature above 51°C results in spherocytosis with consequent increased osmotic and mechanical fragility, and in red cell fragmentation. The cells passing through the burnt area at the time of the burns are thus irreversibly damaged and are destroyed intravascularly, with resultant haemoglobinaemia and haemoglobinuria.

Clinical investigations

Table 8.11 summarizes the clinical investigations that should be carried out in a patient with suspected haemolytic anaemia.

References and further reading

Monographs

Beutler, E. (1978) *Hemolytic Anemia in Disorders of Red Cell Metabolism*, Plenum Medical Book Company, New York.

Dacie, J.V. (1985) The hereditary haemolytic anaemias. In: *The Haemolytic Anaemias*, Vol. 1, Part I, Churchill Livingstone, Edinburgh.

Grimes, A.J. (1980) *Human Red Cell Metabolism*, Blackwell Scientific Publications, Oxford.

Table 8.11. *Summary of the investigation of a patient with suspected haemolytic anaemia*

History
Age, sex
Age at onset of symptoms
Race
Occupation
Jaundice; colour of urine and faeces
Crises
Cholelithiasis
Family history (anaemia, jaundice, splenomegaly, dark urine, cholelithiasis)
Haemoglobinuria; relation to sleep, cold, exercise, or drugs
Symptoms suggestive of disorders causing secondary AIHA
Raynaud's phenomenon
Drug, chemical or alcohol ingestion
Recent travel to tropics

Physical examination
Pallor, cyanosis
Jaundice, splenomegaly, hepatomegaly
General development, facies, presence of congenital abnormalities, leg ulceration, or pigmentation (hereditary haemolytic anaemia)
Signs of disorders causing secondary AIHA, especially lymph node enlargement and purpura

Special investigations

ESSENTIAL INVESTIGATIONS FOR ALL CASES:
Full blood examination, with special reference to:
Morphology of red cells in a well-made and well-stained blood film (note especially spherocytosis, autoagglutination, fragmentation, inclusion bodies)
Reticulocyte count
Plasma haptoglobin
Serum bilirubin
Osmotic fragility test
Direct antiglobulin test
Examination of urine for urobilinogen, haemoglobin, haemosiderin

FURTHER INVESTIGATIONS IN SOME CASES:
Bone marrow aspiration and trephine biopsy (evidence of lymphoma, folate deficiency in AIHA)
Measurement of red cell lifespan (establish haemolytic nature in doubtful cases)
Examination of plasma for haemoglobin and methaemalbumin (intravascular haemolysis)
X-ray of skull, hands, and long bones (hereditary haemolytic anaemia)
Sickle test (sickle-cell anaemias)
Tests for abnormal haemoglobins:
- haemoglobin electrophoresis
- alkali denaturation
- Hb-H inclusions
- heat instability test

Investigation of relatives (hereditary haemolytic anaemia)
Examination of red cells for methaemoglobin and sulphaemoglobin (chemical haemolytic anaemia)
Heinz-body preparation (chemical haemolytic anaemia, hereditary haemolytic anaemia)
Estimation of red cell G6PD and other enzymes (hereditary haemolytic anaemia, chemical haemolytic anaemia)
Cold agglutinins (AIHA)
Investigations to demonstrate aetiology in secondary AIHA, especially LE cell test and lymph node biopsy
VDRL test (paroxysmal cold haemoglobinuria)
Donath–Landsteiner test (paroxysmal cold haemoglobinuria)
Ham's acid serum test, sucrose haemolysis test (paroxysmal nocturnal haemoglobinuria)

Mollison, P.L., Engelfriet, C.P. & Contrenas, M. (1987) *Blood Transfusion in Clinical Medicine*, 8th Ed., Blackwell Scientific Publications, Oxford.

Petz, L.D. & Garratty, G. (1980) *Acquired Immune Hemolytic Anemias*, Churchill Livingstone, Edinburgh.

Mechanisms and diagnosis of haemolysis

Ahuja, S., Lewis, S.M. & Szur, L. (1972) Value of surface counting in predicting response to splenectomy in haemolytic anaemia. *J. Clin. Path.* **25**, 467.

Bentley, S.A. (1977) Red cell survival studies reinterpreted. *Clin. Haemat.* **6**, 601.

Berlin, N.I. & Berk, P.D. (1981) Quantitative aspects of bilirubin metabolism for hematologists. *Blood*, **57**, 983.

Bissell, D.M. (1975) Formation and elimination of bilirubin. *Gastroenterology*, **69**, 519.

Clark, M.R. & Shohet, S.B. (1985) Red cell senescence. *Clin. Haemat.* **14**, 223.

Crosby, W.H. (1981) Reticulocyte counts. *Arch. Int. Med.* **141**, 1747.

Dacie, J.V. & Lewis, S.M. (1984) *Practical Haematology*, 6th Ed., Churchill Livingstone, London.

Deiss, A. & Kurth, D. (1970) Circulating reticulocytes in normal adults as determined by the new methylene blue method. *Am. J. Clin. Path.* **53**, 481.

Ferrant, A. (1983) The role of the spleen in haemolysis. *Clin. Haemat.* **12**, 489.

Godal, H.C., Nyvold, N. & Rustad, A. (1979) The osmotic fragility of red blood cells: a re-evaluation of technical conditions. *Scand. J. Haemat.* **23**, 55.

Hershko, C. (1975) The fate of circulating haemoglobin. *Brit. J. Haemat.* **29**, 199.

Hillman, R.S. & Finch, C.A. (1985) *Red Cell Manual*, 5th Ed., F.A. Davis, Philadelphia.

International Committee for Standardization in Haematology (1980) Recommended method for radioisotope red-cell survival studies. *Brit. J. Haemat.* **45**, 659.

International Committee for Standardization in Haematology (1975) Recommended methods for surface counting to determine sites of red cell destruction. *Brit. J. Haemat.* **30**, 249.

Najean, Y., Cacchione, R., Dresch, C. *et al.* (1975) Methods of evaluating the sequestration site of red cells labelled with ^{51}Cr: a review of 96 cases. *Brit. J. Haemat.* **29**, 495.

Red cell membrane defects

Agre, P., Asimos, A., Casella, J.F. *et al.* (1986) Inheritance pattern and clinical response to splenectomy as a reflection of erythrocyte spectrin deficiency in hereditary spherocytosis. *New Engl. J. Med.* **315**, 1579.

Becker, P.S. & Lux, S.E. (1985) Hereditary spherocytosis and related disorders. *Clin. Haemat.* **14**, 15.

Davidson, R.J., How, J. & Lessels, S. (1977) Acquired stomatocytosis: its prevalence and significance in routine haematology. *Scand. J. Haemat.* **19**, 47.

Glader, B.E., Fortier, N., Albala, M.M. *et al.* (1974) Congenital hemolytic anemia associated with dehydrated erythrocytes and increased potassium loss. *New Engl. J. Med.* **291**, 491.

Kelleher, J.F., Luban, N.L.C., Mortimer, P.P. *et al.* (1983) Human serum 'parvovirus': a specific cause of aplastic crisis in children with hereditary spherocytosis. *J. Pediatr.* **102**, 720.

Lande, W.M. & Mentzer, W.C. (1985) Haemolytic anaemia associated with increased cation permeability. *Clin. Haemat.* **14**, 89.

Palek, J. (1985) Hereditary elliptocytosis and related disorders. *Clin. Haemat.* **14**, 45.

Palek, J. & Lux, S.E. (1983) Red cell membrane skeletal defects in hereditary and acquired hemolytic anemias. *Semin. Hematol.* **20**, 189.

Schrier, S.L. (1985) Red cell membrane biology – introduction. *Clin. Haemat.* **14**, 1.

Wiley, J.S. (1984) Inherited red cell dehydration: a hemolytic syndrome in search of a name. *Pathology*, **16**, 115.

Wolfe, L.C., John, K.M., Falcone, J.C. *et al.* (1982) A genetic defect in the binding of protein 4.1 to spectrin in a kindred with hereditary spherocytosis. *New Engl. J. Med.* **307**, 1367.

Zanella, A., Izzo, C., Rebulla, P. *et al.* (1980) Acidified glycerol lysis test: a screening test for spherocytosis. *Brit. J. Haemat.* **45**, 481.

Zarkowsky, H.S., Mohandas, N., Speaker, C.B. *et al.* (1975) A congenital haemolytic anaemia with thermal sensitivity of the erythrocyte membrane. *Brit. J. Haemat.* **29**, 537.

Glucose-6-phosphate dehydrogenase deficiency and related disorders

Belsey, M.A. (1973) The epidemiology of favism. *Bull. Wld. Hlth. Org.* **48**, 1.

Beutler, E., Blume, K.G., Kaplan, J.C. *et al.* (1979) International Committee for Standardization in Haematology: Recommended screening test for glucose-6-phosphate dehydrogenase (G-6-PD) deficiency. *Brit. J. Haemat.* **43**, 469.

Beutler, E. & Yoshida, A. (1988) Genetic variation of glucose-6-phosphate dehydrogenase: a catalog and future prospects. *Medicine*, **67**, 311.

Blenzle, U. (1981) Glucose-6-phosphate dehydrogenase deficiency. Part I: Tropical Africa. *Clin. Haemat.* **10**, 785.

Dacie, J.V. & Lewis, S.M. (1984) *Practical Haematology*, 6th Ed., Churchill Livingstone, London.

Herz, F., Kaplan, E. & Scheye, E.S. (1970) Diagnosis of erythrocyte glucose-6-phosphate dehydrogenase deficiency in the Negro male despite hemolytic crisis. *Blood*, **35**, 90.

International Committee for Standardization in Haematology (1977) Recommended methods for red-cell enzyme analysis. *Brit. J. Haemat.* **35**, 331.

Keitt, A.S. (1981) Diagnostic strategy in a suspected red cell enzymopathy. *Clin. Haemat.* **10**, 3.

Miwa, S. & Fujii, H. (1985) Molecular aspects of erythroenzymopathies associated with hereditary hemolytic anemia. *Am. J. Hemat.* **19**, 293.

Paglia, D.E. & Valentine, W.M. (1981) Haemolytic anaemia associated with disorders of the purine and pyrimidine salvage pathways. *Clin. Haemat.* **10**, 81.

Panich, V. (1981) Glucose-6-phosphate dehydrogenase deficiency. Part 2: Tropical Asia. *Clin. Haemat.* **10**, 800.

Sansone, G., Perroni, L. & Yoshida, A. (1975) Glucose-6-phosphate dehydrogenase variants from Italian subjects associated with severe neonatal jaundice. *Brit. J. Haemat.* **31**, 159.

Van Noorden, C.J.F. & Vogels, I.M.L. (1985) A sensitive cytochemical staining method for glucose-6-phosphate dehydrogenase activity in individual erythrocytes. II. Further improvements of the staining procedure and some observations with glucose-6-phosphate dehydrogenase deficiency. *Brit. J. Haemat.* **60**, 57.

Pyruvate kinase deficiency and related disorders

Miwa, S. (1981) Pyruvate kinase deficiency and other enzymopathies of the Embden–Meyerhof pathway. *Clin. Haemat.* **10**, 57.

Paglia, D.E. & Valentine, W.N. (1974) Hereditary glucose-phosphate isomerase deficiency: a review. *Am. J. Clin. Path.* **62**, 740.

Valentine, W.N. (1985) Hemolytic anemias and erythrocyte enzymopathies. *Ann. Int. Med.* **103**, 245.

Auto-immune acquired haemolytic anaemia

Atkinson, J.P. & Frank, M.M. (1977) Role of complement in the pathophysiology of hematologic diseases. *Prog. Hematol.* **10**, 211.

Brown, D.L. (1973) The immune interaction between red cells and leucocytes and the pathogenesis of spherocytosis. *Brit. J. Haemat.* **25**, 691.

Chaplin, H. (1982) Lymphoma in primary cold hemagglutinin disease treated with chlorambucil. *Arch. Int. Med.* **142**, 2119.

Crisp, D. & Pruzanski, W. (1982) B-cell neoplasms with homogeneous cold reacting antibodies (cold agglutinins). *Am. J. Med.* **72**, 915.

Dacie, J.V. (1975) Autoimmune hemolytic anemia. *Arch. Int. Med.* **135**, 1293.

Dacie, J.V. & Lewis, S.M. (1984) *Practical Haematology*, 6th Ed., Churchill Livingstone, London.

Engelfriet, C.P., Borne, A.E.G., Beckers, D. *et al.* (1974) Autoimmune haemolytic anaemia: serological and immunochemical characteristics of the autoantibodies; mechanisms of cell destruction. *Ser. Haemat.* **7**, 328.

Frank, M.M. (1985) Assessment of shortened in vivo RBC survival and sites of RBC destruction. In: Chaplin, H. (Ed.) *Immune Hemolytic Anemias. Methods in Hematology*, Vol. 12, Churchill Livingstone, New York.

Freedman, J. (1979) False-positive antiglobulin tests in healthy subjects and in hospital patients. *J. Clin. Path.* **32**, 1014.

Grunwald, H.W. & Rosner, F. (1979) Acute leukemia and immunosuppressive drug use. *Arch. Int. Med.* **139**, 461.

Issitt, P.D. (1985) Serological diagnosis and characterization of the causative autoantibodies. In: Chaplin, H. (Ed.) *Immune Hemolytic Anemias. Methods in Hematology*, Vol. 12 Churchill Livingstone, New York.

Jacobson, L.B., Longstreth, C.F. & Edgington, T.S. (1973) Clinical and immunologic features of transient cold agglutinin hemolytic anemia. *Am. J. Med.* **54**, 514.

Issitt, P.D. (1985) Serological diagnosis and characterization of the causative autoantibodies. In: Chaplin, H. (Ed.) *Immune Hemolytic Anemias. Methods in Hematology*, Vol. 12, Churchill Livingstone, New York.

Jacobson, L.B., Longstreth, C.F. & Edgington, T.S. (1973) Clinical and immunologic features of transient cold agglutinin hemolytic anemia. *Am. J. Med.* **54**, 514.

Liesveld, J.L., Rowe, J.M. & Lichtman, M.A. (1987) Variability of the erythropoietic response in autoimmune hemolytic anemia: analysis of 109 cases. *Blood*, **69**, 820.

Masouredis, S.P. & Chaplin, H., Jr. (1985) Transfusion management of autoimmune hemolytic anemia. In: Chaplin, H. (Ed.) *Immune Hemolytic Anemias. Methods in Hematology*, Vol. 12, Churchill Livingstone, New York.

Parker, A.C., MacPherson, A.I.S. & Richmond, J. (1977) Value of radiochromium investigation in autoimmune haemolytic anaemia. *Brit. Med. J.* **1**, 208.

Petz, L.D. (1982) Red cell transfusion problems in immunohematologic disease. *Ann. Rev. Med.* **33**, 355.

Petz, L.D. & Branch, D.R. (1983) Serological tests for the diagnosis of immune hemolytic anemias. In: McMillan, R. (Ed.) *Immune Cytopenias. Methods in Hematology*, Vol. 8, Churchill Livingstone, Edinburgh.

Petz, L.D. & Branch, D.R. (1985) Drug-induced immune hemolytic anemia. In: Chaplin, H. (Ed.) *Immune Hemolytic Anemias. Methods in Hematology*, Vol. 12, Churchill Livingstone, New York.

Rosse, W.F. (1979) Interactions of complement with the red-cell membrane. *Semin. Hematol.* **16**, 128.

Rosse, W.F. & Adams, J.P. (1980) The variability of hemolysis in the cold agglutinin syndrome. *Blood*, **56**, 409.

Schreiber, A.D., Herskovitz, B.S. & Goldwein, M. (1977) Low-titer cold-hemagglutinin disease. Mechanism of hemolysis and response to corticosteroids. *New Engl. J. Med.* **296**, 1490.

Silverstein, M.N., Gomes, M.R., Elveback, L.R. *et al.* (1972) Idiopathic acquired hemolytic anemia, survival in 117 cases. *Arch. Int. Med.* **129**, 85.

Wolach, B., Heddle, N., Barr, R.D. *et al.* (1981) Transient Donath–Landsteiner haemolytic anaemia. *Brit. J. Haemat.* **48**, 425.

Wortman, J., Rosse, W. & Logue, G. (1979) Cold agglutinin auto-immune hemolytic anemia in nonhematologic malignancies. *Am. J. Hemat.* **6**, 275.

Paroxysmal nocturnal haemoglobinuria

Clark, D.A., Butler, S.A., Braren, V. *et al.* (1981) The kidneys in paroxysmal nocturnal hemoglobinuria. *Blood*, **57**, 83.

Dacie, J.V. & Lewis, S.M. (1972) Paroxysmal nocturnal haemoglobinuria: clinical manifestations, haematology and nature of the disease. *Ser. Haemat.* **5**, 3.

Harruff, R.C. & Rohn, R.J. (1983) Potential errors in the laboratory diagnosis of paroxysmal nocturnal hemoglobinuria. *Am. J. Clin. Path.* **80**, 152.

Hartmann, R.C. & Kolhouse, J.F. (1972) Viewpoints on the management of paroxysmal nocturnal hemoglobinuria. *Ser. Haemat.* **5**, 42.

Hirsch, V.J., Neubach, P.A., Parker, D.M. *et al.* (1981) Paroxysmal nocturnal hemoglobinuria. Termination in acute myelomonocytic leukemia and reappearance after leukaemic remission. *Arch. Int. Med.* **141**, 525.

Jenkins, D.E., Jr. (1972) Diagnostic tests for paroxysmal nocturnal hemoglobinuria. *Ser. Haemat.* **5**, 24.

Leibowitz, A.I. & Hartmann, R.L. (1981) The Budd–Chiari syndrome and paroxysmal nocturnal haemoglobinuria. *Brit. J. Haemat.* **48**, 1.

Nicholson-Weller, A., March, J.P., Rosenfeld, S.I. *et al.* (1983) Affected erythrocytes of patients with paroxysmal nocturnal hemoglobinuria are deficient in the complement regulatory protein, decay accelerating factor. *Proc. Natl. Acad. Sci. U.S.A.* **80**, 5066.

Rosse, W.F., Adams, J.P. & Thorpe, A.M. (1974) The population of cells in paroxysmal nocturnal haemoglobinuria of intermediate sensitivity to complement lysis: significance and mechanisms of increased immune lysis. *Brit. J. Haemat.* **28**, 181.

Rosse, W.F. (1982) Treatment of paroxysmal nocturnal haemoglobinuria. *Blood*, **60**, 20.

Rosse, W.F. & Parker, C.J. (1985) Paroxysmal nocturnal hemoglobinuria. *Clin. Haemat.* **14**, 105.

Sirchia, G. & Lewis S.M. (1975) Paroxysmal nocturnal haemoglobinuria. *Clin. Haemat.* **4**, 199.

Haemolytic anaemia due to drugs, chemicals, and infections

Abdalla, S., Weatherall, D.J., Wickramasinghe, S.N. *et al.* (1980) The anaemia of P. falciparum malaria. *Brit. J. Haemat.* **46**, 171.

Abdalla, S. & Weatherall, D.J. (1982) The direct antiglobulin test in P. falciparum malaria. *Brit. J. Haemat.* **51**, 415.

Caterson, R.J., Savdie, E., Raik, E. *et al.* (1982) Heinz-body haemolysis in haemodialysed patients caused by chloramines in Sydney tap water. *Med. J. Austr.* **2**, 367.

Chan, T.K., Chan, W.C. & Weed, R.I. (1982) Erythrocyte hemighosts: a hallmark of severe oxidative injury in vivo. *Brit. J. Haemat.* **50**, 575.

Davison, R.J.L. (1971) Phenacetin-induced haemolytic anemia. *J. Clin. Path.* **24**, 537.

Fleming, A.F. (1981) Haematological manifestations of malaria and other parasitic diseases. *Clin. Haemat.* **10**, 983.

Goodacre, R.L., Ali, M.A.M., Vanderlinden, B. *et al.* (1978) Hemolytic anemia in patients receiving sulfasalazine. *Digestion*, **17**, 503.

Gordon-Smith, E.C. (1980) Drug-induced oxidative haemolysis. *Clin. Haemat.* **9**, 557.

Kelton, J.G. (1985) Impaired reticuloendothelial function in patients treated with methyldopa. *New Engl. J. Med.* **313**, 596.

Kirtland, H.H., Mohler, D.N. & Horwitz, D.A. (1980) Methyldopa inhibition of suppressor-lymphocyte function. A proposed cause of autoimmune hemolytic anemia. *New Engl. J. Med.* **302**, 825.

Merry, A.H., Looareesuwan, S., Philips, R.H. *et al.* (1986) Evidence against immune haemolysis in falciparum malaria in Thailand. *Brit. J. Haemat.* **64**, 187.

Perrin, L.H., Mackey, L.J. & Miescher, P.A. (1982) The hematology of malaria in man. *Semin. Haemat.* **19**, 70.

Petz, L.D. (1980) Drug-induced haemolytic anaemia. *Clin. Haemat.* **9**, 455.

Salama, A. & Mueller-Eckhardt, C. (1985) The role of metabolite-specific antibodies in nomifensine-dependent immune hemolytic anemia. *New Engl. J. Med.* **313**, 469.

Snyder, E.L. & Spivack, M. (1979) Clinical and serologic management of patients with methyldopa-induced positive antiglobulin tests. *Transfusion*, **19**, 313.

Swanson, M. & Cook, R. (1977) *Drugs, Chemicals and Blood Dyscrasias*, Drug Intelligence Publications, Inc., Hamilton, Illinois.

Ward, P.C.J., Schwartz, B.S. & White, J.G. (1983) Heinz-body anemia: 'Bite-cell' variant—a light and electron microscopic study. *Am. J. Hemat.* **15**, 135.

White, J.M. & Selhi, H.S. (1975) Lead and the red cell. *Brit. J. Haemat.* **30**, 133.

Worlledge, S.M. (1973) Immune drug-induced hemolytic anaemias. *Semi. Hematol.* **10**, 327.

Cardiac haemolytic anaemia

Ducrou, W., Harding, P.E., Kimber, R.J. *et al.* (1972) Traumatic haemolysis after heart valve replacement: a comparison of haematological investigations. *Austr. N.Z. J. Med.* **2**, 118.

Marsh, G.W. & Lewis, S.M. (1969) Cardiac haemolytic anaemia. *Semin. Hematol.* **6**, 133.

Weiss, G.B., Nienhuis, A.W., McIntosh, C.L. *et al.* (1979) Traumatic cardiac hemolytic anemia: a late complication of a Starr-Edwards mitral valve prosthesis. *Arch. Int. Med.* **139**, 374.

Micro-angiopathic haemolytic anaemia

Antman, K.H., Skarin, A.T., Mayer, R.J. et al. (1979) Microangiopathic hemolytic anemia and cancer: a review. *Medicine*, **58**, 377.

Brain, M.C. (1970) Microangiopathic hemolytic anemia. *Ann. Rev. Med.* **21**, 133.

Byrnes, J.J. & Moake, J.L. (1986) Thrombotic thrombocytopenic purpura and the haemolytic-uraemic syndrome: Evolving concepts of pathogenesis and therapy. *Clin. Haemat.* **15**, 413.

Drummond, K.N. (1985) Editorial retrospective. Hemolytic–uremic syndrome—then and now. *New Engl. J. Med.* **312**, 116.

Gasser, C., Gautier, E., Steck, A. *et al.* (1955) Hamolytisch uramische Syndrome: bilaterale Nierenrindennekrosen bei akuten erworbenen hamolytischen Anamien. *Schwiez. Med. Wschr.* **85**, 905.

Goldstein, M.H. Churg, J., Strauss, L. *et al.* (1979) Hemolytic–uremic syndrome. *Nephron*, **23**, 263.

Hayslett, J.P. (1985) Postpartum renal failure. *New Engl. J. Med.* **312**, 1556.

Jacobson, R.J. & Jackson, D.P. (1974) Erythrocyte fragmentation in defibrination syndromes. *Ann. Int. Med.* **81**, 207.

Jaffe, E.A., Nachman, R.L. & Merskey, C. (1973) Thrombotic thrombocytopenic purpura-coagulation parameters in twelve patients. *Blood*, **42**, 499.

Kennedy, S.S., Zacharski, L.R. & Beck, J.R. (1980) Thrombotic thrombocytopenic purpura: analysis of 48 unselected cases. *Semin. Thromb. Hemost.* **6**, 341.

Misiani, R., Apiani, A.C., Edefonti, A. *et al.* (1982) Haemolytic uraemic syndrome: therapeutic effect of plasma infusion. *Brit. Med. J.* **285**, 1304.

Ponticelli, C., Rivolta, E., Imbasciati E. *et al.* (1980) Hemolytic uremic syndrome in adults. *Arch. Int. Med.* **140**, 353.

March haemoglobinuria

Davidson, R.J.L. (1969) March or exertional hemoglobinuria. *Semin. Hematol.* **6**, 150.

Eichner, E.R. (1985) Runner's macrocytosis: a clue to footstrike hemolysis. Runner's anemia as a benefit versus runner's hemolysis as a detriment. *Am. J. Med.* **78**, 321.

Chapter 9
White Cells:
Neutrophilia and Eosinophilia;
Neutropenia and Agranulocytosis;
Infectious Mononucleosis

Physiology of white cells

Sites of production

Granulocyte formation is normally restricted to the bone marrow after birth. The other important components of the myeloid series are the monocytes, which are also produced predominantly in the bone marrow. Monocytes are related to tissue histiocytes, or macrophages, which are present in particular in the spleen, bone marrow, lungs and liver. The process of development of tissue histiocytes is less clearly defined than that of granulocytes and monocytes. Lymphocytes are also produced in bone marrow, and some undergo subsequent modification in other organs, such as the thymus. The majority of lymphocytes are formed outside the bone marrow in lymph nodes, lymphoid collections lining the gastrointestinal tract, and the spleen.

Production and lifespan

Normally, mature forms of the white cell series overwhelmingly predominate in the blood, while precursors are located at extravascular sites. The period spent by the polymorphonuclear neutrophil in the bloodstream averages less than one day, and these cells do not re-enter the blood after they have passed out into the tissues. Lymphocytes and monocytes, on the other hand, do re-enter the bloodstream, and consequently their traffic through the body is more complex than that of the neutrophil.

The pathway by which the segmented neutrophil develops from immature precursors in the bone marrow is described in detail in Chapter 1 (p. 5). Precursors such as myeloblasts and their progeny, the promyelocytes and myelocytes, undergo cell division, and are accordingly classified as the *proliferative compartment* of the neutrophil series. Such cell replication increases the number of neutrophil precursors which, after reaching the stage of the metamyelocyte, cease proliferation and undergo a sequential series of changes leading to the formation of the mature segmented neutrophil. The latter events are said to take place in the *maturation compartment* of the neutrophil series.

Segmented and band neutrophils are the only forms which pass in significant numbers into the circulation under normal circumstances. Approximately one-half of these cells are associated sufficiently closely with vessel walls that they are not present in venous blood obtained by venepuncture. The blood neutrophil count therefore represents only about one-half of the total number of neutrophils in the vascular compartment. Intravenous administration of adrenaline causes many of the neutrophils attached to the endothelium to detach and re-enter the circulating blood. The increase in neutrophil count under these circumstances is rapid, and provides an index of the extent to which neutrophils are present in the attached or 'marginated' state. Corticosteriod administration in amounts equivalent to about 50 mg prednisolone results in a more delayed, but more sustained, rise in the blood neutrophil count. This is due to promotion of the exit of neutrophils from the bone marrow, and accounts for the neutrophil leucocytosis, associated with some immature forms in the blood of patients receiving relatively high doses of corticosteriods.

It is difficult to be certain of the period encompassed by the process of development of the neutrophil from the myeloblast to the time of its entry into the blood, but a currently accepted approximation is about 12 days. The exit of neutrophils from the circulation occurs randomly, and their half-life in the circulation is only of the order of seven hours (Athens *et al.* 1965). The subsequent period spent in the tissues is also considered to be relatively brief. Neutrophils may degenerate following the interaction with microbes which have invaded tissue, and can also be lost from the body by migration into the respiratory or gastrointestinal tracts. Migration of eosinophils into the respiratory tract may assume significant proportions in allergic states affecting the bronchial mucosa.

The lifespan of lymphocytes is extremely variable, as it is very brief in some lymphocyte subsets, while in other subjects the same cell may recirculate for many years.

Metabolic and enzymatic characteristics of white cells

Specific biochemical features account for the specialized functions of the various types of leucocyte.

The granules in the neutrophil represent packages of enzymes which are involved in the killing of ingested microbes and the digestion of phagocytosed material. There are at least two separate types of granule on the basis of differences in enzyme content. The so-called *primary* lightly basophilic staining granules contain, for example, peroxidase plus acid hydrolytic enzymes, while *secondary* granules contain alkaline phosphatase and certain other enzymes. Peroxidase is a major neutrophil protein which catalyses the reaction between the hydrogen peroxide generated in the phagocytosing neutrophil and chloride or iodide ions to chlorinate or iodinate ingested microbes. This process is believed to contribute to the microbicidal function of neutrophils, and deficiency of neutrophil peroxidase has been shown to lessen resistance to mycotic and bacterial infection (Lehrer *et al.* 1969).

A burst of oxygen uptake occurs when neutrophils ingest microbes. The oxygen is reduced by

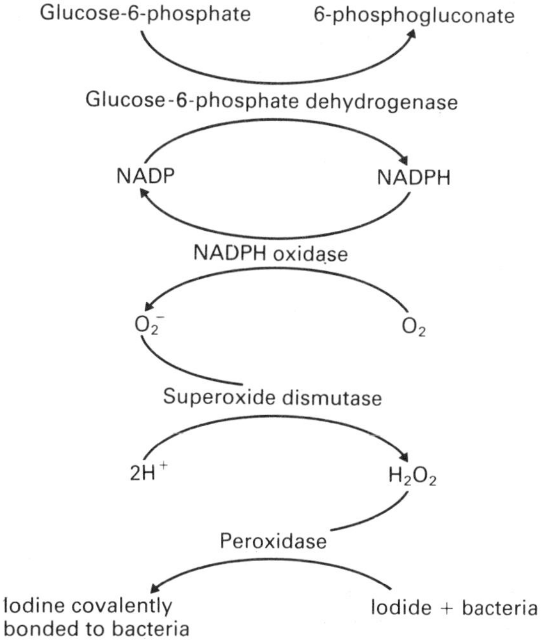

Fig. 9.1. *Outline of the biochemical steps linking the hexose monophosphate shunt and molecular oxygen to oxygen-dependent microbicidal activity in the neutrophil.*

NADPH to generate superoxide radicles (O_2^-), which are weakly microbicidal in their own right. Superoxide undergoes enzymatic 'dismutation' to hydrogen peroxide, which alone, or in the presence of peroxidase as described above, exerts powerful microbicidal activity (Babior 1978a). The sequence of metabolic steps in this process is outlined in Fig. 9.1. The ingested microbes are enveloped in vacuoles into which microbicidal agents are discharged, as illustrated in Fig. 9.2.

Alkaline phosphatase can be demonstrated by cytochemical staining of neutrophils in blood smears. *Neutrophil alkaline phosphatase* activity is derived from the intensity of the microscopically identifiable reaction product of the enzyme within neutrophils, and bears no relation to the activity of alkaline phosphatase in serum. The usual procedure is to examine enzyme activity in 100 consecutive neutrophils, employing a score of 0 for absence of reaction product, 1 for pale diffuse colouration or small areas of granular reaction product, 2 for

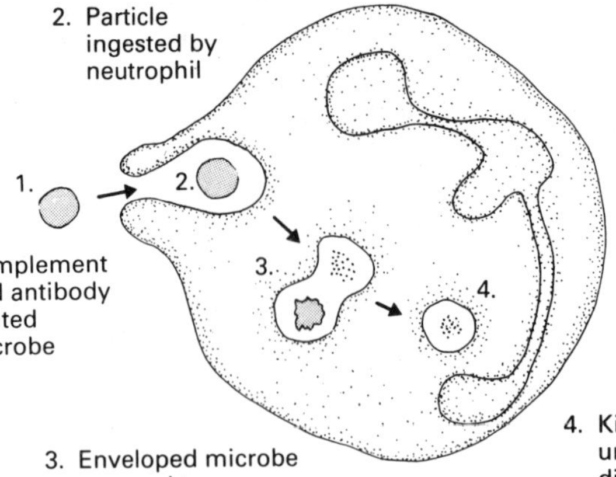

Fig. 9.2. *Sequence of events in microbial killing by the neutrophil.*

unevenly distributed granules, 3 for uniformly distributed granules, and 4 where the cytoplasm is entirely filled with dark reaction product. There is an element of subjectivity in assessment, and some variation with technique, so reference must always be made to the normal range of the laboratory. A typical normal range is 10–100 per 100 neutrophils (Hayhoe & Quaglino 1958).

Elevated values occur as responses to infection, inflammation, and tissue necrosis due to infarction or trauma. Administration of corticosteriods and oral contraceptive preparations can cause elevated values, and the level also rises during pregnancy to reach a maximum at the time of labour. Abnormally high values can also be present in myeloproliferative disorders such as polycythaemia vera and myelofibrosis. High values may also be seen in aplastic anaemia and Down's syndrome.

Subnormal values are so commonly encountered in chronic myeloid leukaemia and paroxysmal nocturnal haemoglobinuria that an abnormally low level is of diagnostic significance. Values are occasionally low in other conditions such as infectious mononucleosis, refractory anaemias, hypophosphataemia, and auto-immune states, including auto-immune thrombocytopenia.

Lysozyme is a hydrolytic enzyme in the granules of neutrophils and monocytes. It splits the muramic acid of bacterial cell walls, and is consequently also referred to as *muramidase*. Lysozyme does lyse certain Gram-positive cocci, but it fails to make a material contribution to bactericidal activity, and evidently is restricted to aiding the digestion of killed organisms, along with other hydrolytic enzymes packaged in cytoplasmic granules. Lysozyme is released into the plasma, where its concentration reflects the mass of lysozyme-containing cells of the body. It is catabolized by the kidney, and is consequently retained in the body in renal failure. In subjects with normal renal function, the serum lysozyme level is of diagnostic value (Wiernick & Serpick 1969, Firkin 1972). Conditions associated with increased turnover of cells of the myeloid series, such as infection, are normally associated with *moderately elevated* levels, although granulomatous states presumably involving large numbers of macrophages, such as sarcoidosis, have been associated in the active phase with *very high* levels. Very high levels, however, most commonly reflect neoplastic involvement of the myeloid series, and are frequently observed in untreated chronic granulocytic leukaemia, and acute or chronic myelomonocytic leukaemia. The level falls when the neoplastic tissue mass decreases in response to therapy. The opposite extreme of a *subnormal* level is seen in states associated with depressed numbers of normal myeloid elements in the body.

Enzymes of particular importance to *lymphocyte* function are also recognized. Proliferating lymphocytes are endowed with relatively high levels of *terminal deoxyribonucleic acid transferase*, and this characteristic can be employed as an aid in the classification of lymphoid neoplastic processes. *Adenosine deaminase* is present in relatively large amounts in T lymphocytes, and is presumably necessary for effective function of a significant subpopulation of cells involved in the immune response, as an inherited deficiency of this enzyme causes as its major clinical consequence a severe combined immunodeficiency state (Polmar 1980).

Function of white cells

Neutrophils are migratory phagocytic cells. They are attracted by *chemotactic factors* to sites of microbial invasion and tissue necrosis, where they congregate by passing out of the bloodstream between the endothelial cells of blood vessels. Neutrophils are the most important cells involved in the body's defences against micro-organisms, and lack of adequate numbers of neutrophils predisposes to infection, particularly by bacteria. Their ability to locate and ingest microbes is enhanced by attachment of antibody and complement to the micro-organism, illustrating the manner in which the various constituents of the body's defences against infection function in a co-operative fashion.

Killing of ingested microbes is mediated by a number of mechanisms, of which the process responsible for the generation of activated oxidative molecules from oxygen is particularly important. Measurement of this mechanism can be performed in the laboratory, using the bonding of radioactive iodide to microbes by neutrophils as an index of their ability to ingest bacteria or yeast, and perform the enzymatic steps culminating in the attachment of iodine to the microbe. Such activity is severely compromised in the potentially fatal disorder of neutrophil microbicidal function, *chronic granulomatous disease*. This is usually an inherited defect in the reaction of molecular oxygen with reduced pyridine nucleotides, and the neutrophils which accumulate at the site of infection ingest but do not readily kill micro-organisms (Babior 1978b).

Microbial killing is also carried out independently by cationic granule proteins, which presumably react with ingested organisms following the secretion of granule contents into the phagocytic vacuole. A more comprehensive measure of microbicidal function is therefore provided by determination of the effectiveness with which neutrophils kill bacteria or yeast.

Eosinophils also possess phagocytic capacity, but do not normally make a significant contribution to the body's defences against invading bacteria. They congregate in tissues affected by allergic reactions, although their role in the allergic process is not fully understood. Production of eosinophils tends to correlate inversely with corticosteroid levels.

Monocytes are also *motile phagocytic cells* endowed with microbicidal mechanisms similar to those of neuthrophils, although monocyte phagocytic and microbicidal activity is considerably less effective than that of the neutrophil. Monocytes and macrophages are predominantly located in the extravascular space, and are particularly involved in the phagocytosis and catabolism of necrotic material.

Lymphocytes are *motile non-phagocytic cells*. There are many subpopulations of lymphocytes which interact with each other and with cells of the monocyte–macrophage series in the maintenance of humoral and cell-mediated immunity (p. 7).

Leucocyte surface antigens

Granulocytes and lymphocytes share surface antigens with many tissues, but they also have their own specific surface antigens.

Neutrophil-specific antigens promote antibody production following transplacental or transfusion-induced immunization of individuals lacking the particular antigen. The major relevance of transplacental immunization is that antibody produced by the mother can cross the placenta and produce neutropenia in the fetus. Surface antigens specific to lymphocytes and to various lymphocyte subsets are discussed in Chapter 1 in relation to the classification of the lymphocytic series (p. 8).

HLA antigens on leucocytes are present on other cell types, and represent the *major* but not sole determinants of *histocompatibility* of tissues. HLA antigens are grouped into four basic systems, HLA-A, HLA-B, HLA-C, and HLA-DR (D related). Each system is represented on the cell surface by an antigen which is the product of an allele of the gene for each system. These genes are located in the major histocompatibility complex on chromosome number 6, and each chromosome therefore directs the formation of one antigen of each system (p. 478). Recognition by the body of cells bearing a foreign HLA pattern underlies the immune-mediated destruction of transplanted or transfused cells that are not histocompatible with those of the recipient. Their relevance to blood transfusion is discussed in Chapter 17 (p. 481).

The HLA genes of each major histocompatibility complex are closely located on the chromosome and are consequently almost always inherited as a single unit. Inheritance follows an autosomal dominant pattern, and this means there is a *one in four chance that any two siblings will share the same maternal and paternal number 6 chromosomes and consequently be HLA identical*, a one in two chance that they will share one parental number 6 chromosome in common, and a one in four chance that they will have no parental number 6 chromosome in common.

The HLA type of an individual is usually determined by studies on peripheral blood lymphocytes. HLA antigens are strongly expressed on these cells, which serve as a conveniently obtainable source of tissue for tissue typing (p. 478). The degree of incompatibility between individuals is also reflected in the degree to which their lymphocytes undergo a proliferative response when exposed to each other in the *mixed lymphocyte reaction*. This reaction is largely dictated by differences at the HLA-DR (D related) gene locus, and serves as a guide to the extent of histocompatibility reactions in transplantation.

Normal white cell values

The values in Table 9.1 illustrate the range in the absolute count of leucocytes encompassed by two standard deviations from the mean, which includes about 95 per cent of normal individuals. White cell counts in infancy and childhood tend to be greater than in adults, with values as high as 25 × 10^9 /l at birth. The count drops over the first seven days of life to about 14 × 10^9 /l. After this time, the absolute neutrophil count falls to approximately the same value as in the adult, although the absolute lymphocyte count remains above adult levels until about 12 years of age.

Table 9.1. *Normal white cell values in peripheral venous blood**

		Absolute count × 10^9 /l
Total leucocyte count		
Adults		4–11
Infants (full-term, at birth)		10–25
Infants (1 year)		6–18
Childhood (4–7 years)		5–15
Childhood (8–12 years)		4.5–13.5
Differential leucocyte count in adults		
Neutrophils	40–75%	2.0–7.5
Lymphocytes	20–50%	1.5–4.0
Monocytes	2–10%	0.2–0.8
Eosinophils	1–6%	0.04–0.4
Basophils	<1%	0.01–0.1

*Dacie & Lewis (1984)

The leucocyte count normally undergoes a minor degree of diurnal variation because of a slight increase in the afternoon. A number of factors, such as the ingestion of food, physical exercise, and emotional stress, can cause an increase in the count.

Values up to 15 × 10^9 /l are common during *pregnancy*, and following parturition the count may rise to 20 × 10^9 /l, although it usually returns to normal within a week.

Pathological variations in white cell values

Neutrophilia

Leucocytosis due to increased numbers of neutrophil series in the blood can occur in a wide variety of conditions. These include physiologically appropriate reactions to extrinsic factors, such as infection or inflammation; responses to pharmacological agents, such as corticosteriods; and excessive production due to neoplastic involvement of the myeloid series. Causes of neutrophilia due to

Table 9.2. *Causes of neutrophilia other than primary disorders of the haemopoietic system*

Infection, particularly acute infection with *cocci*
Tissue injury due to infarction, burns, surgery, and other necrosis-inducing processes
Haemorrhage
Neoplasia
Stress states and hyperactivity such as convulsions, paroxysmal tachycardia, labour, severe colic, delerium tremens
Inflammatory disorders such as certain collagen disorders, gout, rheumatic fever
Metabolic disorders such as diabetic ketoacidosis
Corticosteroid administration
Miscellaneous

extrinsic factors are listed in Table 9.2. It is likely that a relatively limited number of mechanisms is responsible for the increase in production or release of neutrophils from the marginated state or marrow reserve in these conditions.

Infection is the most common cause of neutrophilia, and the degree of neutrophilia is influenced by the type and the severity of the infection. The highest counts are usually associated with infection by Gram-positive cocci (*staphylococci, streptococci, Neisseria*), but high counts can be seen in infections with Gram-negative organisms. More extensive tissue involvement and abscess formation are associated with higher counts. Neutrophilia is not restricted to infections with these organisms, and can occur in some viral infections. Neutrophilia is, however, not a feature of many viral infections, and the development of *neutrophilia late in the course of a viral illness may indicate emergence of secondary bacterial infection.*

In malnourished patients, the neutrophilic response may be blunted, and in chronic infection such as bacterial endocarditis, the increased rate of neutrophil production is not accompanied by significant neutrophilia. *Overwhelming infection can also cause the rate of consumption of neutrophils to outstrip the rate at which they are produced by the bone marrow, and thereby lead to a fall in the neutrophil count to below normal.* This occurs more commonly in neonates and in any age group indicates a serious prognosis.

Increased neutrophil production in infection is usually associated with an increased proportion of less mature neutrophil series in the circulating leucocytes. This usually takes the form of an increase in the percentage of band forms, but metamyelocytes and occasional myelocytes may be present. Such a change is described as a *left shift* in the pattern of neutrophil differentiation. Occasionally the shift to the left may be more pronounced, with the appearance of myeloblasts, to result in a *leukaemoid* blood picture. When this is associated with leucocyte counts as high as 80×10^9 /l, the reaction can resemble certain forms of granulocytic leukaemia. Other changes occur in the neutrophil series in severe infection. The most common is generation of toxic basophilic inclusions in the cytoplasm (*Döhle bodies*). These may be interspersed betwen normal granules, or even replace them. Other cytological features associated with sepsis include pyknotic changes in the nucleus, development of vacuoles in the cytoplasm, and, on rare occasions, the presence of ingested microorganisms.

Non-infectious tissue injury can also cause neutrophilia, and some examples are listed in Table 9.2. Under these circumstances, the presence of neutrophilia is not a reliable index of an infective process. It can, however, be of some value in differentiating, for example, between infarction of the myocardium and other forms of cardiac ischaemia where myocardial necrosis does not occur.

Neutrophilia can develop within hours of *haemorrhage.* The degree of neutrophilia is greater when bleeding occurs into tissues, and may well reflect an aseptic inflammatory response to extravasated blood, comparable to that provoked by tissue necrosis. Major external haemorrhage also results in neutrophilia, the extent of which tends to parallel the degree of blood loss.

Malignant disorders not primarily involving the neutrophil series can cause a reactive neutrophilia, and one condition in which this is relatively common is *Hodgkin's disease.*

Administration of relatively high doses of *corticosterioids* regularly promotes neutrophilia associated with a left shift, and this effect in complex clinical settings can be misinterpreted as an indication of sepsis.

Eosinophilia

The eosinophil count in the peripheral blood of normal subjects ranges from 0.04 to 0.4×10^9 /l, and the percentage of eosinophils among blood leucocytes ranges from 1 to 6 per cent (Dacie & Lewis 1984). Eosinophilia is said to be present when the absolute eosinophil count exceeds 0.4×10^9 /l. Absolute eosinophil counts are more accurately estimated by direct counting in a counting chamber than by extrapolation from the leucocyte differential and the total white cell count. Eosinophil counts are subject to diurnal variation, which has been suggested to be inversely related to the diurnal variation in blood glucocorticoid levels. There is thus a need for standardization, and the value at 8 a.m. is usually taken to represent the basal eosinophil count.

Eosinophilia most commonly occurs as a reaction to extrinsic stimuli, and causes of eosinophilia excluding malignant involvement of the myeloid series are listed in Table 9.3. Increased production of eosinophils in many instances is associated with infiltration by eosinophils of tissues or secretions from tissues affected by allergic reactions. A very rare cause of eosinophila is neoplastic involvement of the myeloid series in which the eosinophil series is the predominant cell line produced. Eosinophilia is a common finding in lympho-proliferative disorders, particularly Hodgkin's disease (p. 283), but also occurs in non-haematological malignancy.

Table 9.3. *Causes of eosinophilia other than primary disorders of the haemopoietic system*

Allergy to extrinsic agents such as vegetable and animal products, parasites, certain other infectious organisms, drugs, and blood products
Neoplasia such as certain lymphoproliferative malignancies and, less commonly, carcinoma
Certain vasculitic and collagen disorders such as polyarteritis nodosa
Dermatological conditions such as pemphigus and dermatitis herpetiformis
Loeffler's syndrome and other forms of pulmonary infiltration
Familial
Post-splenectomy
Miscellaneous

Eosinophilia can range from minor elevation of the eosinophil count to values in excess of 30×10^9/l. It occurs in conditions conventionally regarded as allergic reactions, such as *hay fever, asthma* and *angioneurotic oedema*. Minor elevation of the eosinophil count is far more common in such disorders than marked eosinophilia. Reactions to the presence of *parasites* is a very important cause of eosinophilia, although absence of eosinophilia cannot be assumed to exclude parasitic infestation. Most of the parasites affecting individuals throughout the world, such as *hookworm, ascaris, tapeworm, hydatid, bilharzia, filaria, trichinella, strongyloides, liver fluke,* and visceral larva migrans due to *Toxocara canis,* cause moderate to marked eosinophilia. Eosinophilia can also occur during the less active phase of *malaria,* and in skin infestation with *scabies.* A syndrome initially described as *tropical eosinophilia* evidently represents systemic parasitic infestation, in view of the beneficial response to appropriate drug therapy. The degree of eosinophilia is usually much greater with *tissue invasion* by the parasite, and in many instances migration of parasites through the lungs is accompanied by pulmonary infiltrates on the chest X-ray. It can thus be relatively difficult to distinguish *Loeffler's syndrome* of relatively benign, self-limiting eosinophilia and pulmonary infiltrates from certain forms of parasitic infestation.

Certain microbial infections can also cause eosinophilia, such as those that produce *scarlet fever* and *erythema multiforme. Tuberculosis* is sometimes associated with eosinophilia. The neutrophil leucocytosis that accompanies acute infections is frequently accompanied by a fall in eosinophil count, but in the stage of convalescence when the leucocytosis subsides, the eosinophil count returns to normal, and is sometimes temporarily slightly raised above normal—post-infectious 'rebound' eosinophilia. Eosinophilia may also occur in reactions to *drugs,* which range from subclinical and non-progressive phenomena, to reactions causing serious tissue injury.

Monocytosis

Monocytosis other than in neoplastic involvement of the myeloid series is usually associated with only moderate elevation of the absolute count of monocytes in the blood beyond the upper limit of normal of 0.8×10^9 /l.

Monocytosis can occur as the predominant abnormality in *infections* characteristically associated with a chronic clinical course, such as *tuberculosis, subacute bacterial endocarditis, syphilis, Rickettsia, malaria, etc.* Sometimes *macrophages* are present in the blood in subacute bacterial endocarditis, and are most readily detected in films made from the first drop of blood obtained by puncture of the skin of the ear-lobe. Minor degrees of monocytosis also occur in the recovery phase following acute bacterial infection.

Vasculitis and collagen disorders, non-haematological malignancies, and granulomatous disorders of uncertain but apparently non-infectious aetiology such as *sarcoidosis, ulcerative colitis* and *regional enteritis,* are also associated with monocytosis.

Monocytosis can be a prominent feature in blood dyscrasias involving selective depression of the neutrophil count, and evidently occurs as a response to the infection that occurs under such circumstances. Moderate elevation of the monocyte count in the absence of other disorders can be due to primary disorders of the myeloid series which pursue an indolent neoplastic course and are classified as *chronic myelomonocytic leukaemia,* one of the disorders that is included in the myelodysplastic syndrome (p. 258). The neoplastic nature of such disorders in the early stages of their evolution may be difficult to establish, although detection of a karyotypically abnormal clone of cells in bone marrow serves as an index of a primary haematological neoplasm. Increased monocyte counts are often present in *chronic granulocytic leukaemia* and certain forms of *acute myeloid leukaemia.*

Lymphocytosis

Lymphocytosis is said to ocurr when the absolute count of lymphocytes in the blood exceeds the upper limit of normal of 4×10^9 /l. It is particularly important to recognize that *the upper limit of normal is greater in children, and that it progressively declines towards the adult value with increasing age.* Lymphocytosis refers to elevation of the absolute lymphocyte count in the blood, and the term should not be applied to an increase in the relative proportion of lymphocytes in the absence of an elevated absolute lymphocyte count.

Lymphocytosis is commonly associated with certain infections. A moderate to extreme elevation of the lymphocyte count can occur in children with *pertussis,* and the circulating lymphocytes are essentially normal in appearance. Lymphocytosis with normal morphological features also occurs as an infectious syndrome in which the aetiologic agent or agents are suspected, but not proven, to be viral. This occurs most commonly in children, but can occur in any age group and is called *acute infectious lymphocytosis.* Certain chronic bacterial infections such as *brucellosis, tuberculosis,* and secondary *syphilis* can also be associated with lymphocytosis.

Lymphocytosis associated with *atypical,* enlarged, pleomorphic lymphocytes is encountered in a number of infections which are most frequently due to viruses such as *Epstein–Barr* virus, *cytomegalovirus,* and *infectious hepatitis* viruses. The so-called 'reactive' lymphocyte seen in such conditions may have a sufficiently basophilic cytoplasm to resemble that of the plasma cell, and is referred to as a Turk cell. A persistent absolute lymphocytosis in the absence of an identificable cause can be difficult to differentiate from the early stages of certain neoplastic lymphoproliferative disorders, such as *chronic lymphatic leukaemia* (p. 265) or *well-differentiated non-Hodgkin's lymphoma* (p. 283) with blood spread. A useful approach for distinguishing the latter disorders is evaluation of lymphocyte surface markers (p. 8) which may demonstrate a monotypic population of lymphocytes, suggesting that neoplastic clonal expansion of a specific lymphocytic type has taken place.

Neutropenia and agranulocytosis

Neutropenia is said to be present when the concentration of neutrophils in the blood is below the lower level of normal of 2×10^9/l. The term *agranulocytosis* is not as clearly defined. Literally, it means absence of granulocytes from the peripheral blood. The term was introduced in 1922 by Schultz to describe a clinical syndrome characterized by complete or 'almost complete' absence of neutrophils in the peripheral blood, with severe constitutional symptoms and marked necrotic ulceration, especially of the mouth. The term *agranulocytic angina* is often used to describe the association of ulceration of the throat with severe neutropenia; however, as infection is not necessarily confined to the mouth, the term *agranulocytosis with infection* is to be preferred. Many clinicians use the term agranulocytosis to describe severe neutropenia, irrespective of whether infection is present.

NEUTROPENIA AND THE RISK OF INFECTION

The neutrophil is an essential component of the body's defences against infection, and an inadequate supply of neutrophils profoundly enhances microbial penetration of the tissues. There are factors other than the degree of neutropenia that influence susceptibility to infection, as the neutrophil count does not specifically indicate the number of marginated neutrophils in the vascular compartment, nor the capability of neutrophil precursors in bone marrow to increase production in response to infection. Risk of infection is in fact *not* appreciably increased at neutrophil counts in the range of 1–2 $\times 10^9$ /l in the absence of additional complicating factors. It should also be recognized that a small percentage of the normal population has counts more than two standard deviations below the mean, and thus have counts below the conventionally employed lower limit of normal. Certain racial groups also have a lower limit of normal than Caucasians. Failure to appreciate these factors can result in unnecessary anxiety and investigation in individuals with marginally low neutrophil counts in whom there are no other grounds for suspecting the presence of any clinically significant disorder. The incidence and severity of infection become progressively greater as the neutrophil count falls below 0.5 $\times 10^9$ /l, although in some conditions, such as chronic idiopathic neutropenia, extremely low counts are associated with very much less morbidity and mortality than in individuals undergoing chemotherapy for acute leukaemia, for instance.

Table 9.4. *Causes of neutropenia*

Replacement of normal haemopoietic tissue in bone marrow, especially by haemopoietic or lymphocytic neoplastic states, e.g. acute leukaemia, myelofibrosis, lymphoma, multiple myeloma, myelodysplasia
Infections, especially certain bacterial infections such as typhoid, and early stages of many viral infections such as infectious hepatitis
Overwhelming sepsis in which consumption of neutrophils exceeds production
Megaloblastosis
Cytotoxic therapy
Felty's syndrome
Hypersplenism
Drug or virally induced transient severe neutropenia (agranulocytosis)
Systemic lupus erythematosus
Aplastic anaemia
Neonatal iso-immune neutropenia
Chronic idiopathic neutropenia
Pseudoneutropenia due to an abnormally high proportion of neutrophils in the marginated state
Transient post-haemodialysis neutropenia
Spurious neutropenia in healthy individuals where the count is less than the conventionally stated lower limit of normal
Cyclic neutropenia
Miscellaneous

CAUSES OF NEUTROPENIA

Many conditions are associated with neutropenia, as illustrated in Table 9.4. They range from disorders that affect haemopoietic tissue in general to the neutrophil series in particular, and are discussed in detail in the relevant chapters.

CLINICAL FEATURES

The clinical features of the neutropenic patient reflect those of the *underlying disorder* responsible for the neutropenia, and of *infection*. Patients with acute onset of severe transient neutropenia usually present with infection causing fever and associated constitutional symptoms such as headache, backache, myalgia, and prostration. There is often symptomatic pharyngitis, which is initially diffuse and erythematous, but ulceration develops subsequently. These features reflect the readily visible aspects of infectious involvement of the respiratory and gastrointestinal tract. Tissue invasion can progress to bacteraemia, which is sometimes associated with metastatic lesions in the skin, with pale tender centres surrounded by a zone of erythema. Progression to overt septicaemia under these circumstances is frequently fatal, but in those who survive with severe ongoing sepsis, organ failure such as hepatic dysfunction can develop.

Such a picture of severe bacterial infection can also develop in ongoing neutropenic states such as aplastic anemia and acute leukaemia. A factor that appears to contribute to high morbidity and mortality under these circumstances is inability to increase neutrophil production in response to enhanced utilization of the reduced pool of available neutrophils. *Cognizance of the possibility of underlying neutropenia in a patient presenting with sepsis can be life-saving as a result of immediate institution of intensive therapeutic measures.*

Lesser degrees of neutropenia, particularly of a chronic nature, can be accompanied by recurrent infections in which individual episodes are slow to recover, and the associated constitutional symptoms of malaise and lethargy are out of proportion to mild normochromic normocytic anaemia, often developing as a result of repeated infection. Infected lesions have a tendency to ulcerate and become necrotic. Reduced availability of neutrophils also limits pus formation, and inflammatory exudates are often sero-sanguinous and contain few neutrophils. Infections of the oropharynx and skin are the most prominent lesions. Skin infections such as boils and cellulitis, often with regional lymphadenitis, and infections following minor trauma (e.g. scratches, cuts, and insect bites) or without any obvious cause, are common, especially in the neck, groin, and axilla. Infections of the respiratory tract are also relatively common, and wound healing tends to be delayed.

DRUG-INDUCED NEUTROPENIA AND AGRANULOCYTOSIS

Neutropenia is the most common life-threatening idiosyncratic response of the myeloid series to drugs that do not normally exert cytotoxic action. Transient selective neutropenia which recovers rapidly after withdrawal of the offending agent is a more common drug-idiosyncrasy than the neutropenia occurring as part of the chronic pancytopenia in aplastic anemia.

Large numbers of drugs in differing therapeutic categories have been suspected of causing agranulocytosis, and the most frequently reported agents are listed in Table 9.5. Some drugs are associated with relatively high risk, and the incidence of severe neutropenia has been estimated to be as high as 0.13–0.7 per cent with chlorpromazine, 0.45–1.75 per cent with thiouracils, and 0.86 per cent with amidopyrine (Huguley *et al.* 1966). Dapsone was associated with a sufficiently high incidence of fatal agranulocytosis that it was withdrawn from use for prophylaxis against malaria by the U.S. Army (Ognibene 1970), but it still remains in use for this purpose in some countries.

Table 9.5. *Drugs more commonly associated with idiosyncratic selective neutropenia (agranulocytosis)*

Antipyretic and non-steroidal anti-inflammatory agents
aminopyrine (H), amidopyrine (H), and noramidopyrine (H). These highly effective antipyretics have been withdrawn from sale in certain countries because of the frequency with which they induce agranulocytosis.
phenylbutazone
indomethacin

Tranquillizers
chlorpromazine (H), promazine (H), and other phenothiazines (H)

Anticonvulsants
carbamazepine

Antithyroid drugs
propylthiouracil (H), carbimazole (H) and methimazole (H)

Antibiotics and antimalarials
sulphonamides including combinations with trimethoprim
salicylazosulphapyridine
methicillin
dapsone (H)

Diuretics and antihypertensive agents
thiazides
captopril

H = drugs associated with relatively high risk.

These agents are *high risk drugs*, and a high index of suspicion of underlying agranulocytosis should be exercised with respect to any individual receiving these drugs who develops features of infection. Other drugs, such as phenylbutazone and sulphonamides, are associated with a substantially lower incidence of agranulocytosis, but account for a relatively large proportion of total cases because of their widespread use in the community.

Mechanisms

Agranulocytosis occurs in such an unpredictable and relatively uncommon fashion that predisposing factors must operate in susceptible individuals. One possible mechanism is development of hypersensitivity of an immunological nature, in which only an occasional subject forms antibodies capable of acting alone, or in combination with the drug, to damage neutrophils or their precursors in the bone marrow. The response to amidopyrine in some individuals occurs with such small doses and with sufficient rapidity that it resembles an immune-mediated hypersensitivity reaction (Maddison & Squires 1934, Moeschlin & Wagner 1952), but whether this type of hypersensitivity underlies the idiosyncratic response to other drugs remains to be established. In other instances, neutropenia develops much more slowly, and does not necessarily recur after brief exposure to the drug. For this reason, it is considered that idiosyncratic responses can also be caused by undue susceptibility to a direct toxic effect on neutrophil precursors.

Diagnostic features

The essential feature is extreme depression of the absolute count of neutrophils and band forms in the blood. The absolute count of lymphocytes and monocytes may also occasionally be depressed, although to a lesser extent than the neutrophil series. In the absence of complicating factors, such as infection, the haemoglobin level and platelet count are usually normal, and it is the highly selective nature of the neutropenia that distinguishes agranulocytosis from neutropenia in the alternative type of drug idiosyncratic response, aplastic anaemia. Examination of the *bone marrow* usually reveals *selective* depletion of neutrophil precursors. The type of precursor that is depleted ranges from only the more mature members of the neutrophil series, through to the entire neutrophil series. The marrow cellularity is affected most commonly only by the selective depletion of neutrophil precursors, although in some instances lesser degrees of depletion of megakaryocytes and erythroblasts co-exist. Differentiation from other forms of isolated neutropenia listed in Table 9.4 is usually not difficult when it is evident that the patient is taking, or has stopped taking in the very recent past, a drug known to be associated with agranulocytosis. Occasionally, the relation to a drug is established only in retrospect by the pattern of recovery following the withdrawal of the drug.

Course and prognosis

Most cases present with sepsis which has developed as a result of inadequate production of neutrophils. The thesis has been advanced that serial blood tests in patients taking high risk drugs enable incipient agranulocytosis to be recognized at an early stage, and thereby permit withdrawal of the drug sufficiently early to prevent progression to severe neutropenia. Prospective studies have, however, shown that mild leucopenia develops during administration of antithyroid drugs and sulphonamide compounds, for example, with considerably greater frequency than agranulocytosis. Development of mild leucopenia does not usually presage agranulocytosis during continued administration of the drug, and conversely, agranulocytosis can develop precipitously without a prodromal minor fall in neutrophil count. Serial neutrophil counts therefore do not provide an effective safeguard, and the only measure currently available to limit the incidence of agranulocytosis is avoidance of the use of high risk drugs.

Prognosis in the individual case is particularly dependent on the severity of associated infection and its response to treatment. Death from infection occurred in about 80 per cent of subjects with extreme neutropenia in the pre-antibiotic era, and the most important factor in the marked drop in mortality since that time has been *prompt institution of effective antibiotic therapy*. Despite administration of antibiotics and leucocyte transfusions, the extreme lack of neutrophils prevents control of infection in some instances, such as patients with septicaemic shock, and mortality is currently of the order of 10–20 per cent. The duration of the phase of extreme neutropenia dictates the period of high risk, and is dependent on the rate of recovery of neutrophil production following withdrawal of the offending drug. *Recovery is thus accelerated by prompt recognition and withdrawal of the causative agent*. The subsequent interval before substantial egress of neutrophils takes place into the blood is greatly influenced by the extent to which the depletion of neutrophil precursors proceeds back along the pathway of differentiation (Ruvidic & Jelic 1972). It may be more than a week when precursors are depleted back to the myeloblast stage, or a day or two when only more mature forms are absent from the bone marrow. The rate of recovery does vary with the nature of the drug, and can be slower in the case of phenothiazines, for example. The rate of recovery differs from that in aplastic anaemia and marrow depression during treatment of acute leukaemia, in that recovery of neutrophil production generally occurs more rapidly, sometimes with such exuberance that the marked neutrophilia with left shift usually results in rapid control of infection (Fig. 9.3).

Management

Prompt recognition of the presence of severe neutropenia and its possible *relationship to drug ingestion* is crucial to effective management. It enables a *causative agent to be withdrawn* and thereby permits recovery of neutrophil production to commence. The interval before neutrophils are produced in adequate amounts represents a limited phase of grossly reduced capacity to suppress infection, and *effective antimicrobial therapy* during this time greatly reduces the risk of death. All subjects who have experienced idiosyncratic agranulocytosis must be warned of the likelihood of recurrence on re-exposure and, if possible, carry a warning note to alert all future medical contacts.

No time is to be lost before the institution of antibiotic therapy in an infected agranulocytic subject, as such a person could have bacteraemia capable of progressing to septicaemia. Specimens for microbial culture are first taken from the nose, throat, sputum, exudates from lesions, urine, and *blood*. As the situation represents a medical emergency, broad-spectrum intravenous antibiotic therapy is commenced and later modified, if necessary, according to the antibiotic sensitivity of isolated organisms. Infective agents span a wide range, and are usually not of a hospital-associated multiple antibiotic-resistant nature, unless the agranulocytosis developed in a hospital inpatient. In many instances, invading bacteria are flora of the gastrointestinal tract. Initial antibiotic treatment must therefore be effective against a wide diversity of organisms, and a combination of antibiotics with a wide spectrum of action is employed, often consisting of an aminoglycoside plus a semi-synthetic penicillin or cephalosporin. It is important that the chosen combination be effective against

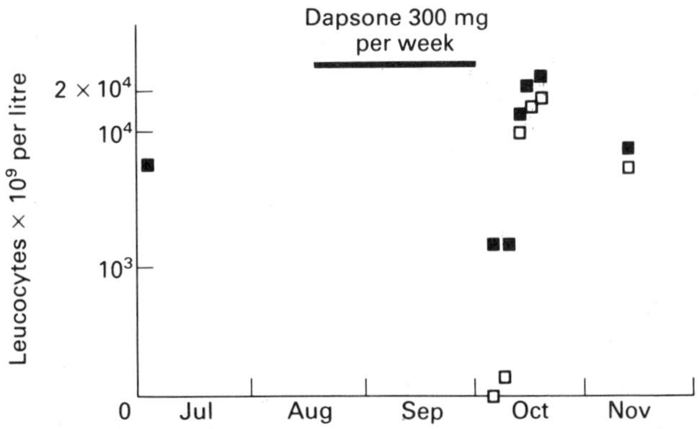

Fig. 9.3. *Counts of total leucocytes (■) and total granulocytic series (□) in the peripheral blood in relation to the period of dapsone ingestion. The total leucocyte count only was determined at the end of June prior to the start of treatment with dapsone.*

Pseudomonas and *Klebsiella* species as well as *E. coli* and *enterococci.*

Steps should be taken to limit the exposure of such a subject to further contact with microbes, particularly those of a multiple antibiotic-resistant nature. Barrier nursing is therefore desirable during the period of increased risk of infection. Nasal spray and mouthwash with antiseptic agents such as chlorhexidine can be employed to limit colonization with external organisms, and oral nystatin or amphotericin administered to limit the gastrointestinal load of yeasts and fungi which are resistant to intravenous antibiotic regimes of the type described above.

In subjects with life-threatening infection the *transfusion of leucocytes* offers the propsect of providing additional support during the period of extreme neutropenia. Leucocytes are isolated by leucapheresis from the blood of donors using intermittent or continuous centrifugation to prepare leucocyte-rich plasma. Large numbers of leucocytes are required before any benefit is obtained, and recovery of transfused neutrophils in the recipient is substantially greater when the donor is a sibling, especially when ABO and HLA antigens are identical to those of the recipient. Survival of the transfused neutrophils is brief, and any increase in the count is sustained for less than one day. An increment is rarely observed in the neutrophil count of *severely* infected recipients following such transfusions, but rapid migration of transfused granulocytes into infected tissue sites has been demonstrated, and it is claimed that morbidity and mortality from infection is reduced (Highby & Burnett 1980). Common practice is for leucocyte transfusions to be given daily for at least several days, which represents a considerable logistic exercise in that each leucapheresis requires several hours. It is thus feasible to provide leucocyte transfusion support during the relatively limited period of profound neutropenia as in agranulocytosis, or following intensive cytotoxic drug therapy, but there is no proven long-term benefit from leucocyte transfusion in states of chronic unremitting severe neutropenia.

Administration of *corticosteroids* has been advocated by some as a possible means for accelerating the restoration of adequate neutrophil counts. In many cases, however, the rate of recovery in the absence of glucocorticoid administration is close to that expected for a wave of unimpeded neutrophil maturation to take place in the bone marrow after the drug is withdrawn, so that there are no strong grounds for the use of glucocorticoids to suppress ongoing immune injury to the neutrophil series once the offending drug is withdrawn. A disadvantage of the use of relatively high doses of glucocorticoids in such a setting is their inhibitory effect on the migration of neutrophils to sites of infection, which further lessens the efficacy of host defences against infection (Bishop *et al* 1968).

Restoration of normal hydration is important in infected subjects as they may have severe fluid depletion.

Attention should also be given to the possible need for parenteral nutrition, as pharyngitis or gastrointestinal tract disturbances can severely limit caloric intake.

Manipulation of ulcerated lesions or instrumentation of any hollow viscus, such as the bladder or the gastrointestinal tract, is associated with a considerable risk of seeding bacteria into the blood, and should be avoided if at all possible during the phase of severe neutropenia.

CHRONIC NEUTROPENIA

Many of the conditions listed in Table 9.4 are associated with persistent rather than transient neutropenia. The underlying cause is usually established from the combination of the clinical and laboratory features, although an exception is chronic idiopathic neutropenia, which is basically diagnosed by exclusion of other specific conditions.

Chronic idiopathic neutropenia is a relatively uncommon disorder, which is usually of an acquired nature, and occurs more commonly in females. Only the neutrophil or the neutrophil plus stab form are depleted from the neutrophil series in the majority of cases, although occasionally less mature precursors are also depleted. In some instances, there is good evidence that the toxic process is auto-immune-mediated injury to the neutrophil series, but procedures for the detection

Table 9.6. *Comparative features of disorders that cause neutropenia*

	Agranulocytosis due to drug idiosyncrasy	Aplastic anaemia	Acute leukaemia and myelodysplastic disorders	Idiopathic neutropenia	Hypersplenism
Frequency	Occasional	Uncommon	Relatively common	Rare	Relatively common
History	Concurrent or very recent drug ingestion	Drug ingestion or exposure to chemicals in about one-half several weeks to several months previously	Rarely exposure to benzene, alkylating agents, or radiation in the past		Features of conditions resulting in splenomegaly
Lymph node enlargement	Absent except in areas draining infected lesions	Absent except in areas draining infected lesions	Sometimes present	Absent except in areas draining infected lesions	Sometimes present as a feature of an underlying disorder
Splenomegaly	Absent	Absent	Sometimes present	Sometimes slightly enlarged	Present
Sternal tenderness	Absent	Absent	Sometimes present	Absent	Absent
Anaemia	Usually absent	Present	Present	Usually absent	Common
Very immature white cells	Usually absent	Absent	Common	Absent	Absent
Thrombocytopenia	Usually absent	Present	Present	Absent	Common
Bone marrow	Granulocytic series hypoplastic. Erythroid series and megakaryocytes usually normal	Hypocellularity of granulocytic, erythroid and megakaryocytic series	Leukaemic or myelodysplastic infiltration	Depletion of some mature granulocytic series. Erythroid series and megakaryocytes normal	Usually hyper- or normocellular

of such activity are not yet in the province of the routine diagnostic laboratory.

The course of the disorder is usually surprisingly benign in view of the very low neutrophil counts that are frequently present (Kyle & Linman 1968). There is thus little or nothing to be gained by speculative trial of immunosuppressive agents in patients in whom infections are not a significant problem. Corticosteroid administration has sometimes been beneficial in others afflicted by recurrent bouts of infection, although occasionally it has been incriminated in predisposing to overwhelming sepsis, presumably because of the impairment of host defence produced by these drugs. Differentiation between the features of this disorder and those of other important causes of neutropenia are outlined in Table 9.6.

Felty's syndrome is the association of chronic neutropenia with splenomegaly and rheumatoid arthritis. Other abnormalities may occur in patients with this condition, including weight loss, pigmentation of the skin, and ulceration of the lower parts of the legs (Fig. 9.4). Felty's syndrome tends to occur in middle age or the elderly, and rheumatoid arthritis usually occurs before the development of neutropenia by many years, although the inflammatory activity of the arthritis may become quiescent before the onset of the neutropenia. Sometimes the detection of a palpable spleen precedes the neutropenia, and sometimes the reverse occurs.

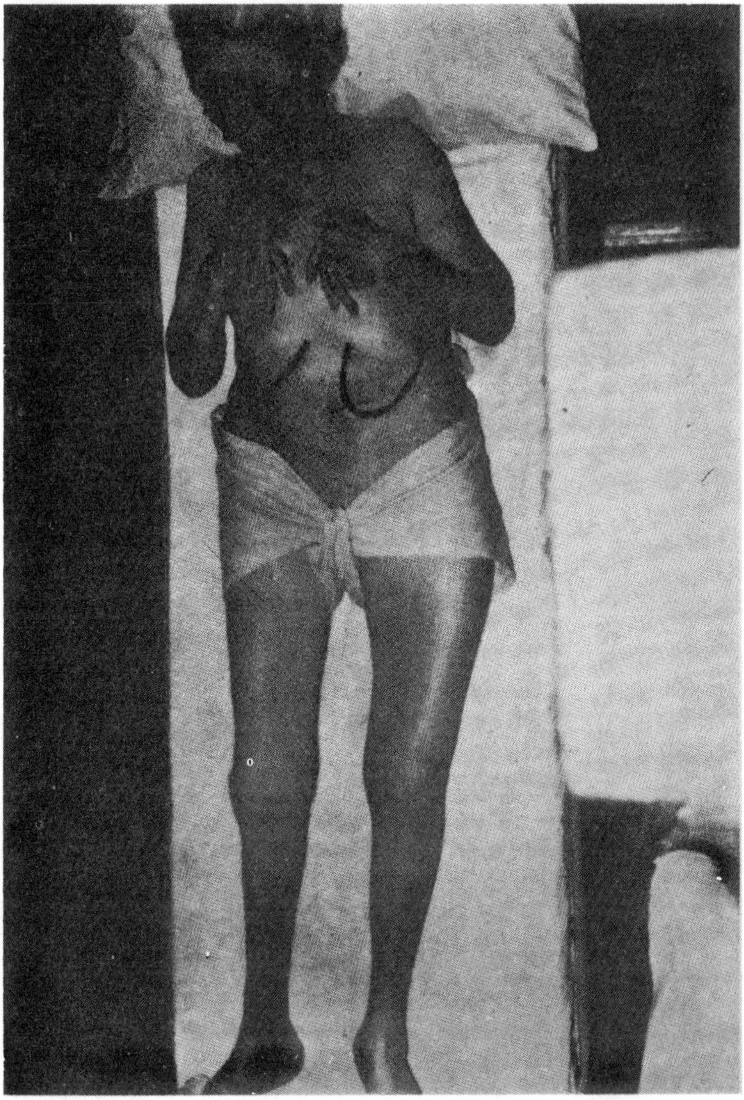

Fig. 9.4. *Photograph of an elderly woman with Felty's syndrome, who presented with chronic leg ulceration, severe rheumatoid arthritic deformities in the hands, splenomegaly, and a minor degree of hepatic enlargement. The Hb level was 10.8 g/dl, WCC 1.7 × 10^9/l, neutrophil count 0.4 × 10^9/l, and platelet count 180 × 10^9/l.*

The mechanism responsible for the neutropenia is uncertain, as different studies have yielded conflicting results, but an unduly large degree of sequestration of neutrophils in the spleen, as well as decreased neutrophil production, appear to contribute (Vincent *et al.* 1974). The leucocyte count is usually 1–4 × 10^9 /l, and the neutrophil count is subnormal. Mild normocytic anaemia and mild thrombocytopenia may also occur. There are varied patterns of change in the granulocyte series in the bone marrow aspirate, including hyperplasia of granulocytic elements, selective depletion of more mature forms, or hypoplasia of the entire granulocytic series. An association exists between the disorder and relatively high titres of rheumatoid factor, the presence of anti-nuclear factor, and evidence of vasculitis.

It is common for neutropenia to persist in the absence of an association with an increased incidence of infection. Under these circumstances, therapeutic intervention offers no benefit to the patient. *Treatment* for patients in whom recurrent infections are a serious problem is usually *splenectomy*. There is frequently a rise in neutrophil count immediately after splenectomy, but the rise is sustained in only about 50 per cent of all subjects subjected to that operation. It has not been possible to identify subjects in whom sustained benefit is achieved, so that splenectomy should not be undertaken lightly, as it may not only be unhelpful, but is also associated with a high incidence of peri-operative morbidity (Moore *et al.* 1971). Administration of corticosteriods may produce some rise in the neutrophil count, but the effect is rarely sustained after the drug is withdrawn, and there is little evidence that treatment with these drugs produces any substantial reduction in infectious problems.

Cyclical neutropenia can occur as an inherited or an acquired disorder. It is commonly difficult to detect because blood counts may be performed in the phase of normal or near-normal neutrophil counts which follows the phase of neutropenia. The overall cycle usually occupies approximately three weeks. The neutropenia in some subjects can be accompanied by bouts of disabling infection, while in others the incidence of infection is not increased (Morley 1967).

Lymphopenia

Lymphopenia is said to occur when the absolute lymphocyte count is below the conventionally employed lower limit of normal of 1.5×10^9 /l. Lymphopenia is usually present in pancytopenia due to any cause, and is common in advanced Hodgkin's disease. It is common in the leucopenic prodromal phase of many viral infections. A selective depletion of blood helper T lymphocytes with or without absolute lymphopenia is very common in the *acquired immune deficiency syndrome* (AIDS). Moderate- to high-dose corticosteroid administration regularly produces lymphopenia.

Infectious mononucleosis

Infectious mononucleosis is caused by infection with *Epstein–Barr virus* (Niederman *et al.* 1968). Many episodes are subclinical or not readily distinguished on clinical grounds from other mild viral infections, but the classical acute infection most commonly recognized in the second or third decade of life is characterized by malaise, fever, pharyngitis, lymphadenopathy, and lymphocytosis with atypical lymphocytes in the blood. This clinical and haematological picture is also seen in infections with *toxoplasma* and *cytomegalovirus*, which for practical purposes comprise, along with Epstein–Barr virus infection, the overwhelming majority of cases of what is sometimes referred to as the *glandular fever syndrome*. Acute Epstein–Barr virus infection is classically differentiated from the other infections by the development of increased titres of heterophile antibodies to sheep, ox, and horse erythrocytes.

Epidemiology and serology

Virtually everyone contracts infectious mononucleosis. Infection can occur from childhood to old age, although the classical acute infection is commonly regarded as an affliction of teenagers and young adults. Most people have been infected by the age of 40 years. The incubation period is probably at least several weeks in duration, and is followed by a period of clinical manifestations usually lasting several weeks. Production of antibody against Epstein–Barr virus capsid antigen commences at this time, and detectable circulating antibody usually persists for life. Production of heterophile antibodies, which also commences at this time, is not sustained. The titre may not be elevated very early in the illness, but is raised in 80–90 per cent of cases in the second to third week, after which it declines. The infectious agent is a DNA virus of the herpes group, and residual intracellular virus persists, possibly for life, and is excreted subsequently in the asymptomatic state. Saliva from such subjects probably serves as an important source of virus, accounting for the sporadic infectious pattern observed in the disorder. It usually does not spread in an epidemic manner.

Clinical features

The florid illness is of relatively abrupt clinical

Table 9.7. *Presenting manifestations and associated complications of infectious mononucleosis*

Common	
Constitutional symptoms of malaise, anorexia, nausea, fatigue	
Fever	
Pharyngitis	
Headache	
Lymphadenopathy	
Splenomegaly	
Intermediate frequency	
Myalgia	
Peri-orbital swelling	
Hepatomegaly or hepatic tenderness	
Mild thrombocytopenia	
Uncommon but important	
Skin rash	
Conjunctivitis	
Purpura or bleeding due to severe thrombocytopenia	
Pneumonitis	
Arthralgia	
Rare	
Splenic rupture	
Haemolysis	
Neurological problems	

onset, and presenting features are listed in Table 9.7.

Malaise, lassitude, headache, and *generalized muscle aching or soreness* are the most common symptoms, and they precede other manifestations such as sore throat and lymph node enlargement. In mild cases, malaise and lassitude may be the only symptoms. Fever occurs in the majority and is commonly present at the onset. It is usually of moderate degree, e.g. below 39°C, but is sometimes higher, especially in patients with extensive pharyngitis, or in sick patients with complications such as meningo-encephalitis. The pulse is often inappropriately slow for the degree of fever. Fever usually lasts 5–10 days, but sometimes persists for several weeks.

Sore throat occurs in over 50 per cent of cases, and *dysphagia* can be a problem and a palatal exanthem may be present. An off-white exudate may also be present, which can be patchy or confluent. Removal of the exudate typically does not cause bleeding. Ulceration may occur, and there may be oedema of the pharynx.

Lymphadenopathy is the most characteristic feature, and virtually always occurs at some stage during the course of the illness. The cervical lymph nodes, particularly the posterior group, are nearly always palpable, and the axillary and inguinal nodes are commonly enlarged. Occasionally, the axillary nodes are enlarged in the absence of cervical enlargement. The nodes are usually palpable when the patient is first seen, but sometimes do not become palpable for another 2–3 weeks. The nodes are moderately enlarged, discrete, mobile, not attached to skin or deeper structures, and are of a rubbery consistency. They are sometimes tender and painful, especially the cervical nodes in patients with pharyngeal involvement, but suppuration does not occur. The enlargement usually subsides over several weeks, commonly with the disappearance of fever, but occasionally some degree of enlargement persists for months, or rarely years.

Anorexia and *nausea* are common, but vomiting and *diarrhoea* are not prominent features. *Abdominal pain* may be due to splenomegaly, in which case it is under the left costal margin, or to mesenteric lymph node enlargement, in which case it is commonly in the right iliac fossa. If the pain in the right iliac fossa is severe, a diagnosis of acute appendicitis or mesenteric lymphadenitis may be made. *Rupture of the spleen* is a rare complication and should be considered if pain under the left costal margin is severe, especially when there is left shoulder tip pain.

Slight to moderate *splenomegaly* occurs in more than 40 per cent of cases, and the tip of the spleen seldom extends more than several centimetres below the costal margin. The spleen is commonly tender, and becomes impalpable as the acute phase of the disease passes, although occasionally it can be felt for several months.

The *liver* is enlarged in about 15 per cent of cases, and may be tender. *Jaundice* develops in 5–10 per cent of cases, usually in the second or third week, and is usually mild and transient. There is commonly biochemical evidence of *hepatocellular damage* even when clinical jaundice is absent, and elevation of plasma transaminase activity can be comparable with that in mild infectious hepatitis.

Skin rashes occur in about ten per cent of cases, usually between the fourth and tenth day of the disease. The rash takes various forms, the most common being macular, but may be rubelliform in young children. Rashes have been reported with much greater frequency in patients given ampicillin, and many instances may therefore reflect an allergic reaction to the drug.

Clinically evident involvement of the nervous system probably occurs only in 1–2 per cent of cases. It can take the form of meningitis, encephalitis, meningo-encephalitis, or polyneuritis. These most commonly develop several weeks after the onset of constitutional symptoms, but may be the presenting problem, or appear at the same time as the constitutional symptoms. Cerebrospinal fluid in neurologically affected individuals contains a moderately increased content of protein and cells, mainly lymphocytes, and the disorder may simulate benign lymphocytic meningitis. Although patients with nervous system involvement may be very ill, full recovery is the most common outcome.

Clinical evidence of *cardiac involvement* is rare, although pericarditis and myocarditis have been reported. Cough with sputum and wheezes or rales occur occasionally. Even less commonly the chest X-ray reveals pneumonitic changes. The most common respiratory problem is *airways obstruction* by tissue hyperplasia in the region of the tonsils or pharynx.

Haematological and serological features

The characteristic finding is atypical lymphocytes in the blood. There is most commonly an absolute lymphocytosis due not only to the presence of these cells, but also to increased numbers of normal lymphocytes. Atypical lymphocytes are generally larger than normal and vary considerably in appearance. The nucleus most commonly departs from the normal round configuration, and while the chromatin has certain features suggestive of an immature pattern, the experienced haematologist is usually able to distinguish these cells without difficulty from those in neoplastic lymphoproliferative disorders. Such cells appear in the blood during the first week of the illness and may initially be present in sufficiently low proportions to resemble the picture encountered in many viral infections. The proportion usually increases to more than 20 per cent of the total leucocytes, and maximum values are achieved during the second week. Atypical cells persist for several weeks to several months, and have been shown to be T lymphocytes with suppressor activity (p. 8), apparently generated as a reaction to infection by virus of other lymphocyte subsets.

Neutrophil counts frequently decline to moderately subnormal values, with a left shift, at a time approximating the peak of the atypical lymphocytosis. On rare occasions, severe neutropenia occurs. The effect on the white cell count of the decline in neutrophil count is offset by the lymphocytosis, to the extent that an absolute leucocytosis occurs in about two-thirds of the patients, and may on rare occasions reach values greater than $20 \times 10^9/l$. Anaemia does not usually occur, but a small percentage of patients develops a mild degree of haemolysis with cold reacting antibodies (p. 197). Minor degrees of thrombocytopenia are very common (Carter 1965), but purpura or bleeding due to severe thrombocytopenia is rare, and this complication tends to occur as a self-limited problem in younger people.

Heterophile antibody causing agglutination of sheep red blood cells occurs in the serum in titres above normal in 80–90 per cent of young adults with infectious mononucleosis. Positive results become more frequent towards the end of the first week, and occur with maximum frequency during the third week. Thus, in a suspected case, the test when negative in the first week should be repeated at a later date. Positive results are less common in younger or older subjects with infectious mononucleosis. Heterophile antibody against ox and horse red blood cells is also produced, and certain currently employed diagnostic procedures employ agglutination of horse red cells for estimation of heterophile antibody.

Differential diagnosis

Differentiation of infectious mononucleosis from other conditions associated with fever, myalgia, lymphadenopathy, pharyngitis, and splenomegaly does not normally present difficulty under circumstances where the major anomaly in the blood is a marked atypical lymphocytosis, and the titre of heterophile antibody is significantly elevated. Difficulties occur when the degree of atypical lymphocytosis is either very low, or sufficiently high to raise concerns about the possibility of a neoplastic lymphoproliferative disorder, but the presence of elevated heterophile antibody levels in such situations is of considerable diagnostic assistance. The major difficulties are when elevation of the heterophile antibody titre does not take place. The most common conditions responsible for an atypical lymphocytosis without elevated heterophile antibody titres are infection with cytomegalovirus, Toxoplasma, Epstein–Barr virus which does not promote a typical heterophile antibody response, and infectious hepatitis.

Acute cytomegalovirus infection can have a clinical course very similar to that of infectious mononucleosis, except that pharyngitis is a less prominent feature. In a greater proportion of cases, the infection is subclinical. The virus does, however, persist in the body after recovery from the acute episode, and can be *passed from the asymptomatic carrier via infected lymphocytes during blood transfusions*, or by excretion of the virus in the sputum or urine. Diagnosis of an acute infection is established by a rise in specific antibody titre of at least fourfold over the course of several weeks.

Another condition which lacks the classical haematological and serological features of infectious mononucleosis, but has certain clinical features in common, is *cat-scratch disease*. There is benign enlargement of regional nodes draining the primary site of infection in up to 50 per cent of cases. In about 90 per cent, there has been close contact with a cat, and in about half there is a history of a cat scratch. The usual incubation period is 1–2 weeks, but there is a wide range from several days up to about 8 weeks.

The primary lesion at the site of inoculation appears as an erythematous nodule or papule, on top of which is a vesicle or pustule which forms a scab. The regional lymph nodes are enlarged, sometimes markedly, and although they may be tender, they are not usually painful. The nodes most often involved are the axillary, but cervical and inguinal nodes may be involved. During the stage of lymph node enlargement there is often fever and malaise which persists for 7–14 days. Occasionally, there is a generalized macropapular rash and rarely encephalitis, pneumonia, thrombocytopenia, and abdominal pain. Diagnosis is based on known exposure to cats, although a scratch may not be recalled, on the clinical picture with tender indurated lymph nodes, and the fact that they follow a single anatomical drainage pattern. The histology of the lymph nodes is characteristic, with giant cells and marked necrosis, but biopsy is generally inadvisable, as sinuses may develop and the wound is usually slow to heal.

Prognosis and management

Infectious mononucleosis is essentially a benign self-limiting disorder in which clinical recovery is virtually complete after two months. Life-threatening complications are very rare and consist mainly of severe thrombocytopenia, neutropenia, hepatocellular damage, neurological damage, respiratory tract obstruction, and rupture of the spleen.

Antibiotics are of no value, except for treatment of superimposed bacterial infection. Rest appropriate for the degree of prostration, plus analgesia and antipyretics, are all that are usually required during the acute phase of the illness. Corticosteroid administration enhances the feeling of well-being and promotes lysis of hyperplastic lymphatic tissue, but the long-term benefits are questionable.

Rupture of the spleen can occur with relatively minor trauma, and for this reason it is recommended that body contact sports be avoided for at least two months, or until the spleen can no longer be palpated.

References and further reading

Athens, J.W., Haab, O.P., Raab, S.O. *et al.* (1965) Leukokinetic studies. XI. Blood granulocyte kinetics in polycythemia vera, infection and myelofibrosis. *J. Clin. Invest.* **44**, 778.

Babior, B.M. (1978a) Oxygen-dependent microbial killing by phagocytes. *New Engl. J. Med.* **298**, 659.

Babior, B.M. (1978b) Oxygen-dependent microbial killing by phagocytes. *New Engl. J. Med.* **298**, 721.

Bishop, C.R., Athens, J.W., Boggs, D.R. *et al.* (1968) Leukokinetic studies. XII. A non-steady-state kinetic evaluation of the mechanism of cortisone-induced granulocytosis. *J. Clin. Invest.* **47**, 249.

Carter, R.L. (1965) Platelet levels in infectious mononucleosis. *Blood*, **25**, 817.

Dacie, J.V. & Lewis, S.M. (1984) *Practical Haematology*, 6th Ed., Churchill Livingstone, London.

Firkin, F.C. (1972) Serum muramidase in haematological disorders: diagnostic value in neoplastic states. *Austr. N.Z. J. Med.* **2**, 28.

Hayhoe, F.G.J. & Quaglino, D. (1958) Cytochemical demonstration and measurement of leucocyte alkaline phosphatase activity in normal and pathological states by a modified azo-dye coupling technique. *Brit. J. Haemat.* **4**, 375.

Highby, D.J. & Burnett, D. (1980) Granulocyte transfusions: current status. *Blood*, **55**, 2.

Huguley, C.M., Lea, J.W. & Butts, J.A. (1966) Adverse hematologic reaction to drugs. In: Brown, E.B. & Moore, C.V. (Eds) *Progress in Hematology*, Vol. V, p.105, Grune & Stratton, New York.

Kyle, R.A. & Linman, J.W. (1968) Chronic idopathic neutropenia. *New Engl. J. Med.* **279**, 1015.

Lehrer, R.I., Hanifin, J. & Cline, M.J. (1969) Defective bactericidal activity in myeloperoxidase-deficient human neutrophils. *Nature*, **223**, 78.

Madison, F.W. & Squires, T.L. (1934) Etiology of primary granulocytopenia (agranulocytic angina). *J. Am. Med. Ass.* **102**, 755.

Moeschlin, S. & Wagner, K. (1952) Agranulocytosis due to the occurrence of leukocyte-agglutinins (Pyramidon and cold agglutinins). *Acta Haemat.* **8**, 29.

Moore, R.A., Brinner, C.M., Sandusky, W.R. *et al.* (1971) Felty's syndrome: long-term follow up after splenectomy. *Ann. Int. Med.* **75**, 381.

Morley, A.A., Carew, J.P. & Baikie, A.G. (1967) Familial cyclical neutropenia. *Brit. J. Haemat.* **13**, 719.

Niederman, J.C., McCollie, R.W., Henle, G. *et al.* (1968) Infectious mononucleosis. Clinical manifestations in relation to EB virus antibodies. *J. Am. Med. Ass.* **203**, 139.

Ognibene, A.J. (1970) Agranulocytosis due to dapsone. *Ann. Int. Med.* **72**, 521.

Polmar, S.H. (1980) Metabolic aspects of immunodeficiency disease. *Semin. Hematol.* **17**, 30.

Ruvidic, R. & Jelic, S. (1972) Haematological aspects of drug-induced agranulocytosis. *Scand. J. Haemat.* **9**, 18.

Vincent, P.C., Levi, J.A. & MacQueen A. (1974) The mechanism of neutropenia in Felty's syndrome. *Brit. J. Haemat.* **27**, 463.

Wiernik, P.H. & Serpick, A.A. (1969) Clinical significance of serum and urinary muramidase activity in leukaemia and other hematologic malignancies. *Am. J. Med.* **46**, 330.

Chapter 10
The Leukaemias

Leukaemias are diseases in which abnormal proliferation of haemopoietic cells causes progressively increasing infiltration of the bone marrow, although in certain forms the lymphatic tissues are particularly affected. The process of differentiation in leukaemic cells is often abnormal, and this commonly results in an immature morphological appearance. Leukaemic cells are usually present in the peripheral blood, where the count ranges from very low to very high values. These cells very commonly have myeloid or lymphocytic characteristics, but occasionally cells with features of erythroid precursors or megakaryocytes are part of the disease process.

The rate of progression varies considerably in different types of leukaemia, but death is the usual outcome in untreated disease as a result of compromised production of mature blood cells. A significant proportion of subjects with acute leukaemia have remissions induced by treatment, and a substantial proportion appear to be cured in certain categories of acute leukaemia. A majority of patients with leukaemia still die as a result of the disease, although the extent to which survival is prolonged by treatment has increased considerably over the past two decades. Therapeutic measures can improve the quality of life in the presence of persisting disease, and significantly prolong life expectancy when remission of the disease is achieved.

Leukaemia accounts for about four per cent of all deaths from malignant disease, although the proportion is greater in childhood.

Aetiology

Leukaemia is generally considered to be a neoplastic disorder originating in a haemopoietic cell which has undergone an intrinsic change, causing it to escape from the normal restraints imposed on proliferative activity. Leukaemic cell populations can consist of cells of one or several different pathways of differentiation.

A critical step in leukaemogenesis appears to be alteration of the structure of DNA in the nucleus of the cell in which the disease is initiated, but the precise nature of the underlying changes at the molecular level in the development of human leukaemia remains to be established. Many contributory factors have been incriminated in the development of neoplastic change, and include inherited predisposition, effects of viruses, and effects of radiation and chemicals.

Molecular biology of leukaemogenesis

There is evidence that leukaemia in humans can be associated with inappropriate expression of certain genes which appear to be involved in regulating basic steps in cell proliferation. The normal counterparts of these genes are referred to as *proto-oncogenes*, and in most instances the precise role played by the gene products in cell behaviour remains to be clarified, although they can, for example, correspond to a receptor for a growth promoting factor, or enzymes involved in pathways that convey information to the nucleus that such receptors have been activated. The name for this group of genes is derived from their capacity to undergo constitutive change to *oncogenes*, characterized by inappropriate expression of the gene in conjunction with neoplastic behaviour of the cell (Pierce *et al.* 1986).

The genetic code for an oncogene is carried in the RNA sequence of certain RNA retroviruses, and is converted into a DNA copy by viral reverse transcriptase after the virus has infected a susceptible strain of animal or bird. The segment of DNA is incorporated permanently into the DNA of the nucleus, and can result in the development of neoplastic behaviour. There is no evidence that retrovirus infection is a common cause of neoplasia in humans, although it does cause a relatively uncommon variant of T lymphocytic leukaemia. There are, however, mechanisms that serve as means for activation of oncogenes, other than introduction of an oncogene into nuclear DNA as the reverse transcript of part of the genome of an infecting retrovirus. These mechanisms include changes as small as *point mutations* in the proto-oncogene, formation of multiple copies of the proto-oncogene, or *gene amplification*, and of particular relevance to human leukaemia, rearrangement of DNA by *translocations of chromosomal material* (Pierce *et al.* 1986).

An example of conversion of a proto-oncogene to an oncogene by chromosome translation is the activation of the Abelson cellular proto-oncogene

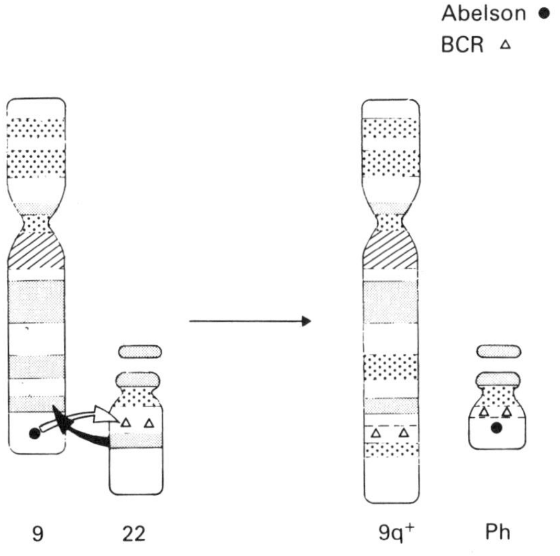

Fig. 10.1. *Formation of the Philadelphia (Ph) chromosome by reciprocal translocation of parts of the long arms of chromosomes 9 and 22. The Ph chromosome and the abnormal chromosome 9q+ persist and are replicated along with the other chromosomes in proliferating chronic myeloid leukaemic cells. The translocation shifts the Abelson gene into the BCR site on chromosome 22, and this alters the regulation of its expression.*

(c-abl) by the translocation which results in the formation of the *Philadelphia chromosome*, recognized many years previously as an association with chronic myeloid leukaemia (Nowell & Hungerford 1961). In this reciprocal translocation between two chromosomes, the c-abl on part of chromosome 9 is transferred into the breakpoint cluster region (BCR) of chromosome 22, as shown in Fig. 10.1. At the same time, part of the long arm of chromosome 22 is transferred onto the long arm of chromosome 9. It appears that segments of c-abl DNA are joined to a DNA sequence in chromosome 22 which results in ongoing production of an Abelson protein with altered structure and function. It is uncertain how this is related to the specific features of chronic myeloid leukaemia, and there appear to be other factors involved in the type of malignant change associated with inappropriate activation of the c-abl proto-oncogene. The Philadelphia chromosome may, for example, be the sole chromosomal abnormality in a form of acute lymphoblastic leukaemia, indicating there are other influences affecting the characteristics of the neoplastic process. Tumours produced in animals by retroviral introduction of this oncogene are also usually different in character from chronic myeloid leukaemia.

It is commonly held that inappropriate activation of other genes involved in critical steps in cellular proliferation may be promoted by other types of chromosome translocation, and result in the genesis of other forms of leukaemia. Another commonly held view is that permanent changes in nuclear DNA occur in a stepwise manner, and that the outcome of the accumulation of abnormalities is malignant behaviour.

Chromosome abnormalities

Chromosome abnormalities are very common in leukaemia, and occur in all major categories of the acute and chronic forms of the disorder. Usually, the abnormality is maintained in a consistent manner in a particular case, in keeping with a defect that is replicated with a high degree of fidelity in the clone of cells arising from the cell in which malignant behaviour first developed. Sometimes, additional changes occur at the time the characteristics of the leukaemia alter, suggesting the abnormalities of the chromosomes are directly involved in abnormal cellular behaviour.

Not all cases of leukaemia have chromosome abnormalities detectable at the microscopic level with currently available techniques. The introduction of banding and specialized staining methods markedly enhanced the precision with which abnormalities in chromosomes could be identified, and it is now possible to recognize translocations between chromosomes which would not have been previously possible. Other types of abnormalities involving chromosomes include addition or deletion of chromosomes, deletion of parts of chromosomes, and formation of chromosomes that are not identifiable as originating from any particular normal chromosome. More than half of all cases of acute leukaemia have chromosome abnormalities, and it is argued that improvement in techniques for delineating chromosome structure are likely to reveal an even higher incidence of deletions, additions, and translocations.

A number of correlations exist between laboratory features or clinical behaviour of leukaemic processes and specific chromosome abnormalities, such as the translocation between the long arms of chromosomes 15 and 17 in acute promyelocytic leukaemia (Fig. 10.2). Other instances are the correlations between specific chromosome abnormalities and disorders with relatively good, or relatively bad, prognosis (Bloomfield *et al.* 1986). Associations between particular types of chromosome abnormality and specific properties of neoplastic processes incriminate chromosome abnormalities as playing an important role in the genesis of specific characteristics of neoplastic activity (Rowley 1984), although it remains to be clarified whether chromosome abnormalities could be secondary consequences of another event which

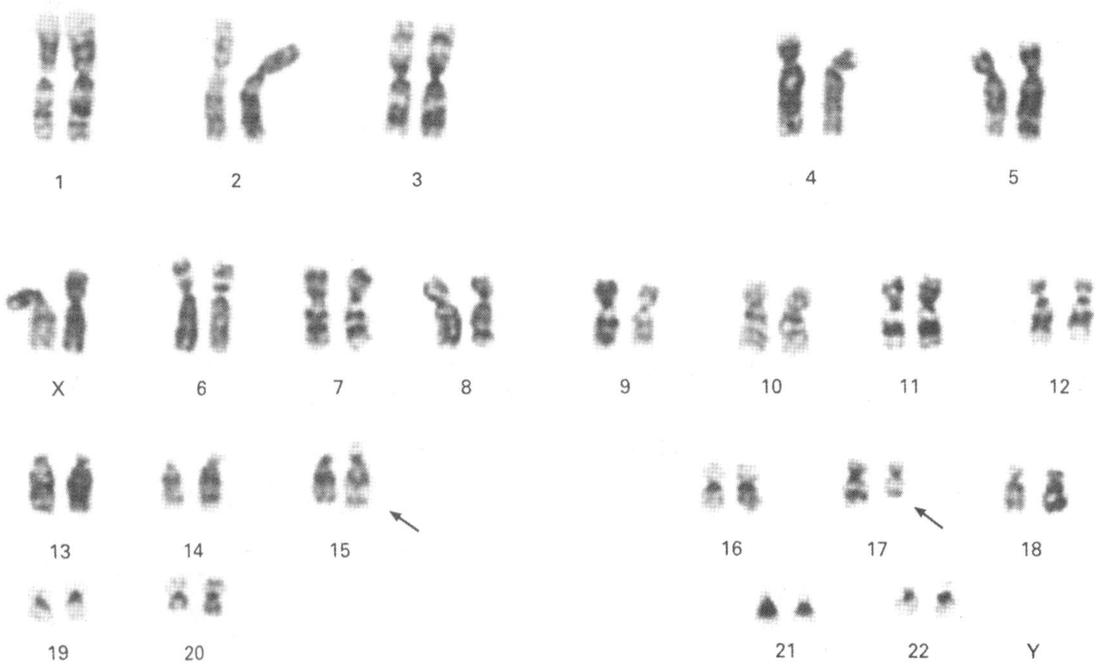

Fig. 10.2. *Chromosomes in acute promyelocytic leukaemia. Giemsa-banded preparation. Arrows indicate addition of material to long arms of one chromosome 15 and loss of material from long arms of one chromosome 17. Result of reciprocal translocation between these chromosomes. This abnormality is difficult to identify with certainty in unbanded preparations. (Courtesy, Department of Cytogenetics, St Vincent's Hospital, Melbourne.)*

is responsible for malignant behaviour. One currently held hypothesis is that changes may occur in DNA which produce a clone of cells predisposed to undergo further change, which in turn results in emergence of an overtly leukaemic cell clone containing particular chromosome abnormalities.

Radiation

There is evidence that ionizing radiation, especially X-irradiation, is leukaemogenic, and that the incidence of leukaemia increases with the cumulative dose received. An increase in the incidence of leukaemia was first noted in irradiated survivors of the atom bomb blast three years after the event, and the incidence peaked after 6–7 years (Bizzozero *et al.* 1966). Patients with ankylosing spondylitis treated with radiotherapy also experienced a dose-related increase in incidence of leukaemia, reaching a maximum incidence of at least several times the average expectancy about six years after irradiation (Court Brown & Abbat 1955). Acute leukaemia and chronic myeloid leukaemia occurred in both irradiated groups. Patients treated with radiotherapy for lymphoma subsequently develop leukaemic or myelodysplastic disorders, but more commonly when cytotoxic chemotherapy is also administered. The incidence of secondary haematological malignancy is relatively high in this group, affecting about three per cent of long-term survivors (Canellos *et al.* 1983). Concern is also expressed over an increased incidence of leukaemia in children who are exposed to diagnostic X-ray *in utero*. The mechanism linking irradiation with development of leukaemia up to many years later is unclear, but it is perhaps relevant that irradiation produces chromosome abnormalities (Buckton *et al.* 1962), although these take the form of random breaks rather than specific abnormalities in chromosome structure.

Chemicals

Leukaemia is more common in people who have been exposed for substantial periods to *benzene* vapour, and the risk of developing leukaemia has been suggested to increase with the extent of cumulative exposure (Rinsky *et al.* 1987). Leukaemia also occurs more commonly in subjects who have taken cytotoxic agents which, as in the case of radiotherapy, produce an increase in the incidence of chromosome breakage. The drugs most commonly implicated are *alkylating agents*, such as chlorambucil, melphalan, procarbazine, and nitrosureas. This problem thus affects patients who have received these drugs for treatment, for example, of multiple myeloma, polycythaemia vera, lymphoma, ovarian cancer, and breast cancer (Rosner & Grünwald 1980, Pedersen-Bjergaard *et al.* 1987).

Viruses

Various forms of leukaemia in animals and birds serve as models for the generation of leukaemia as a result of infection by retroviruses. Leukaemogenic viruses carry their genetic information in RNA, and after infecting a cell, produce a DNA copy by means of the enzyme *reverse transcriptase*, which they contain. The DNA copy, or provirus, is incorporated into the DNA of the nucleus, where it is replicated by the cell along with the host nuclear DNA. Malignant transformation is regularly induced when the viral genome contains an *oncogene*. Oncogenes are believed to be derived from vertebrate proto-oncogenes whose code has been incorporated into infecting retroviral RNA in such a way that it is not normally regulated when reintroduced into inappropriate sites in the DNA of the nucleus, thereby resulting in neoplastic behaviour. Some leukaemogenic retroviruses do not contain oncogenes. Multiple copies of the provirus are inserted into nuclear DNA, and leukaemia develops only in some infected individuals. With this type of virus, development of neoplasia is apparently dependent on chance incorporation of the provirus at an appropriate site (Gallo & Wong-Staal 1982, Weiss & Marshall 1984, Evan & Lennox 1985).

A retrovirus has been identified which can cause an uncommon form of leukaemia in humans. It is designated HTLV-I, for human T cell lymphotrophic virus type I, as it infects T lymphocytes and these cells may evolve into T lymphocytic leukaemia–lymphoma. Infection with the virus is endemic in certain parts of the world, such as southern Japan, the Caribbean, South America, and Central Africa (Sarin & Gallo 1983). The provirus is randomly incorporated into nuclear DNA, and this does not normally result in neoplastic activity. A second event, yet to be clarified, is responsible for development of malignant properties, and a monoclonal T-leukaemic cell population emerges as a result (Broder & Gallo 1985).

Genetic factors

There are occasional clusters of cases of leukaemia in families to suggest genetic factors may be involved, but this is the exception as the disease does not normally occur in an inherited fashion (Gunz & Henderson 1983). A number of disorders in which there are inherited abnormalities of nuclear DNA are, on the other hand, associated with an increased incidence of leukaemia. Children with Down's syndrome, for example, have an increased incidence of leukaemia associated with the presence of the additional chromosome 21 in the cells of the tissues. Inherited disorders such as Fanconi's anaemia, Bloom's syndrome, and ataxia telangiectasia are associated with an increased incidence of leukaemia, and have in common an increased tendency for chromosome breakage, as occurs in irradiated individuals.

Classification

Leukaemia occurs in a number of forms which differ in their clinical, pathological, and haematological features. The two main criteria used in classification are the clinical course of the disease, and the type and degree of differentiation of the predominant leukaemic cell population as revealed by morphological examination of the blood and bone marrow. Leukaemias are therefore classified as *acute and chronic*, according to the clinical course, and *myeloid and lymphoid*, according to the cell line predominantly involved in the leukaemic process. Several other morphologically defined varieties are recognized, and are referred to during the course of this chapter.

Acute leukaemias generally pursue an aggressive clinical course which, unless modified by treatment, rapidly results in death in the great majority of patients. Although the dominant cell is usually an immature 'blast' cell, it is possible to recognize within the myeloid and lymphoid categories, a number of subtypes with characteristic morphological patterns. A group of French, American, and British haematologists has described a classification system which has achieved a high degree of acceptance (the FAB classification), and is based on blood and bone marrow morphological features defined by Romanovsky and cytochemical staining (Bennett *et al.* 1976, 1985). Leukaemia is classified in this system as acute when more than 30 per cent of the bone marrow consists of blast cells. It divides acute myeloid leukaemia into seven subgroups, and acute lymphoblastic leukaemia into three subgroups (Table 10.1)

Chronic leukaemias are also divided basically into lymphoid and myeloid categories, and tend to be more indolent in behaviour. The characteristic cell in chronic lymphocytic leukaemia is the mature lymphocyte, and in chronic granulocytic leukaemia, the myelocyte.

Disorders that do not completely fulfil the criteria for either acute or chronic leukaemia are relatively common. Blast cells are present in smaller proportions, and the course of the disease is less aggressive than acute leukaemia. These conditions are more commonly seen in middle-aged and elderly patients, and have been termed 'indolent acute', or 'smouldering' leukaemia (Greenberg 1983). Conditions of this type form part of the spectrum of disorders collectively referred to as the *myelodysplastic syndrome*, which embraces conditions that are relatively benign, such as acquired refractory sideroblastic anaemia, through to disorders that frequently progress to acute leukaemia.

Incidence

In many parts of the world, increasing numbers of cases of leukaemia have been reported in the past 40 years. While this may be due in part to more accurate diagnosis of leukaemia, there appears to be an increase in the incidence of leukaemia, particularly of acute leukaemia and chronic lymphocytic leukaemia.

Table 10.1. *Acute leukaemia: FAB classification*

Acute myeloid leukaemia (AML) or acute non-lymphoblastic leukaemia (ANLL)

M1 *Myeloblastic leukaemia without maturation*
Myeloblasts with non-granular cytoplasm or rare azurophil granules/Auer rods; more mature myeloid cells not present; some blast cells myeloperoxidase positive.

M2 *Myeloblastic leukaemia with maturation*
Promyelocytes and more mature myeloid cells in addition to myeloblasts; myeloid cells myeloperoxidase positive.

M3 *Hypergranular promyelocytic leukaemia*
Most cells myeloperoxidase-positive promyelocytes with heavy cytoplastic granulation and reniform nuclei; multiple Auer rods, often in parallel bundles ('faggots'); also rare hypogranular type.

M4 *Myelomonocytic leukaemia*
Immature and mature cells of both myeloid (myeloperoxidase positive) and monocytic (non-specific esterase positive) lineage.

M5 *Monocytic leukaemia*
Poorly differentiated type (M5a): non-specific esterase-positive monoblasts with non-granular cytoplasm or rare azurophil granules/Auer rods. Differentiated type (M5b): promonocytes and monocytes in addition to monoblasts.

M6 *Erythroleukaemia*
Erythroblasts >50 per cent of marrow nucleated cells; myeloblasts and promyelocytes increased. Erythroblasts (usually present in peripheral blood) often strongly Periodic-Acid-Schiff stain positive and possess morphological abnormalities.

M7 *Megakaryoblastic leukaemia*
Megakaryoblasts, some with cytoplasmic budding; positive platelet peroxidase reaction on electron microscopy and reactivity to monoclonal antibodies specific for platelet-specific surface antigens.

Acute lymphoblastic leukaemia (ALL)

L1 Homogeneous small lymphoblasts; scanty cytoplasm, regular round nuclei, inconspicuous nucleoli.

L2 Heterogeneous lymphoblasts; variable amounts of cytoplasm, irregular or cleft nuclei, large nucleoli.

L3 Large homogeneous lymphoblasts; basophilic cytoplasm, round nuclei, prominent nucleoli, cytoplasmic vacuolation.

A variable proportion of the lymphoblasts in some cases of ALL L1 and L2 show strong granular PAS positivity. Lymphoblasts in T-cell ALL usually show a focal paranuclear area of positivity when stained for acid phosphatase.

Analysis of early reports on the relative incidence of the acute and chronic forms of the disease suggested that chronic leukaemia was much more common than acute leukaemia, and that acute leukaemia was predominantly a disease of childhood. However, the acute form of leukaemia is now as common as the chronic form, and is more common in adults than in children.

Acute leukaemia

Clinical features

Acute leukaemia may occur at any age. In children, the incidence is highest in the first six years of life; in adults, it occurs at all ages and is not uncommon in middle-aged and elderly persons. Acute leukaemia in children, especially young children, is usually lymphoblastic in type, while in adults it is usually myeloid.

The clinical picture in the principal types is largely indistinguishable, although certain features such as gum hypertrophy and ulcerative lesions of the rectum and vagina are more common in the myelomonocytic (M4) than in the other types. Lymph node enlargement is more common in lymphoblastic leukaemia.

The *onset* of symptoms may be abrupt or insidious. In general, an abrupt onset is more common in children and young adults. The most common mode of presentation is with symptoms of anaemia or haemorrhage, infective lesions of the mouth and pharynx, fever, prostration, headache, and malaise. Presenting problems may occur either singly or in combination, and are listed in Table 10.2. In about one-half of all cases of acute leukaemia in childhood there is a history of infection, frequently respiratory, antedating the apparent onset of leukaemia by several weeks or months.

Bleeding manifestations such as skin petechiae and bruises are common. Bleeding from the gums and nose is also common, and persistent bleeding after tooth extraction or tonsillectomy occasionally first brings the condition to notice. Gastrointestinal, renal tract, uterine, and nervous system haemorrhage commonly occur in the course of the disease. Impairment of vision and deafness or vertigo may result from haemorrhage into the eye and ear respectively. There is a relation between bleeding and fever, the onset of fever sometimes being accompanied by the first appearance of haemorrhage, or by an increase in its severity. Sudden onset of a profound haemorrhagic tendency may be due to development of disseminated intravascular coagulation, a condition associated with acute promyelocytic leukaemia (M3).

Table 10.2. *Presenting manifestations of acute leukaemia*

Common
Anaemia
Fever, malaise
Haemorrhage, bruising, petechiae
Less common
Infection of the mouth and pharynx
Pains in bones and joints (childhood especially)
Upper respiratory tract infection (childhood especially)
Superficial lymph node enlargement (childhood especially)
Occasional
Abdominal pain
Mediastinal obstruction (childhood especially)
Nervous system abnormalities
Skin rash
Gum hypertrophy

Infective lesions of the mouth and throat are frequent. The patient may complain of a sore throat, ulceration of the gums, mouth, or pharynx, or an upper respiratory tract infection. Patients with marked oral sepsis or gingival hypertrophy may first consult a dentist. Lesions in the mouth and pharynx vary in severity from small necrotic ulcers to areas of marked swelling, with extensive necrosis and ulceration. These lesions can be extremely painful. The gums are frequently infected, and necrosis, ulceration, and bleeding may be present. In a few cases there is a true hypertrophy of the gingivae, with marked swelling and heaping up of the gum margin so that the teeth appear almost buried in the gums. This type of gingival hypertrophy is especially characteristic of myelomonocytic (M4) and monocytic leukaemia (M5), although it does occur less commonly in the other forms. It represents tissue infiltration by leukaemia.

Infections are common and may be the presenting feature. They include upper and lower respiratory tract infection, cellulitis, paronychia, bacteraemia, and otitis media. Respiratory tract infection is particularly prominent in children. Susceptibility to infection is due mainly to neutropenia, but a diminished immune response plays a contributing role.

Constitutional symptoms such as fever, malaise, rigors, prostration, and generalized aches and pains are common, especially in patients with infection. However, they may occur in the absence of an obvious site of infection, in which case blood cultures should be performed, as septicaemia may be present. Fever can be especially high in children, temperatures of 39–41°C being not uncommon.

The *liver* and *spleen* can be slightly to moderately enlarged. Enlargement of the spleen below the umbilicus can occur, but is unusual. Enlargement tends to be more pronounced in children than in adults. Ulceration, or even infiltration of the alimentary tract, occasionally results in *abdominal pain* or *diarrhoea*. Ulcerative lesions of the *rectum* and *vagina*, anal fissures, and peri-anal abscesses are relatively common.

The *lymph nodes* may be slightly or moderately enlarged, especially in lymphoblastic leukaemia. However, in many cases they are not palpable, or are only very slightly enlarged when the patient first presents. Enlargement tends to be more pronounced in children. Because of the frequency of oral and pharyngeal sepsis, the cervical nodes are more often enlarged than nodes in other areas, and they are frequently tender.

Pain and tenderness in the bones and about the joints may occur, especially in children. *Tenderness of the sternum*, most marked over the lower end, is occasionally present. Apart from tenderness, there is usually no clinical evidence of bone involvement. In a few cases, the clinical picture of acute osteomyelitis is simulated by the presence of swelling, redness, and tenderness of bones, usually close to the joint. Joint manifestations include migratory joint pain, persistent pain in one or more joints, and the local manifestations of heat, redness, and swelling. The bone pain in children may cause them to stop walking. This picture may resemble acute rheumatic fever. X-ray changes in bones may be present, particularly in children, and consist of destruction of the cortex with thinning and erosion, and periostitis, with periosteal elevation and the formation of new subperiosteal bone, most frequently at the metaphyseal ends of the long bones. Epiphyseal growth may be disturbed.

The most common finding in the *cardiovascular system* is tachycardia, a result of either anaemia or infection, or a combination of both. Pericarditis may occur due to haemorrhage, infiltration with leukaemic cells, or viral or bacterial infection.

Involvement of the *central nervous system* results from either haemorrhage, infection, or infiltration with leukaemia, the latter being a common problem in children. *Intracerebral haemorrhage* represents a very serious event, occurring especially in patients with a rapidly rising white cell count, profound thrombocytopenia, or disseminated intravascular coagulation.

Meningeal involvement (meningeal leukaemia) was seen very commonly in children, often during haematological remission. More adults with acute leukaemia are achieving long remissions, and as a result an increasing incidence is being observed in this group. Meningeal leukaemia is manifested by signs of raised intracranial pressure, with headache, vomiting, papilloedema, meningismus, and irritability; these can occur singly or together. Cranial nerve palsies may develop. The cerebrospinal fluid often is at increased pressure, with an elevated content of protein and cells. Careful examination of the cells with appropriate staining on cytocentrifuge preparations frequently provides the diagnosis. The possibility of meningeal leukaemia should be considered in a patient, especially a child, who develops unexplained headache or vomiting, either in remission or relapse. Less frequently, the patient presents with focal neurological signs. Occasionally, signs of spinal cord compression develop, which may progress to paraplegia. The incidence of meningeal leukaemia is greater in subjects with acute lymphoblastic leukaemia in haematological remission where there has been no effective prophylactic treatment of the central nervous system, than in patients with disease of recent onset.

In the *mucocutaneous* tissues there can be infiltration which can cause irregular hypertrophic lesions.

Haemorrhages into the retina are common. Leukaemic infiltration can also occur and cause perivascular sheathing, and even thickening of the retina, with a change in colour to pale green or orange, has been described.

Urine. A minor degree of albuminuria is common. Microscopic examination may show red cells, as bleeding into the urinary tract can occur because of the haemorrhagic tendency. *Renal insufficiency* can develop especially after treatment, as a result of the various nephrotoxic influences operating in sick individuals experiencing sepsis, exposure to multiple drugs including antibiotics, decreased perfusion, and increased urate excretion.

Blood picture

The 'typical' blood picture is of anaemia and thrombocytopenia, with a moderate or marked increase in white cells, the majority of which are 'blast' cells.

Anaemia is virtually inevitable. It is characteristically progressive and severe, but the rate of progression varies from patient to patient. The red cells usually are moderately anisocytic and poikilocytic, sometimes with mild polychromasia. In some cases, macrocytes are prominent. A moderate increase in reticulocytes up to five per cent can occur, and a small number of nucleated red cells may be seen in the blood film. Nucleated red cells are sometimes a major feature of the blood film in erythroleukaemia (M6).

Thrombocytopenia is also extremely common, often being severe, with platelet counts well below $50 \times 10^9/l$.

The total white cell count ranges between subnormal to markedly elevated values. As a progressive rise in white cell count is usual, counts may exceed $100 \times 10^9/l$, especially in advanced disease. In about 25 per cent of patients, the total white cell count at the onset is reduced, ranging from 1 to $4 \times 10^9/l$. In one large series of patients, the tendency was for white cell counts to be lower in acute myeloid leukaemia categories M2 and M3 (Sultan *et al.* 1981). The majority of leucocytes are usually blast cells, and there is often neutropenia. In occasional patients with low white cell counts, blast cells may be present in very small numbers, and a careful search of the film may have to be made before they are detected. A film made from the buffy coat of centrifuged blood may enable blast cells to be detected more easily under these circumstances. In rare cases, no immature white cells are detected in the blood film after careful inspection. Occasionally, the white cell count remains low, and in very rare cases blast cells cannot be found in the peripheral blood at any stage of the disease.

The very basic morphological features of typical myeloblasts, lymphoblasts, and monoblasts are similar. They are usually cells between 10 and 18 μm in diameter, with a round or oval nucleus, and one or more nucleoli (Fig. 10.3). The cytoplasm is moderately to deeply basophilic, and contains few if any granules. Vacuolation of both cytoplasm and nucleus may occur in certain categories. The cytoplasm of myeloblasts may contain one or more Auer rods, which are red, splinter-shaped inclusions.

In the various forms of acute leukaemia as defined by the FAB classification, the range of cell types in the peripheral blood generally mirrors the abnormal population in the bone marrow. Thus, in acute myeloid leukaemia M1 category, the great majority of nucleated cells in the blood are myeloblasts. More mature myeloid cells are present in addition to myeloblasts in M2, and hypergranular promyelocytes are characteristic of M3. Cells of both myeloid and monocytic lineage are seen in M4, and monocytes, promonocytes, and monoblasts predominate in M5.

The more mature cells in each acute myeloid leukaemia category often contain distinctive morphological abnormalities, for example, reduced or absent secondary granulation, and Pelger–Hüet bilobed nuclear configuration in mature granulocytes. In the acute lymphoblastic leukaemias, in addition to typical blast cells, there are usually some mature lymphocytes, and 'smear' cells, which

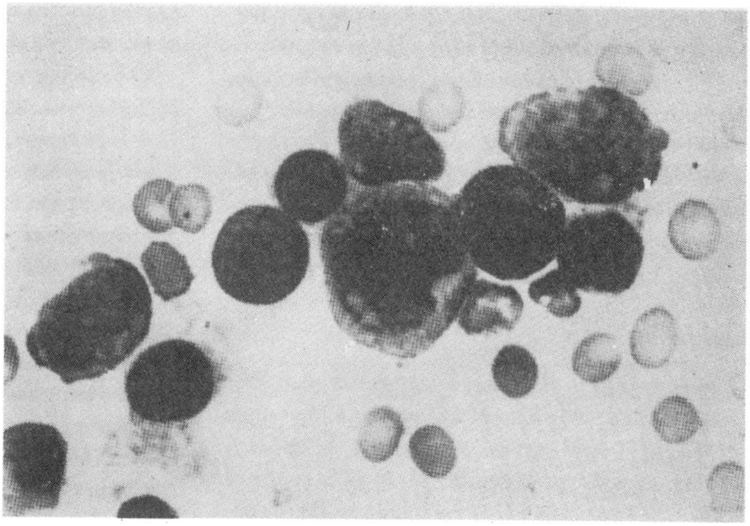

Fig. 10.3. *Acute leukaemia bone marrow aspirate showing several myeloblasts. Protomicrograph (× 520).*

represent cells damaged during preparation of the blood film.

Bone marrow

Morphology. The aspirated marrow fragments in acute leukaemia are characteristically numerous and fleshy. However, because of hypercellularity or associated fibrosis in the marrow, a 'blood tap' is not uncommon, and occasionally a 'dry tap' occurs. In such cases, an imprint of bone marrow cells should be prepared by making appropriate contact between the bone marrow trephine specimen and a glass slide.

Fragments are most commonly, but not always, tightly packed with cells. The cell trails released as the fragments pass along the slide are hypercellular, and although the pattern of cells varies according to the FAB type, blast cells are usually the outstanding feature (see Table 10.1). Cells in mitosis are common. Erythropoietic cells are reduced, and sometimes almost completely absent. Dyserythropoiesis is common—the erythroblasts may be larger than normal, contain nuclear abnormalities, and may have megaloblastic features. Occasionally, substantial numbers of ring sideroblasts (p. 57) are present. Megakaryocytes are usually reduced or absent.

The FAB classification designates a proportion of blast cells of 30 per cent or more as an essential criterion for the diagnosis of acute leukaemia. Similar conditions with less than 30 per cent blast cells are classified as myelodysplastic disorders.

These criteria apply to most cases of acute leukaemia. However, the appearance of the bone marrow is occasionally atypical; thus, it is on occasion hypocellular or normocellular, and in erythroleukaemia (M6) the erythroid series by definition make up a large proportion of the bone marrow cells.

Chromosomes. Examination of bone marrow chromosomes reveals abnormalities in up to 75 per cent of cases, and it has been postulated that improvements in technique which result in greater resolution of chromosome fine structure will enable an even higher proportion of chromosome abnormalities to be detected in acute leukaemia. The nature of the karyotype has a relationship to prognosis, and a number of patterns have been identified which are associated with shorter or longer survival with currently employed chemotherapy (Bloomfield *et al.* 1986, Garson 1988). Presence of the Philadelphia chromosome, or translocations between chromosomes 4 and 11, or chromosomes 8 and 14, for example, have been suggested to be an independent prognostic factor for poor prognosis in acute lymphoblastic leukaemia. A number of other karyotype abnormalities have a high degree of specificity for particular forms of acute leukaemia, such as promyelocytic leukaemia (reciprocal translocation between chromosomes 15 and 17), and a subtype of myelomonocytic leukaemia (internal inversion of part of chromosome 16) (see pp. 237–9).

Diagnosis

In many cases the diagnosis is straightforward. The clinical picture calls for a blood examination which reveals the typical picture of anaemia, thrombocytopenia, and the presence of 'blast' cells, with or without leucocytosis. The diagnosis is then confirmed by marrow aspiration.

TYPE OF LEUKAEMIA

The type of leukaemia is determined by consideration of the morphological features of the leukaemic cells in the blood and marrow as seen in the Romanovsky-stained films. *Cytochemical stains* and estimation of the serum lysozyme give useful supplementary information. *Cell surface markers* defined by reactions with monoclonal antibodies have become particularly useful in classification of leukaemias, as antigens specific for immature lymphoid, erythroid, and megakaryocytic cells can be identified by this means.

Romanovsky stain. The principle features of the various morphological types are summarized in Table 10.1.

Cytochemical stains. Cytochemistry is an adjunct to Romanovsky staining in determining the category of leukaemia. The pattern of staining may indicate whether blasts fit best into the myeloid, lymphoid, or monocyte series. In acute leukaemia, the most useful cytochemical stains and their reaction patterns with immature cells are listed below.

Myeloperoxidase and Sudan Black B. Positive in some immature cells, especially of myeloid and, to a lesser extent, of monocytic series,

Periodic·acid Schiff (PAS). Positive in some immature lymphoid cells and sometimes in erythroblasts in erythroleukaemia (M6);

Non-specific esterase. Positive reaction, inhibited by sodium fluoride, in monocytic series;

Acid phosphatase. Focal positive reaction in T cell acute lymphoblastic leukaemia blast cells, diffuse reaction in monocytic cells.

Cytochemical·stains are discussed in detail by Flandrin & Daniel (1981), and in Dacie & Lewis (1984).

Serum lysozyme (muramidase). Estimation of the serum level of lysozyme is of value in the diagnosis of myelomonocytic (M4) and monocytic (M5) leukaemia, in which the level can be very high (Firkin 1972). Renal failure also causes elevation of the serum lysozyme level, which is accordingly of diagnostic value primarily in patients with a normal plasma creatinine level.

Cell surface markers. Antigens and receptors on the surface of normal haemopoietic cells at various stages of differentiation may also be present on leukaemic 'blast' cells of the same lineage. It is thus possible to classify acute leukaemia not only by conventional morphological criteria, but also in terms of cell surface markers. This has been particularly helpful in the lymphoblastic leukaemias, and several subtypes, each with a particular combination of cell surface and intracellular markers, have been identified. These subtypes do not necessarily conform to the morphologically-defined subgroups in the FAB classification, and the various cell surface marker patterns have clinical and prognostic implications in their own right (Greaves 1981).

Surface markers used for classification of acute lymphoblastic leukaemia are:

1 Immunoglobulin bound to the cell surface membrane (SIg), a B lymphoid cell marker;

2 Sheep erythrocyte (E) rosette formation, a T lymphoid cell surface marker equating with the T11 surface antigen;

3 Surface and internal antigens detected by the use of specific antibodies. These include the common acute lymphoblastic leukaemia (cALL) antigen, T and B lymphoid cell surface antigens, and cytoplasmic μ chains, whose presence in the absence of SIg serves as an index of pre-B cell status. Estimation of

Table 10.3. *Acute lymphoblastic leukaemia: immunophenotypes*

Type	Characteristic features	Frequency
Common	cALL antigen Pan B antigen	+++++
T	E rosette formation Pan T antigen	++/+
pre-T	No E rosette formation Pan T antigen	+
B	SIg	+
pre-B	Cytoplasmic μ chains only	+/−
Null	No definitive markers	++

deoxynucleotidyl transferase (TdT) by immunofluorescence after reaction with monoclonal anti-TdT is also useful in the diagnosis of acute lymphoblastic leukaemia, in which levels are high, in contrast to most cases of acute myeloblastic leukaemia.

With these techniques, acute lymphoblastic leukaemia can be divided into various subtypes as summarized in Table 10.3.

Other diagnostic methods. Electron microscopy is occasionally useful in the diagnosis of undifferentiated leukaemias, and in the identification of megakaryoblastic leukaemia (M7), a rare form in which the blast cells show a characteristic ultrastructural pattern of peroxidase activity (Huang *et al.* 1984). It is, however, a time-consuming procedure and is rarely employed in diagnostic laboratories.

Differential diagnosis

Differentiation must be made from other disorders which present in a similar manner, and from disorders with a blood picture resembling acute leukaemia.

DISORDERS WITH SIMILAR CLINICAL FEATURES

Other causes of ulceration of the throat. A major problem is differentiation from *infectious mononucleosis,* as in both conditions fever, ulceration of the throat, lymphadenopathy and splenomegaly are associated with the appearance of atypical white cells in the blood. Other causes of ulceration of the throat are *acute tonsillitis, Vincent's angina, diphtheria* and *agranulocytic angina,* which are differentiated by haematological and microbiological investigation.

Other causes of joint and bone pain. A diagnosis of *rheumatic fever* may be considered in children presenting with joint pains, as the two conditions have a number of features in common, including joint pains, fever, pallor, anaemia, a systolic bruit, epistaxis, and tachycardia. Polymorph leucocytosis is usual in acute rheumatic fever, whereas neutropenia is the rule is acute leukaemia. Occasionally, when there is marked reddening, swelling, or tenderness of one joint, *osteomyelitis* may be suspected, especially in children.

Other causes of fever and malaise. These include subacute bacterial endocarditis, influenza, upper respiratory tract infections, septicaemia, typhoid fever, brucellosis, and lymphoma.

Cases presenting with *acute abdominal pain, mediastinal obstruction, skin rash,* or *nervous system involvement* must be differentiated from other causes of such conditions.

DISORDERS WITH A SIMILAR BLOOD PICTURE

Myelodysplastic syndromes (p. 258). Significant degrees of anaemia, neutropenia and thrombocytopenia, accompanied by blast cells in the peripheral blood, commonly occur in these disorders, which may be effectively distinguished from acute leukaemia only by a lower proportion of blast cells in the bone marrow aspirate.

A leukaemoid blood picture. The blood picture in infectious mononucleosis (p. 231) is the one most commonly confused with that of acute lymphoblastic leukaemia. Other leukaemoid blood pictures simulating acute leukaemia are uncommon, occurring rarely in infections, including tuberculosis, where the pattern of myeloid precursors in the blood is more in keeping with less fulminant forms of leukaemia (p. 272).

Other causes of pancytopenia must be differentiated from 'subleukaemic' acute leukaemia in which few or no blast cells are observed in the peripheral blood film (p. 244).

Course and prognosis

Before the introduction of antileukaemic therapeutic agents, survival varied from a few weeks to about 10 months, with an average of about 20 weeks in unequivocal acute leukaemia. Longer survivals of 12 months or more occur in untreated disorders which formerly have been classified as acute leukaemia, but would now be designated as myelodysplastic conditions using FAB classification criteria. Spontaneous remissions are very rare, and current experience would indicate the proportion is very much less than considered to be the case three decades ago (Southam *et al.* 1951).

In untreated disease, anaemia is an outstanding feature but can usually be corrected without difficulty by red cell transfusions. It is the infective and haemorrhagic manifestations that eventually produce the major clinical problems, and ultimately are directly responsible for death in the majority of patients.

The most important factor influencing prognosis is whether sustained complete remission is attained by treatment. Prognosis has been greatly altered in childhood lymphoblastic leukaemia by the introduction of effective measures for eradicating disease from the bone marrow and central nervous system. Average survival is greatly extended, and in the L1 form the majority are free of disease five years after presentation. Outcome is less satisfactory in other subtypes of acute leukaemia, including all forms encountered in adults, but the frequency of response to chemotherapeutic agents is sufficiently high to raise the prospect of more prolonged remissions with the introduction of more effective management programmes (Table 10.4).

Treatment

Treatment is considered in the following order:

general considerations;
specific therapeutic agents;
therapy in the individual patient;
symptomatic and supportive therapy.

General considerations

Conservative approaches to the management of acute leukaemia have now been generally superseded by aggressive combination chemotherapy, combined with antibiotic supportive measures and platelet transfusions to combat infection and bleeding, respectively. Such *remission-induction treatment* entails a high degree of morbidity at the time, but the significant prolongation of life that follows successful remission-induction, coupled with the greatly improved quality of life during complete remission, is the reason why it has become accepted as the standard approach to management in the absence of overriding considerations, such as extremes of age or infirmity due to other conditions which have a poor prognosis in their own right. Attainment of *complete remission* entails loss of all abnormal clinical and routine diagnostic laboratory findings attributable to the leukaemia, and return to good health. Peripheral blood and bone marrow parameters return to normal, and therefore morphologically normal blast cells make up fewer than five per cent of cells in the bone marrow aspirate. Substantial but less extensive improvement is classified as *partial remission* when there is return to reasonable physical health, with significant improvement in abnormal physical signs attributable to the leukaemia, a return of at least two of the three peripheral blood elements to normal values, and a significant reduction in the degree of leukaemic cell infiltration in the bone marrow.

The objects of treatment are eradication of the leukaemic process and control of complications, especially those due to inadequate production of normal blood cells, such as anaemia, infection, and haemorrhage.

Eradication of the leukaemic process involves the use of antileukaemic agents, usually in combination, with supplementary measures such as irradiation for destroying disease in sanctuary sites such as the central nervous system. In many forms of acute leukaemia, the amount of neoplastic tissue is greatly reduced, but not completely eliminated by treatment, and relapse occurs in many instances after a phase of haematological normality described as *complete remission*. Considerable efforts are made to prevent relapse of disease, and this aspect of management is currently the subject of intensive investigation.

Centres for treatment. Treatment should be carried out by highly experienced personnel in hospitals with appropriate supportive facilities. This permits the most effective use of antileukaemic agents in a setting where complications of the drugs, especially severe marrow depression, require specialized management skills. Optimum management is unfortunately beyond the capacity of the conventional general medical hospital unit.

Response to treatment varies with the category of leukaemia, and from case to case, so that it is not possible to predict with precision the nature or duration of a response in the individual patient. Factors that influence outcome in adults treated by current chemotherapy programmes are outlined in Table 10.4, and do not take into consideration the impact that bone marrow transplantation is beginning to make in selected categories of this disease. It is evident that the age of the patient and the morphological type of leukaemia are important in influencing the probability of obtaining complete remission. These two factors are to some extent related, as acute leukaemia in children is much more frequently of the L1 lymphoblastic variety than in adults, and in this form the best responses to treatment are obtained. Children under the age of two years do not respond as well as older children. Complete remissions are obtained in more than 90 per cent of children with acute lymphoblastic leukaemia. Remission is less readily achieved in the less common childhood acute myeloid leukaemia. In adults, complete remissions are obtained in about 70 per cent of cases overall. Remissions occur more readily in the lymphoblastic than in the myeloid forms, but there is now no subclass of acute leukaemia in which useful remission rates have not been reported. Those in which remission is least readily achieved or sustained include acute leukaemia evolving during the course of myeloproliferative disorders, myelodysplastic disorders, and chronic myeloid leukaemia, and secondary to irradiation or alkylating agent therapy.

Thus the important consideration in assessment of outcome of any particular form of therapy is the nature of the leukaemic process, as this can radically affect response to current treatment programmes. An improved prognosis in a particular subtype can

Table 10.4. *Treatment response in adult acute leukaemia*

	Acute myeloid leukaemia	Acute lymphoblastic leukaemia
Remission rate	60–80%	70–90%
Median duration of remission	<2 years	2 years
Prolonged disease-free remissions (>3 years disease-free)	10–40%	20–40%
Lower likelihood of remission	Increasing age Prior myelodysplastic or myeloproliferative disorder Certain types of chromosomal abnormality Prior irradiation or alkylating agent treatment	Increasing age Presence of chromosomal abnormality, certain types in particular High WCC Mediastinal mass
Lower likelihood of prolonged remission	Increasing age High initial WCC, FAB M5, M6 subtype Slow clearance of blasts High initial LDH and fibrinogen Certain types of chromosomal abnormality	Increasing age High initial WCC B & T surface markers present FAB L3 subtype

also be related to introduction of more effective management strategies. For example, after attainment of complete haematological remission in L1 acute lymphoblastic leukaemia in children, addition of steps to treat disease sequestered in the central nervous system by radiotherapy and/or chemotherapy has improved life expectancy. Figures are now being reported of greater than 50 per cent 5-year leukaemia-free survival in this particular type of acute leukaemia, and it appears likely that many children free from disease after 5 years will not undergo subsequent relapse.

Outcome of treatment is currently less encouraging in adults. There has, however, been steady improvement since the introduction of treatment with cytosine arabinoside plus daunorubicin, with an increase in median survival to between 18 months and 2 years, and a significant subpopulation of long-term survivors has been accruing since as early as 1968 (Burchenal 1968). There are also indications that allogenic and autologous bone marrow transplantation performed after induction of complete haematological remission can, in certain categories of acute leukaemia, prolong the duration of remission, and thus prolong survival, as relapse of the disease is usually associated with a less satisfactory response to the initially successful treatment regimen.

Specific therapeutic agents

The most commonly employed agents currently in routine use for induction of remission and for the attempted prolongation of remission are summarized in Table 10.5. Remission-induction therapy is most commonly carried out by administration of a combination of drugs, as this has been found in practice to result in synergism of toxic action on leukaemic cells, as indicated by increased incidence of remission, coupled with reduced toxic side-effects when drugs with differing modes of action are employed. There are also theoretical advantages in the early introduction of several different agents, either at the same time or in close sequence, for obtaining the maximum degree of leukaemic cell killing by elimination of subpopulations of cells that are insensitive to one agent but not another (Goldie *et al.* 1982). Less commonly, in clinically indolent disease or in subjects considered unlikely to tolerate intensive combination chemotherapy, treatment with a single agent is administered.

The most effective drugs in the treatment of acute myeloid leukaemia are cytosine arabinoside and the anthracycline antibiotics, daunorubicin and doxorubicin (Adriamycin). A comparatively recent addition, amsacrine (m-AMSA), is also effective and acts with similar efficacy to the anthracyclines in combination with cytosine arabinoside (with or without 6-thioguanine).

Cytosine arabinoside is effective in certain forms of leukaemia when administered intravenously in *low dosage* regimens of approximately 10–20 mg/m^2/day over extended periods of up to 3 weeks. The *conventional dosage* is of the order of 100 mg/m^2/day over 5–7 days, and improved results are considered to be achieved when delivery is by continuous intravenous infusion, although very similar results are obtained by twice-daily subcutaneous injections in ambulatory outpatients. Bone marrow depression is related in degree to dosage and duration of therapy. *High dosage* treatment of the order of 3000 mg twice daily for 3–6 days has a potent effect on leukaemia, and may produce remission in disease which is unresponsive to conventional doses of cytosine arabinoside (Herzig *et al.* 1983, Preisler *et al.* 1983). Such high dosage treatment is accompanied by a high incidence of cerebellar toxicity, conjunctivitis, fever, rash, mucositis, arthralgia, hepatic dysfunction, as well as prolonged severe bone marrow depression.

Daunorubicin is a highly effective anthracycline which is administered intravenously, with considerable caution, as extravasation is associated with local tissue necrosis. It also produces marrow depression and mucositis. A particular problem associated with this drug and the related anthracycline, Adriamycin (doxorubicin), is *cumulative cardiotoxicity*, which can cause irreversible cardiomyopathy when the total dose exceeds about 500 mg/m^2 (von Hoff *et al.* 1982). Cardiotoxic effects are more problematic in subjects with subnormal myocardial functional reserve, and for this reason these drugs are avoided in the elderly and in subjects with

Table 10.5. *Drugs in established use for treatment of acute leukaemia*

Drug	Nature and probable mode of action	Usual mode of administration	More common toxic effects
Cytosine arabinoside (cytarabine)	After phosphorylation, acts as competitive antagonist of pyrimidine nucleotide synthesis and DNA polymerase	Intravenous or subcutaneous infusion or injection	Nausea, marrow depression, rash, arthralgia
Daunorubicin	Antibiotic produced by *Streptomyces caeruleorubidus* (*Strep. peuceticus*). Inhibits replication and transcription of DNA	Intravenous injection	Marrow depression, cardiotoxicity, alopecia, nausea, vomiting
Doxorubicin (Adriamycin)	C-14 hydroxylated daunorubicin derivative	Intravenous injection	As for daunorubicin
6-thioguanine and 6-mercaptopurine	Purine analogues which interfere with *de novo* nucleotide metabolism, salvage, and re-utilization pathways	Oral	Nausea, vomiting, marrow depression
Amsacrine (m-AMSA)	Synthetic amino acridine, intercalates with DNA, preventing DNA replication and transcription	Intravenous injection	Nausea, vomiting, mucositis, marrow depression, alopecia
Vincristine	Alkaloid of complex structure derived from *Vinca rosea*. Acts probably by disruption of the mitotic spindle	Intravenous injection	Motor and sensory peripheral neuropathy, alopecia, abdominal pain and constipation
Prednisolone or prednisone	Synthetic derivative of hydrocortisone. Cause of cytolysis in neoplastic lymphocytic cells unclear	Oral	Susceptibility to infection, mineralocorticoid effects, diabetes, activation of peptic ulcer, osteoporosis
L-asparaginase	Enzyme derived from micro-organisms, degrades L-asparagine to aspartate and ammonia. Asparagine essential to some malignant cells	Intravenous injection	Anaphylaxis and other hypersensitivity reactions, pancreatitis, hepatic dysfunction
Methotrexate	Folic acid analogue. 4-amino-N_{10}-methyl-pteroylglutamic acid. Blocks folate reductase and inhibits DNA synthesis by preventing production of folinic acid	Intravenous infusion or oral	Mucositis, diarrhoea, marrow depression; occasionally alopecia, hepatic fibrosis

cardiac disease. Elimination of the drug is decreased in hepatic insufficiency, when conventional doses can also cause more serious side-effects.

Thioguanine and mercaptopurine are orally administered agents, degraded by xanthine oxidase, and thus less effectively eliminated when given concurrently with allopurinol, a situation associated with potentially serious toxic effects unless the dosage is appropriately reduced.

Amsacrine (m-AMSA) is approximately as effective in acute myeloid leukaemia as the anthracyclines when administered in combination with cytosine arabinoside. The drug is a synthetic acridine analogue which intercalates with DNA, preventing

DNA from serving as a template for DNA replication or transcription. Severe myelosuppression and mucositis are major side-effects, but an advantage over anthracycline drugs is that m-AMSA is not characteristically associated with cumulative cardiotoxicity.

Acute lymphoblastic leukaemia displays a somewhat different pattern of responsiveness, and vincristine (p. 295), corticosteroids, anthracyclines, and L-asparaginase are the most useful drugs currently available. Other agents used to treat this type of leukaemia include cytosine arabinoside and methotrexate.

Therapy in the individual patient

The general aims of antileukaemic therapy are to induce a remission and to prolong the duration of remission.

In general, different agents are used in the attempt to induce remission in childhood and in adult acute leukaemia. This is related largely to the difference, as previously discussed, in the types of leukaemia encountered in these two age groups, with the L1 form of acute lymphoblastic leukaemia predominating in children and constituting only a very small component of cases of acute leukaemia in adults. There is a tendency for children to be treated as for acute lymphoblastic leukaemia, and for adults to be treated as for myeloid leukaemia, when the morphological type of the leukaemia is unclear.

CHILDHOOD ACUTE LEUKAEMIA

Acute lymphoblastic leukaemia

Remission induction. Administration of vincristine and prednisolone has been a widely accepted means of remission induction, and results in remissions in about 90 per cent of cases. It has become increasingly apparent that for remissions to be sustained in a greater proportion of patients, additional leukaemic cell kill during induction therapy is required (Niemeyer *et al.* 1985). To this end an anthracycline (daunorubicin or doxorubicin), or L-asparaginase, or both, is added to the vincristine and prednisolone, as in the representative treatment programme shown in Fig. 10.4.

A dramatic fall in the number of circulating blast cells may occur within 2–3 days in responsive cases, accompanied by reduction in the degree of splenomegaly and lymphadenopathy. Lysis of the malignant cells is sometimes sufficiently rapid to result in profoundly increased production of uric acid. This can cause rapid onset of impaired renal function, with a rapid rise in plasma creatinine, potassium, and phosphate levels, sometimes accompanied by a correspondingly profound depression of the calcium levels. Such rapid and extreme electrolyte disturbances are conducive to promotion of cardiac arrhythmias, which are potentially fatal.

Prophylactic measures should always be instituted before and during remission induction therapy for this reason, a consideration of especial importance when the blood count of leukaemic cells is high, or marked splenomegaly or lymphadenopathy is present. These measures include administration of *allopurinol* in order to depress urate production. Administration of allopurinol is dangerous in subjects receiving 6-mercaptopurine, unless due allowance is made in the dosage of 6-mercaptopurine for the inhibitory action of allopurinol on its catabolism. Another important step under circumstances where there can be rapid cell lysis in response to therapy is the institution of increased fluid input to facilitate removal of purine degradation products in the urine. The solubility of urate can be increased by alkalinization of the urine, so that the likelihood of insoluble urate deposition in the renal tubules under these circumstances is reduced. *Prophylactic measures of this kind should be instituted during treatment of any neoplastic process where rapid lysis of neoplastic cells is a possibility.*

The degree to which the counts of neutrophils and platelets is depressed specifically by *myelosuppressive effects of treatment* is to a considerable extent related to the nature of the agents employed for remission induction, and to the duration that they are administered—there may be relatively little further depression over that already produced by the disease process when prednisolone and vincristine are employed. Myelosuppression is generally much more severe with daunorubicin,

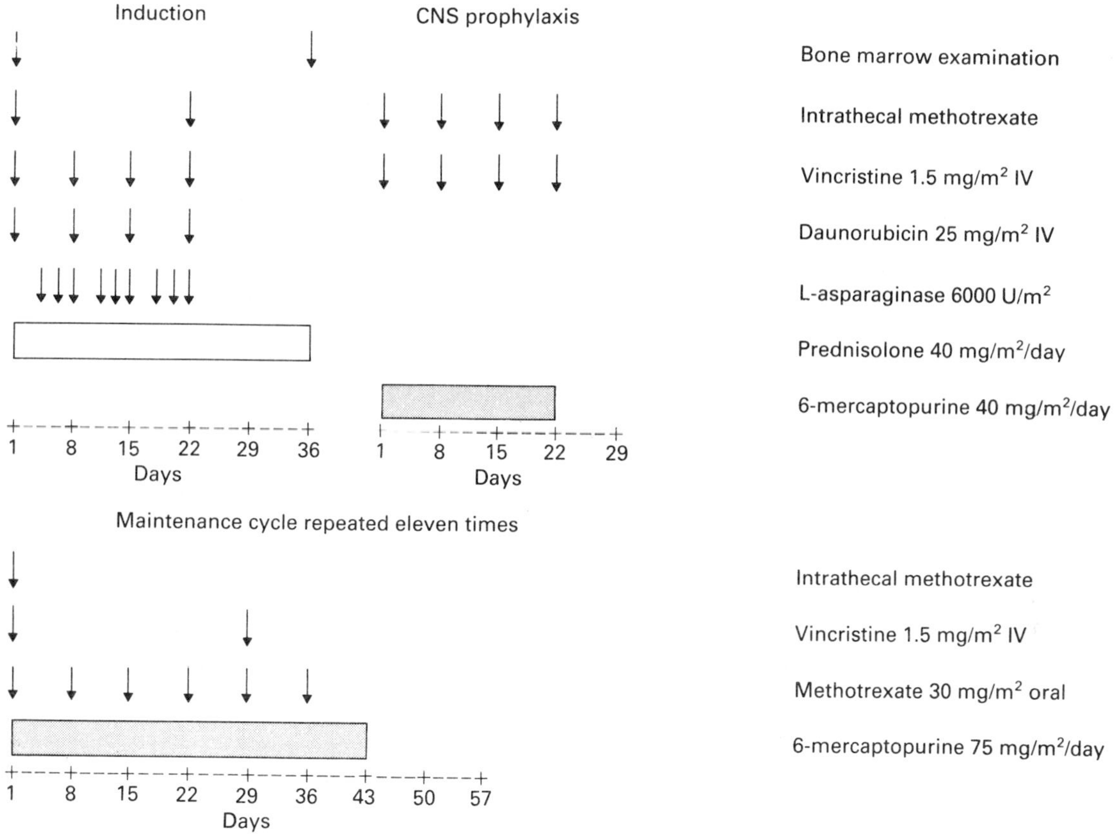

Fig. 10.4. *An example of a protocol used in one large paediatric unit for treatment of acute lymphoblastic leukaemia in children. Note the combination of different types of active agent, and the routine prophylactic treatment of the central nervous system. (Courtesy, Dr H. Ekert, Royal Children's Hospital, Melbourne.)*

doxorubicin, and cytosine arabinoside.

Effects of chemotherapy are monitored by changes in the counts of leukaemic cells, neutrophils, and platelets in the blood, and by changes in the bone marrow—disappearance of leukaemic cells from the blood and bone marrow associated with significant hypocellularity of the bone marrow is generally regarded as an indication for a delay in therapy. Persistence of leukaemic cells is regarded as an indication for continuation of active treatment. The majority of remissions occur after one or two courses of treatment, and are followed by a progressive rise in the counts of neutrophils and platelets, and the level of haemoglobin, to normal values.

Maintenance therapy. Such treatment is usually commenced after the blood picture has returned essentially to normal after induction of complete remission. The driving ambition of the therapist is selectively to eliminate the leukaemic process. A particularly important step in proceeding toward this objective has been the introduction of treatment, after haematological remission has been achieved, to destroy residual leukaemic cells sequestered in the central nervous system. CNS leukaemia is particularly common in childhood acute lymphoblastic leukaemia, and the striking improvement in survival that has followed the introduction of prophylactic treatment to prevent this complication argues strongly for its use as the next step in management following remission induction (Aur *et al.* 1973). Treatment is usually commenced within one month of attaining remission, often by irradiation of the cranium with 24 Gy over 3–4 weeks. Lower doses are used in children under the age of two years. Such treatment, of course, fails to irradiate leukaemic cells in the spinal cord, and for this reason intrathecal methotrexate is given for five doses, twice weekly during the course of cranial irradiation. Approximately the same results are achieved by intrathecal chemotherapy given with sufficiently high doses of parenteral chemotherapy to penetrate the CNS, in an attempt to avoid undesirable effects of cranial irradiation (Bleyer & Poplack 1985) (and see Fig. 10.4).

The other basic concept underlying the approach to therapy after induction of remission is administration of further systemic chemotherapy in an attempt to eradicate or continually suppress any residual leukaemic cells. One approach has been to administer large doses of chemotherapeutic agents as so-called 'consolidation' therapy. This may have merit, especially when the type of acute leukaemia is associated with poor prognostic factors, such as L3 morphologic features, T cell surface antigens, the presence of the Philadelphia chromosome, *etc.*, and the regimen often includes drugs not included in the initial induction therapy (Neimeyer *et al.* 1985).

Present evidence indicates that very intensive chemotherapy is of lesser importance in children who have disease with good prognosis and have been managed with prophylactic CNS treatment, where good results are achieved by maintenance therapy consisting of daily 6-mercaptopurine given by mouth in a dose of 50 mg/m^2, supplemented by a weekly dose of methotrexate, 20 mg/m^2, also given by mouth. On such a regimen, the drug dosage is modified to avoid depression of the leucocyte count below 3×10^9/l. Intermittent courses of vincristine and prednisolone may also be added. Alternative regimens for maintenance chemotherapy have been proposed (Haghbin *et al.* 1980, Niemeyer *et al.* 1985).

Once children who have received prophylactic CNS therapy for leukaemia reach three years without evidence of relapse, there is little evidence that further cytotoxic therapy provides any advantage. Relapse can, however, occur during the phase of maintenance treatment, and management depends on the previous therapeutic history of the patient. If prophylactic CNS therapy was not given, and remission was readily obtained in the first instance with prednisolone and vincristine, maintenance therapy is withheld and the patient treated as on the first occasion. However, if difficulty was experienced in achieving a remission on the first occasion, or remission is not readily obtained with re-treatment, additional agents such as daunorubicin, cyclophosphamide or L-asparaginase should be introduced. A second remission is usually obtained, but remission duration tends to be shorter than following the first remission, and progressively increasing difficulty is experienced in achieving subsequent remissions. Maintenance therapy during second and subsequent remissions should include, where possible, additional chemotherapeutic agents, and if CNS prophylaxis had not been previously administered, this should be performed as leukaemic cells harboured within the CNS may have been the origin of the relapse. Another option in the treatment of children whose disease has relapsed and undergone successful re-induction is allogeneic bone marrow transplantation, if a suitable donor is available. The relapse rate following allogeneic bone marrow transplantation under these circumstances is comparatively high (25–50 per cent), but less than the much higher rate in children treated with chemotherapy alone (Johnson *et al.* 1981, Nesbit *et al.* 1985).

Acute myeloid leukaemia

The principles of treatment are the same as for acute myeloid leukaemia in adults and are discussed in the following section.

ADULT ACUTE LEUKAEMIA

About 20 per cent of cases in adults consist of acute lymphoblastic leukaemia, and in subjects over the age of 25 years, the disease does not respond to treatment as well as acute lymphoblastic leukaemia in children. The remaining cases consist of various categories of acute non-lymphoblastic leukaemia as summarized in Table 10.1, and for convenience in this section are referred to collectively as acute myeloid leukaemia, although it is recognized that the various categories possess specific properties, including different patterns of response to chemotherapy.

Acute lymphoblastic leukaemia

Remission induction. Initial experience with vincristine and prednisolone indicated that these agents could be effective in adult acute lymphoblastic leukaemia, but the frequency with which remission was achieved was less than in children, and, in particular, remissions tended to be of shorter duration. Addition of other drugs such as daunorubicin to the regimen increases the response rate (Blacklock *et al.* 1981). Another regimen which avoids the use of anthracyclines but has a similar remission rate, comparatively well sustained, combines methotrexate with vincristine, L-asparaginase, and dexamethasone (Esterhay *et al.* 1982). This regimen produces comparatively less myelosuppression and, as originally described, included high-dosage methotrexate during remission as an alternative to prophylactic cranial irradiation and intrathecal chemotherapy. The blood levels of methotrexate were sufficiently high to achieve therapeutic concentrations of the drug in the cerebrospinal fluid. Other drug regimens are usually complex and toxic, but have the potential to produce more lasting remissions (Jacobs & Gale 1984, Clarkson *et al.* 1985).

Maintenance therapy. Similar principles as discussed in the case of childhood acute leukaemia apply to the disease in adults. Central nervous system prophylaxis and systemic maintenance therapy appear to be of value, in contradistinction to acute myeloid leukaemia. Consolidation or intensification therapy and allogeneic bone marrow transplantation are therapeutic measures that have been administered in remission, but nonetheless appear less successful in producing sustained remissions as in the typical childhood form of the disease (Jacobs & Gale 1984, Clarkson *et al.* 1985, Champlin & Gale 1987).

Acute myeloid leukaemia

Remission induction. A very commonly employed regimen against which the efficacy of new approaches is compared is a 7-day intravenous infusion of cytosine arabinoside 100 mg/m^2/day plus three daily injections of daunorubicin 45 mg/m^2/day (Rai *et al.* 1981). Important limitations are the cardiotoxic and myelosuppressive effects, which are more serious in the elderly; for this reason, reduction in the daunorubicin dose to 30 mg/m^2/day has been reported to produce an overall better outcome in patients over 60 years of age (Yates *et al.* 1982). Variations on this regimen, such as addition of thioguanine, an increase in the dose of cytosine arabinoside, substitution of doxorubicin for daunorubicin, or substitution of m-AMSA for anthracyclines, have been reported to produce comparable remission-induction rates (Lister & Rohatiner 1982).

Severe myelosuppression during the two weeks following treatment is usual, and assessment of the marrow aspirate three weeks after commencement of treatment generally provides a useful guide to response. About 60 per cent of cases collectively grouped under the title of acute myeloid leukaemia attain meaningful remissions following treatment with this regimen. About two-thirds of these do so after one course. In the remaining one-third, remission is usually attained after a second course of treatment, which is less myelosuppressive as the cytosine arabinoside is administered for five days, and only two injections of daunorubicin are given. Persistence of leukaemia after the second course is usually taken as an indication of refractory disease, and alternative forms of treatment, such as high doses of cytosine arabinoside or other agents, are considered.

Maintenance therapy. There has been disenchantment with the capacity of continuous administration of chemotherapeutic agents during remission to reduce the incidence of relapse, in comparison with the situation in childhood acute lymphoblastic leukaemia. A variety of other regimens has also been employed, including one or more further courses of the successful induction regimen soon after the onset of remission, a course of intensive combination chemotherapy later in the phase of remission, and intermittent courses of moderately intense chemotherapy in which the agents are varied in a cyclical manner. None has met with general acceptance as a means for reducing the rate of recurrence of leukaemia (Gale 1984).

Bone marrow transplantation has been increasingly employed as a form of treatment for acute leukaemia. Transplantation of bone marrow from a histocompatible donor after treatment of the patient with lethal myelosuppressive doses of antileukaemic therapy can occasionally result in long-term remission in patients with overt disease. The most promising results to date are in children or young adults with acute myeloid leukaemia in first remission. There is a reduction in the incidence of relapse in comparison with similar subjects treated by other means, although the benefits from this are counterbalanced to an extent by occurrence of early deaths as a direct consequence of the toxicity of the procedure, or from death due to graft-versus-host disease (Champlin & Gale 1987). Influence on long-term outcome still remains to be clarified, but it is nonetheless clear that this form of therapy is of proven benefit only in younger patients (those less than 40 years old) because graft-versus-host disease becomes more severe with increasing age, and is restricted to subjects who have a histocompatible donor, thus limiting the procedure to the minority of patients with acute leukaemia.

Autologous bone marrow transplantation represents an approach to treatment of patients with acute leukaemia in partial or complete remission, in whom allogeneic bone marrow transplantation is not possible because a histocompatible donor is not available. In this form of therapy, bone marrow is aspirated from the patient in remission, and stored in the frozen state, either without further manipulation or after being subjected to procedures aimed at selectively reducing the content of leukaemic cells. The patient is then exposed to doses of total body irradiation or to antileukaemic agents that would normally be excessively myelotoxic, in the hope of killing residual leukaemic cells. Recovery of haemopoiesis after such treatment is then achieved by re-infusing the stored bone marrow to produce an autograft. Such an approach is still undergoing evaluation, but appears to prolong survival in certain poor prognosis forms of haematological neoplasia.

One of the reasons for the expenditure of such effort to treat the patient after induction of remission is that relapse occurs in the majority of patients managed by conventional approaches within two years, and treatment of relapsed disease is generally less effective in terms of the frequency of remission re-induction and in the duration of further remissions.

Supportive care

There is general acceptance that combination chemotherapy of haematological malignancy, especially acute leukaemia, is ideally managed by specialist units in view of the advantages this provides. Some of these are:

1 The most effective regimens are complex, and the choice of the appropriate combination for a given patient requires *experience* and *judgement*.

2 Duration of remission appears to depend in part on the degree of leukaemic cytoreduction during remission induction, implying that more intensive therapy is overall the most effective. The degree of marrow suppression induced by many therapeutic regimens makes sophisticated *support facilities* essential. Such facilities include experienced physicians and nurses, expert *microbiological* and *virological* services, the availability of isolation *reverse-barrier nursing areas*, and a *cell separator* to provide leucocyte and platelet support. The constant requirement for venous access has resulted in development of long-term *indwelling intravenous catheters* which are surgically implanted, and which require very careful surveillance in neutropenic patients, in particular, to prevent infectious complications of the venous access route.

3 *Psychological and social support* are essential during the prolonged periods of intensive treatment. Support systems become highly developed in specialist units. Mutual confidence leads to increased use of *outpatient* rather than inpatient care.

4 *Cytotoxic drug dispensing* requires specialized equipment and expertise. There are potential mutagenic risks for pharmacists and nursing staff from exposure to cytotoxic drugs, either through contact with skin or from inhalation of aerosol droplets containing drugs. The wearing of gown, mask, and gloves, and the use of biohazard laminar flow equipment, is now routine in the preparation of cytotoxic formulations in specialized units.

5 The concentration of experienced personnel and patients in specialist units makes the development and assessment of new regimens of treatment possible, particularly when the specialist units within a country or region collaborate in the assessment of such new therapy.

Specific aspects of supportive care

Frequent transfusion of red cell concentrate is usually required during remission induction because of the rapid fall in haemoglobin level that commonly occurs at this time with regimens employed for treatment of acute myeloid leukaemia.

Prevention and control of infection is of paramount importance. When patients are severely neutropenic, a reduction in the degree of contact with external pathogens is attempted by confining patients to isolated areas. The cost and labour-intensive nature of these facilities in relation to their marginal advantages have resulted in a tendency to rely more on approaches such as reverse barrier-nursing. Even this measure has not been shown to be particularly effective in preventing infections in leukaemic patients, as many infections are derived from flora in the patient's gastrointestinal tract. Antimicrobial nasal spray and mouth rinse, plus oral administration of nystatin and/or ketoconazole, are generally employed as a means of reducing the load of pathogens in the gastrointestinal tract, and reduce local oropharyngeal infection. Administration of broad-spectrum antibacterial agents is of less certain benefit as a prophylactic measure, although some advantage has been claimed in reduction of opportunistic infection by treatment with co-trimoxazole in conventional dosages (Hughes *et al.* 1985).

Infections are extremely common during treatment, especially during the latter part of the remission-induction phase, when the white cell count is very low. The major principle of treatment of *established* infection is prompt clinical and bacteriological diagnosis, and prompt antibiotic, antifungal, or antiviral therapy appropriate for the organism or organisms responsible for the infection. Onset of fever under such circumstances must be followed by an immediate search for a focus of infection, especially in the mouth, intravenous line, lungs, urinary tract, or skin. *Pseudomonas aeruginosa* and other Gram-negative organisms as well as *organisms that are not common pathogens* can be the cause, especially in patients already treated with antibiotics. Bacteraemia and septicaemia are common, and thus blood cultures should be performed and broad-spectrum antibiotics administered immediately via the intravenous route.

Suitable antibiotic regimes for febrile patients in whom the organism has not yet been isolated usually include a combination of an aminoglycoside plus a broad-spectrum penicillin or cephalosporin. The possibility of infection with yeast or fungus should be considered, especially in patients already treated with corticosteroids and antibiotics. Oral moniliasis can be treated with topical nystatin or amphotericin, but systemic yeast or fungal infection requires parenteral treatment, usually with amphotericin in view of its broad spectrum of activity and the low rate with which resistance to it develops. Patients with severe infection unresponsive to appropriate antibiotics should be treated with the addition of leucocyte transfusion (see p. 228).

Haemorrhage is a very common problem and a frequent cause of death. It is usually a consequence of thrombocytopenia, but a contributing factor can be intravascular coagulation promoted by sepsis or products of certain types of leukaemic cells. Prophylactic transfusions of platelet concentrates are usually given during the remission-induction phase, as it has been shown that prevention of extreme thrombocytopenia is associated with fewer early deaths during treatment. An often employed threshold count, below which platelet transfusions are given, is $20 \times 10^9/l$. Such transfusions can usually be administered every 2–3 days to maintain the platelet count above $20 \times 10^9/l$, but in the presence of infection, bleeding, or antiplatelet antibodies resulting from previous sensitization by allogeneic blood cells or platelets, the requirement is usually greater. Allo-antibodies to platelets can become sufficiently potent effectively to obliterate the benefit of transfusion of platelets from random donors, and under such circumstances selection of partially or completely histocompatible donors can yield platelets that are less damaged after transfusion.

Disseminated intravascular coagulation is a major factor contributing to increased bleeding in acute promyelocytic leukaemia. Prophylactic therapy with heparin has been advocated as a means of suppressing the degree of intravascular coagulation, but it is likely that death from haemorrhage is a consequence of the consumption of coagulation factors and platelets, as active replacement of missing factors reduces mortality from bleeding, which is a particular complication of the treatment of this particular category of acute leukaemia.

Meningeal leukaemia may be present initially or develop during haematological remission in all forms of acute leukaemia. It is far more common in acute lymphocytic than acute myelocytic leukaemia. Antileukaemic agents in common use enter the cerebrospinal fluid in subtherapeutic concentrations when administered systemically in conventional doses, and for this reason about one-half of the episodes of meningeal leukaemia used to occur while systemic disease was in remission in subjects who had not received prophylactic treatment of the central nervous system. The diagnosis is suggested by inappropriate headache or symptoms of central nervous system abnormalities, and may be accompanied by signs of raised intracranial pressure. Confirmation is dependent on examination of the cerebrospinal fluid for the presence of leukaemic cells.

Treatment of meningeal leukaemia is commonly performed by intrathecal instillation of methotrexate in doses of 10 mg/m^2 twice weekly for 2 weeks, and then at weekly intervals until the cerebrospinal fluid is free of leukaemic cells. To avoid bone marrow suppression folinic acid is usually administered concurrently, 15 mg orally 6th hourly for 24 hours. The other commonly used agent is cytosine arabinoside in doses of 30 mg/m^2 at a comparable frequency of administration. Such frequent access to the cerebrospinal fluid is usually a problem, and repeated lumbar punctures can be avoided by inserting a subcutaneous reservoir under the scalp, attached to a catheter which delivers injected material into the third ventricle. Cranial irradiation as described as a prophylactic measure is also performed. It is very difficult to eradicate meningeal leukaemia totally, and for this reason, intrathecal therapy is usually continued at monthly intervals on an ongoing basis (Bleyer & Poplack 1985).

Myelodysplastic disorders

The myelodysplastic disorders are a heterogeneous group of leukaemia-related conditions characterized by various combinations of anaemia, neutropenia, and thrombocytopenia, usually with a normocellular or hypercellular bone marrow. They have several features in common with acute leukaemia, but their clinical course tends to be more chronic, and there is a lesser degree of blast cell infiltration of the bone marrow (less than 30 per cent). Transformation to an acute myeloid leukaemia occurs in some cases. The French-American-British group has classified myelodysplastic disorders into five categories (Bennett *et al.* 1982), employing the basic criteria summarized in Table 10.6.

Clinical features. The great majority of patients are over 50 years of age, and anaemia, recurrent infections or infections that are difficult to eradicate, and haemorrhagic manifestations are the main clinical problems. Transformation to leukaemia results in a clinical picture identical to that of *de novo* acute leukaemia. A secondary form of myelodysplasia is occasionally encountered in persons of any age who have had treatment with radiotherapy, chemotherapy, or a combination of the two.

Table 10.6. *Myelodysplastic disorders: FAB classification*

Type	Bone marrow
Refractory anaemia (RA)	Blasts <5%
Refractory anaemia with ring sideroblasts (RARS)	Blasts <5%, ring sideroblasts >15%
Refractory anaemia with excess of blasts (RAEB)	Blasts 5–20%
Refractory anaemia with excess of blasts in transformation (RAEBT)	Blasts 20–30%
Chronic myelomonocytic leukaemia (CMML)	Peripheral blood monocytes $>1 \times 10^9$/l

Blood picture. There is generally a mild to severe normocytic, or mildly macrocytic, anaemia. The red cells may be dimorphic, both hypochromic and normochromic cells being present, particularly in refractory anaemia with ring sideroblasts. Other red cell abnormalities include basophilic stippling and the presence of nucleated red cells (often with dyserythropoietic changes). Neutropenia of variable degree is usually present. Sometimes there is a shift to the left in the neutrophil series, and occasionally blast cells are seen. Hypogranular or agranular granulocytes, and granulocytes with bilobed Pelger–Hüet nuclear configuration are commonly encountered. An increase in monocytes is characteristic of chronic myelomonocytic leukaemia. Platelets are usually reduced, in some cases to very low levels, and are often dysfunctional.

Bone marrow. The marrow aspirate is normocellular to hypercellular, and there is morphological evidence of disordered development of all cell series. The proportion of erythroid precursors varies considerably, but dyserythropoietic features are common and include asynchrony between maturation of cytoplasm and nucleus, megaloblastoid changes, multinuclearity, nuclear fragmentation, cytoplasmic vacuolation, basophilic stippling, and Howell–Jolly bodies. Marrow iron stores are usually increased, and ring sideroblasts are often present, being by definition very prominent in refractory sideroblastic anaemia (p. 58). Changes of dysgranulopoiesis include aberrant staining of the primary granules of myeloid precursors, hypogranular granulocytes, Pelger–Hüet-type cells, and the presence of a variably increased proportion of blast cells. Micromegakaryocytes and large monolobular megakaryocytes are also seen.

Management approaches vary widely because these disorders not only vary widely in the extent of abnormal behaviour within a particular category, but the different categories possess substantially different patterns of behaviour. In many conditions, the clinical consequences can be sufficiently mild for no active therapeutic steps to be required. In situations where anaemia is the sole clinical problem of significance, transfusion alone may produce a good quality of life for many years, to the extent that transfusion-induced haemochromatosis can develop unless iron chelation therapy is administered to prevent toxicity from chronic iron overload. Refractory anaemia with ring sideroblasts equates with primary acquired refractory sideroblastic anaemia, and is discussed in further detail in Chapter 3. Progression of chronic myelomonocytic leukaemia can be suppressed or reversed by administration of relatively non-toxic agents such as mercaptopurine or hydroxyurea.

In refractory anaemia with excess blasts, other major problems that can be encountered are infection and haemorrhage, due to inadequate numbers, or disordered function, of neutrophils and platelets. Transformation to overt acute myeloid leukaemia occurs with moderate frequency in this disorder, and more frequently in refractory anaemia with excess blasts in transformation. Response to treatment after transformation is less satisfactory even than in *de novo* acute myeloid leukaemia. Sometimes there is very substantial improvement in cytopenia, tantamount to remission of these disorders, following treatment with low doses of cytosine arabinoside for extended periods of up to three weeks (Tricot *et al.* 1984), but responses to intensive treatment are generally less satisfactory than in the case of acute myeloid leukaemia.

Chronic granulocytic leukaemia

Chronic myelocytic leukaemia, chronic myeloid leukaemia, and chronic myelogenous leukaemia are synonyms for chronic granulocytic leukaemia.

Clinical features

Chronic granulocytic leukaemia (CGL) is a disease predominantly of middle life, the majority of cases occurring between the ages of 30 and 60 years, with a maximum incidence around the age of 45 years. It is rare under the age of 20. In older children, the disorder resembles that of adults, but a distinctive juvenile variety occurs in younger children. The sex incidence is approximately equal.

Onset is usually insidious, symptoms often having been present for many months before diagnosis. The majority of patients first seek medical advice because of symptoms due to anaemia, splenic enlargement, or raised metabolic rate, either alone or in combination. Presenting manifestations are listed in Table 10.7.

The most prominent symptoms are those of *anaemia*—fatigue, weakness, pallor, and dyspnoea.

Constitutional symptoms due to the raised metabolic rate are common in relatively advanced disease and include malaise, weight loss, and night sweats. Malaise, sometimes with marked exhaustion and prostration, is often a prominent symptom, especially in patients with high or rapidly rising white counts.

Symptoms resulting from *splenomegaly*, when it is marked, include a feeling of weight, dragging, or actual pain under the left costal margin, gastrointestinal symptoms, especially dyspepsia, flatulence and easy satiety after eating, and swelling of the abdomen. In some cases there is little or no gastrointestinal disturbance, despite marked splenomegaly. The accidental discovery of an enlarged spleen by the patient is sometimes the presenting manifestation. Acute pain over the spleen may occur following *splenic infarction*, and may mimic an acute abdominal emergency.

Haemorrhagic manifestations. Easy bruising, sometimes with the occurrence of haematomas, can occur, although severe bleeding is unusual.

Non-specific *skin lesions*, herpes zoster, and leukaemic infiltration are much less common than in chronic lymphocytic leukaemia. Pruritus without

Table 10.7. *Presenting manifestations of chronic granulocytic leukaemia*

Common
Anaemia
Splenomegaly
Fatigue
Weight loss
Moderately common
Night sweats
Minor bruising
Occasional
Joint pain
Bone pain
Amenorrhoea
Priapism
Accidental discovery on routine blood examination

any obvious skin changes occurs occasionally. Leukaemic skin infiltration is of unfavourable prognostic significance.

Bone and joint pains occur occasionally, and the sternum is sometimes, but not usually, tender to pressure. Radiological changes in the bones are uncommon, but localized areas of cortical destruction, or less frequently of sclerosis, are occasionally seen. The blood uric acid is frequently raised, but gout is relatively uncommon.

Amenorrhoea is a frequent complication in advanced disease, whilst *menorrhagia* may occur if the platelet count falls. *Priapism* due to obstruction to blood flow in the corpus cavernosum is an occasional but distressing complaint which is difficult to treat.

Infiltration of the *nervous system* is uncommon, and nervous system manifestations for the most part are due to haemorrhage. The nature of these manifestations depends on the site and the extent of the haemorrhage. Haemorrhage into the ocular fundus may cause impairment of vision, and haemorrhage into the internal ear, deafness and vertigo.

Fever is usually not a marked feature until the later stage of the disease, when it is common, but it is often absent in the early stages.

On *examination* at the time of diagnosis, *splenomegaly* is the outstanding physical sign, and apart from pallor and slight to moderate wasting, it is frequently the only abnormal finding. The spleen can be enlarged to below the level of the umbilicus. It sometimes extends into the left iliac fossa, and occasionally even to the right. It is firm and retains its normal contour, and the notch is easily felt. Following infarction, a rub may be felt or heard over the spleen. The spleen often becomes impalpable after treatment, and in rare cases it is not palpable at the time of diagnosis, for example when the condition is detected by routine blood examination. Smooth, moderate *hepatomegaly* is usual. *Lymph node enlargement* is much less common than in chronic lymphocytic leukaemia.

The degree of *wasting* increases with progression of the disease. *Bruising* is sometimes present, but purpura is uncommon, as are haemorrhages into the fundus oculi.

Juvenile type. This rare disorder in children

(usually under three years) bears certain resemblances to chronic granulocytic leukaemia (Hardisty *et al.* 1964) but tends to involve greater lymph node enlargement, less marked splenomegaly, more frequent infections, facial rash, and more haemorrhagic manifestations. The total leucocyte count is usually not as high, the total monocyte count is increased, thrombocytopenia is usual, and the disorder is Philadelphia-chromosome negative in contrast to the adult type. It tends to run a relatively shorter course, with a worse response to chemotherapy than the adult type, and bone marrow transplantation, where possible, offers long-term remission and cure (p. 265).

Blood picture

The typical blood picture in chronic granulocytic leukaemia at the time of presentation with clinical features of the disorder is of moderate anaemia, and a markedly elevated total white cell count with a full spectrum of cells of the granulocyte series, including 20 per cent or more of myelocytes. The platelet count can be normal, although it is raised in about one-half of cases, sometimes markedly.

At the time of diagnosis, the anaemia is usually of moderate degree, with haemoglobin levels from 8 to 10 g/dl. As the disease progresses, anaemia becomes more severe. Red cells are usually normocytic and normochromic, and a small proportion of erythroblasts are occasionally present.

The leucocyte count ranges up to 500×10^9 /l, or even higher. Segmented neutrophils and myelocytes constitute the majority of cells. Neutrophils vary in size, giant and dwarf forms being common. Myelocytes are the characteristic cells and comprise 10–50 per cent of the white cells. The vast majority are neutrophilic, although a few are eosinophilic and basophilic. Myeloblasts comprise up to ten per cent, but can rapidly increase in proportion when 'blast crisis' occurs (p. 262). An increase in the proportion of basophils (2–10 per cent) is a characteristic feature and can increase further as the disorder progresses towards transformation to acute leukaemia. The neutrophil alkaline phosphatase activity is markedly reduced.

Changes of only minor degree may be present when the disorder is detected by routine blood examination, as would be expected for the disease at a relatively early stage in its evolution.

The serum vitamin B_{12} level and unsaturated vitamin B_{12} binding capacity are frequently increased.

Bone marrow

Marrow aspiration yields hypercellular fragments with complete or partial replacement of fat spaces. The cell trails are hypercellular. The cells are mainly of the myeloid series, the myelocyte being the predominant cell, although promyelocytes and myeloblasts are also increased. The differential count of myeloid cells is similar to that of cells in the blood, although there is further shift to the left. Erythropoiesis is normoblastic, but sometimes dyserythropoietic. The myeloid : erythroid ratio is increased, due mainly to the white cell hyperplasia, but in the later stages there may be an actual reduction in erythropoietic tissue. Megakaryocytes are often prominent and are usually smaller than normal. Increased *fibrosis* is a notable feature of histological sections of the marrow in some cases.

Chromosome findings. Cytogenetic examination of bone marrow and blood cells has shown that a specific abnormality, the Philadelphia chromosome, is characteristically associated with the neoplastic cells in chronic granulocytic leukaemia. It is an abnormally small chromosome produced, as described previously, by reciprocal translocation between parts of the long arms of chromosomes 22 and 9 in nearly all instances (p. 237). The abnormalities of chromosomes 9 and 22 are illustrated in the banded chromosome preparation depicted in Fig. 10.5. Following conventional treatment, the Philadelphia chromosome usually cannot be detected in the peripheral blood when the immature cells have disappeared, but it persists in the bone marrow cells. With the onset of blastic transformation, additional chromosome changes may develop. A relatively common occurrence is the appearance of additional Philadelphia chromosomes.

Course of disorder

For most of its course, the disease behaves as a chronic process and responds predictably to

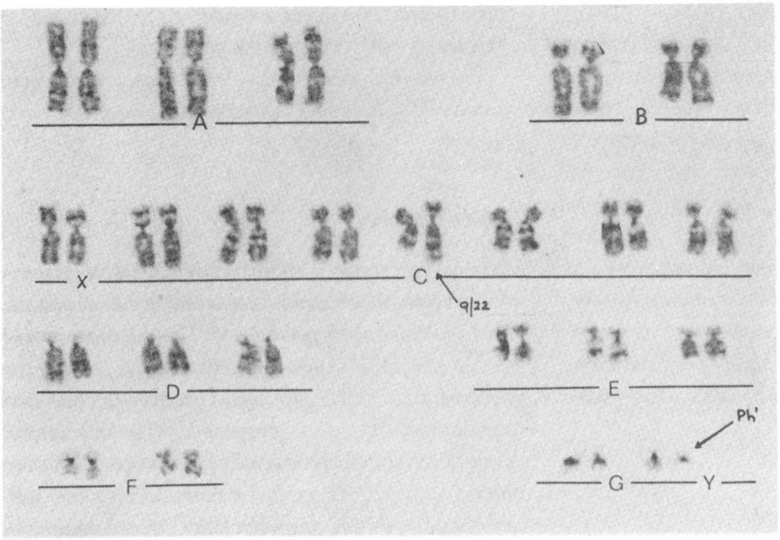

Fig. 10.5. *Chronic granulocytic leukaemia. Banded karyotype showing the* Ph^1 *chromosome as a 9/22 translocation.*

therapy. The most frequent termination of the chronic phase is blastic transformation, where the characteristics of the disease usually alter radically to that of acute leukaemia with a rapidly fatal course, usually with survival of less than six months. About 80 per cent of patients with chronic granulocytic leukaemia die as a result of blastic transformation, while the remainder die from intercurrent disease.

Prognosis is difficult to predict in an individual case, as death, especially in younger subjects, is usually a consequence of blastic transformation, an event that occurs with a probability of about 25 per cent per year. The average duration of survival from the time of detection is therefore 3–4 years. However, there is considerable individual variation in survival, from less than one year to ten years or more.

Blastic transformation ('blast crisis'). Blastic transformation may be suspected clinically because it is commonly associated with *symptoms* of malaise, fatigue, anorexia, night sweats, bone pain, and splenic discomfort. The patient may feel markedly unwell before any overt changes appear in the peripheral blood or even in the none marrow. Important physical *signs* are weight loss, pallor, pyrexia, sternal tenderness, progressively increasing splenomegaly, and the appearance of lymphadenopathy, which typically is absent in the chronic phase of the disease. Death usually results from haemorrhage or infection, or a combination of both, in disease unresponsive to treatment.

The most common change in the peripheral blood is a rapidly rising white cell count, appearance of a large proportion of blast cells, a falling haemoglobin level, and development of thrombocytopenia. The spectrum of white cell precursors characteristic of the chronic phase of the disease is lost, and a cell distribution typical of acute leukaemia occurs, often with a predominance of blast cells and some segmented neutrophils. In most cases, the blast cells are myeloid in type, but in 20–30 per cent the blast cells have lymphoblastic features (Griffin *et al.* 1983). Examination of the bone marrow aspirate reveals an increased proportion of blast cells, which may constitute 80 per cent or more of the cells.

Some instances of clinical deterioration are atypical in that the course is not a fulminating one, and blood examination may reveal no increase in immature cells. The bone marrow may appear unchanged or even hypoplastic, and a 'dry' or 'blood' tap is not uncommon. The diagnosis of this 'accelerated phase' of the disorder may be difficult to establish even in the presence of severe symptoms. Estimation of the neutrophil alkaline phosphatase level may be of assistance, as it may rise after transformation has occurred. The development of new chromosome abnormalities may also be of diagnostic value.

Chloroma

Chloroma is a term used to describe the occurrence of localized subperiosteal leukaemic tumour masses. The tumours are found most frequently in the skull, but they also occur in other bones, particularly the sternum, ribs, vertebrae, and sacrum. Chloroma develops both in acute myeloid leukaemia and in chronic granulocytic leukaemia, although in the latter it frequently denotes the onset of blastic transformation. The cells of the tumour masses usually contain sufficient porphyrin to give the tumour a green colour, which rapidly fades on exposure to light. Tumour masses also occur in other organs and tissues. Sometimes the tumours antedate the appearance of frank leukaemic features by months or even a year or more. Temporary regression of tumour masses may occur after radiotherapy; otherwise, treatment is that of acute myeloid leukaemia.

Differential diagnosis of chronic granulocytic leukaemia must be made from conditions which can cause a similar type of blood picture. Of these, the most important are uncommon leukaemic processes in which the Philadelphia chromosome is negative, and *myelofibrosis*, in which the clinical picture may be similar, splenomegaly being the outstanding feature (Table 10.8). A 'leukaemoid' blood picture

Table 10.8. *Comparsion of myelofibrosis and chronic granulocytic leukaemia*

	Myelofibrosis	Chronic granulocytic leukaemia
Clinical features		
History	Possible preceding phase of polycythaemia vera. Occasional history of splenomegaly for years	
Splenomegaly	Usually marked	Moderate to marked
Fever	Uncommon	Common in uncontrolled advanced disease
Blood examination		
Anaemia	Often slight to moderate despite marked splenic enlargement	Anaemia usually appreciable when splenomegaly marked
Red cell morphology	Poikilocytosis with oval and tear-shaped cells prominent	Poikilocytosis not usually prominent
White cell count	Normal, raised, or low. When raised, seldom more than $50 \times 10^9/l$	Usual range $20–500 \times 10^9/l$
Nucleated red cells	Almost invariable and often numerous	Present in small numbers or absent
Neutrophil alkaline phosphatase	Normal, raised, or reduced	Reduced
Bone-marrow aspiration	'Dry' or 'blood' tap without marrow fragments usual. Occasionally normocellular or hypocellullar	Hyperplastic fragments with absence of fat spaces
Chromosomes	Philadelphia-chromosome negative	Philadelphia-chromosome positive
Bone-marrow trephine	Numerous fibroblasts. New bone formation common. Megakaryocytes often prominent. Collagen present as well as increased reticulin	Granulocytic hyperplastic replacement of fat spaces
Course	Chronic course over many years common	Chronic course unless blastic transformation occurs

associated with severe infection or secondary malignancy of bone may also cause difficulty when the spleen is palpable (p. 272).

Treatment of chronic phase disease

There is no curative treatment for chronic granulocytic leukaemia, apart from allogeneic bone marrow transplantation. Treatment is usually palliative and symptomatic, the object being to effect the longest possible active, useful, and comfortable life for the patient. With adequate palliative treatment, it is usually possible to achieve not only a short increase of the actual time of survival but, more importantly, a significant lengthening of the comfortable and useful period of the patient's life. Thus, many patients who without treatment would spend most of their remaining life as chronic invalids are able to continue their normal occupations until a relatively short time before death occurs as a consequence of blastic transformation. The main form of palliative treatment is chemotherapy with busulphan. Splenic irradiation, which was the first effective form of treatment for this disease, has now been replaced by chemotherapy, as life expectancy has been shown to be superior with the latter treatment (MRC trial 1968). The simplicity and ease of administration of chemotherapy, given adequate supervision, also argues strongly for this as standard treatment unless more effective eradicative measures are available (p. 265).

CHEMOTHERAPY

A number of chemotherapeutic agents cause temporary suppression of activity in chronic granulocytic leukaemia. They include dibromomannitol, busulphan, thioguanine and hydroxyurea. Of these, busulphan causes control of a more predictable nature than the other agents, and the effects tend to last longer. Busulphan has therefore been the most often used chemotherapeutic agent.

Busulphan is a sulphonic acid ester which is an orally absorbed alkylating agent, and is usually administered to adults in a dose of 4–6 mg per day. In general, there is progressive fall in white cell count, relief of symptoms, rise in haemoglobin level, and regression of splenomegaly (Fig. 10.6). Usually, improvement is not apparent for 2–3 weeks, and satisfactory control requires treatment for 2–4 months. Treatment is relatively free from side-effects and does not cause nausea or vomiting. Neutropenia and thrombocytopenia are possible toxic effects, but are uncommon with the recommended dosage provided treatment is ceased at an appropriate time, such as when the leucocyte count has fallen to 15–20 $\times 10^9$ /l. Blood examination should be performed every 1–2 weeks until satisfactory control is achieved, and then monthly.

When an essentially normal blood count is achieved, a decision must be made about whether to continue busulphan at a lower dose, or cease treatment until increased activity recurs, when a further course is given. Intermittent therapy is

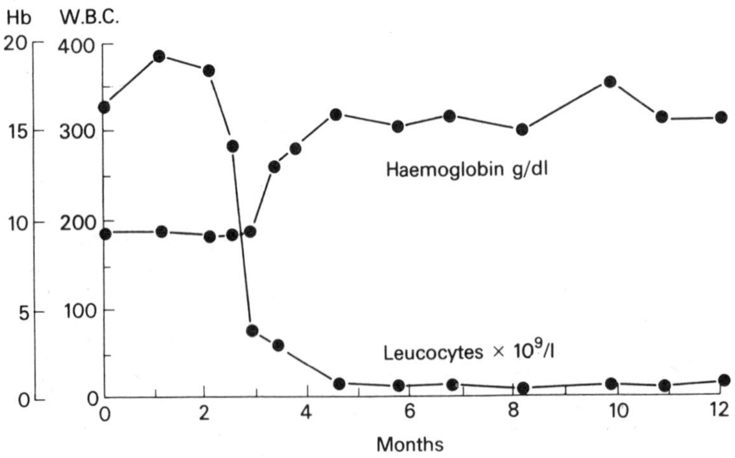

Fig. 10.6. *Response to busulphan administered for two months in a dose of 6 mg/day to a patient with chronic granulocytic leukaemia. Note eventual normalization of leucocyte count and haemoglobin level, which persisted without re-introduction of treatment during the following ten months.*

commonly employed, and criteria for continuous therapy are discussed by Galton (1959). He recommends intermittent therapy when the doubling time of the leucocyte count exceeds 70 days, and continuous therapy when it is less. The dose of busulphan required for continuous therapy must be sought by trial and error, but it is useful to begin with 2 mg daily, and to make adjustments according to the trend of the leucocyte count.

Side-effects

The main undesirable effect of busulphan is excessive myelosuppression, and this is more likely to occur if the initial dose exceeds 4 mg daily. Some patients are unusually sensitive to this dose, and there is a precipitous fall in white cell count. Treatment should be immediately discontinued if this occurs, but it may be resumed later at a lower dose. Severe myelosuppression occurs more commonly in patients on continuous maintenance therapy.

Apart from bone marrow depression, side-effects are few. The most common are skin pigmentation and amenorrhoea. More serious is a syndrome with features resembling Addison's disease. Pulmonary fibrosis can also occur. These side-effects are more likely to develop with prolonged treatment. The syndrome resembling adrenal cortical insufficiency is characterized by weight loss, severe weakness, fatigue, anorexia, nausea, and pigmentation.

OTHER FORMS OF TREATMENT

Other chemotherapeutic agents that have been widely used with effective suppression of disease activity include dibromomannitol, hydroxyurea and thioguanine. Chlorambucil is also effective, but more likely to induce thrombocytopenia and immunosuppression.

Leucapheresis enables the leucocyte count to be lowered rapidly under conditions where vascular perfusion may be compromised by increased viscosity of the blood due to effects of extremely high leucocyte counts, a problem referred to as *leucostasis*. Effects of leucapheresis are transient, and this form of treatment is usually coupled with measures for suppressing proliferative activity of the disease.

Bone marrow transplantation has become increasingly employed in younger subjects where a histocompatible bone marrow donor is available. This procedure can result in complete remission of chronic myeloid leukaemia, an outcome not achieved by any routinely employed form of treatment with chemotherapy alone. Allogeneic bone marrow transplantation is associated with considerable immediate morbidity and mortality (p. 256), but the threat to survival is less in fit young subjects than that of the almost inevitable transformation of the disorder to acute leukaemia. Long-term survival following transplantation is now of the order of 50 per cent.

Treatment of blast crisis

Refractoriness to treatment with the drug that had previously been effective in the chronic phase of the disease is often one of the first indications of blastic transformation, and agents used to suppress chronic phase disease are generally unsatisfactory after blastic transformation has taken place. Combination chemotherapy is also less effective in inducing remission than in the corresponding forms of acute leukaemia which have arisen *de novo*, although it is frequently possible to obtain remission of a relatively transient nature in the acute lymphoblastic variety of blastic transformation. Under the latter circumstance, reversion usually occurs to chronic phase disease, and it is under such conditions in particular that allogeneic *bone marrow transplantation* offers the prospect of 20 per cent long-term remission in younger subjects, when a histocompatible donor is available.

Chronic lymphocytic leukaemia

Clinical features

Chronic lymphocytic leukaemia (CLL) is a disease predominantly of the middle and older age group, the majority of cases being detected between 45 and 75 years, with a maximum incidence at about 55 years. It is very uncommon under the age of 30 years. Males are affected twice as frequently as females.

The *onset* is characteristically insidious. Most patients present with enlargement of superficial lymph nodes, or with gradually increasing weakness and fatigue due to anaemia, but not uncommonly the condition is accidentally discovered when the patient seeks medical advice for some other reason. Presenting manifestations are listed in Table 10.9

Enlargement of the superficial lymph nodes is the outstanding clinical feature, with several—if not all—sites being involved, unless the disorder has been accidentally discovered by routine blood examination early in its course. The degree of enlargement varies. It is usually moderate but may be marked, especially in the later stages, when the nodes may exceed 5 cm in diameter. The nodes are firm, discrete, not usually attached to the skin or superficial structures, and are usually painless, as in the case of the lymphomas. Lymphadenopathy can produce a variety of signs and symptoms, depending on the position of the enlarged glands. Such a form of presentation is similar to that in lymphomas except that the enlarged lymph nodes are usually more widespread when the patient presents.

Anaemia invariably develops later in the course of the disease, and commonly anaemic symptoms, such as slowly increasing weakness, fatigue, pallor, and effort dyspnoea, are the presenting symptoms. However, anaemia is not present in patients with early stage disease. An important complication in approximately ten per cent of cases is *acquired haemolytic anaemia*. This is sometimes the first manifestation of chronic lymphatic leukaemia. It should be suspected when the degree of anaemia is inappropriately severe for the degree of lymph node and splenic enlargement, the degree of lymphocytosis, or when spherocytes or agglutination are present in the blood film. The importance is that if haemolytic anaemia is not recognized, the patient may be thought to be in an advanced stage of the disease, and usually effective treatment for acquired haemolytic anaemia will not be instituted.

Constitutional symptoms due to raised metabolic rate, namely malaise, anorexia, fever, sweats, and weight loss, occasionally develop in advanced disease, but are usually absent for many months or years after diagnosis.

Splenomegaly is usually present at the time of diagnosis, and is usually less marked than in chronic myeloid leukaemia, enlargement to below the umbilicus being uncommon. Nevertheless, the spleen is sometimes considerably enlarged and may extend into the left iliac fossa. In such cases, the patient may complain of a mass or of compression effects on the gastrointestinal tract. Mild to moderate *hepatomegaly* develops in most patients.

Purpura and other haemorrhagic manifestations usually occur in the later stages of the disease, but are uncommon at the onset. Occasionally the patient presents with spontaneous bleeding into the skin or with other haemorrhagic manifestations, such as persistent bleeding following trauma or tooth extraction. The cause of thrombocytopenia can be a syndrome resembling idiopathic thrombocytopenic purpura, which tends to respond to corticosteroids or splenectomy in a similar manner to auto-immune thrombocytopenia (p. 381). Thrombocytopenia can also develop as a consequence of impaired platelet production due to haemopoietic tissue replacement by the disease, or from myelosuppressive effects of agents used for therapy of the disorder.

Respiratory and other infections. Infections such as bronchitis and pneumonia are common in chronic

Table 10.9. *Presenting manifestations of chronic lymphocytic leukaemia*

Common
Lymph node enlargement
Anaemia
Accidental discovery on clinical or haematological examination
Occasional
Predisposition to infection
Haemorrhagic manifestations
Acquired haemolytic anaemia
Splenomegaly
Gastrointestinal symptoms
Skin infiltration
Nervous system manifestations
Bone or joint pains
Mediastinal pressure or obstruction
Disturbances of vision or hearing
Tonsillar enlargement

lymphocytic leukaemia, and infections at other sites are also increased in frequency, especially in advanced disease. The production of normal immunoglobulin is often impaired, and this abnormality progresses through the course of the disease to result in increasing susceptibility to infection. Moderately reduced levels of IgG, IgA and IgM are relatively frequent findings. Neutropenia and corticosteroid administration are other factors that contribute to predisposition to infection, particularly to fungi and viruses, and infection is one of the most common direct or contributory causes of death.

Lesions of the skin are more common in chronic lymphatic than in chronic myeloid leukaemia, and direct involvement may take the form of circumscribed, raised, brownish or purple–red nodules of varying sizes, or of generalized infiltration with desquamation and thickening of the skin. There may be widespread erythema in patients with generalized infiltration by certain particular forms of lymphatic leukaemia.

Tonsillar enlargement may occur, and occasionally enlargement of the lachrymal and salivary glands gives the picture of Mickulicz's syndrome.

Nervous system manifestations may result from infiltration of the nervous system, from pressure of enlarged node masses, or, in the later stages, from haemorrhage.

Blood picture

The haemoglobin level ranges from normal values in virtually all cases of very early stage disease, through to moderate or severely depressed values in advanced chronic lymphocytic leukaemia with extensive haemopoietic tissue replacement. Anaemia is usually normochromic and normocytic under the latter conditions. When anaemia is due to haemolysis, it usually has the typical features of auto-antibody-mediated red cell destruction, with spherocytosis, a positive Coombs' test, and a reticulocytosis if the erythropoietic capability of the bone marrow is not impaired by infiltration of disease or by myelosuppressive effects of treatment.

The typical feature is a raised lymphocyte count, which at the time of diagnosis usually ranges from 50 to 200 $\times$ 10^9/l, although it is occasionally greater. When the disorder is detected by routine blood examination at an early stage in its development, the count can be appreciably less than 50 $\times$ 10^9/l, sometimes less than 10 $\times$ 10^9/l. Usually, 90 per cent or more of the leucocytes are mature lymphocytes, mostly small with a thin rim of cytoplasm, although in some cases the lymphocytes are of medium size. The cells in the blood film tend to have a monotonous appearance, although some may be disrupted during the preparation of the film and are referred to as 'smear' cells (Fig. 10.7). The

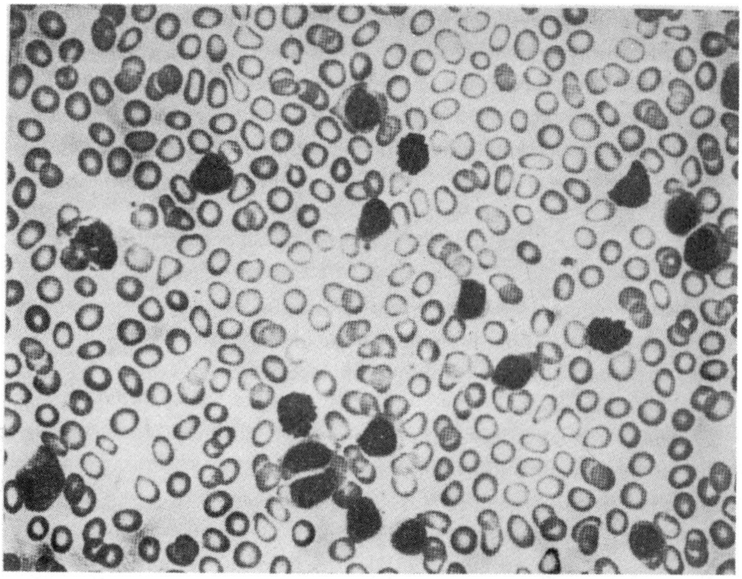

Fig. 10.7. *Photomicrograph of blood film in chronic lymphocytic leukaemia showing monotonous picture of small lymphocytes interspersed with occasional smear cells (× 430).*

absolute neutrophil count is usually in the normal range until the later stages of the disease, when it becomes depressed as a consequence of several factors, including replacement of normal haemopoietic tissue by the disorder, hypersplenic effects of an enlarged spleen, or myelosuppression by therapeutic agents.

In *classical* chronic lymphatic leukaemia, the disorder is caused by monoclonal expansion of a B-lymphocyte population with a relatively low density of surface immunoglobulin. These cells have the relatively unusual and diagnostically useful property of forming rosettes with mouse, but not sheep, erythrocytes. *There are a number of important variants in which the neoplastic lymphocytes are T cells.* These conditions are considerably less common, except that one type occurs relatively frequently in certain geographic areas such as parts of Japan. Such disorders tend to pursue a more malignant course, be associated more commonly with infiltration of the skin, and respond differently to chemotherapeutic agents than the more common B-cell form of chronic lymphatic leukaemia.

The platelet count initially is normal or moderately reduced, but, in the later stages, marked thrombocytopenia with counts of less than $50 \times 10^9/l$ is common.

Bone marrow

The typical findings in the bone marrow aspirate are an increase in lymphocytes and a corresponding reduction of megakaryocytes, myeloid precursors, and erythroid precursors, the extent of normal haemopoietic tissue replacement increasing as the disorder progresses.

Diagnosis

Diagnosis is usually straightforward. Detection of enlarged superficial lymph nodes or an enlarged spleen calls for a blood examination, which is essentially diagnostic.

Diagnostic difficulty can occur when there is a minor degree of absolute lymphocytosis but the white cell count is less than $10 \times 10^9/l$ and the bone marrow is not extensively infiltrated with lymphocytes. Repeated examination over a long period may be necessary in such cases before a definite diagnosis can be made. The diagnosis may be overlooked in patients presenting with skin disorders, nervous system manifestations, and gastrointestinal symptoms, especially when superficial lymph node enlargement is not prominent. Differentiation from lymphoma with blood spread is sometimes difficult, but B cells in the latter condition generally have a greater density of surface immunoglobulin, and do not form rosettes with mouse erythrocytes. Differentiation from states associated with reactive lymphocytosis can also occasionally be difficult, but the B cells under these circumstances form a polyclonal population, and the lymphocytosis often regresses with the passage of time.

Course and prognosis

The average duration of life from time of diagnosis is 3–4 years, although individual survival varies from less than one year to ten years or more. Survival in general is greatly influenced by the stage to which the disease has advanced at diagnosis and by the rate of the progression.

Staging systems have been devised to provide an indication of prognosis (Rai *et al.* 1975, Binet *et al.* 1981) as summarized in Table 10.10. There are limitations in such a system, which for practical purposes is simple and cannot take every factor into consideration. For example, the influence on prognosis of enlargement of a single organ is not included, nor is the influence of immune *versus* non-immune cytopenia (particularly thrombocytopenia) taken into account (Gale & Foon 1985).

Table 10.10. *Relation of stage of chronic lymphocytic leukaemia to prognosis**

Stage	Characteristics	Median survival
0	Peripheral blood lymphocytosis	>10 years
I	With lymphadenopathy	>8 years
II	With hepatosplenomegaly	<7 years
III	With anaemia	2–5 years
IV	With thrombocytopenia	<2 years

*Rai *et al.* (1975).

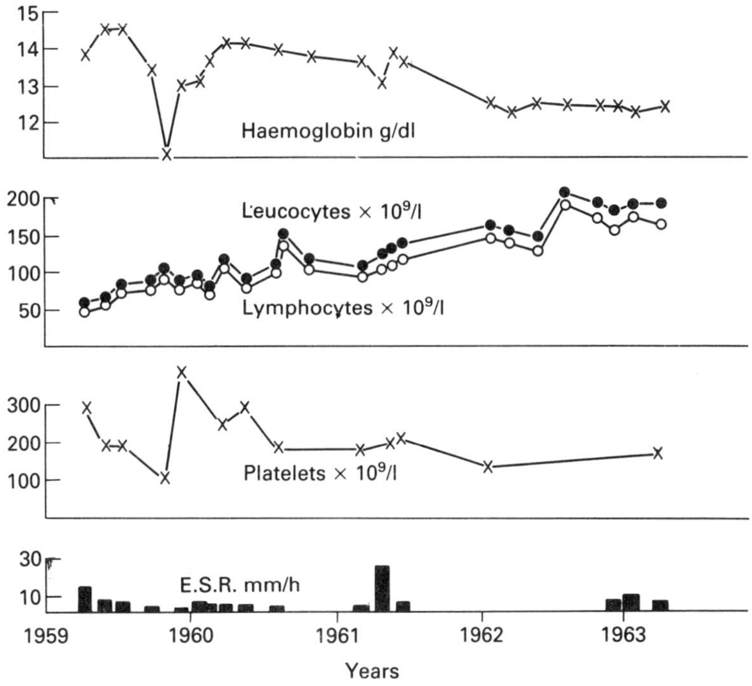

Fig. 10.8. *Indolent course of chronic lymphatic leukaemia in a patient who was not receiving treatment. Treatment was not initiated until 1967.*

In many patients, the condition causes little or no disability and may progress relatively slowly over many years. It is usually characterized initially by only slight to moderate lymph node and splenic enlargement, minimal or no anaemia, and only a moderate lymphocytosis, e.g. 10–60 $\times$ 10^9/l, although exceptions occur (Fig. 10.8). In such patients, it is not uncommon for the condition to be discovered accidentally, either when routine clinical examination reveals symptomless lymph node enlargement, or when blood examination reveals lymphocytosis. The disorder nonetheless progresses over potentially extremely long periods to cause increasing lymph node and splenic enlargement, anaemia, neutropenia, and thrombocytopenia.

Many patients die from unrelated complications encountered in old age, but others die from consequences of bone marrow replacement by the disease, which causes anaemia, neutropenia, and thrombocytopenia. Death usually results from cachexia and infection, often pneumonia.

Acquired haemolytic anaemia or immune thrombocytopenia may develop at any point in the course of the disease, and, as treatable and reversible complications, should always be considered when anaemia or thrombocytopenia is inappropriately severe for the stage of the disease.

Treatment

No treatment for eradication of chronic lymphocytic leukaemia is known. Treatment is consequently palliative and symptomatic, the object being to effect the longest possible active, useful, and comfortable life for the patient with the minimum amount of treatment. With optimum management, the patient can often lead a relatively normal life for many years. Approaches for suppression of disease activity include alkylating agents, corticosteroids, and radiotherapy. Splenectomy can be helpful especially in subjects with immune cytopenia, and parenteral γ globulin in subjects with infectious problems due to hypogammaglobulinaemia.

RADIOTHERAPY

Radiotherapy is mainly used for treatment of an enlarged spleen or lymph node masses. It frequently produces substantial reduction in the volume of bulky tissues and can be useful for relieving obstructive effects, but even when radiotherapy is confined to one area, it may produce a surprising degree of myelosuppression in unirradiated sites, and thus should be employed with caution.

CHEMOTHERAPY

Chlorambucil is still considered to be the most satisfactory chemotherapeutic agent for the treatment of chronic lymphocytic leukaemia. Galton *et al.* (1961) found just over one-half of all patients treated for the first time obtained benefit, and most responded equally well to one or two further courses. The recommended initial daily dose was 0.15 mg/kg, or about 10 mg/day for a 70 kg adult. Blood counts should be performed weekly, and administration should be discontinued when the leucocyte count has returned to near normal levels. In most cases it is necessary to discontinue the drug 4–6 weeks after starting treatment, and to allow 2–4 weeks for observation of the leucocyte counts, before resuming treatment at a lower dose of 5 mg/day or less, until a satisfactory response has been obtained. Response is manifested by a fall in lymphocyte count, sometimes followed by a rise in haemoglobin level and platelet count, and regression in size of enlarged lymph nodes and spleen. Neutropenia is the most serious toxic effect, and treatment should be ceased if the neutrophil count falls below 1×10^9/l. Thrombocytopenia may also be induced, and the drug must be administered with caution if the patient has thrombocytopenia before treatment is commenced. It may be possible to withhold treatment for many months or even years after a satisfactory response to treatment has been obtained.

Cyclophosphamide can also cause regression of the disorder and is useful in patients with significant thrombocytopenia. The usual dose is 100–200 mg/day, and cross-resistance with chlorambucil is usually not encountered, so that cyclophosphamide may be effective in patients with disease refractory to chlorambucil. It does, however, have a tendency to cause neutropenia and therefore must be administered with caution (Wall & Conrad 1961).

CORTICOSTEROIDS

When administered in sufficiently high doses, such as 25–100 mg prednisolone daily, there is often reduction in the activity of the disorder, with a decrease in size of lymph nodes and spleen, and a rise in haemoglobin level and platelet count. Beneficial effects can occur in disease refractory to chemotherapy or irradiation, as well as in combination with relatively lower doses of chlorambucil in patients in whom severe thrombocytopenia or neutropenia otherwise precludes treatment with alkylating agents. The dose of corticosteroid should be reduced as rapidly as possible because of the associated increase in susceptibility to infection. Sometimes, instances of the disorder refractory to chlorambucil alone achieve clinical benefit from a dose of prednisolone of approximately 10 mg/day, together with relatively low doses of chlorambucil.

CHOICE OF THERAPY

The approach to management depends on the stage and activity of the disease, and whether autoimmune cytopenic complications are present.

Early stage chronic lymphocytic leukaemia (stages 0–II) requires no treatment. The patient should be encouraged to lead a normal life and undergo clinical and haematological assessment about every three months. Treatment is not required until signs of more active disease develop, which may not be for a number of years. This approach is being investigated by controlled trial of therapy in early disease, but there is no evidence as yet to justify a change in attitude.

Actively progressive, more advanced stage chronic lymphocytic leukaemia. Anaemia, systemic symptoms, pressure or obstruction from lymph node enlargement, and marked splenomegaly are indications for treatment. The choice between radiotherapy and chemotherapy is not always easy. Most commonly, treatment is instituted with *chlo-*

rambucil, but radiotherapy can be considered when enlarged lymph nodes produce local compressive effects. Disease refractory to chlorambucil with or without prednisolone may benefit from combination chemotherapy with drugs including doxorubicin, cyclophosphamide, vincristine, and prednisolone, the former given in relatively low doses because of the high risk of myelosuppressive side-effects.

SYMPTOMATIC AND SUPPORTIVE THERAPY

Anaemia is sometimes relieved by specific treatment of the disease, but in the later stages severe anaemia is a common problem which responds relatively poorly to transfusion, even when it is not caused by auto-antibody-mediated haemolytic anaemia. Corticosteroids sometimes produce relief, and occasionally surgical removal of an enlarged spleen results in reduction of transfusion requirements, although the procedure is accompanied by a high incidence of complications in such patients.

Patients in the later stages of the disease are more susceptible to *infection*, which should thus be treated promptly with appropriate antibiotics. Respiractory tract infections are especially common, and persistent chronic bronchitis may be particularly troublesome in the winter. In patients with recurrent infections, the administration of intravenous γ globulin can be helpful in subjects with hypogammaglobulinaemia.

Management of auto-antibody-mediated haemolytic anaemia or thrombocytopenia follows similar principles as for the idiopathic forms of these disorders, except that attempts are also made to suppress the activity of the leukaemic process.

Other chronic lymphoproliferative disorders

Hairy cell leukaemia

Hairy cell leukaemia is an uncommon disorder of middle and late adult life, characterized by the presence in bone marrow, spleen, and peripheral blood of abnormal mononuclear cells with hairy cytoplasmic projections, and best detected by phase-contrast microscopy. Males are affected more frequently than females. Most patients have marked splenomegaly, and lymphadenopathy is unusual.

The *blood picture* is often that of mild normocytic normochromic anaemia with neutropenia and moderate thrombocytopenia. The proportion of hairy cells varies widely, but is usually in the order of 10–50 per cent, and only occasional patients have a high leucocyte count with numerous hairy cells. Marrow aspiration is frequently difficult due to an increase in marrow reticulin, but in patients from whom a satisfactory specimen is obtained, extensive replacement of normal haemopoietic tissue with hairy cells is apparent. Infiltration is readily detected in trephine biopsies of bone marrow. The nature of the hairy cells varies, but most cases belong to the B-lymphocyte lineage.

Patients with minor degrees of cytopenia can be asymptomatic, and therapeutic intervention may be deferred if careful monitoring reveals an indolent clinical course. Clinical complications or overt progression of the disorder is regarded as an indication for intervention, especially the bleeding, infection, or anaemia that occur commonly in advanced disease. Splenectomy is usually regarded as the treatment of first choice when splenomegaly is present, as splenectomy produces partial or even complete correction of cytopenia. It fails to produce any benefit in about 20 per cent of cases. In the responders, the improvement is not sustained, although it may take many years for the cytopenias to recur as a result of bone marrow infiltration. Treatment at any stage of the illness with cytotoxic agents, such as chlorambucil in doses similar to those used in chronic lymphocytic leukaemia, can sometimes produce substantial regression of the disease, and improvement in the degree of cytopenia, but with a high risk of infectious complications. More satisfactory responses have been obtained with long-term subcutaneous injections of *alpha interferon*, which produce marked and sustained regression of hairy cell leukaemia, and reduce or eliminate its clinical manifestations in more than one-half of patients with advanced disease (Golomb 1987). The enzyme inhibitor *deoxycoformycin* also produces marked regression of the disease in a majority of patients (Spiers *et al.*

1987), so that prognosis in advanced disease has improved substantially in recent years due to the introduction of new therapeutic agents.

Prolymphocytic leukaemia

This is a rare form of lymphocytic leukaemia in which the circulating lymphoid cells are larger and less mature in appearance than lymphocytes in chronic lymphocytic leukaemia, but more mature than in acute lymphoblastic leukaemia. It occurs more often in elderly males, and is associated with splenomegaly, but not particularly with lymphadenopathy. The prolymphocyte count in the peripheral blood can be greatly increased, as high as $200 \times 10^9/l$, and the abnormal cell population in most cases has the surface phenotype of B cells.

The disease tends to progress more rapidly than typical chronic lymphocytic leukaemia, and treatment is indicated at an early stage, although response to alkylating agents and corticosteroids is usually poor. Splenectomy, splenic irradiation, leucapheresis, and combination chemotherapy have been tried with varying and often little success in small numbers of patients, and the final place of these modalities in treatment is still uncertain (Oscier *et al.* 1981).

Leukaemoid blood picture

The term *leukaemoid reaction* is used to describe the occurrence of a peripheral blood picture resembling that of leukaemia in a subject who does not have leukaemia. The blood picture may suggest the presence of leukaemia because of marked elevation of the total white cell count, or the presence of immature white cells, or both. Leukaemoid reactions may be either myeloid or lymphoid. In general, a particular disorder causes only one type of reaction, but some may cause either a myeloid or a lymphoid leukaemoid reaction.

The diagnostic problem

The conditions causing leukaemoid blood reactions fall into two groups:

1 Conditions in which the blood picture suggests leukaemia, but the clinical features of the underlying disorder causing the leukaemoid reaction are obvious and suggest the correct diagnosis. The majority of cases fall into this group, and present little difficulty in diagnosis when both the clinical and haematological features are considered carefully;

2 Conditions in which both the blood picture and clinical features resemble leukaemia, so that it is difficult to distinguish the leukaemoid reaction from leukaemia. These include cases in which there is splenic or lymph node enlargement, haemorrhagic manifestations, fever in the absence of any obvious infective process, and cases in which the percentage of immature cells in the blood is high.

Table 10.11 lists certain differences between leukaemoid reactions and leukaemia which help in differential diagnosis. However, in the individual case, diagnosis can be difficult, especially when the underlying disorder causing the leukaemoid reaction is not obvious. In such cases, further observation or investigation may reveal the true nature of the illness. Marrow aspiration and trephine biopsy are usually diagnostic, as the marrow changes in leukaemoid reactions are seldom sufficiently marked to suggest leukaemia. Cytogenetic studies may be helpful in the exceptional situation where an abnormal karyotype will establish that the process is of a neoplastic nature.

Myeloid leukaemoid reactions

A myeloid leukaemoid blood picture may be defined arbitrarily as one in which the total white count exceeds $50 \times 10^9/l$ and myelocytes and/or myeloblasts appear in the peripheral blood. This is the usual type of myeloid leukaemoid reaction, but occasional cases are seen in which immature granulocytes are present although the total white count is within normal limits.

CAUSES OF MYELOID LEUKAEMOID REACTIONS

Infections. Leukaemoid reactions due to infection are more common in children than in adults. With severe infections, the total leucocyte count may exceed $50 \times 10^9/l$, and a few myelocytes and

Table 10.11. *Comparison of leukaemoid reactions and leukaemia*

	Leukaemoid reactions	Leukaemia
Clinical features	Clinical features of the causative disorder often obvious	Splenomegaly, lymph node enlargement, and haemorrhage more common than with leukaemoid reactions
Blood examination		
Total white cell count	Increase usually only moderate; seldom exceeds $100 \times 10^9/l$	Can exceed $100 \times 10^9/l$
Proportion of immature cells	Usually small or moderate. Myelocytes seldom exceed 5–15 per cent, and 'blasts' 5 per cent	Usually numerous
White cell morphology	Toxic changes may be seen in infective cases	Cells often atypical as well as immature. Toxic changes uncommon
Anaemia	May occur, but often slight or absent	Usually present and progressive
Nucleated red cells	Frequent in leuco-erythroblastic anaemia due to marrow infiltration	Less frequent
Platelets	Mainly normal or increased, but reduced in leuco-erythroblastic anaemia and intravascular coagulation	Decreased, except in chronic granulocytic leukaemia
Bone marrow	White cell hyperplasia may be present but seldom to same degree as in leukaemia	Hyperplastic with potentially large proportion of immature cells
Autopsy	Infiltration of organs and tissues absent	Leukaemic infiltration of organs and tissues

promyelocytes, and even an occasional myeloblast, may be seen in the peripheral blood. Leukaemoid reactions can occur, for example, following splenectomy when there is associated bleeding, haemolysis, or infection.

Most cases can be distinguished from leukaemia on careful consideration of the clinical and haematological features: (a) the cause of the infection is usually obvious; (b) the percentage of the immature cells is small, e.g. 5–10 per cent; (c) anaemia is slight or absent except in the presence of a complicating feature such as haemolysis or haemorrhage; (d) there may be toxic changes in the neutrophils as seen in infection; and (e) the neutrophil alkaline phosphatase tends to be normal or increased in leukaemoid reactions, which is useful in differentiating them from chronic granulocytic leukaemia in which the value is subnormal.

Rare cases of disseminated tuberculosis simulating acute myeloid leukaemia have been described.

Secondary to non-haematological malignancy. A moderate neutrophil leucocytosis of 15–30 $\times 10^9/l$ with a 'shift to the left can occur in malignancy, especially with necrotic tumours or when there is complicating infection. Occasionally, the white count exceeds $50 \times 10^9/l$, and a small percentage of myelocytes and myeloblasts are found. There is seldom any confusion with leukaemia.

Acute haemolysis. Leucocytosis with total white counts of $30 \times 10^9/l$ or more, with the appearance of myelocytes in the blood, may occur in acute haemolytic anaemia. Superficially, anaemia, splenomegaly, and the presence of nucleated red cells may suggest leukaemia, but appropriate investigation establishes the haemolytic nature of the disorder.

Leuco-erythroblastic blood picture

The term leuco-erythroblastic blood picture is used to describe the presence of immature myeloid and nucleated red cells in the peripheral blood, often as a consequence of disturbance of the bone marrow architecture by abnormal tissue.

Causes of a leuco-erythroblastic picture are:

secondary carcinoma of bone; this is the most common cause;

myelofibrosis;

thalassaemia major, especially after splenectomy;

active haemolytic anaemia;

multiple myeloma (uncommon);

lymphoma (uncommon);

Gaucher's and Niemann–Pick disease (rare);

marble bone disease (rare).

Characteristics of anaemia associated with this abnormality vary somewhat with the disorder infiltrating the bone marrow, and are detailed in the appropriate sections. There are nonetheless certain general features. Anisocytosis and poikilocytosis (particularly tear-shaped cells) are usual, and are often marked. A key feature is the presence of nucleated red cells, which are often numerous and disproportionately high compared with the number of reticulocytes. They commonly number up to 10 or more per 100 white cells. A moderate increase in reticulocytes, e.g. from 3 to 10 per cent, is usual. The white cell count is usually normal or moderately raised, but is sometimes reduced. The other key feature is that the leucocyte differential count shows a shift to the left, irrespective of the total white count, usually with the appearance of metamyelocytes, a few myelocytes, e.g. from 5 to 10 per cent, and sometimes even an occasional myeloblast. The platelet count is normal or reduced, although it may be increased in myelofibrosis.

It should be remembered that immature red and white cells sometimes occur in the blood in disorders that are neither neoplastic nor diseases of bone, e.g. acute haemolytic anaemias, megaloblastic anaemias, and thalassaemia major.

CAUSES OF LYMPHATIC LEUKAEMOID REACTIONS

Infectious mononucleosis and *cytomegalovirus* infection (p. 231).

Pertussis may cause a marked absolute lymphocytosis which must be differentiated from that of chronic lymphocytic leukaemia. In pertussis, the lymphocytes are usually normal and mature, and the haemolgobin level and platelet count are normal. Occasionally, the lymphocyte count in *measles* and *chickenpox* is high enough to simulate chronic lymphocytic leukaemia.

Rare cases of *tuberculosis* with either a lymphocytic or lymphoblastic blood picture have been reported. Most have occurred with disseminated tuberculosis, in which the lymph nodes, liver, and spleen were enlarged. Blood lymphocytes counts of over 50×10^9/l have been recorded. In the bone marrow, there can be a reduction in normal haemopoietic elements, either with or without an increase in lymphocytes.

Rare cases of *carcinoma* are associated with a marked rise in total lymphocyte count, e.g. to 20×10^9/l or more. The lymphocytes may all be mature, but sometimes a small proportion of lymphoblasts is present. In such cases, diagnosis from lymphocytic leukaemia may be difficult in the absence of a clinically obvious primary tumour.

References and further reading

Basic biology

Bizzozero, O.J., Jr, Johnson, K.G. & Ciocco, A. (1966) Radiation-related leukaemia in Hiroshima and Nagasaki, 1946–1964. I. Distribution, incidence and appearance time. *New Engl. J. Med.* **274**, 1905.

Broder, S. & Gallo, R.C. (1985) Human T-cell leukaemia viruses (HTLV): a unique family of pathogenic retroviruses. *Ann. Rev. Immunol.* **3**, 321.

Buckton, K.E., Jacobs, P.A., Court Brown W.M. *et al.* (1962) A study of the chromosome damage persisting after X-ray therapy for ankylosing spondylitis. *Lancet*, **ii**, 676.

Canellos, G.P., Come, S.E. & Skarin, A.T. (1983) Chemotherapy in the treatment of Hodgkin's disease. *Semin. Hematol.* **20**, 1.

Conen, P.E. & Erkman, B. (1966) Combined mongolism and leukaemia: report of eight cases with chromosome studies. *Am. J. Dis. Child.* **112**, 429.

Court Brown, W.M. & Abbat, J.D. (1955) The incidence of leukaemia in ankylosing spondylitis treated with X-rays. *Lancet*, **ii**, 1283.

Evan, G.I. & Lennox, E.S. (1985) Retroviral antigens and tumours. *Brit. Med. Bull.* **41**, 59.

Gallo, R.C. & Wong-Staal F. (1982) Retroviruses as etiologic agents of some animal and human leukemias and lymphomas and as tools for elucidating the molecular mechanisms of leukemogenesis. *Blood*, **60**, 545.

Gunz, F.W. & Henderson, E.S. (1983) *Leukemia*, 4th Ed., Grune & Stratton, New York.

Holland, W.W., Doll, R. & Carter, C.O. (1962) Mortality from leukaemia and other cancers among patients with Down's syndrome (mongols) and among their parents. *Brit. J. Cancer*, **16**, 177.

MacMahon, B. (1962) Prenatal X-ray exposure and childhood cancers. *J. Nat. Cancer Inst.* **82**, 1173.

Nowell, P.C. & Hungerford, D.A. (1961) Chromosome studies in human leukaemia. II. Chronic granulocytic leukemia. *J. Nat. Cancer Inst.* **27**, 1013.

Pedersen-Bjergaard, J., Larsen, S.O., Struck, J. *et al.* (1987) Risk of therapy-related leukaemia and preleukaemia after Hodgkin's disease. *Lancet*, **ii**, 83.

Pierce, J.H., Eva, A. & Aaronson, S.A. (1986) Interactions of oncogenes with haemopoietic cells. *Clin. Haemat.* **15**, 573.

Rinsky, R.A., Smith, A.B., Horning, R. *et al.* (1987) Benzene and leukemia. *New Engl. J. Med.* **316**, 1044.

Rosner, F. & Grünwald, H.W. (1980) Cytotoxic drugs and leukaemogenesis. *Clin. Haemat.* **9**, 663.

Rowley, J.D. (1984) Biological implications of consistent chromosome rearrangements in leukemia and lymphoma. *Cancer Res.* **44**. 3159.

Sarin, P.S. & Gallo, R.C. (1983) Human T-cell leukemia-lymphoma virus (HTLV). *Prog. Hemat.* **13**, 149.

Sawitsky, A., Bloom, D. & German, J. (1966) Chromosome breakage and acute leukemia in congenital telangiectatic erythema and stunted growth. *Ann. Int. Med.* **65**, 485.

Uchida, I., Holungar, R. & Lawler, C. (1968) Maternal radiation and chromosomal aberrations. *Lancet*, **ii**, 1045.

Weiss, R.A. & Marshall, C.J. (1984) Oncogenes. *Lancet*, **ii**, 1138.

Acute leukaemia

Aur, R.J.A., Hososa, M.S., Wood, A. *et al.* (1973) Comparison of two methods for preventing central nervous system leukaemia. *Blood*, **42**, 349.

Bennett, J.M., Catovsky, D., Daniel, M.T. *et al.* (1976) Proposals for the classification of the acute leukaemias. *Brit. J. Haemat.* **33**, 451

Bennett, J.M., Catovsky, D., Daniel, M.T. *et al.* (FAB co-operative group) (1982) Proposals for the classification of the myelodysplastic syndrome. *Brit. J. Haemat.* **51**, 189.

Bennett, J.M., Catovsky, D., Daniel, M-T. *et al.* (1985) Criteria for the diagnosis of acute leukemia of megakaryocytic lineage (M7). A report of the French-American-British Cooperative Group. *Ann. Int. Med.* **103**, 460.

Blacklock, H.A., Matthews, J.R.D., Buchanan, J.G. *et al.* (1981) Improved survival from acute lymphoblastic leukemia in adolescents and adults. *Cancer*, **48**, 1931.

Bleyer, W.A. & Poplack, D.G. (1985) Prophylaxis and treatment of leukemia in the central nervous system and other sanctuaries. *Semin. Oncol.* **12**, 131.

Bloomfield, C.D., Goldman, A.I., Alimena, G. (1986) Chromosome abnormalities identify high-risk and low-risk patients with acute lymphoblastic leukemia. *Blood*, **67**, 415.

Burchenal, J.H. (1968) Long-term survivors in acute leukaemia and Burkitt's tumour. *Cancer*, **21**, 595.

Champlin, R. & Gale, R.P. (1987) Bone marrow transplantation for acute leukemia: recent advances and comparison with alternative therapies. *Semin. Hematol.* **24**, 55.

Clarkson, B., Ellis, S., Little C. *et al.* (1985) Acute lymphoblastic leukemia in adults. *Semin. Oncol.* **12**, 160.

Dacie, J.V. & Lewis, S.M. (1984) *Practical Haematology*, 6th Ed., Churchill Livingstone, London.

Esterhay, R.J., Wiernik, P.H., Grove, W.R. *et al.* (1982) Moderate dose methotrexate, vincristine, asparaginase, and dexamethasone for treatment of adult acute lymphocytic leukemia. *Blood*, **59**, 334.

Evans, A.E., Gilbert, E.S. & Zandstra, R. (1970) The increasing incidence of central nervous system leukaemia in children *Cancer*, **26**, 404.

Farber, S., Diamond, L.K., Mercer, R.D. *et al.* (1948) Temporary remissions in acute leukemia in children produced by folic acid antagonist 4-amino-pteroylglutamic acid (Aminopterin). *New Engl. J. Med.* **238**, 787.

Firkin, F.C. (1972) Serum muramidase in haematological disorders: diagnostic value in neoplastic states. *Austr. N.Z. J. Med.* **2**, 28.

Flandrin, G. & Daniel, M-T. (1981) Cytochemistry in the classification of leukemias. In: Catovsky, D. (Ed.) *The Leukemic Cell*, Churchill Livingstone, Edinburgh.

Foon, K.A., Schroft, K.A. & Gale, R.P. (1982) Surface markers on leukemia and lymphoma cells: recent advances. *Blood*, **60**, 1.

Fourth International Workshop on Chromosomes in Leukemia (1984) A prospective study of acute non-lymphocytic leukemia. *Cancer Genet. Cytogenet.* **11**, 249.

Gale, R.P. (1984) Progress in acute myelogenous leukemia. *Ann. Int. Med.* **101**, 702.

Garson, O.M. (1988) Cytogenetics of leukemic cells. In: Henderson, E. & Lister, J. (Eds) *Leukemia*, 5th Ed., Grune & Stratton, New York.

Goldie, J.H., Coldman, A.J. & Gudauskas, G.A. (1982) Rationale for the use of alternating non-cross-resistant chemotherapy. *Cancer Treat. Rep.* **66**, 439.

Greaves, M.F. (1981) Analysis of the clinical and biological significance of lymphoid phenotype in acute leukaemia. *Cancer Res.* **41**, 4752.

Greenberg, P.L. (1983) The smouldering myeloid leukemic states: Clinical and biological features. *Blood*, **61**, 1035.

Haghbin, M., Murphy, M.L., Tan, C.C. *et al.* (1980) A long-term clinical follow-up of children with acute lymphoblastic leukemia treated with intensive chemotherapy regimens. *Cancer*, **46**, 241.

Hersh, E.M., Wong, V.G. Henderson, E.S. *et al.* (1966) Hepatotoxic effects of methotrexate. *Cancer*, **19**, 600.

Herzig, R.H., Wolff, S.N. Lazarus, H.M. *et al.* (1983) High-dose cytosine arabinoside therapy for refractory leukemia. *Blood*, **62**, 361.

Huang, M., Li, C-Y., Nichols, W.L. *et al.* (1984) Acute leukemia with megakaryocytic differentiation: a study of 12 cases identified immunocytochemically. *Blood*, **64**, 427.

Hughes, W.T., Feldman, S., Gigliotti, F. *et al.* (1985) Prevention of infectious complications in acute lymphoblastic leukaemia. *Semin. Oncol.* **12**, 180.

Jacobs, A.D. & Gale, R.P. (1984) Recent advances in the biology and treatment of acute lymphoblastic leukemia in adults. *New Engl. J. Med.* **311**, 1219.

Janossy, G., Hoffbrand, A.V., Greaves, M.F. *et al.* (1980) Terminal transferase enzyme assay and immunological membrane markers in the diagnosis of leukaemia: a multiparameter analysis of 300 cases. *Brit. J. Haemat.* **44**, 221.

Johnson, F.L., Thomas, E.D., Clark, B.S. *et al.* (1981) A comparison of marrow transplantation with chemotherapy for children with acute lymphoblastic leukemia in second or subsequent remission. *New Engl. J. Med.* **305**, 846.

Juneja, S.K., Imbert, M., Jouault, H. *et al.* (1983) Haematological features of primary myelodysplastic syndromes (PMDS) at initial presentation: a study of 118 cases. *J. Clin. Path.* **36**, 1129.

Kerkhofs, H., Hagemeijer, A., Lecksma, C.H.W. *et al.* (1982) The 5q–chromosome abnormality in haematological disorders. A collaborative study of 34 cases from the Netherlands. *Brit. J. Haemat.* **52**, 365.

Lister, T.A. & Rohatiner, A.Z.S. (1982) The treatment of acute myelogenous leukemia in adults. *Semin. Hematol.* **19**, 172.

May, S.J., Smith, S.A., Jacobs, A. *et al.* (1985) The myelodysplastic syndrome: analysis of laboratory characteristics in relation to the FAB classification. *Brit. J. Haemat.* **59**, 311.

McKenna, R.W., Parkin, J., Bloomfield, C.D. *et al.* (1982) Acute promyelocytic leukaemia: a study of 39 cases with identification of a hyperbasophilic microgranular variant. *Brit. J. Haemat.* **50**, 201.

Mufti, G.J., Oscier, D.G., Hamblin, T.J. *et al.* (1983) Low doses of cytarabine in the treatment of myelodysplastic syndrome and acute myeloid leukemia. *New Engl. J. Med.* **309**, 1653.

Nesbitt, M.E., Woods, W.G., Weisdorf, D. *et al.* (1985) Bone marrow transplantation for acute lymphocytic leukemia. *Semin Oncol.* **12**, 149.

Niemeyer, C.M., Hitchcock-Bryan, S. & Sallan, S.E. (1985) Comparative analysis of treatment programs for childhood acute lymphoblastic leukemia. *Semin. Oncol.* **12**, 122.

Nies, B.A., Bodey, G.P., Thomas, L.B. *et al.* (1965) The persistence of extramedullary leukemia infiltrates during bone marrow remission of acute leukemia. *Blood*, **26**, 133.

Preisler, H.D., Early, A.P., Raza, A. *et al.* (1983) Therapy of secondary acute non-lymphocytic leukemia with cytarabine. *New Engl. J. Med.* **308**, 21.

Rai, K.R., Holland, J.F., Glidewell, O.J. *et al.* (1981) Treatment of acute myelocytic leukemia: A study by cancer and leukemia Group B. *Blood*, **58**, 1203.

Solal-Celigny, P., Desaint, B., Herrera, A. *et al.* (1984) Chronic myelomonocytic leukemia according to FAB classification: analysis of 35 cases. *Blood*, **63**, 634.

Southam, C.M., Craver, L.F., Dargeon, H.W. *et al.* (1951) A study of the natural history of acute leukaemia. *Cancer*, **4**, 39.

Sultan, C., Deregnaucourt, J., Ko, Y.W. *et al.* (1981) Distribution of 250 cases of acute myeloid leukaemia (AML) according to the FAB classification and response to therapy. *Brit. J. Haemat.* **47**, 545.

Tricot, G., de Bock, R., Dekker, A.W. *et al.* (1984) Low dose cytosine arabinoside (Ara C) in Myelodysplastic Syndromes. *Brit. J. Haemat.* **58**, 231.

Von Hoff, D.D., Rozencweig, M. & Piccart, M. (1982) The cardiotoxicity of anticancer agents. *Semin. Oncol.* **9**, 23.

Yates, J., Glidewell, O., Wiernik, P. *et al.* (1982) Cytosine arabinoside with daunorubicin or adriamycin for therapy of acute myelocytic leukemia: a CALGB study. *Blood*, **60**, 454.

Zwaan, F.E. & Jansen, J. (1984) Bone marrow transplantation in acute non-lymphoblastic leukemia. *Semin. Hematol.* **21**, 36.

Chronic granulocytic leukaemia

Galton, D.A.G. (1959) Treatment of chronic leukaemias. *Brit. Med. Bull.* **15**, 78.

Griffin, J.D. Todd, R.F., Ritz, J. *et al.* (1983) Differentiation patterns in the blastic phase of chronic myeloid leukemia. *Blood*, **61**, 85.

Hardisty, R.M., Speed, D.E. & Till, M. (1964) Granulocytic leukaemia in childhood. *Brit. J. Haemat.* **10**, 551.

MRC Working Party for Therapeutic Trials in Leukaemia (1968) Chronic granulocytic leukaemia: comparison of radiotherapy and busulphan therapy. *Brit. Med. J.* **1**, 201.

Rowley, J.D. (1973) A new consistent chromosomal abnormality in chronic myelogenous leukaemia identified by quinacrine fluorescence and Giemsa staining. *Nature*, **243**, 31.

Wiernik, P.H. & Serpick, A.A. (1970) Granulocytic sarcoma (chloroma). *Blood*, **35**, 361.

Chronic lymphocytic leukaemia

Binet, J.L., Auquier, A., Dighiero, G. *et al.* (1981) A new prognostic classification of chronic lymphocytic leukemia derived from a multivariate survival analysis. *Cancer,* **48**, 198.

Boggs, D.R., Sofferman, S.A., Wintrobe, M.M. *et al.* (1966) Factors influencing the duration of survival of patients with chronic lymphocytic leukaemia. *Am. J. Med.* **40**, 243.

Catovsky, D. (1977) Hairy-cell leukaemia and prolymphocytic leukaemia. *Clin. Haemat.* **6**, 245.

Enno, A., Catovsky, D., O'Brien, M. *et al.* (1978) "Prolymphocytoid" transformation of chronic lymphocytic leukaemia. *Brit. J. Haemat.* **41**, 9.

Gale, R.P. & Foon, K.A. (1985) Chronic lymphocytic leukemia: recent advances in biology and treatment. *Ann. Int. Med.* **103**, 101.

Galton, D.A.G., Wiltshaw, E., Szur, L. *et al.* (1961) The use of chlorambucil and steroids in the treatment of chronic lymphocytic leukaemia. *Brit. J. Haemat.* **7**, 73.

Golomb, H.M. (1987) The treatment of hairy cell leukemia. *Blood,* **69**, 979.

Golomb, H.M., Catovsky, D. & Golde, D.W. (1978) Hairy cell leukemia. A clinical review based on 71 cases. *Ann. Int. Med.* **89**, 677.

Jansen, J., Schmit, H.R.E., Meyer, C.J.L.M. *et al.* (1982) Cell markers in hairy cell leukemia studied in cells from 51 patients. *Blood,* **59**, 52.

Oscier, D.G., Catovsky, D., Errington, R.D. *et al.* (1981) Splenic irradiation in B-prolymphocytic leukaemia. *Brit. J. Haematol.* **48**, 577.

Rai, K.R., Sawitsky, A., Cronkite, E.P. *et al.* (1975) Clinical staging of chronic lymphocytic leukemia. *Blood,* **46**, 219.

Spiers, A.S., Moore, D., Cassileth, P.A. *et al.* (1987) Remissions in hairy cell leukemia with pentostatin (2'-doxycoformycin). *New Engl. J. Med.* **316**, 825.

Wall, R.L. & Conrad, F.G. (1961) Cyclophosphamide therapy. *Arch. Int. Med.* **108**, 456.

Leukaemoid reactions

Annotation (1967) Leukaemoid reactions. *Lancet,* **ii**, 408.

Chapter 11
Tumours of Lymphoid Tissues; The Paraproteinaemias

Neoplastic proliferation of cells of the lymphoid series can give rise to solid tissue tumours, the *malignant lymphomas*, and to tumours of plasma cells which are generally categorized as *multiple myeloma*. In multiple myeloma, there is usually production of large amounts of identical immunoglobulin molecules, and, as this differs from the heterogeneous pattern of immunoglobulin molecules produced in a normal immune reaction, the monoclonal protein produced in multiple myeloma is called a *paraprotein*. Occasionally, lymphoproliferative disorders give rise to high molecular weight paraproteins, and this clinical syndrome, which has different histological features and natural history from multiple myeloma, is termed *macroglobulinaemia*. Abnormal cellular and humoral immunity is common in malignant disorders of the lymphoid system.

The malignant lymphomas

Classification

The two major categories of malignant lymphoma are Hodgkin's disease, representing slightly less than half of all cases, and non-Hodgkin's lymphomas, which make up the remainder.

Hodgkin's disease is characterized by the presence of binucleate Sternberg–Reed giant cells, with prominent nucleoli, and variable numbers of lymphocytes, plasma cells, and eosinophils, which are considered to be reactive to the disease rather than part of the neoplastic process. Fibrosis is often present, and can produce the commonly observed nodular sclerosing histological pattern. Four subtypes (Table 11.1) are recognized on basic histological characteristics in the widely used Rye classification (Lukes *et al.* 1966). The neoplastic process tends to involve adjacent lymph nodes early, with spread to distant areas occurring at a later stage.

Non-Hodgkin's lymphomas are a more heterogeneous group of disorders, the classification of which has been the subject of much controversy in recent years. The widely employed classification system of Rappaport (Table 11.1) is based on the presumed identity, degree of differentiation, and growth pattern of the primary cell type as observed microscopically in involved lymph nodes. The presence of well-differentiated cells and a nodular growth pattern is generally associated with a more favourable prognosis. Although it is now apparent that the nomenclature used in the Rappaport classification is, in some instances, inappropriate (e.g. the 'histiocyte' of histiocytic lymphoma is, in reality, a transformed lymphocyte usually of B-cell derivation), the system retains wide popularity among clinicians and pathologists.

Recent advances in knowledge of the anatomy and physiology of the immune system have led to the development of functional classifications based on immunological analysis of the neoplastic cell population. Using cell surface markers similar to those employed in the acute leukaemias (pp. 246–7), it has been shown that the majority of non-Hodgkin's lymphomas are of monoclonal B-cell origin, a lesser number being T cell or non-T, non-B in type. The classifications of Lukes and Collins (Table 11.1) and Lennert *et al.* (1975) combine this newer immunological data with traditional mor-

Table 11.1. *Classification of the lymphomas*

Hodgkin's disease

RYE CLASSIFICATION (Lukes *et al.* 1966)
Lymphocyte predominant
Nodular sclerosing
Mixed cellularity
Lymphocyte depleted

Non-Hodgkin's lymphoma

RAPPAPORT CLASSIFICATION (1966)

Nodular
Lymphocytic, well differentiated
Lymphocytic, poorly differentiated
Lymphocytic and histiocytic, mixed

Diffuse
Lymphocytic, well differentiated
Lymphocytic, poorly differentiated
Lymphocytic and histiocytic, mixed
Histiocytic
Undifferentiated
Burkitt's lymphoma
Lymphoblastic

LUKES–COLLINS CLASSIFICATION (1974)

B cell
Small lymphocytic
Plasmacytoid lymphocytic
Follicular centre cell (follicular or diffuse)
  Small cleaved
  Large cleaved
  Small non-cleaved
  Large non-cleaved
Immunoblastic sarcoma

T cell
Small lymphocytic
Convoluted lymphocytic
Cerebriform lymphocytic
Immunoblastic sarcoma

Histiocytic

Undefined

phological concepts. A number of other classification systems are used in various countries, and in an attempt to promote a more uniform approach and permit translation between the systems, a group of pathologists sponsored by the National Cancer Institute has recently proposed a 'working formulation for clinical usage' (the non-Hodgkin's lymphoma pathologic classification project, 1982).

In many instances of malignant lymphoma, the histology becomes less well differentiated as the disease progresses; treatment by radiation or chemotherapy may modify the histological appearance, particularly by eradication of differentiated lymphoid cells. As the natural history of the disease in any given patient correlates best with the initial histological pattern, and this assessment forms the basis of many subsequent decisions relating to management, the utmost care must be taken to ensure adequate histological assessment at the outset in each instance and to preserve histological specimens for future reference.

Diagnostic approach in malignant lymphoma

The initial approach to a patient with a lymphoid tumour is to consider the possibility that this might be due to some infective, inflammatory, or chemical cause. Common non-neoplastic causes of lymph node enlargement are listed in Table 11.2. Clinical inquiry may reveal evidence suggesting a systemic infective process such as infectious mononucleosis (p. 231), toxoplasmosis or, less commonly, cytomegalovirus infection. These three conditions present a very similar clinical picture with pyrexia, lymph node enlargement, usually generalized, and characteristic atypical lymphocytes in the peripheral blood.

Acquired immunodeficiency syndrome (p. 488) and, in particular, the *lymphadenopathy syndrome*, associated with human immunodeficiency virus (HIV) infection should be excluded by appropriate investigations. Clinical suspicion should be aroused if the patient belongs to a 'high-risk' group, a homosexual or bisexual male, a haemophiliac, an intravenous drug user, or one who has received a blood transfusion within the past few years. The protean manifestations include weight loss, respiratory infections, diarrhoea, and thrombocytopenia, which are common to lymphoma and may not help differentiation. The presence of circulating antibody to HIV is of infection and may be diagnostic

Table 11.2. *Causes of lymph node enlargement resembling malignant lymphoma*

Bacterial
Acute bacterial infections
Tuberculosis
Viral
Infectious mononucleosis
Cytomegalovirus
Acquired immunodeficiency syndrome
Other infections
Toxoplasmosis
Cat-scratch fever
Chemical
Hydantoin pseudolymphoma
Other
Sarcoidosis
Auto-immune diseases
Angio-immunoblastic lymphadenopathy
Non-specific reactive hyperplasia in chronic dermatitis
Infiltration with other neoplastic processes

associated with evidence of severe immunodepression, and the reversal of the helper to suppressor T-lymphocyte ratio in the peripheral blood. On occasions, however, lymph node biopsy may be required to exclude lymphoma.

A less common infective cause of lymph node enlargement which sometimes causes difficulty in diagnosis is that associated with *cat-scratch fever*. Here, there may be evidence that the patient has a cat as a pet, although frequently a specific episode of scratching is not recollected. Lymph node enlargement is most commonly found in the epitrochlear group, and to a lesser extent in the adjacent axilla, but sometimes it is seen in the posterior triangle or inguinal region. Usually the lymph nodes are hot, tender, and somewhat indurated. *Tuberculosis* of lymph nodes is becoming less common, but still must be considered in differential diagnosis, particularly when the lymph node mass is in the vicinity of the tonsillar or jugulodigastric lymph node. Substantial enlargement of lymph nodes sometimes arises in association with *rheumatoid arthritis*, but usually in the vicinity of inflamed joints; similar lymph node enlargement may be seen in association with other collagen diseases, particularly *systemic lupus erythematosus*.

An important condition always to be considered in differential diagnosis of lymph node or splenic enlargement is *sarcoidosis*. Clinical features which may be helpful in its diagnosis are the presence of any manifestation of inflammation in the uveal tract such as iritis or iridocyclitis; the presence of parotid enlargement; the association of erythema nodosum with hilar lymph node enlargement seen on X-ray; and the finding on investigation of hyperglobulinaemia, hypercalcaemia, or an increase in urinary calcium excretion. The histological appearance of a lymph node is generally diagnostic.

An unusual, but important, problem in differential diagnosis from lymphoma is *lymphadenopathy induced by anticonvulsant drugs*. This is sometimes termed *pseudolymphoma* as both the clinical and histological pictures loosely mimic some forms of histiocytic non-Hodgkin's lymphoma; the history of exposure to the drugs is very important in establishing the diagnosis. It occurs most commonly with the drug mesantoin, usually in patients who have been receiving the drug for many months. However, it has also been described with phenytoin. The patient may have fever and skin rash in addition to marked lymph node enlargement, and occasionally the spleen may be enlarged. Histologically, there is considerable disturbance of normal architecture in the lymph nodes with hyperplasia of 'histiocytic' cells. Sometimes, focal necrosis is also seen. Several cases are now recorded, however, in which this lymph node reaction has gone on to the development of true malignant lymphoma (Hyman & Sommers 1966).

Angio-immunoblastic lymphadenopathy is a more recently described syndrome, occurring mostly in older patients and characterized by marked immunological disturbance (Frizzera *et al.* 1975, Lukes & Tindle 1975, Cullen *et al.* 1979). The disease is characterized by lymphadenopathy, and there is often an associated transitory skin rash, arthralgia, and immune haemolytic anaemia. Usually there is a marked polyclonal increase in serum immunoglobulin, on occasion with a superadded monoclonal paraprotein. Recurrent respiratory infections are a feature and may eventually prove fatal. The relationship of this syndrome to malignant lymphomas remains uncertain as occasional cases appear to resolve completely, whilst other patients die from their disease within 12–24 months, or progress to frank malignant lymphoma (immunoblastic). Many cases respond for a time to corticosteroid therapy, or chemotherapy as employed for non-Hodgkin's lymphoma.

Thus in every case of suspected *malignant lymphoma*, the establishment of a tissue diagnosis is mandatory to exclude non-malignant causes of lymph node enlargement, and to determine the subgroup of lymphoma to which the patient's disease belongs.

Clinical features

HODGKIN'S DISEASE

Hodgkin's disease has a wide age incidence from childhood through to old age. However, its most frequent incidence is in the 20–40 age group. Males are affected approximately twice as commonly as females.

The presenting manifestations are listed in Table 11.3. Most commonly the disease presents with involvement of a single group of lymph nodes, and where these are in a prominent external situation, such as in the neck, systemic symptoms are less common than when the disease develops in the mediastinum or para-aortic lymphatic chain. *Superficial lymph nodes* are involved in approximately 90 per cent of patients at presentation, and approximately 70 per cent of these are in the cervical region. Most commonly, the enlargement is asymptomatic, but on occasion tenderness of the nodes occurs, associated with histological findings of tissue necrosis, which is a common feature of Hodgkin's disease.

Table 11.3. *Clinical manifestations of Hodgkin's disease*

Common
Lymphadenopathy
Mediastinal involvement
Fever, night sweats
Weight loss
Malaise
Less common
Pruritus
Abdominal pain
Alcohol-induced pain
Anaemia
Occasional
Nerve root compression
Local compression or obstruction by tumour mass
Bone pain
Skin infiltration

Mediastinal Hodgkin's disease is found in approximately 10 per cent of patients at presentation, but is reported in as many as 60 per cent at some stage during the course of the disease (Moran & Ultmann 1974). It is particularly common in the nodular sclerosing form of the disease. In patients with mediastinal disease, involvement of the right supraclavicular lymph node group is common. Obstruction of the superior vena cava may develop and cause distension of the veins of the neck and upper chest wall. Encroachment on the trachea and major bronchi may cause cough and dyspnoea, and occasionally symptomatic oesophageal obstruction develops. Findings of superior mediastinal obstruction represent an emergency demanding immediate treatment.

Intra-abdominal Hodgkin's disease is most commonly represented by involvement of the spleen and para-aortic lymph nodes. Clinical detection of such disease when the patient first presents may be difficult unless the disease is extensive. Although staging laparotomy (pp. 289–90) has shown an incidence of up to 40 per cent of abdominal involvement in untreated patients (Moran & Ultmann 1974), symptoms of involvement, such as splenic discomfort, pain from abdominal masses, or disturbance of bowel habit, occur in only a few per cent of untreated patients. Systemic disturbance, particularly anorexia and weight loss, nausea, fever, and pruritus carry a strong association with retroperitoneal lymph node enlargement.

Involvement of nasopharynx and tonsil (Waldeyer's ring) is unusual in Hodgkin's disease but, when present, often causes symptoms of nasal congestion or disturbance of swallowing.

Spinal cord and nerve root compression, whilst uncommon, are important to recognize, as spinal cord compression may progress to cause paraplegia.

X-ray of the spine may show a dense (sclerotic) vertebral body, but, most commonly when spinal cord compression develops, the deposit of tumour is epidural in situation and computerized tomography or myelogram may be required for anatomical localization. Most common sites of involvement are the lower dorsal and upper lumbar spine. Root pain, paraesthesiae, weakness and stiffness of the legs, and disturbance of micturition are the most common symptoms. Once spinal cord compression has developed, a delay of 24 hours may result in permanent damage.

Intracerebral involvement is much less common than involvement of the spinal cord. Meningeal invasion does occur and presents with headache, slight neck stiffness, and raised intracranial pressure; cranial nerve palsies are less common. The cerebral cortex may be compressed by tumour masses from without, but primary infiltration of the brain is exceedingly rare. Intra-orbital deposits occur at times, but are more common in non-Hodgkin's lymphoma.

Bone involvement may occur at many sites. Most commonly, this is within the bone marrow where the disease may become widespread. This may rarely result in pancytopenia, but by far the most common cause of anaemia in Hodgkin's disease is normochromic anaemia of the type seen in chronic inflammatory disorders. Localized deposits involving bone sometimes result in pain and disability. Radiologically, the lesions are generally sclerotic, but may be osteolytic in part. Vertebrae, pelvis, ribs, humeri, scapulae, and femora are the most common sites. Serum alkaline phosphatase is commonly raised in the presence of widespread involvement of bone.

Skin manifestations are common; they are usually nonspecific and include pruritus, pigmentation, and purpura. *Pruritus* is the most common of these complaints and is often intense and persistent. Herpes zoster occurs, especially when vertebrae are involved, and sometimes precedes an exacerbation of the disease. Brownish pigmentation of the skin, either localized or generalized, is an occasional manifestation. *Infiltration* of the skin by Hodgkin's disease is uncommon, but, when it occurs, may take the form either of single or multiple discrete non-tender nodules or plaques which are commonly purplish-red or brown, but occasionally skin coloured. Ulceration of the infiltrated area may occur.

Infiltration of viscera other than the spleen and axial lymphatic lymph node groups indicates advanced disease. The *liver* is the most commonly involved non-lymphatic organ, and infiltration may present with jaundice, discomfort, or pain. Involvement of *lung* parenchyma is usually asymptomatic and detected on X-ray, but invasion of *pleura* may give rise to chest pain or breathlessness associated with the development of pleural effusion. Direct invasion of the *heart* (myocardial infiltration) occasionally causes congestive cardiac failure or arrhythmias, bundle branch block, and other electrocardiographic changes. *Pericarditis* with effusion sometimes develops.

Systemic manifestations may be apparent at presentation in Hodgkin's disease and commonly arise at a later stage in unresponsive or relapsed disease. The most common are *fatigue, malaise, fever, sweats, pruritus, anorexia,* and *weight loss.* They carry a strong association with widespread disease and hence are an unfavourable prognostic feature; however, they may all occur in association with a single large lymph node mass, and all subside on successful treatment of local disease. Fever and pruritus are particularly associated with involvement of upper retroperitoneal nodes.

The type of fever varies. It is often moderate and intermittent in nature, but is occasionally more hectic with a remittent course swinging between normal and 40°C or higher. In other patients the 'Pel–Ebstein pattern' is seen, with regularly recurring periodic elevation of temperature extending over some days to even a week or longer.

Metabolic disturbance may be seen in the form of *hyperuricaemia.* This may be manifested as clinical gout, as renal colic associated with the passage of urate deposits from the kidneys, or occasionally as renal failure associated with crystal deposition within the kidneys.

Alcohol-induced pain occurs in approximately one patient in six with Hodgkin's disease. The pain is usually related to an area of active disease, and the interval between drinking and the onset of pain varies between five minutes and several hours. The pain may be severe and prostrating, and may persist from 20 minutes up to 24 hours. Occasionally, it is the first indication of an undiscovered site of involvement which is otherwise asymptomatic.

Defects in *cellular immunity*, as a consequence of the disease and compounded by chemotherapy, are manifested by susceptibility to viral, fungal, and protozoal infections. Anergy, with failure to exhibit delayed-type hypersensitivity to recall antigens, is common as the disease progresses.

Blood picture. At the time of diagnosis, a significant minority of patients have a mild normocytic normochromic anaemia, often with an elevated ESR. Anaemia is extremely common in advanced disease. A mild increase in white cell count is a frequent finding, and some patients have an eosinophilia, which rarely may reach 40–50 per cent. Lymphopenia is also common in advanced disease. The platelet count is usually normal, but occasional patients have a thrombocytosis. Trephine biopsy of the marrow shows involvement with Hodgkin's disease in 5–10 per cent of patients at the time of diagnosis.

NON-HODGKIN'S LYMPHOMA

Like Hodgkin's disease, non-Hodgkin's lymphoma may arise at any age. As in Hodgkin's disease, males are affected approximately twice as commonly as females. In general, the clinical pictures are similar to those of Hodgkin's disease but there are certain broad differences with respect to sites commonly involved. This group of lymphomas varies widely in its rapidity of onset and spread, but there is less tendency to be confined to the axial lymph node structures than with Hodgkin's disease at presentation, and involvement of nasopharynx, tonsil, inguinal, and mesenteric structures is very much more common, as is involvement of the bone marrow.

Character of the lymph nodes. The rate of enlargement of the nodes is extremely variable. In the most benign forms, enlargement may gradually develop over months or years, whilst at the other extreme, tender, fleshy masses may develop, causing obstruction and pressure symptoms in a matter of weeks. Pain may occur when growth is rapid or extension outside the node capsule causes infiltration of other structures. Local invasion and tissue destruction are prominent in the poorly differentiated non-Hodgkin's lymphomas. Involvement of epitrochlear lymph nodes is sometimes seen in nodular lymphocytic lymphomas, although less commonly in diffuse types. It is extremely rare in Hodgkin's disease.

Involvement of the nasopharynx, tonsil and gastrointestinal tract is much more common in non-Hodgkin's lymphoma than in Hodgkin's disease. At autopsy, involvement of the gastrointestinal tract is observed in 50–70 per cent of non-Hodgkin's lymphomas, the most common sites being mesenteric lymph nodes, peritoneum, liver, and small bowel. At presentation, about five per cent of cases have symptoms due to nasopharyngeal or tonsillar involvement—soreness or pain in the throat, nasal obstruction or bleeding, a lump in the throat, or dysphagia. In such cases, regional nodes are usually palpable.

Large masses involving stomach, small bowel, or large bowel may be the presenting feature of the disease, and occasionally, in such instances, surgical resection is successful in producing a sustained remission when no extension into draining lymph nodes has occurred. Such patients generally present with gastrointestinal bleeding, abdominal pain, vomiting, or weight loss, and have been suspected of some other form of neoplastic disease. Rarely, steatorrhoea develops as a result of direct invasion of the bowel, or blockage of lacteals by the tumour. Tumour masses occur in the caecum and rectum, but these are very much less frequent than those in the ileum, which can present with features of intestinal obstruction. Massive enlargement of the spleen is not uncommon and is frequently associated with involvement of the liver. Presentation with ascites may indicate extensive peritoneal deposits or invasion of the thoracic duct, in which case the ascites is generally chylous. Such features are relatively common in the nodular varieties of non-Hodgkin's lymphoma, and may occur at a stage in which the disease is readily amenable to treatment.

Patients with *coeliac disease* are known to be at greater risk than normal for the development of malignancy, usually in the small bowel, and malignant lymphoma constitutes about half of these cases. The predominant histological subgroup is large cell (histiocytic) lymphoma (Swinson *et al.* 1983).

Systemic features are generally less common than in Hodgkin's disease. Pruritus is uncommon, except in the presence of skin involvement, and *pyrexia* more often indicates secondary infection consequent on *depressed immune function* — these patients occasionally have hypogammaglobulinaemia, rendering them susceptible to bacterial infection. Cellular immunity may also be impaired, creating a predisposition to viral and fungal infections.

Most patients have normal haematological parameters early in the course of their illness. As progression occurs, the haemoglobin level falls, and there may be thrombocytopenia and neutropenia. Marrow involvement, detected by trephine biopsy, is present in 30–70 per cent of patients. This group of patients is more prone to develop spread of lymphoma cells to the peripheral blood and central nervous system.

Auto-immune disorders are more common in non-Hodgkin's lymphoma than in Hodgkin's disease, and may give rise to acquired haemolytic anaemia (p. 191) and thrombocytopenia (p. 377).

Metabolic complications occur in non-Hodgkin's lymphoma, as in Hodgkin's disease. The more aggressive forms are particularly prone to *hyperuricaemia*, especially during response to cytotoxic drugs or radiation therapy. *Hypercalcaemia* sometimes occurs, and is more common in advanced disease. Long-term control is usually attained, as in multiple myeloma, only by effective treatment of the underlying disease.

Cutaneous T-cell lymphomas constitute a specific clinical entity. In contrast to other forms of non-Hodgkin's lymphoma, those presenting with skin infiltration are more commonly, but not inevitably, of T-cell origin. They include *mycosis fungoides, Sézary syndrome, and lymphomatoid papulosis.*

Mycosis fungoides is an uncommon chronic lymphoproliferative disorder with characteristic clinical and histological features. The progress of the disease, which runs a course of 3–4 years from diagnosis, have been conveniently divided into three stages. In *stage I*, there are widespread, patchy, scaly, and erythematous eruptions, which may be present for many years before diagnosis. There is often severe pruritus. This stage is called premycotic, and is commonly misdiagnosed as eczema or psoriasis. Progression to *stage II* is accompanied by tumour-like lesions and infiltrated plaques in the skin. Some lesions may regress, leaving pigmented macules. Lymphadenopathy may develop. In *stage III*, the skin tumours ulcerate and fungate. Visceral involvement is evident, with hepatosplenomegaly and deterioration in the general condition of the patient. Median survival is about one year from the development of systemic disease.

The disease has a number of reported associations which may have a bearing on aetiology. These include an increased prevalence of HLA-DR5, occupational exposure to petrochemicals and other solvents, and cytogenetic abnormalities. During the course of the disease, lymphopenia develops, with changes in the circulating T-cell population. There is an increase in suppressor to helper T cell ratio. The malignant T cells in the skin, however, usually possess the surface antigens characteristic of helper T cells.

The diagnosis is made on histological examination of the skin infiltrate, which contains characteristic pleomorphic lymphocytes, often in clusters termed Pautrier's micro-abscesses.

When the disease is confined to the skin, total body electron-beam therapy in doses up to 40 Gy may result in prolonged disease-free remissions. Topical nitrogen mustard and ultraviolet irradiation after ingestion of UV-activated drugs may result in definite but transitory responses. In stage III disease, combination chemotherapy (p. 297) can produce significant remissions, and some authors have suggested that chemotherapy should be administered after total body electron-beam therapy.

Sézary syndrome is closely related to mycosis fungoides; ultrastructurally, the abnormal lymphocyte in both disorders is indistinguishable. There is generalized exfoliative erythroderma and pruritus, and plaques, nodules, tumours, and ulcers develop. The diagnostic feature, apart from the histology of the skin lesions, is the appearance of characteristic atypical lymphocytes (Sézary cells) in the peripheral blood.

These disorders are reviewed in detail by Safai &

Good (1980), Edelson (1980) and Epstein (1980).

Diagnosis

The first step in diagnosis of a patient with lymph node enlargement is the consideration of possible non-malignant as well as malignant causes of lymph node enlargement (p. 279). Inquiry should be made into possible infective causes, exposure to anticonvulsant drugs, and any symptoms that may indicate specific inflammatory disease processes. Once obvious non-malignant causes have been excluded, either on the history or by relevant tests, or where doubt remains as to the cause, the next step is to establish a tissue diagnosis by means of biopsy. Wherever possible, this is performed on palpable superficial lymph nodes.

LYMPH NODE BIOPSY

Since so much depends on the histological appearance of the biopsied node, it is of the utmost importance that the clinician should assist the pathologist by sending the nodes which have been carefully selected and excised without trauma.

Choice of node. Whenever possible, the inguinal and upper deep cervical (tonsillar) nodes should be avoided as they often reveal non-specific inflammatory changes resulting from previous infections, which may mask any specific changes present. Posterior triangle, supraclavicular, and epitrochlear nodes are satisfactory; they are easily accessible, and can if necessary be excised under local anaesthetic. Axillary nodes are usually histologically satisfactory, but they are not always easily accessible, and general anaesthesia is usually necessary for adequate biopsy. The nodes excised should be the larger nodes from the main mass of an involved chain, avoiding the small outlying nodes.

Excision and fixation. The aim is to excise at least one complete node, and preferably more. The incision should allow adequate inspection of the biopsy site, and permit excision of the node without trauma. Traction and crushing by forceps must be particularly avoided, as they can cause sufficient distortion of the tissues to make histological interpretation difficult or even impossible. The capsule of the excised nodes should be intact, as study of the capsule and adjacent tissues is a most important part of the histological examination. Prompt examination is essential, and the node should be transferred to the histopathology laboratory, fresh and *unfixed*, immediately after excision. Imprints from the cut surface made on a clean microscope slide are of considerable diagnostic value, as the morphology of neoplastic lymphoid cell types is well demonstrated by Giemsa staining. Cell-surface antigens (markers) can be identified with immunocytochemistry or fluorescence-activated cell sorting, using a panel of monoclonal antibodies. This can be useful in establishing whether a monoclonal population of lymphoid cells consistent with a neoplastic process is present, and in providing an indication of the lineage of any abnormal cells.

Interpretation. In most cases, a diagnosis can be made from the appearance of the biopsied node. However, sometimes, especially in the early stages or when a small node has been excised, the changes are not definitive and differentiation from an inflammatory reaction may be impossible. In particular, early Hodgkin's disease may be difficult or impossible to distinguish from chronic reactive sinus hyperplasia associated with chronic inflammatory disorders. In cases of doubt, a repeat biopsy may be required. A further difficulty may arise because distinction between a poorly differentiated tumour of lymphoid tissue and anaplastic metastatic carcinoma in a lymph node can be difficult or impossible to make on morphological grounds, especially when there is no obvious primary carcinoma. In these cases, immunocytochemical detection of specific lymphoid cell surface markers on the abnormal cells may enable the distinction to be made.

DIAGNOSIS WHEN SUPERFICIAL NODES ARE NOT ENLARGED

Diagnostic difficulty occurs in patients without superficial lymph node enlargement. When examination suggests involvement of the bone marrow or liver, *trephine biopsy of the bone marrow* (Fig. 11.1) or *liver biopsy*, respectively, may yield a diagnostic biopsy specimen, which by definition is indicative of extranodal disease. When mediastinal

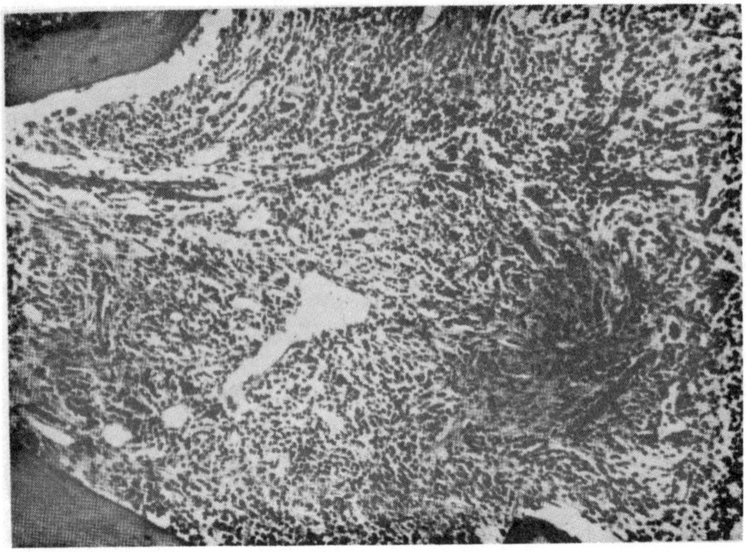

Fig. 11.1. *Photomicrograph of a bone marrow trephine biopsy revealing the presence of a focus of Hodgkin's disease. The marrow aspirated from an adjacent site did not contain any diagnostic material. Sternberg–Reed cells must be present for an unequivocal diagnosis of Hodgkin's disease to be established.*

involvement is the only feature, *scalene node biopsy* sometimes establishes the diagnosis. If this is not diagnostic, it may be necessary to consider diagnostic thoracotomy or mediastinoscopy.

When biopsy at the above sites is not diagnostic, it may be necessary to wait until a superficial lymph node becomes sufficiently large to biopsy. Occasionally, a diagnostic laparotomy must be performed without initial proof of diagnosis of malignant lymphoma. In such cases, the surgeon should be requested to proceed as when performing a *staging laparotomy* (p. 289).

Assessment of extent of the disease (staging)

Once a histological diagnosis of malignant lymphoma has been established, the next question to be resolved is the extent of the disease, so that an appropriate plan of treatment may be designed. The overriding consideration is to determine whether *all* of the disease in the body is amenable to intensive radiation therapy, which provides one of the most convenient approaches to obtaining a cure. Generally, this means disease restricted to sites that can be treated by high radiation dosages. The presence of disease in organs, especially the lung, or in widespread bone marrow sites precludes curative radiotherapy, and the alternative approach to curative therapy in such cases must be planned chemotherapy.

Classification of the extent of disease has been the subject of debate. The classification of the stage of the disease summarized in Table 11.4 represents a simplified version of the classification adopted by the Rye conference (Carbone *et al.* 1971) for

Table 11.4. *Staging of extent of disease in lymphoma*

Stage	Extent of disease
I	Nodal involvement within one region
II	Nodal involvement within two or more regions limited to above or below the diaphragm
III	Nodal involvement both above and below the diaphragm
IV	Involvement of one or more extralymphatic structures
In Hodgkin's disease, each stage is further subdivided into:	
A	No systemic symptoms
B	Documented fever or loss of more than ten per cent bodyweight

Note

1 'Nodal' involvement includes structures of Waldeyer's ring or spleen.

2 Later modifications permit inclusion in I, II, or III if a single extranodal site is involved, with the suffix E followed by identification of the site.

Hodgkin's disease, and can also be applied to non-Hodgkin's lymphoma. Stage I represents localized nodal involvement in one region and is modified to stage I_E for extralymphatic involvement at a single site which is still amenable to surgery or radiotherapy. Stage II implies nodal involvement in two or more non-contiguous regions limited to either above or below the diaphragm, and, again, II_E in the Ann Arbor classification is when one of those sites is extranodal but still amenable to local therapy. Stage III is disease both above and below the diaphragm, and extranodal or splenic involvement may be denoted by the suffix E or S. Stage IV is disseminated disease with involvement of one or more extranodal sites.

In Hodgkin's disease, a further subdivision is made into categories A and B according to the presence of constitutional symptoms. Where there has been weight loss of more than ten per cent of body weight, or documented fever, the suffix B is added as this denotes a worse prognosis and consequently has some bearing on choice of therapy. Pruritus is a common systemic symptom, but is now known to correlate only poorly with prognosis and is thus not employed as a criterion for B-type status (Carbone *et al.* 1971).

SPECIAL INVESTIGATIONS IN STAGING

The investigations employed in the staging process are set out in Table 11.5. The extent of superficial lymph node enlargement is documented in every patient, and the size of the spleen and liver should be noted. Thoracic computerized tomography (CT) provides the most sensitive non-invasive assessment of mediastinal lymph node involvement, but a routine chest X-ray is usually adequate to assess the mediastinum. In cases of doubt, tomograms should be performed when parenchymal lung shadows may represent infiltration. Examination of the peripheral blood should be performed in every case to identify any haematologic abnormality, and particular attention should be paid to the differential white cell count, evidence of haemolysis, and thrombocytopenia. However, as extensive focal infiltration of bone marrow may occur without any abnormality in the peripheral blood picture, bone

Table 11.5. *Clinical assessment of a patient with lymphoma*

History
Rate of onset
Constitutional symptoms (anorexia, weight loss, fatigue, sweats, fever, pruritus)
Symptoms of anaemia
Symptoms suggesting compression or obstruction by mediastinal, abdominal, axillary, pelvic, and femoral lymph nodes
Symptoms suggesting involvement of extranodal sites—nasopharynx, bone, gastrointestinal tract
Symptoms of spinal cord involvement
Examination
Superficial lymph node enlargement—site and degree
Splenomegaly and hepatomegaly
Abdominal masses
Signs of obstruction or pressure by mediastinal, abdominal, axillary, pelvic, and femoral lymph nodes
Signs of involvement of nasopharynx, bone, gastrointestinal tract
Signs of spinal cord involvement
Skin—rash, infiltration, herpes zoster, purpura
Jaundice
Special investigations
Lymph node biopsy
Full blood examination, including platelet count
Liver function tests
Serum creatinine, urea and uric acid
Serum protein electrophoresis
Bone marrow aspiration and trephine (at least two sites)
Liver/spleen scan
X-ray of chest
X-ray of nasopharynx
CT scan of abdomen and pelvis
Further investigations required in some cases
The following investigations may be required when clinical evidence suggests involvement of particular lymph nodes or organs:
Laryngoscopy or bronchoscopy
Skeletal X-ray
Intravenous or retrograde pyelogram
Venography (inferior vena cava)
Barium meal or barium enema
Quantitation of immunoglobulins
Gallium scan
Liver biospy
Thoracic CT scan
Lymphangiography

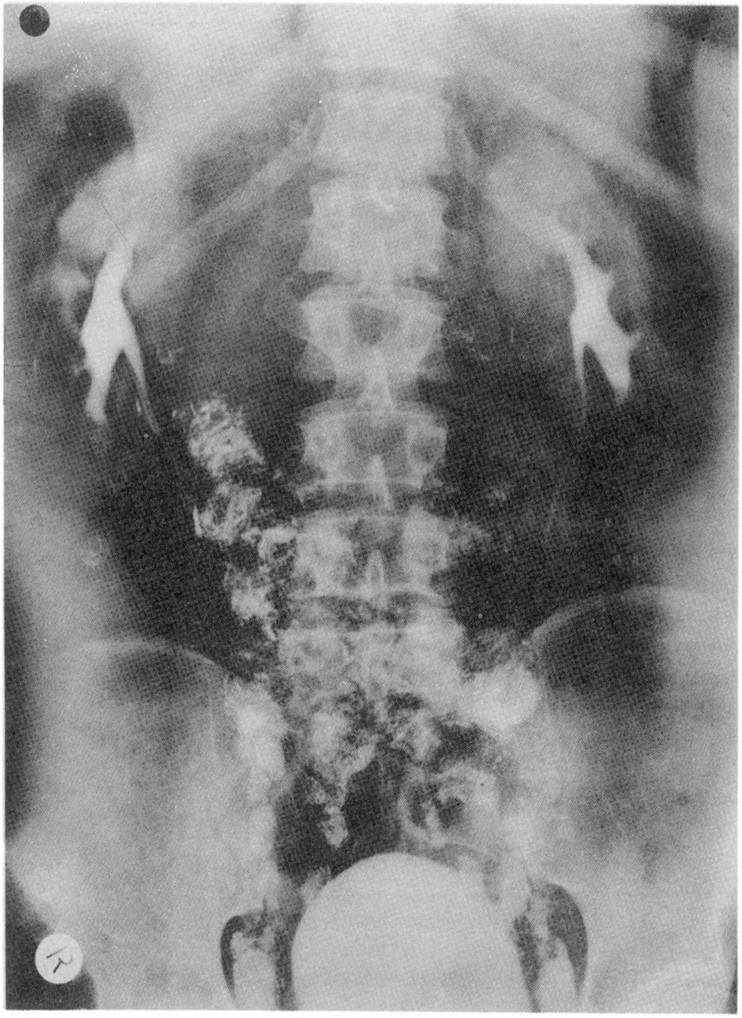

Fig. 11.2. *Bilateral lower limb lymphangiogram indicating extensive enlargement of para-aortic lymph nodes with abnormal architecture characteristic of involvement by disease in a patient with Hodgkin's disease. Note failure of this procedure to indicate the presence of extensively enlarged para-aortic nodes high in the abdomen.*

marrow aspiration and trephine biopsy should be performed in every patient. (Aspiration is simpler, but gives a lower yield of positive results in lymphoma compared with trephine biopsy.)

The occurrence of lymphoma below the diaphragm may be obvious on clinical grounds, but must be extensive for this to be the case. The introduction of *lower limb lymphangiography* greatly improved the accuracy of diagnosis of involved retroperitoneal lymph nodes, particularly those in the lower para-aortic chains and pelvis. An example of a positive result is shown in Fig. 11.2. However, in most instances, *CT scanning* of the pelvis and abdomen provides adequate accuracy in diagnosing intra-abdominal disease (Fig. 11.3). It has advantages over lymphangiography in detecting enlarged nodes in the high para-aortic, pre-aortic, and mesenteric groups, and lacks the discomfort of lymphangiography. In addition, the size of the liver and spleen are also gauged, as is the presence of deposits in these organs, providing these are reasonably extensive. The greater precision of lymphangiography in showing abnormal architecture in nodes that are only slightly enlarged is one advantage over CT scanning. *Gallium-67 scanning* is another imaging technique which is not widely employed but has been advocated as an additional means for localization of disease.

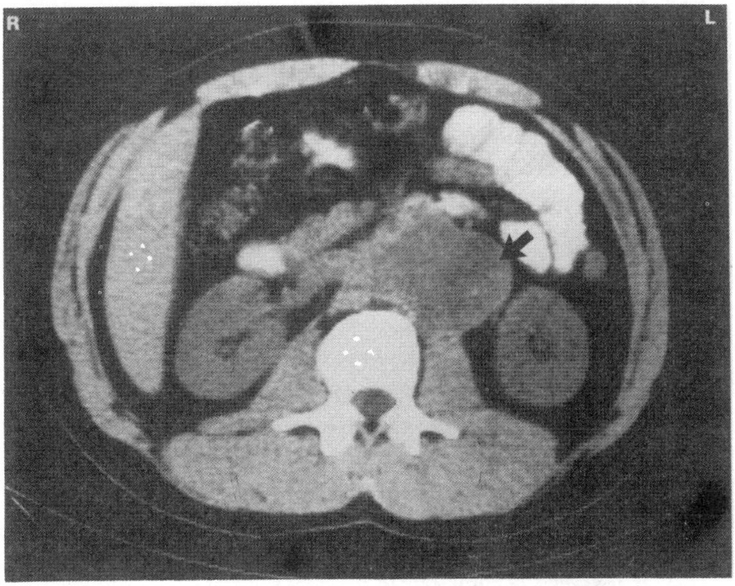

Fig. 11.3. *CT scan of abdomen illustrating an abnormally enlarged lymph gland mass (arrow) at the level of the renal pedicle. Such a technique can detect impalpable enlarged glands in the abdomen, and is particularly suited for detecting abnormalities of this type in the upper abdomen where lymphangiography may be unreliable.*

Involvement of the liver may be suspected on the basis of hepatic enlargement or because of abnormal biochemical liver function tests. However, this may reflect non-specific reactive responses which are relatively common in Hodgkin's disease. A better index of abnormal tissue structure is provided by CT scan, ultrasound, and scans with radioactive colloid. The presence of hepatic involvement has been generally held to exclude radiotherapy as potential curative treatment, and definitive evidence is sought by percutaneous needle biopsy.

Estimation of serum creatinine and urea should be performed in every case, because infiltration of kidneys or obstruction of ureters can be caused by lymphoma.

Further radiological examinations indicated in some cases include skeletal survey, contrast X-rays of the nasopharynx to assess involvement of Waldeyer's ring, and intravenous pyelography to evaluate whether the ureters are compressed or displaced by para-aortic lymph node enlargement. Barium studies of the gastrointestinal tract are of relatively little value unless symptoms or signs point to local involvement by lymphoma.

Tests of immune function, such as serum protein electrophoresis to assess total immunoglobulin and the presence of paraproteins, are readily performed and may be of value both in diagnosis and in the assessment of susceptibility to infection.

STAGING LAPAROTOMY

Staging laparotomy, initially a controversial issue but subsequently accepted by most, has again became a source of contention. The concept that the extent of disease could be more accurately ascertained in patients with Hodgkin's disease by laparotomy was introduced by Kaplan and his colleagues. Whilst it was seen initially as a radical approach when applied to patients presenting with disease confined apparently to the neck, the demonstration that 20 per cent or more of such patients suffer from disease in the spleen or liver that could not be detected by other means established that the procedure does have an important place in the assessment of such patients (Rosenberg *et al.* 1971, Jones 1980). When the investigations outlined above clearly demonstrate that the site(s) of disease do not permit radiotherapy to be curative, there is no purpose in proceeding with a staging laparotomy.

Staging laparatomy is a rational step when employed to provide greater precision in evaluating the extent of disease in order to define the subgroup of patients in whom there is a high probability that all disease is restricted to sites that can be treated by potentially curative doses of radiation. This is important, as patients treated by extensive radiotherapy with disease outside the fields of treatment will inevitably suffer recurrence of the disease.

Others argue that staging laparotomy can be omitted because of: (a) the morbidity and occasional mortality associated with the procedure; (b) the ability to extend the field of radiotherapy to the level of L4 and include the spleen if not removed; (c) the comparatively good response to chemotherapy of patients who relapse after radiotherapy (Lacher 1983, Gomez *et al.* 1984); and (d) the lack of demonstrable survival advantage in subjects who have undergone staging laparotomy (Haybittle *et al.* 1985).

Staging laparotomy should be performed only by surgeons fully conversant with the requirements of the procedure. It involves resection of the spleen and careful pathological examination of both this organ and associated nodes in the splenic pedicle. Para-aortic nodes should be explored and biopsied as enlargement on CT scan or on lymphangiography may occur as a reactive state and, at times, para-aortic nodes involved with Hodgkin's disease are not well outlined. Needle and wedge biopsy of the liver should be obtained, and mesenteric nodes carefully inspected. Where it is anticipated that radiation therapy will be applied to the lateral walls of the pelvis in female patients, the ovaries should be moved at laparotomy to a more central position.

Complications following such laparotomy are few in experienced hands. Splenectomy results in elevation of the platelet count postoperatively, and care should be taken to ensure rapid mobilization of the patient wherever possible. In most debilitated patients, widespread disease is detected by other means, so that in the majority of cases wound healing is rapid, and definitive treatment for the disease may be undertaken shortly after surgery. In view of a possible disadvantage in the efficacy of clearance of microbes from the circulation, these subjects are usually immunized with multivalent pneumococcal vaccine prior to removal of the spleen.

Principles of treatment in lymphoma

GENERAL CONSIDERATIONS IN TREATMENT

Advice to patient and relatives

Explanation of the situation to the patient is a major responsibility of the physician, and the temptation to shrink from explaining the nature of the disease should be resisted other than under exceptional circumstances. If patients are to undertake a prolonged course of treatment requiring tolerance of side-effects and co-operation with drug therapy, they must be able to comprehend the reasons for the discomfort, and be motivated to seek recovery from the disease. Anxieties on the part of the patient with respect to family responsibilities and personal and financial worries may present real problems in management, and should be explored as far as possible in the early stages of the illness. Explanation to the patient and relatives should cover both the nature of the disease and the grounds for optimism based on the known results of therapy. The nature of side-effects that are likely to be experienced should be discussed to allay anxiety when they arise, and to ensure the fullest co-operation when supportive measures are necessary. The patient should be encouraged to lead a normal active life within the limitations of treatment, and every attempt should be made to keep hospitalization to a minimum.

Objects of therapy

The knowledge that a significant proportion of patients with lymphoma may be cured means that careful assessment must be made in every patient, both with respect to histological diagnosis and extent of disease, so that the most appropriate therapy is undertaken. The basic choice falls between radiotherapy and chemotherapeutic approaches, but within the second of these alternatives a choice must be made between aggressive combination chemotherapy, with its promise of long-term remission and cure, and simple palliative approaches. The decision between radical treatment, palliative therapy, or observation with no

Table 11.6. *Treatment options for Hodgkin's disease*

Pathological stage	DXRT		Chemotherapy (CT)
IA & IIA	Upper or lower field (subtotal)		If there is bulky disease, e.g. mediastinal mass, CT may be added
IB & IIB	Total lymphoid	or	CT
IIIA	Total lymphoid	or	CT
IIIB & IV	—		CT

active therapy in each case is one of considerable importance and is influenced by assessment of the patient's capacity to tolerate radical treatment, given all appropriate supportive assistance.

Radical radiotherapy is the treatment of choice in localized *Hodgkin's disease*. It is very often curative in non-bulky disease which is localized to regions to which appropriately high doses of radiation can be delivered. Chemotherapy is, on the other hand, the treatment of choice for widespread or recurrent disease. The choices are outlined in Table 11.6. In *non-Hodgkin's lymphoma*, chemotherapy is the mainstay of management, and radiotherapy has a limited curative role.

RADIATION THERAPY

Mega-voltage X-ray is the usual form of radiation, providing least in the way of local and constitutional disturbances. Local X-ray therapy may be administered solely to involved regions, but generally treatment is planned to cover what is termed an upper or lower mantle field or both (total nodal irradiation). Only one mantle field is treated in a single course of therapy. An upper mantle field represents irradiation above the diaphragm with shielding to the lungs and much of the heart; it includes the deep and superficial lymphatic chains in the neck, supraclavicular and axillary regions, and mediastinal structures. It may be extended upwards to include Waldeyer's ring where appropriate, and down to the level of L4 to include the upper para-aortic nodes, and also to include the spleen if staging laparotomy is not performed.

A lower mantle field has the shape of an inverted Y, with shielding covering the lateral structures such as liver and kidneys, and the midline pelvic structures and gonads. During the course of therapy, patients ordinarily develop inflammation affecting the pharynx and oesophagus with upper mantle treatment, as well as some discomfort to the skin at the front and back. In lower mantle therapy, marked gastrointestinal disturbance is common. An acute radiation pneumonitis affects 5–10 per cent of patients subjected to upper mantle radiotherapy, and a course of corticosteroids may be required to suppress the inflammation. General radiation sickness may occur, but is modified by the administration of anti-emetic therapy. Typically, older patients suffer a greater degree of systemic upset with radiation therapy than the young, and this may rarely influence the choice or extent of treatment in individual patients.

Radical radiation therapy of this kind (ordinarily to a dose of 35–40 Gy) invariably suppresses bone marrow proliferation in the irradiated area, and sometimes this necessitates temporary cessation of treatment. A rest period is usually required between upper and lower mantle treatment to allow haemopoietic recovery to occur, and should there be evidence during this period of spread of disease to sites not amenable to radiation, the treatment plan should be reconsidered and chemotherapy undertaken before further bone marrow damage results from radiotherapy. Rapid spread of this kind, however, is uncommon.

In some cases, it is appropriate to administer both radical radiotherapy and combination chemotherapy as initial treatment. The combined approach offers a better chance of cure (Wiernik *et al.* 1979, Hoppe *et al.* 1979) in stage II Hodgkin's disease with a bulky tumour (e.g. mediastinal). The treatment may be administered by alternating several courses of chemotherapy with radiotherapy

(Hoppe *et al.* 1979). However, the combination of both modes of treatment increases the risk of a second tumour developing in the future, especially acute leukaemia (Canellos *et al.* 1983).

Response to radiation therapy

Hodgkin's disease is a highly radiosensitive tumour, and long-term survival rates relate very much to the extent of disease when treatment is first undertaken. Results have improved enormously in the past 30 years; in a comparison of patients treated between 1948 and 1964 with those treated between 1969 and 1973, the proportion of patients alive 5 years after diagnosis improved from 34 to 87 per cent (Aisenberg & Qazi 1976). In patients with disease of stage IA and IIA on presentation (patients without systemic symptoms and disease confined to treatable areas on one side of the diaphragm), figures relating to recurrence and survival at 5 years show a high probability of cure in the great majority of cases. Projected 10-year survival was greater than 80 per cent, particularly where initial assessment included staging laparotomy to pick up the significant number in whom otherwise undetectable splenic disease would have been missed. Results of treatment in stage IB, IIB and IIIB disease are less satisfactory, and practice varies in different centres as to whether such patients receive radiation or chemotherapy. Results in stage IIIB disease are little different from stage IV, making it unsuitable for radiotherapy, whilst stage IIIA, particularly if of a favourable histological subgroup, may be effectively treated by radiation (Hoppe 1980, Haybittle *et al.* 1985).

Non-Hodgkin's lymphoma is also highly radiosensitive, but the rate of recurrence following radiation treatment varies considerably with the histological type, and can be much greater than in Hodgkin's disease. Lymphocytic types have a rapid response but have a tendency to recur in untreated regions. Histiocytic or poorly differentiated types may respond rapidly but high radiation dosages are required to prevent recurrence in treated areas.

CHEMOTHERAPY

As in the chemotherapy of the infectious diseases, chemotherapy in neoplastic diseases is based upon the principle of selective toxicity. The ideal antineoplastic drug would be one with no action upon the normal body tissues but with a powerful toxic action upon the tumour. However, it is far more difficult to find an ideal antineoplastic drug than it is to find a suitably selective antibiotic, for, whereas bacterial cells are foreign to the body and have metabolic processes differing profoundly from those of human cells, the cells of malignant tumours are not truly foreign, and the metabolic differences so far detected are, in the main, quantitative. Consequently there is no ideal antineoplastic agent known. All the agents at present in use inflict damage of varying degree upon normal body tissues. As would be expected, the normal tissues most likely to be affected are those which proliferate most actively — the bone marrow, gonadal tissue, the epithelium of the alimentary tract, and the fetus, although exceptions occur. The agent of choice for a given neoplastic disease is the one that has the highest ratio of therapeutic to toxic effects, i.e. the greatest target specificity.

Responses to given agents vary greatly from one type of tumour to another. Even with a single type of tumour there are individual variations in degree of response from one patient to another; also the susceptibility to toxic side-effects varies from patient to patient. In order to gain additive antitumour effects and to minimize side-effects, effective cytotoxic drugs are generally given in combination in such a way that they have as few additive side-effects as possible on normal tissues, although bone marrow suppression is the usual dose-limiting factor.

General principles for use of chemotherapeutic agents

Cytotoxic drugs were initially used as palliative therapy in patients with advanced disease, but the introduction of aggressive combination chemotherapy for patients with Hodgkin's disease of stages III and IV by de Vita *et al.* (1970) revolutionized the approach to drug treatment of lymphomas. Not only may the disease be arrested, but cures are achieved in a significant number of patients hitherto facing inevitable death from their disease. Chemotherapy provides a varying, and sometimes considerable, meaningful prolongation of life in patients who have no chance of cure by radiotherapy, and is in fact becoming the most frequent means by which cure is attained in neoplastic disorders of this type.

Use of cytotoxic drugs in combination requires knowledge of the pharmacodynamics, effects, and side-effects of each drug, and experience with the effects of the drugs used in combination. The experience of others is available to a considerable extent when a *protocol* is employed, the dosage and timing of drug administration being laid down in a manner which, from previous extensive experience, has been found to be safe and predictable. Many such protocols contain instructions concerning modification of dosage required in the event of the development of bone marrow depression or other side-effects, but in all forms of chemotherapy, close clinical and haematological supervision are essential. Careful documentation of response of the tumour and the occurrence of side-effects, especially changes in the red cell, white cell, and platelet counts must be maintained throughout the period of treatment.

Susceptibility to side-effects of drugs is variable. Bone marrow is particularly susceptible to depression for months following intensive irradiation, or for some weeks following previous chemotherapy in patients with infiltration of the bone marrow.

Many side-effects of drugs are potentiated by renal or hepatic failure, and are more prominent in the elderly, requiring diminution of dosage or sometimes the withholding of particular drugs when side-effects become troublesome.

Palliative chemotherapy may be undertaken as the appropriate course in a patient unable or unwilling to tolerate more rigorous combination chemotherapy. In such instances, a single drug effective by the oral route, or combinations of drugs in doses less than those employed in intensive treatment, may be used. Such an approach may be appropriate in patients over the age of 70 years, but it must be remembered that cumulative side-effects may still arise, depending on the drug used, and careful monitoring is still necessary.

Agents used in treatment of lymphomas

Many chemotherapeutic agents are now available. The principal drugs may be grouped under the headings of alkylating agents (e.g. nitrogen mustard, cyclophosphamide, chlorambucil, nitrosoureas), vinca alkaloids (vincristine and vinblastine), procarbazine and dacarbazine (agents with actions similar to the alkylating agents), antibiotics with antitumour effects (e.g. Adriamycin and bleomycin), the folate antagonist methotrexate, and corticosteroids. Only those currently most widely used are discussed below.

NITROGEN MUSTARD

Nitrogen mustards are nitrogen analogues of sulphur mustard (mustard gas), a vesicant gas used in the First World War. The nitrogen mustard now widely used in therapeutics is bis(2-chlorethyl) methylamine hydrochloride (HN_2).

Mode of action. Nitrogen mustard (HN_2) reacts chemically with the DNA molecule and is especially active against proliferating cells, both normal and neoplastic. Lymphoid tissue and bone marrow are particularly susceptible to its action, and tumours of cells of the lymphoid series are relatively responsive to HN_2 therapy. Because of the similarity of its action on growing cells to that of X-rays, it is classed as a 'radiomimetic' agent. HN_2 is stable as a dried powder, but once in solution forms the chemically reactive unstable ethylene immonium cation which is capable of reacting with a variety of chemical radicals, replacing the hydrogen in the reacting chemical by an alkyl group. This chemical reaction is known as alkylation.

Dose and administration. HN_2 is administered intravenously. It is extremely irritant to extravascular tissues and hence is administered into the tubing or side-arm of a fast-flowing intravenous infusion of saline. Because of the common occurrence of nausea, premedication should be given, and further anti-emetic treatment may be necessary. Anti-emetic regimens vary considerably, but 10 mg metoclopramide intravenously immediately before chemotherapy, followed by 10 mg orally every 6 hours, is often effective. Alternatively, lorazepam, haloperidol, or chlorpromazine may be used. Most of the combinations of chemotherapy currently in use for lymphoma treatment require anti-emetic treatment.

The toxicity of HN_2 is directly related to dosage. Acute gastrointestinal upset, including nausea, vomiting, anorexia, and sometimes diarrhoea, may begin within a few minutes of injection, and is generally much less after 4–6 hours. With high dosages, however, anorexia may persist for several days. The nadir of bone marrow depression, in terms of the degree of neutropenia and thrombocytopenia, is usually reached 10–14 days after a single large dose of HN_2, and recovery to normal counts occurs in most instances by about 4 weeks.

CYCLOPHOSPHAMIDE

This substance has the same alkylating groups as nitrogen mustard, attached to a cyclic phosphorus compound, but becomes active only after enzymatic cleavage of the ring structure. Such enzyme activity is high in many malignant tumours and may produce a high local alkylating effect at the tumour site compared with other tissues. However, enzyme activity is also present in liver and other normal tissues. Cyclophosphamide can be administered orally, directly into serous cavities, or injected into veins without special precautions.

Dosage and administration. The drug is supplied in ampoules as it is stable in solution, or in coated tablets of 50 mg. It is often injected intravenously in doses of 750–1500 mg/m^2, and causes less nausea in comparison with HN_2. Leucopenia regularly occurs, and generally reaches a nadir approximately ten days after such administration. Erythropoiesis is also suppressed, but platelets generally decrease less with this drug than with other alkylating agents. Alopecia is very common and may be total. With either regular or very high-dose administration there is a tendency to develop haemorrhagic cystitis. This complication is less common if the drug is administered early in the day and the patient is given a large fluid intake together with a diuretic such as frusemide to flush the toxic metabolites from the bladder.

Oral administration of the drug on a long-term basis is generally in a dose of 50–100 mg/m^2, but the dose is titred according to the marrow tolerance of the individual patient. With such treatment, the onset of haemorrhagic cystitis may be gradual, and may be foreshadowed by the development of nocturia, reflecting fibrosis of the bladder wall and submucosal tissues.

CHLORAMBUCIL

This alkylating agent is restricted to oral usage. It is usually given in a regular daily dose of 0.05–0.2 mg/kg bodyweight, depending on haemopoietic tissue tolerance. Chlorambucil seldom causes gastrointestinal upset. Its principal side-effect is bone marrow depression, which is less readily reversible than in the case of cyclophosphamide or HN_2. Anaemia, leucopenia, and thrombocytopenia, when they occur, tend to develop slowly with continuous daily therapy, and after the drug is withdrawn, only slow improvement in peripheral blood count can be expected over periods of up to several months.

Chlorambucil is most commonly administered as a single agent, or in combination with corticosteroids, for treatment of relatively well-differentiated lymphoma where suppression of disease activity results in substantial clinical benefit. Because of the prolonged nature of the marrow depressant effects it is not commonly used in combination chemotherapy.

MELPHALAN

This drug is administered by the oral route, and is associated with only minor gastrointestinal side-effects except when used in high dosage, when such symptoms may be troublesome in occasional patients. It is available in 2 mg and 5 mg tablets, and a convenient method of administration is intermittent courses at relatively high dosages of 9 mg/m^2/day for 4 days, every 4–6 weeks. The ensuing neutropenia reaches a nadir in 2–3 weeks, and should recover before another course is administered at the same dosage. Melphalan may also be given on a daily basis in a dosage of 0.05–0.1 mg/kg.

The drug has few serious side-effects, apart from the reversible bone marrow depression noted above, and a definite association with *secondary leukaemia*. It is often effective in plasmacytoid lymphocytic neoplasia, and is used in the treatment of multiple myeloma.

NITROSOUREAS

The nitrosoureas—1,3-bis(2-chlorethyl)-l-nitrosourea (BCNU) and 1-(2-chlorethyl)-3-cyclohexyl-1-nitrosourea (CCNU)—have been incorporated into combination chemotherapy as they have a spectrum of activity similar to nitrogen mustard and cyclophosphamide. They function as bifunctional alkylating agents. Two specific features are their ability to cross the blood–brain barrier, and their tendency to cause delayed and rather prolonged myelosuppression. Following a single dose, the nadir of neutropenia and thrombocytopenia may be up to six weeks. BCNU is administered by intravenous infusion in doses of 100–200 mg/m^2 as a single agent, and in about half this dose when administered in combination with other cytotoxic drugs. CCNU is administered as a single oral dose of 130 mg/m^2, the dose also being reduced when the drug is used in combination with other cytotoxic agents.

VINCA ALKALOIDS

The vinca alkaloids, vincristine and vinblastine, are two of a variety of antineoplastic alkaloids derived from the periwinkle flower, *Vinca rosea*. They are very similar in their action, and one of the toxic effects is disruption of the mitotic spindle, causing metaphase arrest in dividing cells.

Vincristine is readily soluble in aqueous solution, and is stable as a freeze-dried powder. The usual dosage is up to 1.4 mg/m^2 for adults, and 2 mg/m^2 for children. It is available in 2 mg ampoules ready for reconstitution and may be given by direct intravenous injection, although great care should be taken as there is considerable irritant action if extravasation occurs. The compound is rapidly cleared from the circulation with a half-life of only a few minutes. Toxicity to the bone marrow is relatively minor compared with other cytotoxic drugs, and the major limiting factor is neurological toxicity. Alopecia is also a troublesome complication. Loss of deep tendon reflexes develops most prominently in the legs, and is usually seen only after three or four weekly doses of 2 mg in adults of normal size. However, occasionally unpleasant paraesthesiae and signs of neuropathy develop even after the first dose, and such side-effects appear to be more common in older patients. Abdominal pain and constipation may also occur as manifestations of autonomic neuropathy, and disturbance of bladder function is also seen in a small proportion of patients. Variable and often complete recovery of neurological function occurs after cessation of treatment.

Vinblastine is a similar drug which is administered at about five times the dosage of vincristine. It is equally effective against lymphoid tumours, but at the dosage employed causes a greater degree of bone marrow suppression than vincristine. Neurological disturbance is less common with vinblastine than with vincristine, but the drug is slightly more irritant than vincristine and more inclined to induce nausea shortly after injection. Like vincristine, it is available as a freeze-dried powder, and ampoules contain 10 mg. When used as a single agent, it is ordinarily administered in a dose of 0.1–0.15 mg/kg, or 3.7 mg/m^2.

Both of these alkaloids are widely used in combination chemotherapy because of the relatively slight bone marrow toxicity they cause. Dosages and schedules for use, therefore, are governed by the drugs with which they are combined. It is advisable to use them not more than once every 7–10 days so that neurological toxicity may be evaluated before a further injection is given.

EPIPODOPHYLLOTOXINS

VP-16 (etoposide) and VM-26 (teniposide) are semi-synthetic derivatives of podophyllotoxin, itself a mitotic inhibitor with unacceptable gastrointestinal toxic effects. VP-16 appears to arrest cells in late S or G2 phases of the cell cycle, while VM-26 prevents cells from entering mitosis. The drugs are administered by intravenous infusion, usually diluted in normal saline. Marrow suppression is the principal toxic effect, but hypotension may be associated with rapid administration. Fever and nausea are mild side-effects. VM-26 can replace vincristine in combination chemotherapy regimens for treatment of lymphoma with comparable efficacy and reduced neurological side-effects (Ding *et al.* 1986).

PROCARBAZINE

This compound is a derivative of methylhydrazine and acts in a manner that closely resembles the alkylating agents. It is effective when given by mouth, and is employed most commonly in a dosage of 50–150 mg/m^2/day (1–2.5 mg/kg) for periods of two or more weeks at a time. In addition to bone marrow suppression, which appears to be fully reversible on withdrawal of the drug, it produces central nervous system symptoms. Drowsiness, depression, nausea, and vomiting are not uncommon, particularly in the elderly. As the drug is a monoamine oxidase inhibitor, care must be taken to avoid foods such as cheese and chocolate. The drug also interferes with metabolism of alcohol, and patients should abstain from alcohol whilst on treatment.

A related drug is *imidazole carboxamide*, also known as dacarbazine (DTIC), a triazene alkylating agent. DTIC is administered intravenously and is employed in the 'ABVD' regimen for Hodgkin's disease (Bonodonna *et al.* 1975). DTIC causes severe nausea and vomiting, as well as significant myelosuppression.

OTHER DRUGS

Other drugs commonly employed in the chemotherapy of lymphomas are Adriamycin (doxorubicin) (p. 250), cytosine arabinoside (p. 250), methotrexate (p. 251) and corticosteroids. Interferon has produced some occasional beneficial responses and is undergoing further evaluation.

Combination chemotherapy for Hodgkin's disease

The most commonly used form of combination therapy is the *MOPP* regimen (Table 11.7). Usually six cycles of MOPP therapy are administered, and there is no evidence that further benefit is obtained from administration of further cycles (Coltman 1980). This particular protocol was introduced by de Vita *et al.* (1970), and produced complete remission in 81 per cent of the previously untreated patients in their study with advanced disease considered unsuitable for radiation treatment. Subsequent experience has confirmed that this regimen can produce very long, complete remissions consistent with cure in at least one-half of patients with advanced stage Hodgkin's disease, nearly all of whom would have died in the past when available therapy was limited to radiotherapy or single chemotherapeutic agent administration. The MOPP regimen has become the benchmark against which other measures for treatment of Hodgkin's disease are compared.

Table 11.7. *MOPP combination chemotherapy (de Vita et al. 1970)*

Drug	Dosage
Nitrogen mustard	6 mg/m^2 intravenously daily on days 1 and 8
Vincristine	1.4 mg/m^2 intravenously daily on days 1 and 8
Procarbazine	100 mg/m^2 orally daily from days 1 to 14 inclusive
Prednisone (with 1st and 4th courses)	40 mg/m^2 orally daily from days 1 to 14 inclusive

Six cycles are given with two weeks rest between completion of one cycle and commencement of the next. Modification of drug dosage may be necessary because of leucopenia or thrombocytopenia, as described in the original reference.

Myelosuppression is very commonly encountered during treatment with the MOPP regimen, and attenuation of the dosage of NH_2 and procarbazine is often necessary, especially in the latter cycles of treatment. Another very common side-effect is induction of sterility. Males are almost always rendered sterile by a full course of treatment, and sterility develops in some females, usually in the older of the susceptible subjects.

Alternative chemotherapy protocols which produce similar results include ABVD (Adriamycin, bleomycin, vinblastine, and DTIC) introduced by Bonadonna and colleagues (1975), and variations to the MOPP protocol, such as addition of bleomycin or replacement of nitrogen mustard with chlorambucil. Alternation of courses of MOPP and ABVD (Santoro *et al.* 1982), or alternation of chemotherapy and radiation therapy appear to be promising approaches (Wiernik *et al.* 1979), but definitive studies are still required to establish whether any represent a significant advance over MOPP therapy alone.

There is, however, good evidence that therapy such as the ABVD regimen can produce sustained remissions with apparent cure in Hodgkin's disease which is unresponsive to MOPP therapy. ABVD treatment is also recommended for advanced stage disease which undergoes early relapse after MOPP therapy, but there is no evidence that ABVD is superior for disease which undergoes relapse after more than 12 months.

Chemotherapy for non-Hodgkin's lymphoma

The management options in non-Hodgkin's lymphoma are less clearly established than in Hodgkin's disease. Differing responses to treatment of the various histological subtypes have led to approaches that vary according to the histology, clinical state, age, and general condition of the patient. The sites of involvement with tumour and the size of tumour masses also influence the approach to treatment.

Some generalizations can be made. The *favourable prognosis* non-Hodgkin's lymphomas (the histological subtypes of nodular lymphocytic or nodular mixed cell, and diffuse well-differentiated), while having a generally benign natural history and good response to therapy, are curable only in the minority of cases. There is no logic in employing aggressive chemotherapy or radiotherapy of the type currently available, with their significant morbidity and even mortality, if the quality of life and survival of the patient is not influenced beneficially. This has led to widespread use of the following approach. The rather uncommon stages I and II in good-prognosis non-Hodgkin's lymphomas are treated with local intensive radiotherapy. More extensive stage III and IV disease is treated with chemotherapy aimed at suppression of disease activity and alleviation of symptoms.

Sometimes, disease that shows no apparent progression in more elderly patients is kept under observation, and treatment is not instituted unless acceleration of disease activity takes place. Progressive or symptomatic disease is most commonly treated by cycles of combination chemotherapy such as the CVP regimen (Table 11.8), or by continuous oral administration of chlorambucil until a maximum response is obtained. It has not been established that maintenance treatment provides any additional benefit after a complete remission has been carefully documented by staging procedures.

The approach to the treatment of poor-prognosis histological subtypes is quite different. They usually progress rapidly, and advanced-stage unresponsive disease is frequently fatal within six months of diagnosis. Rapid cell turnover renders these tumours susceptible to 'cycle-specific' cytotoxic drugs and to radiotherapy.

Diffuse, poorly differentiated lymphocytic, diffuse mixed cell, and the 'histiocytic' or large cell lymphomas fall into this category. Stage I disease responds well to high-dose radiotherapy. A large proportion, particularly of the diffuse large cell variety, can be cured (Sweet *et al.* 1981). The best results in stages II, III and IV disease are with combination chemotherapy. The CHOP regimen (McKelvey *et al.* 1976) has been widely employed

Table 11.8. *CVP therapy for non-Hodgkin's lymphoma (Bagley et al. 1972)*

Drug	Dosage	Timing
Cyclophosphamide	400 mg/m^2 orally*	days 1–5
Vincristine	1.4 mg/m^2 intravenously	day 1
Prednisone	100 mg orally	days 1–5

Cycles of treatment are given every 3 weeks in the dosages stated. Neutropenia reaches a nadir on days 7–14. The dosage of cyclophosphamide is modified, if necessary, according to white cell and platelet counts at the commencement of the next cycle.

*The 5 days of oral cyclophosphamide can be replaced by a single intravenous injection of 750 mg/m^2 cyclophosphamide on the first day of each cycle.

Table 11.9. *CHOP regimen for poor prognosis non-Hodgkin's lymphoma*

Drug	Dose	Day
Cyclophosphamide	750 mg/m^2 *iv*	1
Adriamycin	50 mg/m^2 *iv*	1
Vincristine	1.4 mg/m^2 *iv*	1
Prednisolone	100 mg orally	1–5

The regimen is repeated every three weeks, and these dosages may require modification according to bone marrow toxicity.

with *overall* complete response rates of about 65 per cent (39–83 per cent in different series) and an *overall* median survival time of 2 years (Table 11.9). More aggressive regimens have been developed and are being evaluated. Inclusion of bleomycin, methotrexate, and cytarabine, and alternating the administration of drugs, may increase the efficacy of those already contained in the CHOP protocol, as exemplified by the results claimed for the MACOP-B regimen (Klimo *et al.* 1985), although the superiority of such alternative regimens must be established by further clinical trial (Miller *et al.* 1988).

A specific subcategory of diffuse, poor-prognosis lymphoma is *T cell lymphoblastic lymphoma* (Nathwani *et al.* 1976). This disease mostly affects young males, is T-cell derived, and presents with a mediastinal mass. Very aggressive treatment with regimens akin to acute lymphoblastic leukaemia protocols is recommended for the therapy of this disorder (Streuli *et al.* 1981).

The chemotherapy of non-Hodgkin's lymphoma is reviewed by Portlock (1983) and in a recent volume of *Seminars in Hematology* (1988).

Autologous bone marrow transplantation is currently undergoing evaluation as a means for enabling more intensive myelosuppressive chemotherapy to be administered to patients with lymphoma (Singer & Goldstone 1986). Bone marrow from the patient is cryopreserved and then returned by intravenous infusion after normally lethal dosages of chemotherapeutic agents have been administered. The re-infused marrow restores haemopoietic tissue over the ensuing few months, and remissions have been obtained by this approach in lymphoma unresponsive to conventional dosages of chemotherapy.

Outcome in malignant lymphoma

The markedly improved prognosis that follows radical radiation or chemotherapeutic management in responsive instances of this group of diseases has been described. Prognosis in *Hodgkin's disease* depends to an extent on the stage of disease when it presents. Patients with stage IA and IIA disease established by staging laparotomy, and who subsequently receive a full course of radiotherapy, have a survival at 5 years in excess of 85 per cent, and although some relapses may occur for up to 10 years, the majority of these patients may be regarded as cured (Aisenberg & Qazi 1976, Hoppe 1980, Haybittle *et al.* 1985). Poor responses are commoner with lymphocyte depleted but no essential difference has been noted in remission rates between the other histological subtypes of the disorder. Adverse prognostic factors are disease in relapse after prior chemotherapy, the presence of a large mediastinal mass, advanced age, and the presence of B symptoms.

Patients presenting with extensive Hodgkin's disease not amenable to radiation therapy, but treated with intensive combination chemotherapy, have complete remission rates of 75–85 per cent after 6 months of MOPP treatment (de Vita *et al.* 1970). Persistence of remission with values for survival at 5 years as high as 86 per cent have been reported (Young *et al.* 1972), but most centres obtain values for disease-free survival of 50–60 per cent in patients with extensive disease.

Non-Hodgkin's lymphoma has a much more variable outcome, and this is related to histological type. Nodular and diffuse well-differentiated lymphocytic lymphomas have a relatively indolent course even in the untreated state, and in nodular lymphoma amenable to radiation treatment, median survival uncorrected for age is reported to be approximately 7.5 years (Jones 1974).

Stage I and IE diffuse large-cell lymphoma treated by intensive radiotherapy also has a comparatively good prognosis, and approximately 75 per cent of cases may be cured (Bush *et al.* 1977, Sweet *et al.* 1981). More extensive disease may be cured by chemotherapy, but the overall prognosis is worse, the median survival ranging from 23 to 50 months with current regimens. More extensive and bulky disease, and increasing age are adverse prognostic factors, with stage IV large-cell lymphoma having a median survival of less than 12 months.

Myeloma and other paraproteinaemias

Disorders characterized by abnormal proliferation of immunoglobulin-producing cells and abnormal production of immunoglobulin represent part of the spectrum of disease due to neoplastic behaviour of the B-lymphocyte series (Table 11.10). Synonyms used to describe these disorders include *paraproteinaemia, monoclonal gammopathy,* and *plasma cell dyscrasia.* A basic knowledge of the synthesis and structure of normal immunoglobulins is essential for the understanding of these disorders.

Table 11.10. *Disorders associated with paraproteinaemia*

Multiple myeloma
Waldenström's macroglobulinaemia
Chronic lymphatic leukaemia
Non-Hodgkin's lymphoma
Benign monoclonal gammopathy
Heavy chain disease
Primary amyloidosis

Structure of the immunoglobulins

The antibody molecules of normal human serum comprise five distinct classes of immunoglobulins which have been designated IgG, IgA, IgM, IgD, and IgE. The basic unit of all immunoglobulin molecules consists of four polypeptide chains: two identical heavy chains (MW 60 000) and two identical light chains (MW 20 000). The heavy chains of IgG, IgA, IgM, IgD, and IgE are referred to as gamma (γ), alpha (α), mu (μ), delta (δ), and epsilon (ε) respectively. Four subclasses of IgG, two subclasses of IgA, and two subclasses of IgM are recognized. There are two types of light chains, kappa (κ) and lambda (λ), each immunoglobulin molecule having either two kappa or two lambda light chains. Amino-acid sequence analyses of light chains have shown that the amino-terminal half of the chain is characterized by a variable amino-acid sequence (the variable region or V_L) and the carboxyl-terminal half by a constant sequence (the constant region or C_L). Heavy chains have a similar variable region (V_H) and three or four constant regions (C_H^1, C_H^2, C_H^3, and C_H^4. IgM occurs in serum as a pentamer of five linked IgM monomeric molecules, although small amounts of the monomer

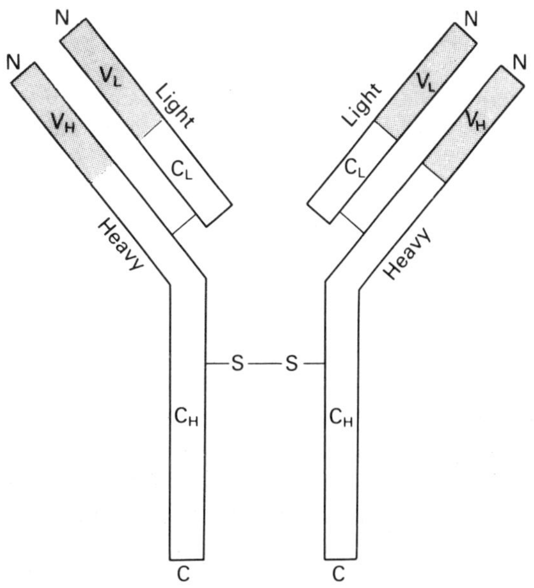

Fig. 11.4. *The basic immunoglobulin molecule consists of two heavy and two light chains, linked by disulphide bonds. Each chain consists of a variable (V) and constant (C) region. N represents the amino-terminal amino acid, and C the carboxyl-terminal amino acid of each polypeptide chain.*

Table 11.11. *Human immunoglobulins*

	IgG	IgA	IgM	IgD	IgE
Heavy chain					
Class	γ	α	μ	δ	ε
Subclass	IgG_1, IgG_2, IgG_3, IgG_4	IgA_1, IgA_2	IgM_1, IgM_2		
Light chain					
Class	$\kappa_1\lambda$	$\kappa_1\lambda$	$\kappa_1\lambda$	$\kappa_1\lambda$	$\kappa_1\lambda$
Molecular formulae	$\gamma_2\kappa_2$	$(\alpha_2\kappa_2)_n$	$(\mu_2\kappa_2)_n$	$\delta_2\kappa_2$	$\varepsilon_2\kappa_2$
	$\gamma_2\lambda_2$	$(\alpha_2\lambda_2)_n$	$(\mu_2\lambda_2)_n$	$\delta_2\lambda_2$	$\varepsilon_2\lambda_2$
Molecular weight	160 000	170 000 x n*	900 000	180 000	200 000
Sedimentation co-efficient (S_{20}, w)	7	7	19	7	8
Half-life in circulation (days)	21	6	5	3	2
Mean normal serum concentration (g/l)	12	2	1	0.03	0.0002
Intravascular fraction (%)	45	40	80	75	50
Complement fixation capability	+	0	+	0	0
Placental transfer	+	0	0	0	0

*n = 1, 2, 3.

may be present. IgA is largely present as a monomer, but polymers also occur. There are two antigen-binding sites on each immunoglobulin monomer, and these are located at the apposed N-terminal regions of the light and heavy chains. The basic structure of the immunoglobulin molecule is depicted schematically in Fig. 11.4, and the properties of the various immunoglobulins are summarized in Table 11.11.

Synthesis

Immunoglobulin is normally synthesized and incorporated into the outer membrane of resting B lymphocytes. It is predominantly IgD or monomeric IgM, and serves as the means for recognition of specific antigen. Presentation of such an antigen to the B cell by the helper–inducer cell network results in cell proliferation and subsequent differentiation into a clone of plasma cells. These cells synthesize large amounts of antibody specific for the antigen, and secrete the antibody into the extracellular fluid.

The means by which cells are able to generate antibody to molecules to which the body has not been previously exposed is by rearrangement of segments of DNA in the genes that code for the individual chains of immunoglobulin molecules. The basic unrearrranged 'germ-line' genes in a previously unexposed B lymphocyte contain many individual segments, from which certain segments are selected, rearranged, and rejoined in such a manner as to produce a gene coding for an immunoglobulin with a binding site that is specific for the foreign antigen to which the cell has been exposed. The very large number of possible combinations of DNA segments involved in such a process is believed to account for the enormous diversity of different antigen-binding sites on antibodies which can be produced by the immune system (Tonegawa 1985).

Messenger RNA for the light and heavy chains is translated into protein by the abundant polyribosomes of the plasma cell. The chains are then linked together covalently and carbohydrate attached before the complete immunoglobulin molecule is secreted.

It is usual for more than one clone of plasma cells to be generated in response to exposure of the body to a foreign antigen, and the precise antigen-binding characteristics and the properties of the immunoglobulin molecule tend to vary from clone to clone. The net result of stimulation of the immune system by a particular foreign antigen is production of many similar, but not identical, antibody molecules directed against that antigen. About 70 per cent of IgG antibodies to a particular antigen have κ, and 30 per cent λ light chains. The polyclonal nature of the immunoglobulins produced in the normal antibody response gives rise to the diffuse band in the γ globulin region of the serum protein electrophoretogram.

Abnormal synthesis

Abnormal synthesis of secreted immunoglobulin occurs when an abnormally large monoclonal population of plasmacytic or lymphocytic cells develops from a single precursor cell. This cell population produces identical molecules of immunoglobulin, or identical fragments of the immunoglobulin molecules. As the protein is homogeneous, the molecules migrate during serum electrophoresis as a discrete monoclonal (M) protein spike or band, and it is commonly referred to as a *paraprotein*. The presence of a paraprotein is one of the most common features of neoplastic plasma cell disorders, and also occurs in some instances of lymphocytic neoplastic activity.

Imbalance between light and heavy chain synthesis is common in such disorders. In myeloma, the most common abnormality is production of an excess of light over heavy chains. The excess light chains are secreted into the extracellular fluid, but pass readily through the glomerulus and are thus not retained in the circulation as effectively as are paraproteins consisting of intact immunoglobulin molecules. Light chains are catabolized by the renal tubular cells, but when present in excess pass into the urine as *Bence Jones protein*. In about 25 per cent of myelomas, only light chains are secreted by the neoplastic plasma cells, and this disorder is referred to as Bence Jones myeloma. In heavy chain disease, fragments or intact molecules of the heavy chain are secreted by the neoplastic cells (p. 312).

Myeloma

Myeloma is a chronic, progressive, and fatal malignant condition in which the fundamental abnormality is a neoplastic proliferation of plasma cells which infiltrate the bone marrow, and often other body tissues. The plasma cells are usually abnormal and immature in appearance. Occasionally, they appear in the peripheral blood in large numbers, and the disorder is then referred to as plasma cell leukaemia. Myeloma is uncommon, but not rare, and is being recognized with increasing frequency.

Pathological physiology

The pathological and clinical features of myeloma are predominantly due to tissue infiltration, production of large amounts of paraprotein, and impairment of immunity.

Bone infiltration causes destruction of medullary and cortical bone due to the stimulation of osteoclast activity by a factor released by the myeloma cells (Josse *et al.* 1981), usually designated *osteoclast-activating factor*. This leads to osteoporosis, and more frequently to localized lytic lesions and pathological fractures. Increased resorption of bone results in hypercalcaemia in a significant minority of cases. Abnormal cells form intra- and extra-osseous tumours, and infiltration of the bone marrow ultimately results in defective haemopoiesis.

Production of large amounts of paraprotein results in a wide variety of abnormalities as indicated in Table 11.12. Some of these abnormalities reflect the extensive increase in plasma volume due to the presence of large amounts of paraprotein, which causes a dilutional effect on the concentration of albumin and red cells in the blood. Toxic effects of light chains on the renal tubules make a major contribution to the development of the irreversible renal failure, which is one of the important poor prognostic factors in this disease.

Clinical features

Myeloma is predominantly a disease of middle and old age, with a maximum incidence between the

Table 11.12. *Pathophysiological effects of paraproteins*

Raised serum globulin level
Hypoalbuminaemia
Hyponatraemia
Dilutional anaemia
Raised ESR, rouleaux in blood film
Hyperviscosity
Interference with platelet function and coagulation pathway
Proteinuria
Renal failure
Amyloidosis
Cryoglobulinaemia

ages of 50 and 70 years. It is uncommon under the age of 40 years.

Presentation. The majority of patients present with bone pain, symptoms of anaemia, skeletal deformity, tumour formation, spontaneous fractures, or nervous system manifestations, either singly or in combination. Less common presenting manifestations are a bleeding tendency, renal insufficiency, and pulmonary infections.

Bone pain is the presenting manifestation in about 70 per cent of patients, and is usually the outstanding symptom. Nevertheless it may be absent, occasionally, throughout the whole course of the disease. Pain is most frequent in the lumbar, sacral, and thoracic spine, then in the rib cage, but it also occurs in the hips, legs, shoulders, and arms. It is uncommon in the skull. Tenderness of the bones is common, and these problems are basically due to *pathological fracture, lysis* or *compression.*

Tumour formation is not uncommon and may occur on any bone, but especially on the ribs. Tumours vary in size, sometimes being quite large. They are generally firm and often tender. Occasionally, when the cortex is very thin, characteristic 'egg shell' cracking is felt and the tumours are fluctuant. *The disorder sometimes presents with a single prominent tumour of bone, and occasionally the appearance of this apparently solitary growth precedes overt involvement of other bones by months or even years.* In rare cases, there is a large single destructive tumour of bone, with the histological appearance of a plasmacytoma, which is cured by amputation or irradiation and is not followed by involvement of the skeleton elsewhere — solitary plasmacytoma of bone. Rarely, isolated extra-osseous plasmacytomas occur, and are more likely to be cured by excision or intensive irradiation than plasmacytomas involving bone.

Nervous system involvement is common. Most frequently it is due to compression by collapsed vertebrae or myeloma tissue. Compression of the spinal cord and nerve roots is the most frequent neurological complication, and may result in paraplegia or quadraplegia. Isolated peripheral neuropathy is a rare complication and its cause is unknown. Blunting of mental function occurs in the *hyperviscosity syndrome.* Disturbance of brain function ranging from drowsiness to seizures can be produced by *hypercalcaemia,* and the development of hypercalcaemia must be suspected under such circumstances.

Anaemia almost invariably occurs at some stage in the illness, and in advanced cases is frequently severe. It is relatively common at presentation, and an important contributing factor is the dilutional effect of large amounts of paraprotein in the circulation.

Renal insufficiency. Chronic renal insufficiency frequently develops during the course of the disease, and occasionally is the initial manifestation. Retinal abnormalities are uncommon, and unless there is co-existent essential hypertension the blood pressure is normal. For this reason, myeloma should be considered as a possible cause in any patient with chronic renal insufficiency and a normal blood pressure.

The most important pathological changes in the kidney take the form of atrophy and dilatation of the tubules with cast formation in the tubular lumen. These are the characteristic of 'myeloma' kidney. The casts are composed of a mixture of normal plasma proteins and precipitated Bence Jones protein. Multinucleate epithelial cells are often found adjacent to the casts. Bence Jones protein is also believed to damage renal tubules directly. Other factors in the genesis of renal failure include deposition of myeloma proteins, dehydration, local infection, hyperuricaemia, hypercalcaemia, and plasma cell infiltration of the kidney. Acute renal failure in the absence of previous renal impairment is less frequent, but may follow the hypovolaemia and dehydration associated with some forms of intravenous pyelography. The Fanconi syndrome of renal tubular malabsorption can be associated with Bence Jones proteinuria, and may precede the development of overt myeloma by several years.

Bleeding manifestations occasionally bring the disorder to notice. Epistaxis and bleeding from the gums or into the skin are the most common bleeding manifestations, but melaena, haematuria, retinal and other haemorrhages may occur (Lackner 1973). Several factors contribute to the pathogenesis of the bleeding, the most important being the presence of the abnormal protein. An effect on platelets by the paraprotein often leads to abnormal platelet function, with prolongation of the bleeding time and defective adhesion, aggregation, and platelet factor 3 availability. Thrombocytopenia may also contribute as it can occur in advanced disease.

The paraprotein may also act as an anticoagulant and inhibit some steps in the coagulation pathway. The most common abnormality is inhibition of fibrin monomer polymerization, which results in prolongation of the thrombin clotting time and defective clot retraction. Rare cases of interference with factor VIII activity have been described. Hyperviscosity also contributes to abnormal bleeding and bruising, but occurs more commonly in macroglobulinaemia (p. 310).

Infections are common in myeloma. They may be the presenting feature, and are an important cause of morbidity and mortality in myeloma (Kyle 1975). Chest infection with *Streptococcus pneumoniae* does occur, but infections with a wide variety of other Gram-positive and Gram-negative organisms are more common and involve virtually any part of the body. This predisposition to infection is multifactorial in nature. There are usually subnormal levels of normal immunoglobulins, and suppression of the normal antibody response, in particular the primary response. Neutrophils may function suboptimally, and their concentration in the blood is frequently depressed by interference with haemopoiesis due to marrow infiltration by myeloma, by cytotoxic chemotherapy, and even by the occasional development of myelodysplastic disorders later in the course of the illness.

Amyloidosis. Amyloidosis develops in up to ten per cent of patients. The distribution of the amyloid follows that of primary amyloid disease, in skin, heart, skeletal muscle, tongue, and gastrointestinal tract. Kidneys, liver, and spleen may also be involved. Renal involvement may lead to the nephrotic syndrome. The carpal tunnel syndrome is an occasional complication. The evidence that immunoglobulin light chains are the major protein component of amyloid fibrils in myeloma is described by Glenner *et al.* (1973).

Visceral involvement. Infiltration of the liver, spleen, lymph nodes, and other organs is commonly found at post mortem, but rarely causes major clinical problems. The spleen and lymph nodes are occasionally palpable, especially in cases of plasma cell leukaemia. Moderate enlargement of the liver is more common.

Cryoglobulinaemia. Five per cent of myeloma proteins are cryoglobulins which reversibly gel in the cold and cause symptoms of cold intolerance. Cryoglobulinaemia may precede the development of overt myeloma by several years.

Clinical features in relation to immunoglobulin class. The different immunochemical classes of myeloma have a tendency to have certain characteristic clinical features (Hobbs 1969). IgG myeloma is associated with a higher level of paraprotein, a greater reduction of normal immunoglobulin levels, and more frequent infections than other types. Amyloidosis and hypercalcaemia are less frequent. IgA myeloma is often complicated by hypercalcaemia, and heavy Bence Jones proteinuria is usual. Amyloidosis is not uncommon, but infection is less frequent. IgD myeloma is reputed to occur more commonly in younger patients, and hypercalcaemia and renal failure are frequent. Heavy Bence Jones proteinuria is usual. Amyloidosis and extra-osseous tumours may occur. Bence Jones myeloma also occurs in a slightly younger age group, and is particularly characterized by osteolytic lesions, hypercalcaemia, renal failure, and amyloidosis.

Blood picture

The blood picture in myeloma is not diagnostic. Nevertheless, the diagnosis is often suggested by the presence of certain features—marked red-cell rouleaux formation (Fig. 11.5), the presence of atypical plasma cells, an abnormally blue-stained background in the blood film, and a greatly increased ESR.

Anaemia is often present at diagnosis, or it develops during the course of the disease. The anaemia is usually *normochromic* and *normocytic* in nature. A dilutional effect of the expanded plasma volume in patients with high concentrations of paraprotein contributes to the lowering of the haemoglobin concentration. Depression of erythropoiesis due to infiltration of the bone marrow, and the effects of cytotoxic chemotherapy are additional important factors. Other factors that can cause or contribute to anaemia are renal failure, chronic

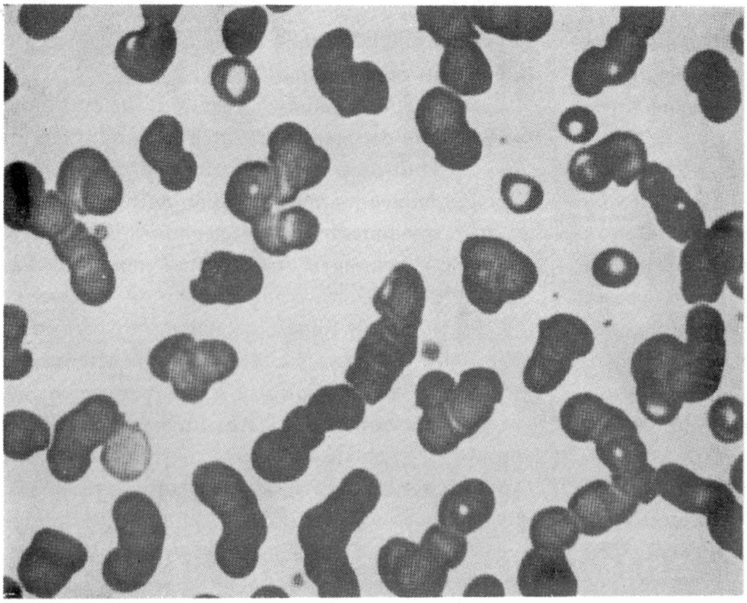

Fig. 11.5. *Peripheral blood film in myeloma. Photomicrograph showing marked rouleaux formation by red cells. This patient presented with anaemia and chronic renal insufficiency without bone pain or abnormal bone X-rays. Myeloma was suspected because of the marked rouleaux formation, and was confirmed by marrow aspiration (× 710).*

infection, bleeding, and development of myelodysplastic or leukaemic disorders.

The *white cell count* may be normal, raised, or moderately reduced, but moderate leucopenia is the most common, especially in advanced disease and in association with cytotoxic therapy. A leuco-erythroblastic picture with the appearance of immature red cells and granulocytes develops in about ten per cent of patients. Small numbers of myeloma cells appear in the blood in about 20 per cent of patients. Rarely, they appear in large numbers, when the condition is referred to as *plasma cell leukaemia*. The *platelet count* is often reduced in myeloma.

The ESR is very often raised. Values frequently exceed 100 mm/hour and sometimes 150 mm/hour. However, the ESR can be normal or raised by only a moderate degree in those patients with Bence Jones myeloma, in whom a paraprotein is absent from the blood. Blood grouping and cross-matching may be difficult because of red-cell rouleaux formation.

Bone marrow

Bone marrow aspiration and trephine biopsy establish the diagnosis in most cases. Usually, infiltration with myeloma cells is diffuse, so that aspiration at any of the usual sites yields typical cells, but occasionally the lesions are focal, with areas of normal marrow between the tumour masses. In such cases, if the needle enters normal marrow the myeloma cells will be missed. Sometimes, diagnostic foci of myeloma cells are present in a trephine biopsy of bone marrow adjacent to a region from which the aspirate is not diagnostic. Biopsy of a radiologically abnormal or tender site is usually diagnostic, although sometimes a dry or blood tap is obtained when the aspiration needle enters a mass of myeloma tissue. If the overall features are suggestive of myeloma, a biopsy should be performed at an alternative site if the initial biopsy appearance is within normal limits.

The bone marrow fragments are usually hypercellular, and the cell trails usually contain myeloma cells. These cells commonly constitute 15–30 per cent of the differential count, but higher percentages may occur. Myeloma cells vary in appearance from small, mature, differentiated cells resembling typical plasma cells, to large, immature, undifferentiated cells of 20–30 per μm diameter. Many cells have intermediate characteristics (Fig. 11.6). The cytoplasm of the mature cells is basophilic, sometimes with a perinuclear halo. The nucleus is

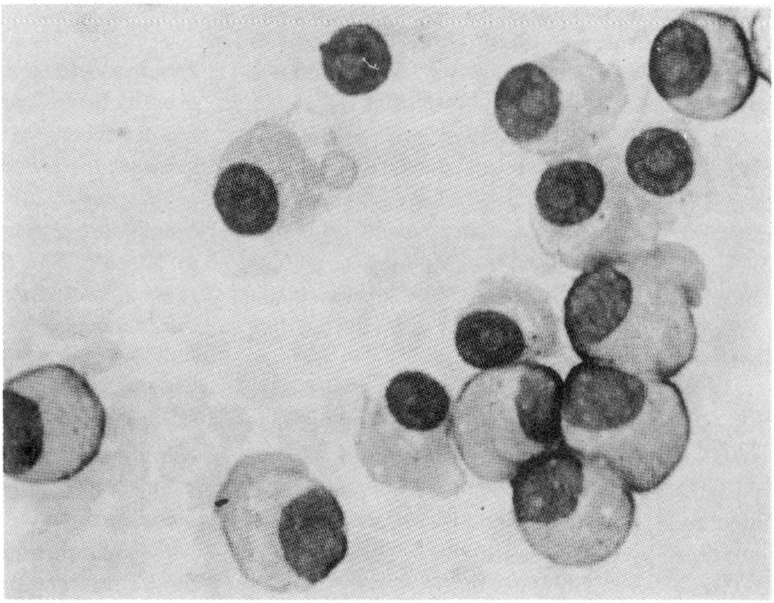

Fig. 11.6. *Numerous abnormal plasma cells in the bone marrow aspirate of a subject with myeloma.*

commonly eccentric, and the chromatin is arranged in coarse strands, although it seldom shows the typical cartwheel arrangements which may be seen in the classical plasma cell. The cytoplasm of the more immature cells is abundant, light blue, and may show a perinuclear halo, vacuolation, and Russell bodies; the nucleus is more vesicular, with finer and evenly distributed chromatin. Nucleoli are common in the immature cells. Multinucleated cells are common, and mitoses are sometimes seen.

At post mortem in advanced disease, the marrow commonly has a grey gelatinous appearance, often with haemorrhage, and there is erosion and destruction of cortical bone.

Increased proportions of plasma cell are present in the bone marrow in some other disorders. These includes aplastic anaemia, rheumatoid arthritis, hepatic cirrhosis, sarcoidosis, secondary carcinoma, systemic lupus erythematosus, and chronic inflammation. However, the plasma cells are usually mature and are seldom present in excess of ten per cent. In most cases, the diagnosis is obvious from the clinical and laboratory features. Occasionally, differentiation is more difficult, and diagnosis based on the appearance of individual plasma cells present in small numbers may not be reliable.

Blood chemistry

Total serum protein concentration is often increased due to the presence of paraprotein. However, a reduction in albumin concentration is common and tends to offset the effect of the increased amount of paraprotein. Total serum protein commonly ranges from 70 to 120 g/l, but may be higher.

The paraprotein usually appears as a single narrow homogeneous M-band on the serum electrophoretogram. Very rarely, there are two bands. Commonly, the concentration of normal γ globulin is moderately to profoundly reduced. The position of the band on the strip varies from case to case. It is usually in the γ globulin region, but occasionally is in the β globulin region. An obvious paraprotein band is not evident in Bence Jones myeloma or non-secretory myeloma, which make up 20–30 per cent of all myelomas. In these instances, the serum protein electrophoretogram is normal or shows a reduction in γ globulin.

Immunoelectrophoresis shows that the paraprotein is IgG in about 50 per cent of cases, IgA in 25 per cent, and IgD in 1 per cent. From 50 to 70 per cent of these patients have Bence Jones proteinuria when tested for by sensitive techniques (see below).

In the patients in whom there is no obvious M-band on the serum protein electrophoretic strip, Bence Jones proteinuria is nearly always present, and free light chains can usually be identified in the serum by immunoelectrophoresis. These cases are referred to as *Bence Jones myeloma*. In rare instances, in spite of clear-cut clinical and morphological evidence of myeloma, paraproteins or paraprotein fragments are not found in either serum or urine in the so-called *non-secretory myelomas*. Other very rare types of myeloma are those associated with IgM and IgE paraproteins.

The serum calcium concentration is often raised. The concentration of phosphate is normal but rises when renal insufficiency develops. Serum alkaline phosphatase is normal or slightly raised, a point of importance in differentiation from hyperparathyroidism and secondary carcinoma of bone, in which significant elevation is usual. The serum uric acid concentration is often raised, even in the absence of renal insufficiency.

The plasma volume and serum viscosity are elevated in about 80 per cent of patients. Viscosity does not usually reach a level sufficient to cause symptoms of the hyperviscosity syndrome (p. 310), but hyperviscosity can occur in occasional cases of IgA myeloma and IgG myeloma of IgG_1 and IgG_3 subclasses.

Urine

Free monoclonal κ or λ light chains appear in the urine as Bence Jones protein, and their detection is one of the bases of the diagnosis of myeloma. Bence Jones protein was originally described in terms of its unique behaviour on heating. Urine containing Bence Jones protein flocculates when heated slowly to 50–60°C. The flocculated protein dissolves on boiling, and reappears on cooling below 60°C. Unfortunately, heat test is unreliable, especially with low concentrations of Bence Jones protein. The most reliable means for the detection of Bence Jones protein is electrophoresis of a concentrated urine specimen on cellulose acetate. The monoclonal light chains usually migrate as a marrow band in the globulin region.

Electrophoretic methods detect Bence Jones protein in the concentrated urine of 50–70 per cent of myeloma patients with a serum paraprotein, and in nearly all patients who do not have a serum paraprotein.

More sensitive immunological techniques detect small amounts of free light chains in most normal urines, but these are polyclonal rather than monoclonal, and show broad electrophoretic mobility on electrophoresis. True Bence Jones proteinuria is practically pathognomonic of myeloma, although it

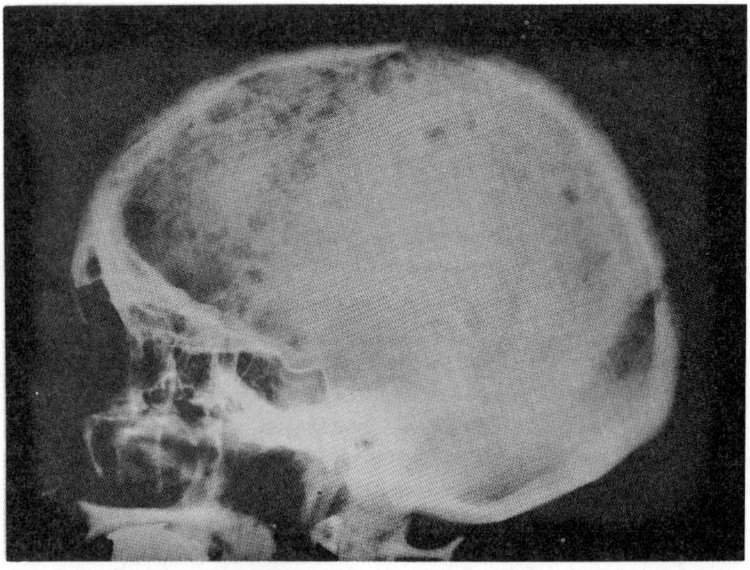

Fig. 11.7. *X-ray of skull in a patient with myeloma, illustrating multiple punched-out areas.*

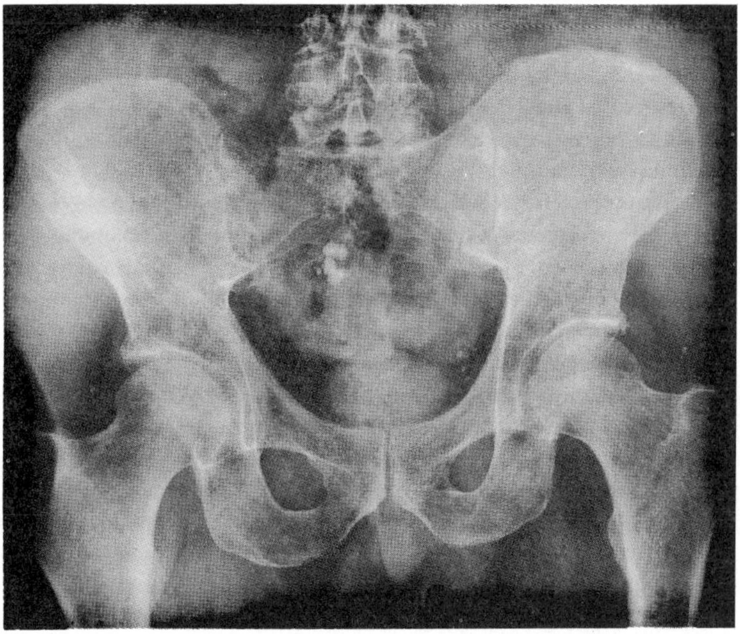

Fig. 11.8 *X-ray of pelvis and upper femora in a patient with myeloma. Note generalized osteoporosis and localized punched-out areas.*

may occasionally occur in macroglobulinaemia, amyloidosis, lymphoma, and leukaemia (Solomon 1976).

Bone X-ray

Bone X-ray changes occur in about 90 per cent of patients at some stage in the course of the illness. Thus absence of bone change does not exclude myeloma. Bone changes consist of either diffuse decalcification or localized areas of bone destruction, or a combination of the two (Figs 11.7 & 11.8). The localized osteolytic lesions usually appear as multiple, rounded, discrete, punched-out areas with no sclerosis at the margin. They occur most frequently in bones normally containing red marrow, and are especially common in the skull. Diffuse osteoporosis is especially common in the spine, where wedge-shaped compression fractures are frequent.

Diagnosis

Diagnosis is straightforward when the combination of diffuse osteoporotic or multiple osteolytic lesions, infiltration of the bone marrow with plasma cells, and a serum or urinary M-protein is present. Each of these abnormalities can occur individually in other conditions, which must therefore not be confused with myeloma. Increased proportions of plasma cells occur in the bone marrow, for example, in chronic infection, hepatic cirrhosis, and certain chronic inflammatory states. Such reactive plasmacytosis of the bone marrow can usually be distinguished from myeloma because the serum immunoglobulins are polyclonal in nature, and monoclonal Bence Jones protein is not present in the urine. Osteolytic lesions can also be caused by metastatic cancer, but the presence of surrounding sclerosis tends to differentiate such lesions from those caused by myeloma.

The most difficult disorder to differentiate from myeloma is *benign monoclonal gammopathy*, because the difference is essentially of a quantitative rather than a qualitative nature. An important difference is that the level of paraprotein and degree of normal immunoglobulin suppression tends to be less in benign monoclonal gammopathy, but the critical distinction is the lack of progression and lack of injurious clinical manifestations in benign monoclonal gammopathy. Such a distinction may only be established by serial observations over a considerable period. These observations should be continued indefinitely, as about five per cent of patients so classified progress to active myeloma each year. It remains a very important distinction because cytotoxic chemotherapy basically contributes only its adverse effects to the patient with benign monoclonal gammopathy.

A high index of suspicion increases the chance of early diagnosis of myeloma in certain settings, such as severe osteoporosis or vertebral collapse, unexplained proteinuria or renal impairment, a very high ESR, rouleaux in the blood film, normochromic normocytic anaemia, or unexpectedly severe or frequent infections.

Management

Active therapeutic measures are warranted in progressive disease, and although treatment almost invariably does not eradicate myeloma, it can often suppress disease activity for many years and result in meaningful prolongation of life and relief of symptoms.

Life expectancy bears an inverse relationship to myeloma tumour mass at the time that treatment is commenced, and thus the *clinical stage* of the disease is an indicator of prognosis in view of its correlation with the total tumour cell burden in the body. Staging criteria suggested by Durie & Salmon (1975) classify *stage I* disease as lack of significant anaemia, normal plasma calcium, normal bone structure, and paraprotein levels below certain thresholds (IgG <50 g/l, IgA <30 g/l, urine Bence Jones protein < 4 g/24 hours). Increasing stage of disease correlates with increasing myeloma cell mass, through an intermediate stage II to *stage III* disease, the latter characterized by the presence of one or more of the following: haemoglobin <8.5 g/dl; hypercalcaemia, more than 3 bone lytic lesions; or high paraprotein levels (IgG >70 g/l, IgA >50 g/l, urine Bence Jones protein >12 g/24 hours). Patients are subclassified on the basis of renal function, with those with a plasma creatinine <0.18 mM/l designated as subgroup A, and those with creatinine levels >0.18 mM/l are designated as subgroup B.

SYMPTOMATIC MEASURES

Some patients become very ill at some stage during the course of the illness because of *hypercalcaemia*. Treatment by rehydration with intravenous fluids is particularly important, and often results in improvement of the reversible element of renal impairment produced by the hypercalcaemia. Depression of the excessive plasma calcium concentration can be promoted by increasing the urinary excretion of calcium with certain diuretics such as frusemide, although other diuretics such as thiazides can have the opposite effect. Corticosteroids are particularly useful in suppressing the underlying osteolytic process, and doses of 50–100 mg prednisone or prednisolone daily often produce substantial benefit, and may result in restoration of normal plasma calcium concentrations. *The most important measure in obtaining sustained control of the hypercalcaemia is suppression of the myelomatous process by chemotherapy.*

Anaemia may require correction by transfusion with packed red cells. Administration of oxymetholone has been shown in some studies to increase the level of haemoglobin.

Hyperviscosity can be corrected by plasmapheresis if this complication is causing clinical problems. Because circulating red blood cells contribute to blood viscosity, it is especially important to consider correction of hyperviscosity before blood transfusion, or to perform plasmapheresis during the transfusion.

Local pain, especially in bone, is a very common and serious problem in myeloma. Myeloma tissue is generally sensitive to *radiotherapy*, and as localized areas of bone pain are usually due to local infiltration, radiotherapy is often very helpful in producing a gradual reduction in pain and arresting the progression of the disorder in the irradiated area.

Nervous system compression is a relatively common problem, and localized compressive effects by myeloma tissue may be reversed by radiotherapy, or by laminectomy when there is an urgent need to reduce pressure on the spinal cord.

CHEMOTHERAPY

Three agents have been used extensively in view of their ability to reverse the progression of myeloma when administered by the oral route, either singly or in combination. The most commonly employed drug is the alkylating agent *melphalan* (L-phenylalanine mustard). It can be administered *continuously* in a dose of 1–3 mg/day, but is more commonly given *intermittently* in a dose of 9 $mg/m^2/day$ for 4 days every 4–6 weeks. Melphalan is myelotoxic, and as its absorption is variable the dosage must be adjusted either up or down according to the degree of myelosuppression indicated by serial monitoring of the blood count. Evidence that the proportion of patients who undergo an objective response is almost doubled by concurrent administration of *corticosteroid* (e.g. prednisone 100 $mg/m^2/day$ for 4 days) is summarized by Bersagel & Rider (1985).

Cyclophosphamide is about as effective in producing an objective response as melphalan. It does, however, tend to produce alopecia and chemical cystitis, but it can be effective in myeloma that is unresponsive to melphalan. It can be administered *continuously* in a dose of 1–3 mg/kg/day or *intermittently* in doses of 1000 mg/m^2 every 3 weeks.

High doses of *corticosteroids* such as prednisone or prednisolone 60 $mg/m^2/day$ for 5 days, administered every 8th day for 3 courses, can produce objective responses as single-agent therapy, even in myeloma refractory to other drug treatment (Alexanian *et al.* 1983). Combinations including other agents are also employed. Additional drugs that are effective against myeloma include vincristine, Adriamycin, BCNU, CCNU and procarbazine. Most combinations include one or more of these drugs with corticosteroids plus melphalan and/or cyclophosphamide, and while they represent a more intensive chemotherapeutic attack on the disease (Case *et al.* 1977), they have yet to be unequivocally proven to produce a substantial increase in median survival over that obtained with melphalan and prednisolone (Bersagel & Rider 1985). *Interferon* shows some promise in the treatment of myeloma.

RADIOTHERAPY

Intensive radiotherapy may eradicate localized extra-osseous plasmacytomas, but the usual widespread infiltration of the bone marrow in myeloma makes it difficult to utilize radiotherapy for treatment of the overall disease process.

Response to treatment: prognosis

The outcome in an individual patient with myeloma is profoundly influenced by a number of factors. There is an overall longer median survival in patients with stage I than stage III disease from the time of institution of chemotherapy. This, however, may reflect the earlier stage of progression of the disease process and the lack of osseous, haematological, and renal complications in stage I patients. Significant *irreversible renal impairment* is in particular associated with a poor prognosis (MRC 1973, Bersagel *et al.* 1979). *A dominant prognostic factor is the nature of the response to chemotherapy.* Patients who obtain a very good response have a substantially longer median survival than those who are refractory to treatment. Objective responses to current treatment regimens occur in 50–70 per cent of patients, and a considerable proportion of the responders live for many years longer than the median survival of about 18 months in untreated disease.

Although the extent of the tumour burden bears an inverse relation to survival, the outcome is nonetheless influenced by the rate of progression of the myelomatous process. In some untreated subjects in whom the parameters of the disease satisfy the diagnostic criteria of myeloma, the disorder may progress very slowly and exhibit a plateau-like phase of activity. Under such conditions, chemotherapy offers no significant benefit. *Plateau-phase* behaviour is commonly observed after an objective response is achieved with chemotherapy, where the condition remains basically in a static, non-progressive state in the absence of further chemotherapy for up to many years.

The plateau phase of the disease is almost always terminated by recommencement of actively progressive myeloma. Such a development is associated with a poor prognosis when the patient is currently receiving chemotherapy, but further objective responses, even with the initially successful chemotherapeutic regimen, are relatively frequently attained when the patient has not been receiving chemotherapy during the plateau phase. It has been argued that median survival is not increased by continuation of chemotherapy during the established plateau phase in myeloma. The generally accepted approach is that administration of chemotherapy is required in either previously untreated or previously responsive disease when the disorder is undergoing active progression.

Progressive disease may be obvious from clinical manifestations such as worsening osteolysis or marrow depression, but useful laboratory indices of progressive disease are progressive elevation of serum β_2 microglobulin (Bataille *et al.* 1984, Garewal *et al.* 1984), and increasing levels of paraprotein in serum or urine.

Currently available chemotherapeutic regimens tend to reduce the bulk of myeloma tissue and may substantially prolong life, but virtually never eliminate the disorder. Death from myeloma usually occurs from complications of progressive disease unresponsive to treatment, either at presentation or after recurrence of activity following an initial objective response. Common terminal events include complications of pancytopenia and immunosuppression, such as infection or haemorrhage, and complications of renal failure. An emerging, but less common, cause of death is the sequelae of myelodysplastic or acute leukaemic disorder, which appear to be largely secondary to exposure to the alkylating agents used in the treatment of myeloma (p. 258).

Waldenström's macroglobulinaemia

This is an uncommon neoplastic proliferation of B lymphocytes which produce IgM paraproteins, called macroglobulins because of their high molecular weight. The pathological and clinical features of the disorder are due to infiltration by the disease, causing marrow failure and enlargement of the liver, spleen, and lymph nodes, and to the consequences of the paraprotein in the blood, which may markedly increase viscosity, interfere with haemostasis, and exhibit cryoglobulin behaviour by gelling at reduced temperature.

Clinical features

The disorder usually occurs between the ages of 50 and 70 years, and is more common in males. The most prominent features are weakness, a bleeding tendency, recurrent infections, and visual disturbances. A degree of hepatosplenomegaly and lymph node enlargement occurs in the majority. Bone pain and tenderness are rare, and, while bone X-rays may show osteoporosis, focal areas of destruction as in myeloma are atypical. Neuropathy occurs occasionally.

Many of the clinical features are due to an increase in *serum viscosity*. When the serum viscosity as measured by the Ostwald viscometer exceeds 4.0 (normal 1.4–1.8), which usually corresponds to an IgM level of 30–50 g/l, a characteristic set of symptoms and signs may ensue, referred to as the *hyperviscosity syndrome* (Bloch & Maki 1973). The main features of the hyperviscosity syndrome, which occurs in 30–50 per cent of patients with Waldenström's macroglobulinaemia, include ocular changes, mucous membrane bleeding, neuropsychiatric manifestations, and congestive cardiac failure. Ocular symptoms range from minor blurring of vision to complete blindness. Fundal abnormalities can be striking, with stasis of blood in grossly distended and tortuous retinal veins, punctate haemorrhages, exudates, and even papilloedema on rare occasions. Recurrent epistaxes and bleeding from the mucous membrane of the mouth and gums in the absence of thrombocytopenia are common. Abnormalities of coagulation and platelet function similar to those seen in myeloma (pp. 302, 367) contribute to the bleeding diathesis, but increased viscosity itself probably interferes with the microcirculation. Neuropsychiatric manifestations include lassitude, headache, cerebellar dysfunction, confusion, coma, and convulsions.

Blood picture

Normochromic normocytic anaemia is common and may be marked. The red cell mass is usually mildly reduced, and there is often a substantial increase in plasma volume. The white cell count is usually normal or slightly decreased. The differential count is usually within normal range, but a lymphocytosis may be present. Platelets are normal or decreased. The outstanding feature is marked rouleaux formation in the blood film and an increased ESR, which is often over 100 mm/hour.

Bone marrow

There is a marked increase in the proportion of lymphocytes, many of which can be damaged and lose cytoplasm during the preparation of the film of the marrow aspirate. Forms intermediate between lymphocytes and plasma cells are seen in some cases. A decrease in erythroid, myeloid, and megakaryocytic series is common. Mast cells are often prominent, particularly around and within the marrow fragments. Marrow architecture is usually better appreciated in a bone marrow trephine biopsy, which is essential in the occasional patient in whom no marrow particles can be obtained by aspiration. Affected *lymph nodes* are moderately enlarged and show characteristic infiltration with lymphocytes and plasma cells, the normal reticulin pattern of the node being retained.

Blood chemistry

There is usually an increase in total protein concentration due to the increase in the concentration of macroglobulin, which usually exceeds 20 g/l and rarely may be as high as 120 g/l. Serum protein electrophoresis reveals a discrete M-band in the β- or γ-globulin region, similar to that seen in myeloma. Immunoelectrophoresis confirms its IgM nature. Bence Jones protein is present in small amounts in the urine of at least half of the patients, but the amount is typically much less than in myeloma. Normal immunoglobulin levels in the serum are not reduced to the same extent as in myeloma.

Treatment

Waldenström's macroglobulinaemia is often an indolent condition, and chemotherapy may not be necessary for much of the course of the disorder. Troublesome symptoms can be due to hyperviscosity, and *plasmapheresis* is very effective in rapidly reducing viscosity. IgM is largely located in the intravascular compartment and thus its concentration is efficiently reduced by exchange of the patient's plasma with normal plasma-protein preparations during this procedure. In some patients, the increase in serum viscosity is slow, and intermittent plasmapheresis may control troublesome symptoms.

Chlorambucil and cyclophosphamide are the most commonly employed therapeutic agents, and produce objective improvement and a fall in the serum concentration of IgM in about half of the patients. The initial daily dose of chlorambucil is 6–10 mg, and the maintenance dose 2–6 mg. Care must be taken to monitor dosage as the initial dose ultimately causes severe marrow depression in most subjects.

Care must also be exercised in the transfusion of such patients, as a rise in red cell count above a certain point can, in the presence of substantial concentrations of paraprotein, result in clinically significant hyperviscosity.

Paraproteins associated with other lymphocytic neoplastic states

Waldenström's macroglobulinaemia represents part of a spectrum of lymphoplasmacytic neoplasms in which paraprotein production may occur. In most instances, the paraprotein is IgM, and the two other most common conditions are *chronic lymphatic leukaemia* and diffuse *non-Hodgkin's lymphoma*. Paraproteins are detected in up to 10 per cent of the latter disorders, but the concentration in the serum is typically lower than in Waldenström's macroglobulinaemia (Alexanian 1975). The distinction from Waldenström's macroglobulinaemia is usually not difficult, although in some instances there may be condiserable overlap of features in some cases of non-Hodgkin's lymphoma. Therapy is that considered appropriate for the underlying disorder, and objective responses to treatment are accompanied by a fall in the serum paraprotein concentration.

Benign monoclonal gammopathy

The *prevalence* of benign monoclonal gammopathy in the community is considerably greater than that of myeloma or malignant lymphoplasmacytic disorders. Detection of paraproteins in otherwise well persons becomes progressively more common with increasing age, and prevalence of such paraproteins is of the order of several per cent in individuals over the age of 70 years. The paraproteins are mostly IgG, but IgM paraproteins are not uncommon. It is fundamental to the diagnosis of benign monoclonal gammopathy that neither significant progression of the condition, nor malignant features of myeloma or lymphoplasmacytic neoplasms are present. There are thus no symptoms due to the presence of the monoclonal protein; the liver, spleen, and lymph nodes are not enlarged; osteolytic lesions are absent; and the bone marrow aspirate does not contain a significant increase in the proportion of lymphocytes or plasma cells. As the presence of a paraprotein may be the sole abnormality in the early stages of myeloma or Waldenström's macroglobulinaemia, it is necessary to keep a patient with a provisional diagnosis of benign monoclonal gammopathy under regular clinical and haematological surveillance indefinitely in order to ensure that the disorder is truly benign—about five per cent per year evolve into a malignant disorder.

Although the passage of time is necessary to confirm the benign character of the disorder, several biochemical features are of value in differentiating benign from malignant paraprotein-related disorders. The presence of Bence Jones proteinuria, subnormal levels of normal serum immunoglobulins, paraprotein levels in serum exceeding 10 g/l, and a progressive rise in paraprotein level, all point to the diagnosis of a malignant disorder (Hobbs 1967), as does an increased serum β_2 microglobulin level. Chemotherapy is not indicated in benign monoclonal gammopathy.

Heavy chain disease

This disorder consists of a group of uncommon neoplastic conditions characterized by production of a paraprotein consisting only of part or all of a heavy chain of the immunoglobulin molecule. The conditions in which the heavy chain corresponds either to the γ or the α heavy chain tend to follow a course similar to malignant lymphoma, and Mu heavy chain disease is strongly associated with infiltration of the intestine by the neoplastic cells. Mu heavy chain disease is even more rare, and is found uncommonly in association with what otherwise appears to be typical chronic lymphatic leukaemia.

Amyloidosis

Paraproteins are detected in serum or urine of nearly 90 per cent of patients with primary amyloidosis. Such patients have no histological or radiological evidence of myeloma or macroglobulinaemia, although the organ distribution of amyloid resembles that of myeloma-associated amyloidosis (Kyle & Bayrd 1975). In both myeloma and primary amyloidosis, a major constituent of the amyloid protein is derived from light chains. Chemotherapy with agents similar to those employed in the treatment of myeloma has been reported to halt the progression of the disease occasionally, and in some instances produces partial recovery of the function of infiltrated organs.

Miscellaneous disorders

Paraproteins are occasionally identified in the serum of patients with *cold agglutinin syndrome*. They have also been detected in association with a variety of other inflammatory or neoplastic conditions, but most authorities consider that the latter associations are fortuitous, the prevalence of paraproteinaemia being no greater than in the general population.

Transient paraproteinaemia is occasionally encountered in acute infections and drug reactions, but the paraprotein does not usually display antibody specificity.

References and further reading

Lymphomas: pathology and immunology

Bartl, R., Frisch, B., Burkhardt, R. *et al.* (1982) Assessment of bone marrow histology in the malignant lymphomas (non-Hodgkin's): classification and staging. *Brit. J. Haemat.* **51**, 1551.

Lennert, K., Mohri, N., Stern, H. *et al.* (1975) The histology of malignant lymphomas. *Brit. J. Haemat.* (Suppl.) **31**, 193.

The non-Hodgkin's lymphoma pathologic classification project (1982) National Cancer Institute sponsored study of classifications of non-Hodgkin's lymphomas. Summary and a description of a working formulation for clinical usage. *Cancer,* **49**, 2112.

Leong, A.S-Y. & Forbes, I.J. (1982) Immunological and histochemical techniques in the study of the malignant lymphomas: a review. *Pathology,* **14**, 247.

Lukes, R.J., Craver, L.F., Hall, R.C. *et al.* (1966) Report of the nomenclature committee. *Cancer Res.* **26**, 1311.

Lukes, R.J., Taylor, C.R., Parker, J.W. *et al.* (1978) A morphologic and immunologic surface marker study of 299 cases of non-Hodgkin's lymphomas and related leukaemias. *Am. J. Pathol.* **90**, 461.

Lukes, R.J. & Collins, R.D. (1974) Immunologic characterization of human malignant lymphomas. *Cancer,* **34**, 1488.

Mintzer, D.M. & Hauptman, S.P. (1983) Lymphosarcoma cell leukemia and other non-Hodgkin's lymphomas in leukemia phase. *Am. J. Med.* **75**, 110.

Rappaport, H. (1966) Tumors of the hemopoietic system. In: *Atlas of Tumor Pathology,* Section III. Fascicle 8. Armed Forces Institute of Pathology, Washington DC.

Sutcliffe, S.B. (1985) *Immunology of the Lymphomas,* CRC Press, Florida.

Classification, clinical features, complications and diagnosis

Aisenberg, A.C. (1966) Manifestations of immunologic unresponsiveness in Hodgkin's disease. *Cancer Res.* **26**, 1152.

Berard, C., O'Connor, G.T., Thomas, L.B. *et al.* (1969) Histopathological definition of Burkitt's tumour. *Bull. Wld. Hlth. Org.* **40**, 601.

Block, J.B., Edgcomb, J., Eisen, A. *et al.* (1963) Mycosis fungoides' natural history and aspects of its relationship to other malignant lymphomas. *Am. J. Med.* **34**, 228.

Crowther, D., Fairley, G.H. & Sewell, R.L. (1969) Significance of the changes in the circulating lymphoid cells in Hodgkin's disease. *Brit. Med. J.* **2**, 473.

Cullen, M.H., Stansfeld, A.G., Oliver R.T.D. *et al.* (1979) Angio-immunoblastic lymphadenopathy: report of ten cases and review of the literature. *Quart. J. Med.* **48**, 151.

Dolman, C.L. & Cairns, A.R.M. (1961) Leucoencephalopathy associated with Hodgkin's disease. *Neurology,* **11**, 349.

Edelson, R.L. (1980) Cutaneous T-cell lymphoma: mycosis fungoides, Sézary syndrome, and other variants. *J. Am. Acad. Dermat.* **2**, 89.

Epstein, E.H. (1980) Mycosis fungoides: clinical course and cellular abnormalities. *J. Invest. Dermat.* **75**, 103.

Frizzera, G., Moran, E.M. & Rappaport, H. (1975) Angio-immunoblastic lymphadenopathy. *Am. J. Med.* **59**, 803.

Gams, R.A., Neal, J.A. & Conrad, F.G. (1968) Hydantoin-induced pseudo-pseudo-lymphoma. *Ann. Int. Med.* **69**, 557.

Garrison, C.O., Dines, D.E., Harrison, E.G.Jr. *et al.* (1969) The alveolar pattern of pulmonary lymphoma. *Proc. Mayo Clin.* **44**, 260.

Hyman, G.A. & Sommers, S.C. (1966) The development of Hodgkin's disease and lymphoma during anticonvulsant therapy. *Blood,* **28**, 416.

Jones, S.E. (1974) Clinical features and course of the non-Hodgkin's lymphomas. *Clin. Haemat.* **3**, 131.

Lukes, R.J. & Tindle, B.H. (1975) Immunoblastic lymphadenopathy. *New Engl. J. Med.* **292**, 1.

McCormick, D.P., Ammann, A.J. Ishizaka, K. *et al.* (1971) A study of allergy in patients with malignant lymphoma and chronic lymphocytic leukaemia. *Cancer,* **27**, 93.

Moran, E.M. & Ultmann, J.E. (1974) Clinical features and course of Hodgkin's disease. *Clin. Haemat.* **3**, 91.

Mullins, G.M., Flynn, J.P.G., El-Mahdi, A.M. *et al.* (1971) Malignant lymphoma of the spinal epidural space. *Ann. Int. Med.* **74**, 416.

Olumide, A.A., Osunkoya, B.O. & Ngh, V.A. (1971) Superior mediastinal compression: a report of five cases caused by malignant lymphoma. *Cancer,* **27**, 193.

Patchefsky, A.S., Brodovsky, H.S., Mendyke, H. *et al.* (1974) Non-Hodgkin's lymphomas: a clinicopathologic study of 293 cases. *Cancer,* **34**, 1173.

Pirofsky, B. (1968) Autoimmune haemolytic anaemia and neoplasia of the reticuloendothelium. *Ann. Int. Med.* **68**, 109.

Plager, J. & Stutzman, L. (1971) Acute nephrotic syndrome as a manifestation of active Hodgkin's disease. *Am. J. Med.* **50**, 56.

Qazi, R., Aisenberg, A.C. & Long, J.C. (1976) The natural history of nodular lymphoma. *Cancer,* **37**, 1923.

Safai, B. & Good, R.A. (1980) Lymphoproliferative disorders of the T-cell series. *Medicine,* **59**, 335.

Schein, P.S., Chabner, B.A., Canellos, G.P. *et al.* (1974) Potential for prolonged disease-free survival following combination chemotherapy of non-Hodgkin's lymphoma. *Blood,* **43**, 181.

Swinson, C.M., Slavin, G., Coles, E.C. *et al.* (1983) Coeliac disease and malignancy. *Lancet,* **i**, 111.

Ultmann, J.E. & Moran, E.M. (1973) Clinical course and complications of Hodgkin's disease. *Arch. Int. Med.* **131**, 332.

Young, R.C., Corder, M.P., Haynes, H.A. *et al.* (1972) Delayed hypersensitivity of Hodgkin's disease. A study of 103 untreated patients. *Am. J. Med.* **52**, 63.

Staging

Anderson, K.C., Leonard, R.C.F., Canellos, G.P. *et al.* (1983) High-dose gallium imaging in lymphoma. *Am. J. Med.* **75**, 327.

Carbone, P.P., Kaplan, H.S., Musshoff, K. *et al.* (1971) Report of the committee on Hodgkin's disease staging classification. *Cancer Res.* **31**, 1860.

Glatstein, E. & Goffinet, D.R. (1974) Staging of Hodgkin's disease and other lymphomas. *Clin. Haemat.* **3**, 77.

Goffinet, D.R., Castellino, R.A., Kim, H. *et al.* (1973) Staging laparotomies in unselected previously untreated patients with non-Hodgkin's lymphoma. *Cancer*, **32**, 672.

Gomez, G.A., Reese, P.A., Nava, H. *et al.* (1984) Staging laparotomy and splenectomy in early Hodgkin's disease: No therapeutic benefit. *Am. J. Med.* **77**, 205.

Haybittle, J.L., Hayhoe, F.G.J., Easterling, M.J. *et al.* (1985) Review of British national lymphoma investigation studies of Hodgkin's disease and development of prognostic index. *Lancet*, **i**, 967.

Jones, S.E. (1980) Importance of staging in Hodgkins Disease. *Semin. Oncol.* **7**, 126.

Kadin, M.E., Glatstein, E. & Dorfman, E.F. (1971) Clinicopathologic studies of 117 untreated patients subjected to laparotomy for the staging of Hodgkin's disease. *Cancer*, **27**, 1277.

Lacher, M.J. (1983) Routine staging laparotomy for patients with Hodgkins disease is no longer necessary. *Cancer Invest.* **1**, 93.

Rosenberg, S.A. (1971) A critique of the value of laparotomy and splenectomy in the evaluation of patients with Hodgkin's disease. *Cancer Res.* **31**, 1737.

Rosenberg, S.A., Boiron, M., de Vita, V.T. *et al.* (1971) Report of the committee on Hodgkin's disease staging procedures. *Cancer Res.* **31**, 1862.

Vinciguerra, V. & Silver, R.T. (1971) The importance of bone marrow biopsy in the staging of patients with lymphosarcoma. *Blood*, **38**, 804.

Webb, D.I., Ubogy, G. & Silver, R.T. (1970) Importance of bone marrow biopsy in the clinical staging of Hodgkin's disease. *Cancer*, **26**, 313.

Treatment and prognosis

Advances in chemotherapy for Hodgkin's and non-Hodgkin's lymphoma (1988) *Semin. Hemat.* **25**, Suppl. 2, 1.

Aisenberg, A.C. & Qazi, R. (1976) Improved survival in Hodgkin's disease. *Cancer*, **37**, 2423.

Bagley, C.M., Jr, de Vita, V.T., Jr, Berard, C.W. *et al.* (1972) Advanced lymphosarcoma: intensive cyclical combination chemotherapy with cyclophosphamide, vincristine and prednisone. *Ann. Int. Med.* **76**, 227.

Bonadonna, G., Zucali, R., Monfardino, S. *et al.* (1975) Combination chemotherapy for Hodgkin's disease with adriamycin, bleomycin, vinblastine and imidazole carboxamide versus MOPP. *Cancer*, **36**, 252.

Bush, R.S., Gospodarowicz, M., Sturgeon, J. *et al.* (1977) Radiation therapy of localised non-Hodgkin's lymphoma. *Cancer Treat. Rep.* **61**, 1129.

Canellos, G.P., Come, S.E. & Skerin, A.T. (1983) Chemotherapy in the treatment of Hodgkin's disease. *Semin. Hematol.* **20**, 1.

Canellos, G.P., de Vita, V.T., Arseneau, J.C. *et al.* (1975) Second malignancies complicating Hodgkin's disease in remission. *Lancet*, **i**, 947.

Canellos, G.P., Young, R.C., Berard, C.W. *et al.* (1973) Combination chemotherapy and survival in advanced Hodgkin's disease. *Arch. Int. Med.* **131**, 388.

Coltman, C.A. (1980) Chemotherapy of advanced Hodgkin's disease. *Semin. Oncol.* **7**, 155.

De Vita, V.T., Serpick, A.A. & Carbone, P.P. (1970) Combination chemotherapy in the treatment of advanced Hodgkin's disease. *Ann. Int. Med.* **73**, 881.

Ding, J.C., Cooper, I.A., Firkin, F. *et al.* (1986) Investigation of additive potential of teniposide and vincristine in non-Hodgkins lymphoma. *Cancer Treat. Rep.* **70**, 985.

Hoppe, R.T. (1980) Radiation therapy in the treatment of Hodgkin's disease. *Semin. Oncol.* **7**, 144.

Hoppe, R.T., Kushlan, P., Kaplan, H.S. *et al.* (1981) Treatment of advanced stage favourable histology non-Hodgkin's lymphoma: A preliminary report of a randomized trial comparing single agent chemotherapy, combination chemotherapy, and whole body irradiation. *Blood*, **58**, 592.

Hoppe, R.T., Portlock, C.S., Glatstein, E. *et al.* (1979) Alternating chemotherapy and irradiation in the treatment of advanced Hodgkin's disease. *Cancer*, **43**, 472.

Kaplan, H.S. (1966) Long-term results of palliative and radical radiotherapy of Hodgkin's disease. *Cancer Res.* **26**, 1250.

Kaplan, H.S. (1970) On the natural history, treatment and prognosis of Hodgkin's disease. In: *The Harvey Lectures*, 1968–69, p. 215, Academic Press, New York.

Klimo, P. & Connors, J.M. (1985) MACOP-B chemotherapy for the treatment of diffuse large cell lymphoma. *Ann. Int. Med.* **102**, 596.

Koziner, B., Little, C., Passe, S. *et al.* (1982) Treatment of advanced diffuse histiocytic lymphoma: an analysis of prognostic variables. *Cancer*, **49**, 1571.

McKelvey, E.M., Gottlieb, J.A., Wilson, H.E. *et al.* (1976) Hydroxyldaunomycin (adriamycin) combination chemotherapy in malignant lymphoma. *Cancer*, **38**, 1484.

Miller, T.P., Dana, B.W., Weick, J.K. *et al.* (1988) Southwest Oncology Group clinical trials for intermediate- and high-grade non-Hodgkin's lymphomas. *Semin. Hemat.* **25**, Suppl. 2, 17.

Nathwani, B.N., Kim, H. & Rappaport, H. (1976) Malignant lymphoma, lymphoblastic. *Cancer*, **38**, 964.

Olumide, A.A., Osunkoya, B.O. & Ngh, V.A. (1971) Superior mediastinal compression: a report of five cases caused by malignant lymphoma. *Cancer*, **27**, 193.

Patchefsky, A.S., Brodovsky, H.S., Mendyke, H. *et al.* (1974) Non-Hodgkin's lymphomas: a clinicopathologic study of 293 cases. *Cancer*, **34**, 1173.

Pirofsky, B. (1968) Autoimmune haemolytic anaemia and neoplasia of the reticuloendothelium. *Ann. Int. Med.* **68**, 109.

Portlock, C.S. (1983) "Good risk" non-Hodgkin's lymphomas: Approaches to management. *Semin. Haemat.* **20**, 25.

Qazi, R., Aisenberg, A.C. & Long, J.C. (1976) The natural history of nodular lymphoma. *Cancer,* **37**, 1923.

Santoro, A., Bonadonna, G., Bonfante, V. *et al.* (1982) Alternating drug combinations in the treatment of advanced Hodgkin's disease. *New Engl. J. Med.* **306**, 770.

Schein, P.S., Chabner, B.A., Canellos, G.P. *et al.* (1974) Potential for prolonged disease-free survival following combination chemotherapy of non-Hodgkin's lymphoma. *Blood,* **43**, 181.

Singer, C.R. & Goldstone, A.H. (1986) Clinical studies of autologous bone marrow transplantation in non-Hodgkins lymphoma. *Clin. Haemat.* **15**, 105.

Streuli, R.A., Kaneko, Y., Variakajis, D. *et al.* (1981) Lymphoblastic lymphoma in adults. *Cancer,* **47**, 2510.

Sweet, D.L., Kinzie, J., Gaeke, M.E. *et al.* (1981) Survival of patients with localised diffuse histiocytic lymphoma. *Blood,* **58**, 1218.

Swinson, C.M., Slavin, G., Coles, E.C. *et al.* (1983) Coeliac disease and malignancy. *Lancet,* **i**, 111.

Ultmann, J.E. & Moran, E.M. (1973) Clinical course and complications of Hodgkin's disease. *Arch. Int. Med.* **131**, 332.

Wiernik, P.H., Gustafson, J., Schimpff, S.C. *et al.* (1979) Combined modality treatment of Hodgkin's disease confined to lymph nodes: Results eight years later. *Am. J. Med.* **67**, 183.

Young, R.C., Corder, M.P., Haynes, H.A. *et al.* (1972) Delayed hypersensitivity in Hodgkin's disease. A study of 103 untreated patients. *Am. J. Med.* **52**, 63.

Immunoglobulins: structure and synthesis

Natvig, J.B. & Kunkel, H.G. (1973) Human immunoglobulins: classes, sub-classes, genetic variants and idiotypes. *Adv. Immunol.* **16**, 1.

Solomon, A. (1976) Bence–Jones proteins and light chains of immunoglobulins. *New Engl. J. Med.* **204**, 17.

Tonegawa, S. (1985) The molecules of the immune system. *Sci. Am.* **253** (No. 4), 104.

Myeloma

Acute Leukemia Group B (1975) Correlation of abnormal immunoglobulin with clinical features of myeloma. *Arch. Int. Med.* **135**, 46.

Alexanian, R., Haut, A., Khan, A.U. *et al.* (1969) Treatment for multiple myeloma. Combination of chemotherapy with different melphalan dose regimens. *J. Am. Med. Ass.* **208**, 1680.

Alexanian, R., Balcerzak, S., Bonnet, J.D. *et al.* (1975) Prognostic factors in multiple myeloma. *Cancer,* **36**, 1192.

Alexanian, R., Yap, B.S. & Bodey, G.P. (1983) Prednisone pulse therapy in myeloma. *Blood,* **62**, 572.

Bartl, R., Frisch, B., Burkhardt, R. *et al.* (1982) Bone marrow histology in myeloma; its importance in diagnosis, prognosis, classification and staging. *Brit. J. Haemat.* **51**, 361.

Bataille, R. & Sany, J. (1981) Solitary myeloma. Clinical and prognostic features of a review of 114 cases. *Cancer,* **48**, 845.

Bataille, R., Durie, B.G. & Grenier, J. (1983) Serum beta$_2$-microglobulin and survival duration in multiple myeloma: a simple reliable marker for staging. *Brit. J. Haemat.* **55**, 439.

Bataille, R., Grenior, J.Q. & Sany, J. (1984) Beta$_2$-microglobulin in myeloma: optimal use for staging, prognosis, and treatment—a prospective study of 160 patients. *Blood,* **63**, 468.

Bayrd, E.D. (1948) The bone marrow on sternal aspiration in multiple myelom. *Blood,* **3**, 987.

Bersagel, D.E., Bailey, A.J., Langley, G.R. *et al.* (1979) The chemotherapy of plasma cell myeloma and the incidence of acute leukaemia. *New Engl. J. Med.* **301**, 743.

Bersagel, D.E. & Rider, W.D. (1985) Plasma cell neoplasms. In: de Vita, V.T., Hellman, S. & Rosenberg, S.A. (Eds) *Cancer. Principles and Practice of Oncology,* 2nd Ed. pp. 47, 1768, Lippincot, Philadelphia.

Bloch, K.J. & Maki, D.G. (1973) Hyperviscosity syndromes associated with immunoglobulin abnormalities. *Semin. Hematol.* **10**, 113.

Carter, P.M., Slater, L., Lee, J. *et al.* (1974) Protein analyses in myelomatosis. *J. Clin. Path.* **28**, Suppl.(Ass. Clin. Path.) **6**, 45.

Case, D.C., Lee B.J. & Clarkson, B.D. (1977) Improved survival times in multiple myeloma treated with melphalan, prednisolone, cyclophosphamide, vincristine, and BCNU: M-2 protocol. *Am. J. Med.* **63**, 897.

Cohen, J.H. & Rundles, R.W. (1975) Managing the complications of plasma cell myeloma. *Arch. Int. Med.* **135**, 177.

Costa, G., Engle, R.L., Jr, Schilling, A. *et al.* (1973) Melphalan and prednisone: an effective combination for the treatment of multiple myeloma. *Am. J. Med.* **54**, 589.

Defronzo, R.A., Humphrey, R.C. Wright, J.R. *et al.* (1975) Acute renal failure in multiple myeloma. *Medicine,* **54**, 209.

Dreicer, R. & Alexanian, R. (1982) Nonsecretory multiple myeloma. *Am. J. Hematol.* **13**, 313.

Durie, B.G. & Salmon, S.E. (1975) A clinical staging system for multiple myeloma. Correlation of measured myeloma cell mass with presenting clinical features, response to treatment and survival. *Cancer,* **36**, 842.

Durie, B.G., Salmon, S.E. & Moon, T.E. (1980) Pretreatment tumor mass, cell kinetics and prognosis in multiple myeloma. *Blood,* **55**, 364.

Fishkin, B.G., Orloff, N., Scaduto, L.E. *et al.* (1972) IgE multiple myeloma: a report of the third case. *Blood,* **39**, 361.

Garewal, H., Durie, B.G., Kyle, R.A. *et al.* (1984) Serum beta$_2$-microglobulin in the initial staging and subsequent monitoring of monoclonal plasma cell disorders. *J. Clin. Oncol.* **2**, 51.

George, R.P., Poth, J.L., Gordon, D. *et al.* (1972) Multiple myeloma—intermittent, combination chemotherapy compared to continuous therapy. *Cancer*, **29**, 1665.

Hobbs, J.R. (1967) Paraproteins, benign or malignant? *Brit. Med. J.* **3**, 699.

Hobbs, J.R. (1969) Immunochemical classes of myelomatosis. *Brit. J. Haemat.* **16**, 599.

Jancelewicz, Z., Takatsuki, K., Sugai, S. *et al.* (1975) IgD multiple myeloma. Review of 133 cases. *Arch. Int. Med.* **135**, 87.

Josse, R.G., Murray, T.M., Mundy, G.R. *et al.* (1981) Observations on the mechanism of bone resorption induced by multiple myeloma marrow culture fluids and partially purified osteoclast-activating factor. *J. Clin. Invest.* **67**, 1472.

Kyle, R.A. (1975) Multiple myeloma. Review of 869 cases. *Proc. Mayo Clin.* **50**, 29.

Kyle, R.A., Maldonaldo, J.E. & Bayrd, E.D. (1974) Plasma cell leukemia. Report on 17 cases. *Arch. Int. Med.* **133**, 813.

Lackner, H. (1973) Hemostatic abnormalities associated with dysproteinemias. *Semin. Hematol.* **10**, 125.

Levi, D.F., Williams, R.C. & Lindstrom, F.D. (1968) Immunofluorescent studies of the myeloma kidney with special reference to light chain disease. *Am. J. Med.* **44**, 922.

Maldonaldo, J.E., Velosa, J.A. Kyle, R.A. *et al.* (1975) Fanconi syndrome in adults. A manifestation of a latent form of myeloma. *Am. J. Med.* **58**, 354.

Medical Research Council's Working Party for Therapeutic Trials in Leukaemia (1971) Myelomatosis: comparison of mephalan and cyclophosphamide therapy. *Brit. Med. J.* **1**, 640.

Medical Research Council's Working Party for Therapeutic Trials in Leukaemia (1973) Report on the first myelomatosis trial. Part I. Analysis of presenting features of prognostic importance. *Brit. J. Haemat.* **24**, 123.

Meyers, B.R., Hirschman, S.Z. & Axelrod, J.A. (1972) Current patterns of infection in multiple myeloma. *Am. J. Med.* **52**, 87.

Pruzanski, W. & Russell, M.L. (1976) Serum viscosity and hyperviscosity syndrome in IgG multiple myeloma: the relationship to Sia test and to concentration of M component. *Am. J. Med. Sci.* **271**, 145.

Rosner, F. & Grunwald, H. for Acute Leukemia Group B (1974) Multiple myeloma terminating in acute leukemia. Report of 12 cases and review of the literature. *Am. J. Med.* **57**, 927.

Stone, M.J. & Frenkel, E.P. (1975) The clinical spectrum of light chain myeloma. A study of 35 patients with special reference to the occurrence of amyloidosis. *Am. J. Med.* **58**, 601.

Zlotnick, A. & Rosenmann, E. (1975) Renal pathologic findings associated with monoclonal gammopathies. *Arch. Int. Med.* **135**, 40.

Macroglobulinaemia

Bartl, R., Frisch, B., Mahl, G. *et al.* (1983) Bone marrow histology in Waldenstrom's macroglobulinaemia. Clinical relevance of subtype recognition. *Scand. J. Haemat.* **31**, 359.

Dutcher, T.F. & Fahey, J.L. (1959) The histopathology of the macroglobulinemia of Waldenstrom. *J. Nat. Cancer Inst.* **22**, 887.

Hobbs, J.R., Carter, P.M., Cooke, K.B. *et al.* (1974) IgM paraproteins. *J. Clin. Path.* **28**, Suppl. (Ass. Clin. Path.) **6**, 54.

McCallister, B.D., Bayrd, E.D., Harrison, E.G. *et al.* (1967) Primary macroglobulinemia; review with a report on 31 cases and notes on the value of continuous chlorambucil therapy. *Am. J. Med.* **43**, 394.

MacKenzie, M.R., Brown, E., Fundenberg, H.H. *et al.* (1970) Waldenstrom's macroglobulinemia: correlation between expanded plasma volume and increased serum viscosity. *Blood*, **35**, 394.

MacKenzie, M.R. & Fundenberg, H.H. (1972) Macroglobulinemia: an analysis of forty patients. *Blood*, **39**, 874.

MacKenzie, M.R. & Babcock, J. (1975) Studies on the hyperviscosity syndrome. II. Macroglobulinemia. *J. Lab. Clin. Med.* **85**, 227.

Solomon, A. & Fahey, J.L. (1963) Plasmapheresis therapy in macroglobulinemia. *Ann. Int. Med.* **58**, 789.

Heavy chain disease, other paraproteinaemias, and amyloidosis

Alexanian, R. (1975) Monoclonal gammopathy in lymphoma. *Arch. Int. Med.* **135**, 62.

Axelsson, U., Bachmann, R. & Hallen, J. (1966) Frequency of pathological proteins (M-components) in 6995 sera from an adult population. *Acta Med. Scand.* **179**, 235.

Axelsson, U. & Hallen, J. (1972) A population study on monoclonal gammapathy: follow up after 5½ years on 64 subjects detected by electrophoresis of 6995 sera. *Acta Med. Scand.* **191**, 111.

Frangione, B. & Franklin, E.C. (1973) Heavy chain diseases: clinical features and molecular significance of the disordered immunoglobulin structure. *Semin. Hematol.* **10**, 53.

Glenner, G.G. (1973) Immunoglobulin and amyloid fibril proteins. *Brit. J. Haemat.* **24**, 533.

Glenner, G.G., Terry, W.D. & Isersky, C. (1973) Amyloidosis—its nature and pathogenesis. *Semin. Hematol.* **10**, 65.

Grey, H.M. & Kohler, P.F. (1973) Cryoimmunoglobulins. *Semin. Hematol.* **10**, 87.

Isobe, T. & Osserman, E.F. (1974) Patterns of amyloidosis and their association with plasma-cell dyscrasias, monoclonal immunoglobulins and Bence–Jones proteins. *New Engl. J. Med.* **290**, 473.

Kim Hun, Heller, P. & Rappaport, H. (1973) Monoclonal gammopathies associated with lymphoproliferative disorders: a morphologic study. *Am. J. Clin. Path.* **59**, 282.

Kyle, R.A. & Bayd, E.D. (1975) Amyloidosis: review of 236 cases. *Medicine,* **54**, 271.

Kyle, R.A. (1982) Monoclonal gammopathy of undetermined significance (MGUS): a review. *Clin. Haemat.* **11**, 123.

Kyle, R.A. (1982) Amyloidosis. *Clin. Haemat.* **11**, 151.

Kyle, R.A. (1984) 'Benign' monoclonal gammopathy. A misnomer? *J. Am. Med. Ass.* **251**, 1849.

Ritzzmann, S.E., Loukas, D., Sakai, H. *et al.* (1975) Idiopathic (asymptomatic) monoclonal gammopathies. *Arch. Int. Med.* **135**, 95.

Vodopick, H., Chaskes, S.J., Solomon, A. *et al.* (1974) Transient monoclonal gammopathy associated with cytomegalovirus infection. *Blood,* **44**, 189.

Williams, R.C., Jr, Bailly, R.C. & Howe, R.B. (1969) Studies of 'benign' serum M-components. *Am. J. Med. Sci.* **257**, 275.

Zawadzki, Z.A. & Edwards, G.A. (1972) Nonmyelomatous monoclonal immunoglobulinemia. In: Schwartz, R.S. (Ed.) *Progress in Clinical Immunology,* Vol. 1, Grune & Stratton, New York.

Chapter 12
Polycythaemia; Myelofibrosis

Polycythaemia

The term polycythaemia, strictly speaking, implies elevated levels of all cellular elements of the blood, although it is usually used when there is elevation of the red cell count alone, or in combination with elevation of granulocyte or platelet numbers. An increase in red cell count is typically accompanied by an increase in the haemoglobin concentration and haematocrit (PCV). If the mean corpuscular volume is subnormal, the increases in haemoglobin and PCV are proportionately less than the increase in red cell count.

Polycythaemia may result from an increase in the total number of red cells in the body (true polycythaemia), or from a reduction in plasma volume relative to the volume of red cells (spurious or relative polycythaemia). True polycythaemia may be due to a primary disorder of haemopoietic tissue which produces excessive numbers of red cells (polycythaemia vera), or secondary to excessive stimulation of normal erythroid precursors by the physiological regulator, *erythropoietin*, in states such as chronic hypoxaemia (secondary erythrocytosis).

Polycythaemia is suspected when the haemoglobin concentration is above the normal range. In true polycythaemia, the total volume of red cells in the body is above normal, while in relative polycythaemia, it is within the normal range. Except where clinical and peripheral blood parameters are absolutely diagnostic of polycythaemia vera, it is mandatory to estimate the total red cell volume in order to establish whether true polycythaemia is present. A difficult diagnostic situation exists, however, when the effect of excessive numbers of red cells in true polycythaemia is *masked* by appreciable reduction in mean corpuscular volume as a consequence of iron deficiency.

Total *red cell volume* is usually measured by isotope dilution methods (ICSH 1980). Normal *total blood volume* for both men and women is 70 ± 10 ml/kg bodyweight. Normal *red cell volume* for *men* is 30 ± 5 ml/kg, and for *women* is 25 ± 5 ml/kg, these figures representing the mean ± 2 standard deviations, encompassing values in 95 per cent of normal individuals (Dacie & Lewis 1984).

The causes of polycythaemia are listed in Table 12.1.

Secondary polycythaemia (erythrocytosis)

Secondary polycythaemia, or erythrocytosis, is the term applied to an elevated total red cell volume resulting from increased stimulation of normal erythroid precursors, usually as a consequence of lowering of the increased erythropoietin production due to oxygen saturation of arterial blood. A minority of cases are due to disorders where erythropoietin production is increased despite a normal arterial oxygen saturation.

Secondary erythrocytosis due to tissue hypoxia

PATHOGENESIS

The fundamental factor in this type of erythrocytosis is subnormal tissue oxygen delivery, which acts as a stimulus to erythrocyte production (p. 10). In general, the degree of erythrocytosis is proportional to the degree of reduction in arterial oxygen

Table 12.1. *Causes of polycythaemia*

True polycythaemia
Polycythaemia vera
Secondary polycythaemia (erythrocytosis)
SECONDARY TO TISSUE HYPOXIA
High altitude
Congenital heart disease
Chronic pulmonary disease
Miscellaneous (uncommon or rare):
acquired heart disease
disorders associated with alveolar hypoventilation
central: cerebral disorders
peripheral: mechanical impairment of chest movement
abnormalities of haemoglobin reductive mechanisms
increased oxygen affinity haemoglobins
chronic mild carbon monoxide exposure, e.g. in smokers
SECONDARY TO INAPPROPRIATELY INCREASED ERYTHROPOIETIN PRODUCTION
Non-neoplastic kidney disease: cysts, hydronephrosis
Tumours: kidney, liver; miscellaneous: cerebellar haemangioblastoma, phaeochromocytoma, adrenal adenoma, uterine myoma, virilizing ovarian tumour
Benign familial polycythaemia
Relative polycythaemia
Dehydration
Redistribution of body fluids
Spurious polycythaemia (polycythaemia of 'stress')

saturation, but wide individual variation occurs.

Lowered arterial oxygen delivery by the blood may be due to:

1 *Inadequate oxygenation of blood in pulmonary capillaries.* This may result from lowering of the partial pressure of oxygen in the inspired air; alveolar hypoventilation, i.e. reduction in the volume of air passing into the alveoli per unit time; or from changes that interfere with the diffusion of oxygen across the alveolar membrane into capillaries, such as fibrosis, infiltration, or reduction in the total area of alveolar membrane.

2 *A shunt between the venous and arterial circulations,* resulting in mixing of unsaturated systemic venous blood with arterial blood.

3 *Decreased oxygen transporting capacity of the haemoglobin in red cells.*

CLINICAL FEATURES

The clinical features of secondary hypoxic polycythaemia are those of the causative disorder, together with cyanosis of varying degrees. The depth of the cyanosis depends on the degree of oxygen desaturation and the severity of the polycythaemia. With mild polycythaemia, cyanosis may be absent. The spleen is typically not enlarged but occasionally it is palpable, particularly in cyanotic congenital heart disease.

BLOOD PICTURE

In secondary polycythaemia, the red cells alone are increased in number, the white cell and platelet counts being normal in the absence of complicating factors. The haemoglobin, RCC, and PCV values are increased. The bone marrow shows a selective hyperplasia of erythroblasts or is normal in appearance. The total blood volume is raised as a result of the increased total red cell volume, but the plasma volume is usually normal or slightly lowered.

CAUSES OF HYPOXIC SECONDARY ERYTHROCYTOSIS

High altitude

The compensatory erythrocytosis that develops in residents at high altitudes is due to inadequate oxygenation of blood as a result of the low atmospheric partial pressure of oxygen. The degree of change is proportional to the degree of reduction in arterial oxygen saturation, which in turn is related to the altitude. Red cell counts of 7–8 $\times 10^{12}/l$, or even higher, have been recorded in the Indians of the Peruvian Andes. The increase in red cell count and haemoglobin is greater in patients with chronic altitude sickness than in otherwise healthy residents at the same altitude. When newcomers arrive at high altitudes, there is an initial increase in the red cell count due to haemoconcentration, but within a matter of weeks the total red cell mass increases as a result of increased erythropoiesis. Return to sea-level is followed by a fall in haemoglobin levels to normal (Lenfant & Sullivan 1971).

Congenital heart disease

Secondary polycythaemia develops in cyanotic congenital heart disease because of shunting of blood from the right to the left side of the heart; this results in a proportion of the venous blood by-passing the lungs and not being oxygenated. In general, the degree of erythrocytosis increases as the volume of shunted blood increases. The commonest cause of cyanotic congenital heart disease in adults is the tetralogy of Fallot; less common causes are Eisenmenger's complex and transposition of the great vessels. Cyanosis may also develop with atrial septal defect, ventricular septal defect, and patent ductus arteriosus when there is reversal of the shunt due to the development of pulmonary hypertension. Sometimes, the reversed shunt does not occur until adult life, and thus the cyanosis is not noted until then.

Red cell counts usually range from 6.5 to 8 $\times 10^{12}$/l, but values of 9–10 $\times 10^{12}$/l or more may occur in severe cases. Clubbing of the fingers, retarded growth, and varying degrees of dyspnoea are commonly associated with the cyanosis. However, dyspnoea is not always a marked symptom, even when quite definite cyanosis is present.

Repeated phlebotomy has a limited place in the management of such patients (Rosenthal *et al.* 1970).

Chronic pulmonary disease

Secondary erythrocytosis may develop in certain chronic diseases of the lung in which structural changes interfere with oxygenation of pulmonary capillary blood, and so produce a lowered arterial oxygen saturation. Emphysema and pulmonary fibrosis are the most common causes.

Other causes of hypoxic polycythaemia

Central (cerebral) causes include the usual type of non-erythropoietin producing cerebral tumours, cerebral ischaemia, Parkinson's disease, encephalitis lethargica, and lesions of the hypothalamus and the pituitary. In about 50 per cent of cases of Cushing's syndrome, the haemoglobin level is at the upper normal limit or is slightly raised. This, however, may be a relative rather than a true erythrocytosis.

Peripheral causes that compromise inspiration include massive *obesity*, in which erythrocytosis may be relieved by weight loss; others are severe spondylosis, kyphoscoliosis, poliomyelitis, and myotonic dystrophy.

These conditions are all characterized by moderately reduced arterial oxygen tension, but it should be noted that the degree of saturation whilst awake and at rest may be considerably greater than that which occurs during exercise or sleep. The diagnosis, therefore, hinges both on the presence of some underlying cause and reduced arterial oxygen saturation (less than 90 per cent).

Decreased availability of functional haemoglobin in erythrocytes

Carboxyhaemoglobinaemia can cause mild erythrocytosis in heavy smokers (Smith & Landaw 1978). Methaemoglobin and sulphaemoglobin are also incapable of carrying oxygen (p. 20). Spectroscopic examination of the blood is diagnostic (Dacie & Lewis 1984).

Increased haemoglobin oxygen affinity. Familial erythrocytosis (p. 333) may be secondary to increased affinity of haemoglobin for oxygen. This may be due either to inherited abnormalities of haemoglobin structure (p. 153) or of 2,3-DPG metabolism (p. 19). Oxygen dissociation studies reveal an increased affinity for oxygen under both circumstances.

Secondary erythrocytosis due to inappropriate erythropoietin production

It is being increasingly recognized that polycythaemia may result from an excess production of erythropoietin. There are two broad groups of causes—non-neoplastic renal disease and tumours, of which the most common are renal carcinoma and hepatoma. Quite often, elevated levels of erythropoietin have been demonstrated in the plasma or urine, and less frequently in the causative tumour or cyst. Furthermore, return of plasma erythropoietin levels to normal and disappearance of erythrocytosis has been described following resection of the abnormal tissue responsible for the inappropriate production of erythropoietin. The literature is reviewed by Thorling (1972) and Hammond & Winnick (1974).

The erythrocytosis is usually mild to moderate, with packed cell volumes of 0.55–0.66, but occasionally higher. Red cell morphology is normal. In uncomplicated cases, the leucocyte count, platelet count, and neutrophil alkaline phosphatase value are normal. Splenomegaly is usually absent. Arterial oxygen saturation is normal. Treatment is that of the causation disorder.

NON-NEOPLASTIC RENAL DISEASE

Erythrocytosis occurs occasionally in a number of non-neoplastic renal conditions. They include hydronephrosis, cystic disease (polycystic, multilocular, and single cysts), and ischaemia, e.g. renal artery stenosis. In cystic disorders, one postulate is that the expanding cyst compresses renal vessels, causing local tissue anoxia, and so stimulates erythropoietin formation in the same way as general anoxia.

Transient polycythaemia with increased levels of urinary erythropoietin has been described following renal transplantation. It is considered likely that the source of erythropoietin is the transplanted kidney, and that the cause of the increase is ischaemia or damage to the donated kidney.

TUMOURS

In these disorders, the tumour is generally considered to be the source of the erythropoietin, although with large renal tumours, interference with renal blood supply may be a contributing factor.

Renal carcinoma is probably the commonest cause of polycythaemia associated with renal disease. In one series of 350 patients with renal carcinoma, polycythaemia occurred in 2.6 per cent of patients, and conversely carcinoma of the kidney was found in 4.4 per cent of 205 patients with polycythaemia (Damon *et al.* 1958).

Primary carcinoma of the liver is not uncommonly accompanied by mild to moderate erythrocytosis. Brownstein & Ballard (1966) found that about 3 per cent of patients had haemoglobin levels of about 18 g/dl, and that 9.4 per cent had haemoglobin levels above 16 g/dl; they suggest that in patients with hepatic disease haemoglobin levels above 16 g/dl may be a clue to the co-existence of hepatoma. The actual increase in red cell mass may be greater than indicated by the haemoglobin level and PCV, as an increase in plasma volume in cirrhosis of the liver is common. Erythrocytosis has also been reported in association with a hamartoma of the liver.

Miscellaneous. (Modan 1971) Erythrocytosis, usually mild, has also been described in association with *cerebellar haemangioblastoma, phaeochromocytoma, adrenal adenoma, uterine myoma,* and *virilizing ovarian carcinoma.* There is good evidence that erythrocytosis associated with cerebellar haemangioblastoma and phaeochromocytoma is due to the production of erythropoietin by the tumour. In cases of uterine myomata, it has been suggested that, as tumours in all the reported cases were very large, the erythrocytosis is caused by mechanical interference with either the blood supply to the kidneys or the urinary flow, resulting in an increased renal erythropoietin production (Thorling 1972).

Polycythaemia with cerebellar tumour must be differentiated from polycythaemia vera with prominent cerebral manifestations, particularly headache and papilloedema.

Polycythaemia vera

Erythraemia, Vaquez–Osler disease, and polycythaemia rubra vera are synonyms for polycythaemia vera, which is a chronic, progressive, and ultimately fatal disease, in which the fundamental abnormality is an excess production of the formed elements of the blood by a hyperplastic bone marrow. The marrow hyperplasia is not secondary to any recognized bone marrow stimulus, and studies using isoenzymes for glucose-6-phosphate dehydrogenase indicate that the affected cells are members of a clone that has arisen from a single progenitor (Adamson *et al.* 1976, Fialkow 1980). Progenitors of red cells in polycythaemia vera are unusually responsive to erythropoietin (Prchal *et al.* 1978), and there is an apparent appropriate reduction in the plasma concentration of erythropoietin in response to the elevated PCV (Koeffler & Goldwasser 1981). Polycythaemia vera may be regarded as a relatively benign type of neoplasm of haemopoietic tissue, in which the dominant clinical manifestations are due to the abnormal increase in red cell precursor activity. The occasional occurrence of cytogenetic abnormalities in bone marrow cells, particularly trisomy 9, emphasizes its neoplastic nature (Lawler 1980). Similar features exist in myelofibrosis and essential thrombocythaemia, emphasizing the relationship between these disorders. Polycythaemia vera is classified as one of the myeloproliferative disorders and commonly evolves into myelofibrosis.

Pathological physiology

The fundamental abnormality is hyperplasia of the precursors of the red cells, granulocytes, and platelets in the bone marrow, with resultant excess production of these cells. The overproduction of red cells results in an increase in the total red cell volume, sometimes to twice its normal value, or even more. This results in an increase in the number of red cells per litre of blood, and thus an elevated PCV, and in an absolute increase in the total blood volume of the body. The increased blood volume is due predominantly to the increase in total red cell volume, the plasma volume generally being within the normal range, although it is sometimes increased. The increased blood volume is accommodated mainly by capillary dilatation; at post mortem all the organs of the body are engorged with blood. Table 12.2 sets out the red cell, plasma, and blood volumes in various forms of polycythaemia.

Overproduction of red cells is responsible for most of the symptoms of polycythaemia vera, and, together with the excess number of platelets, for the vascular insufficiency which causes much of the morbidity and mortality (Schafer 1984). The increased blood volume causes a diversity of symptoms, the most prominent being cerebral. The increase in PCV, and the associated increase in viscosity of the blood, tends to slow the rate of blood flow, and predisposes to the thrombosis that

Table 12.2. *Blood volume studies in polycythaemia vera, secondary polycythaemia, and pseudopolycythaemia*

	Haemoglobin (g/dl)	PCV	Total blood volume (ml/kg)	Red cell volume (ml/kg)	Plasma volume (ml/kg)
Polycythaemia vera Typical case. Male aged 47 years	24	0.74	120	78	42
Polycythaemia vera with polycythaemia 'masked' by plasma volume increase due to congestive cardiac failure plus iron deficiency anaemia due to gastrointestinal bleeding. Male aged 60 years	11.7	0.45	129.9	52.8	77.1
Polycythaemia vera with polycythaemia 'masked' by plasma volume increase not due to congestive cardiac failure. Female aged 60 years	15.2	0.47	100	42.1	57.9
Secondary polycythaemia due to emphysema with pulmonary fibrosis. Arterial oxygen saturation 78 per cent. Male aged 64 years	19	0.64	82.6	49.5	33.1
Pseudopolycythaemia Male aged 45 years	20	0.60	64.8	34.2	30.6
Normal values					
Male	13–18	0.40–0.54		25–35	40–50
Female	11.5–16.5	0.37–0.47		20–30	40–50

so commonly occurs. Increased platelet adhesiveness may also contribute (Shield & Pearn 1969).

A haemorrhagic tendency also occurs. The cause is incompletely understood, but it is probable that several factors contribute, namely vascular engorgement and defects of platelet function similar to those of essential thrombocythaemia (Schafer 1984).

Clinical features

Polycythaemia vera is primarily a disease of middle and old age, the majority of cases occurring between 40 and 80 years, with onset most frequently at about 60 years. It occurs occasionally in younger adults, and rare cases in the second decade have been described. Males are affected a little more commonly than females. The incidence is higher in Jews of European origin, and is lower in Negroes.

The clinical picture is influenced by the severity and rate of progress of the disorder, and by the number and type of complications. Symptoms are caused mainly by the increased blood volume and by the thrombotic and haemorrhagic complications. The increased blood volume causes engorgement and slowing of the circulation in many organs; therefore, symptoms may be referred to a number of systems.

The *onset* is usually insidious, often with vague symptoms referred to one or more of the systems mentioned below. The most common presentation is with cerebral symptoms. Occasionally, an acute thrombotic or haemorrhagic complication causing a medical or surgical emergency is the presenting manifestation. When asymptomatic, the disorder is sometimes accidentally discovered on routine physical examination. Table 12.3 lists the presenting manifestations.

Central nervous system. Cerebral symptoms occur in most patients, and are the commonest presenting manifestation. Headache, fullness in the head, and dizziness are the usual complaints, but visual symptoms, tinnitus, syncope, loss of memory, inability to concentrate, and irritability also occur. Headache may be mild or severe, frequent or occasional, and varies in location from frontal to occipital. It may be worse on awakening in the morning or on lying down. *Depression* and other

Table 12.3. *Presenting manifestations of polycythaemia vera*

Common
Cerebral symptoms, especially headache and dizziness
Cardiovascular symptoms
Development of red face or bloodshot eyes
Weakness, lassitude, and tiredness
Gastrointestinal symptoms, especially dyspepsia
Visual disturbances
Pruritus
Thrombotic complications
Haemorrhagic manifestations
Peripheral vascular disease
Accidental discovery on routine examination
Occasional
Splenomegaly
Gout
Incidental discovery in investigation of other medical problems
Psychiatric manifestations

psychiatric disturbances occur occasionally.

Cerebrovascular accidents vary from mild attacks causing transient weakness of a limb, loss of consciousness or dysphasia, to the classical picture of a major cerebral thrombosis or haemorrhage. They are a common cause of death.

Weakness, lassitude, fatigue, and weight loss are common symptoms.

Cardiovascular system. Cardiac symptoms are frequent, dyspnoea being the most common. Because of the age group in which polycythaemia occurs, degenerative arterial disease and essential hypertension are frequent associations, and probably contribute largely to the cardiovascular manifestations. Hypertension is present in about one-half of cases, but because it is corrected in only a few cases after adequate therapy, it is probably due to essential hypertension, the increased blood volume making relatively little contribution. In the normotensive patient, the heart is usually of normal size. Angina of effort, coronary insufficiency, and cardiac failure are important and common complications.

Peripheral vascular disorders of varying types are frequent. They result from slowing of the circulation, thrombosis, and associated atherosclerosis. Erythromelalgia, arterial thrombosis, thromboangiitis obliterans, superficial and deep venous thrombosis, and Raynaud's phenomenon may occur. Pain in the extremities, including intermittent claudication, may be a prominent symptom. Arterial occlusion may result in gangrene.

Gastrointestinal symptoms, especially dyspepsia and flatulence, occur frequently. Symptoms are due mainly to the vascular engorgement of the alimentary tract, but about ten per cent of cases have a radiologically or endoscopically demonstrable peptic ulcer, usually duodenal. Abdominal pain may result from peptic ulceration, splenic enlargement, or infarction, or occasionally from mesenteric thrombosis. Haemorrhage from the congested mucosa of the stomach and bowel, or from a peptic ulcer, is not uncommon. Occasionally, the patient actually presents with anaemia resulting from occult gastrointestinal bleeding (see Table 12.2). Mild weight loss is common.

Visual disturbances are common; they result from engorgement of retinal veins and sometimes from thrombosis or haemorrhage. Scotomata, spots before the eyes, and transient dimness of vision are most common, but temporary blindness or diplopia may occur.

Thrombosis and haemorrhage, particularly thrombosis, are important causes of both morbidity and mortality. Thrombotic manifestations include cerebral and coronary thrombosis, mesenteric thrombosis, thrombosis of peripheral arteries, and pulmonary thrombosis. Postoperative thrombosis is common. Wasserman & Gilbert (1966) have estimated that more than 75 per cent of *patients with uncontrolled polycythaemia develop bleeding or thrombotic complications following major surgery, and elective procedures should never be undertaken prior to control of the polycythaemia.* Thrombosis and haemorrhage occur more frequently in patients over the age of 70 years (Tartaglia *et al.* 1986).

Gout occurs in about 10 per cent of cases, and elevated plasma urate in more than 50 per cent; the gout may be temporarily exacerbated by treatment. The first attack of gout may precede the diagnosis of polycythaemia vera by some years. Uric acid nephropathy with diffuse deposition of uric acid crystals through the kidney may occur, and in some cases there is calculus formation. *Bone pain* also occurs occasionally.

Generalized pruritus, often worse on the palms and soles, and aggravated by hot baths, occurs in about half the cases; it is an important symptom in diagnosis, especially in differential diagnosis from secondary polycythaemia in which it rarely, if ever, occurs. The pruritus is considered to be due to liberation of histamine from the basophil granulocytes (Gilbert *et al.* 1966). *Paraesthesiae* with numbness and tingling may also occur.

Obstetric and gynaecological problems in women of child-bearing age are discussed by Harris & Conrad (1967).

Physical examination

On examination, the outstanding features are the red colour of the skin and mucous membranes, congestion of the conjunctival vessels, and engorgement of the retinal veins. Splenomegaly is present at the time of diagnosis in some 70 per cent of cases.

Skin and mucous membranes. The red colour of the skin and mucous membranes is a striking feature in most, but not all, patients. The skin in florid cases is typically a brick-red colour, often with a dusky cyanotic hue which is more marked in cold weather. The high colour results from the marked engorgement and distension of the superficial capillaries. Easily recognized telangiectasia on the cheeks is common. The nail beds and palms of the hands are useful sites for assessment of the degree of plethora. The skin is warm, and the superficial veins are often distended. The mucous membranes of the mouth and tongue are often a deep red colour.

The *conjunctival vessels* are usually injected. Excess lacrimation may occur, but pain or soreness of the eyes is rare. It is not uncommon for the patient to present complaining of bloodshot eyes, or to give a history of having been treated for conjunctivitis. *Ophthalmoscopic examination* reveals a deeply coloured retina with engorged, tortuous veins. Retinal thrombosis and haemorrhage are sometimes seen.

Splenomegaly is present in 70 per cent of cases initially, and may subsequently develop in others. It is usually only of mild to moderate degree, although it is occasionally marked. The spleen is smooth and firm, and relatively rapid enlargement suggests the development of myelofibrosis or leukaemia. Infarction of the spleen may cause perisplenitis with pain and sometimes a friction rub. *Hepatomegaly*, either slight or moderate, is often present.

Chest X-ray. The chest X-ray may show prominent pulmonary vessels. The large number of visible 'end on vessels may produce mottling, particularly in the lower and mid-zones of the lungs, well out to the periphery. Previous pulmonary infarction may have resolved completely, or may have left areas of plate atelectasis or linear scars.

Blood picture

Blood obtained by venepuncture is dark, thick, viscous, and clots readily. The increased viscosity may make the spreading of satisfactory films difficult.

The red cell count is raised, usual values being 8–10 $\times 10^{12}/l$, and with counts up to 12 $\times 10^{12}/l$ occurring occasionally. The haemoglobin level is usually in the range of 18–24 g/dl, although it may be higher. The MCH is often slightly reduced, and thus the relative increase in haemoglobin level may be a little less than the degree of increase in red cell count. The PCV is raised, usually 0.60–0.70, and sometimes higher. The MCV is usually in the lower normal range, but may be reduced, especially when there has been gastrointestinal bleeding.

In the film of an uncomplicated case, the red cells usually appear normal. There is sometimes slight anisocytosis and microcytosis. A few round polychromatic macrocytes and an occasional nucleated red cell may be seen. Reticulocytes are 1.5 per cent or above in half the cases. In patients who have had repeated venesections or spontaneous bleeding, features of iron deficiency may be prominent.

Leucocytosis is present in nearly half the cases at presentation, the white count usually being from 12 to 20 $\times 10^9/l$, though occasionally counts up to 50 $\times 10^9/l$ occur. There is usually a shift to the left with metamyelocytes and stab forms, and often occasional myelocytes.

The neutrophil alkaline phosphatase is increased in more than 70 per cent of cases, but correlates poorly with the white cell count (Berlin 1975).

The platelet count is above 400 $\times 10^9/l$ in nearly two-thirds of cases, most frequently ranging from 400–800 $\times 10^9$, but occasionally reaching several thousand $\times 10^9/l$. Macrothrombocytes may be seen. The blood clotting time is not prolonged, but the clot is bulky and may be fragile. The bleeding time is usually normal, but is occasionally prolonged.

The *sedimentation rate is very often low*, usually being not more than 1 mm/hour. The serum bilirubin value is commonly at the upper limit of normal, but is sometimes slightly raised. Plasma iron and ferritin levels may be decreased, and are especially so after venesection. The serum level of vitamin B_{12}, unsaturated B_{12}-binding capacity, and lysozyme are commonly elevated. Reduction in serum folate levels may occur occasionally, a reflection of mild deficiency secondary to erythroid hyperplasia. Blood histamine values are often raised, and the activity of the enzyme histidine decarboxylase, which is responsible for histamine synthesis, is increased in leucocyte-rich blood fractions.

The plasma protein levels, including the fibrinogen concentration, are usually normal. The serum uric acid is raised in over 50 per cent of cases. The serum lactic dehydrogenase activity is usually normal, as is the serum haptoglobin level.

When the disorder evolves into *myelofibrosis*, the peripheral blood picture of that condition develops (p. 337). The haemoglobin level progressively falls, moderate to marked anisocytosis and poikilocytosis appear, and the number of myelocytes and normoblasts increases, together with the degree of polychromasia. There may be an elevated total white cell count, with a shift to the left, but at times the white count falls and leucopenia develops. The platelet count sometimes remains high, but often falls to normal, or less than normal, as the disease evolves.

Bone marrow

Bone marrow hyperplasia is evident on *trephine biopsy*. There is replacement of fat cells in the usual sites of haemopoiesis, giving the marrow a darker red appearance than normal, and an extension of the red marrow down the shafts of the long bones which normally contain yellow marrow. Trephine specimens commonly show some increase in reticulin. In a recent study, 25 per cent showed a slight increase at presentation, whilst in 11 per cent the increase was moderate or marked (Ellis *et al.* 1986).

Aspirated marrow usually contains numerous fragments, which low-power examination shows to be densely cellular and to contain either no fat or much less fat than normal. The cell trails are usually hypercellular. Erythropoiesis is normoblastic, and numerous clumps of developing normoblasts are prominent. Granulopoiesis is active, and since it shares in the hyperplasia, the myeloid:erythroid ratio is usually within normal limits, although it is sometimes reduced. Megakaryocytes are increased in number, and because of their size, are a prominent feature of the marrow. They often occur in clumps of 2–5 or even more, and are most obvious in the region of marrow fragments and at the margins of the film. Many megakaryocytes have platelet masses attached. *Sometimes, aspiration of particles is difficult or impossible, and this is not uncommonly related to more extensive development of reticulin, or extreme hypercellularity of the marrow.*

Diagnosis

In fully developed cases, the diagnosis is usually obvious from the presence of the *classical triad*—a dusky brick-red colour of the face ('ruddy cyanosis'), splenomegaly, and an elevated haemoglobin level with leucocytosis and thrombocytosis. However, it must be remembered that splenomegaly, leucocytosis and thrombocytosis are absent in a proportion of cases (p. 324). Pruritus for which there is no other obvious cause in a polycythaemic patient strongly suggests polycythaemia vera. Similarly, a raised neutrophil alkaline phosphatase in a polycythaemic patient also strongly suggests polycythaemia vera, provided that infection and other causes of increased alkaline phosphatase are absent (p. 218).

Total red cell mass should be measured in most cases in order to exclude relative polycythaemia (p. 334).

Diagnostic difficulty may occur in those cases in which the red cell values are only slightly increased, or are in the upper normal range. This may occur in the *early* stages, or when the polycythaemia is *'masked'* by a complicating factor, such as consequences of occult intestinal bleeding. An increase in plasma volume occasionally masks polycythaemia and occurs typically in cases complicated by congestive cardiac failure, but may occur without cardiac failure (Table 12.2).

Rare cases actually present with anaemia due to gastro-intestinal bleeding (Fig. 12.1). The anaemia may be either normochromic, or hypochromic due to iron deficiency. Such a situation must be differentiated from anaemia due to the development of myelofibrosis.

Differential diagnosis

Differentiation must be made from other disorders with similar clinical manifestations, and from other causes of a raised haemoglobin level.

In cases with an insidious onset, the vague and often somewhat indefinite symptoms such as headache, dizziness, fullness in the head, weakness, and lassitude may not suggest a specific diagnosis. On the other hand, when symptoms point mainly to one system or organ, diagnosis of primary disease of that system or organ may be made and the underlying polycythaemia overlooked (Table 12.3). Thus, a primary diagnosis of *congestive cardiac failure, essential hypertension, coronary artery disease, peptic ulcer, functional dyspepsia, peripheral vascular disease, phlebothrombosis or thrombophlebitis, cerebrovascular accident, mesenteric infarction, conjunctivitis*, or *gout* may be made.

Pseudopolycythaemia may be confused with polycythaemia vera, especially early and 'masked' cases, in which the red cell count is not markedly raised (Table 12.4). The plethoric facies of the two conditions may be indistinguishable. Pseudopolycythaemia lacks certain clinical features of polycythaemia vera—the typical ruddy colour of the mucous membranes, marked engorgement of retinal veins, splenomegaly, pruritus, leucocytosis, thrombocytosis, and raised neutrophil alkaline phosphatase; however, as any or all of these may be absent in polycythaemia vera, especially in the early

Table 12.4. *Comparison of polycythaemia vera, secondary polycythaemia, and pseudopolycythaemia*

	Polycythaemia vera	Hypoxic secondary erythrocytosis	Secondary erythrocytosis without hypoxia	Pseudopolycythaemia
Aetiology	Neoplastic	Hypoxia due to underlying disorder—pulmonary and cardiac disease commonest causes	Inappropriately increased erythropoietin production—associated with renal and certain other tumours	Unknown. Anxiety state, hypertension, obesity commonly associated
Clinical features				
Facies	Brick-red colour	Bluish cyanosis in more severe cases	Brick-red colour in more severe cases	Brick-red colour in more severe cases
Oral mucous membranes	Ruddy cyanosis	Bluish cyanosis	Normal or ruddy cyanosis	Normal
Conjunctival vessels	Injected	Injected in more severe cases	Injected in more severe cases	Injection absent or slight
Retinal vessels	Engorged	Engorged in severe cases	Engorged in severe cases	Not engorged
Spleen	Palpable (3/4 cases)	Usually impalpable	Usually impalpable	Usually impalpable
Pruritus	Common	Absent	Absent	Absent
Blood examination				
Red cell count, haemoglobin, and PCV	Mild through to marked increase	Increase usually mild to moderate	Increase usually mild to moderate	Increase usually mild
White cell count	Raised (3/4 cases)	Normal	Normal	Normal
Platelet count	Raised (2/3 cases)	Normal	Normal	Normal
Sedimentation rate	1 mm/hour or less	About 1 mm/hour except in severe cases	About 1 mm/hour except in severe cases	About 1 mm/hour
Neutrophil alkaline phosphatase	Usually but not invariably increased	Normal (may be increased by infection)	Normal	Normal
Arterial oxygen saturation	Normal	Reduced	Normal	Normal
Blood volume studies				
Red cell volume	Increased	Increased	Increased	Normal
Plasma volume	Usually normal, but may be reduced or increased	Normal or slightly reduced	Normal or slightly reduced	Reduced

stages, distinction can often be made with certainty only by red cell and plasma volume determinations. If blood volume determinations cannot be performed, careful clinical and haematological observations over a period of months or years may be necessary. In pseudopolycythaemia, the blood parameters remain relatively static, while in polycythaemia vera the haematological changes progress, and typical features appear in time. The usual error is for pseudopolycythaemia to be diagnosed as polycythaemia vera and treated as such.

Secondary hypoxic erythrocytosis can usually be distinguished by the presence of clinical manifestations of an underlying cause of hypoxia (most often a pulmonary or cardiac lesion), by the normal white cell and platelet counts, and by the absence of splenomegaly. When doubt exists as to whether the spleen is enlarged, an isotopic liver/spleen scan is of value. The white cell count may be raised by a complicating infection, especially in pulmonary disease.

Difficulty arises where central cyanosis is not prominent at rest. It may become more so on exercise. This occurs most commonly with pulmonary disease such as emphysema and pulmonary fibrosis, particularly in obese patients. It should be remembered that in some cases of congenital heart disease associated with reversed shunt, and in some cases of pulmonary arteriovenous fistula, cyanosis and polycythaemia do not develop until adult life.

Estimation of the arterial oxygen saturation is important in diagnosis; it is usually normal in polycythaemia vera, and below 90 per cent in secondary polycythaemia. Once it is established that the polycythaemia is of the secondary type, appropriate investigations can be carried out to determine the cause of the hypoxia if it is not obvious.

Renal erythrocytosis. The possibility of a renal cause should be considered in all patients with erythrocytosis but no leucocytosis, thrombocytosis, splenomegaly, or hypoxia. It should especially be considered in the polycythaemic patient with haematuria, although it must be recognized that haematuria can occur as a complication of polycythaemia vera. Pruritus is absent in renal polycythaemia, and the neutrophil alkaline phosphatase is normal unless a sizeable renal carcinoma is present.

Erythrocytosis with cerebellar tumour. Polycythaemia vera with headache and papilloedema, or with cerebellar signs due to vascular accident, must be differentiated from the rare association of erythrocytosis with cerebellar haemangioblastoma. The tumour is uncommon, but 15–20 per cent have some degree of elevated haemoglobin level.

Course and prognosis

The natural history without treatment is of a chronic, progressive, and ultimately fatal disorder. It can be divided into three phases.

1 The *onset phase*, before the red cell volume has been much increased, is relatively asymptomatic and usually lasts for some years. A careful history at the time of diagnosis commonly reveals that mild symptoms have been present for several years prior to diagnosis.

2 The *erythraemic phase*, when the classical signs and blood picture develop, shows considerable individual variation in both severity of symptoms and rate of progress. In the majority of untreated cases, symptoms and signs slowly progress, but the course may be punctuated by acute episodes due either to thrombosis or haemorrhage, which can be fatal. In a few cases, the clinical manifestations and haematological picture remain relatively stationary for some years. This second phase lasts from several years to ten years or more.

3 The *spent* or *'burnt-out' phase*, which ultimately occurs in patients who survive the vascular complications of the second stage, is associated with the development of myelofibrosis which not uncommonly is complicated by leukaemia.

Myelofibrosis is a common terminal event, but may develop early in some cases. There is frequently a leuco-erythroblastic anaemia with anisocytosis and poikilocytosis, and a progressive and usually marked enlargement of the spleen. Occasionally, the blood picture is that of pancytopenia (p. 337). The onset is usually relatively slow, the patient having been in remission for some time following the last course of treatment. Marrow aspiration yields a 'dry' or 'blood' tap, and marrow trephine biopsy shows the typical picture of myelofibrosis (p. 338).

Leukaemia is estimated to develop in at least ten

per cent of cases, and is considered to be largely the result of the use of radioactive phosphorus (^{32}P) or alkylating agents. However, it also occurs, uncommonly, in patients treated by phlebotomy alone. It is usually of the acute myeloid variety, although the picture can resemble that of certain of the myelodysplastic disorders.

The major *causes of death* are thrombosis and haemorrhage (especially cerebral thrombosis and haemorrhage, coronary occlusion, and gastrointestinal haemorrhage), congestive cardiac failure, marrow failure, and leukaemia. Occasionally death occurs from some unrelated disorder, e.g. carcinoma. Before the introduction of ^{32}P treatment, the average duration of survival after diagnosis was 5–7 years, the usual causes of death being thrombosis and haemorrhage. With the use of ^{32}P, or busulphan or other alkylating agents, and the consequent reduction of vascular complications, the average period of survival was lengthened to 10–15 years. Studies by the Polycythaemia Vera Study Group suggest that even further improvement may be achieved through the avoidance of both radioactive and alkylating agents (Berk *et al.* 1986, Kaplan *et al.* 1986).

Treatment

It has been pointed out that the majority of symptoms and complications of polycythaemia vera are due to two factors, namely the increased blood volume, and the tendency to thrombosis and haemorrhage, factors which are a direct result of the excess production of red cells and platelets by the hyperplastic marrow. Therefore, *the principle of treatment is reduction in the red cell mass by venesection, followed by suppression of bone marrow cell production.* When suppression of blood cell production has been achieved, symptoms are alleviated and the incidence of vascular complications falls from more than 40 to less than 5 per cent (Wasserman & Gilbert 1966).

Suppression of bone marrow activity can be achieved either by intravenous injections of radioactive phosphorus (^{32}P), or by chemotherapy with myelosuppressive drugs. Venesection to reduce the red cell mass is the most urgent initial treatment in a severely polycythaemic patient, as it can rapidly reduce blood viscosity before a response to any other definitive treatment can be achieved.

PLAN OF THERAPY IN THE INDIVIDUAL PATIENT

When the diagnosis of polycythaemia vera is made, three basic approaches to therapy are available: (a) venesection plus measures to depress marrow activity; (b) therapy to depress bone marrow activity; and (c) venesection alone.

The choice of treatment is based on two main factors: the degree of increase in red cell mass as judged by its effect on the haematocrit, plus the symptoms and signs that it produces; and the degree of thrombocytosis.

When the platelet count is raised and the patient has symptoms, marrow suppressive therapy should be used. When the PCV is increased above 0.55, or if symptoms are troublesome, preliminary venesection should be performed. The majority of patients at the time of diagnosis require repeated venesection followed by marrow suppressive therapy. In the occasional patient with mild erythrocytosis and a normal platelet count, venesection alone may be sufficient for a considerable period of time before active progression of the disease warrants the introduction of myelosuppressive therapy.

The same considerations apply when active progression of the disease resumes after a phase of effective myelosuppression. However, with careful follow-up, the increase in activity is detected early, and sometimes there is only a moderate increase in PCV and no thrombocytosis. In such cases, venesection alone may be sufficient treatment for months or even years.

It is important that myelosuppressive therapy be given as soon as a marked increase in platelet count occurs, as some studies suggest the incidence of thrombotic complications is greater in patients with thrombocytosis (Dawson & Ogston 1970).

CHOICE OF MARROW DEPRESSIVE AGENT

Radioactive phosphorus is the simplest form of myelosuppressive therapy. Its advantages include ease of administration, simple follow-up, and more certain prediction of the effects resulting from a particular dose. The disadvantage is the higher incidence of leukaemia in long-term survivors in comparison with patients who receive no agents with mutagenic potential. It remains the treatment of choice for patients aged over 60 years with a requirement for myelosuppressive treatment.

Chemotherapy. The cytotoxic agents most used have been chlorambucil, busulphan, and hydroxyurea. The initially postulated advantage of chemotherapy over ^{32}P was a possibly lower incidence of leukaemia, but it is now established that chlorambucil therapy is significantly associated with the development of leukaemia (Bert *et al.* 1981). Busulphan therapy is probably associated with an incidence of leukaemia approaching that seen with ^{32}P (Brodsky 1982), and it is too early to be certain whether hydroxyurea is similar in this respect (Donovan *et al.* 1984, Kaplan *et al.* 1986). Chemotherapy has certain disadvantages: the patients must take tablets for weeks or months, and the response to a given dose is less predictable than with ^{32}P. Blood counts must be performed frequently, especially in the initial stages, so that dosage can be adjusted. The dosage of the drugs is usually slightly less than that used for treatment of chronic granulocytic leukaemia (p. 264).

In summary, when myelosuppressive therapy is required, ^{32}P is the agent of choice in patients over the age of 60 years, while chemotherapy should be considered in younger patients. Chemotherapy is indicated in patients who develop resistance to ^{32}P.

RADIOACTIVE PHOSPHORUS

Control of disease activity by ^{32}P was introduced by Lawrence in 1938, and has proved an effective and generally non-toxic method of treatment. Following its administration, radiation of the marrow cells results from the uptake of ^{32}P into the nucleic acids of mitotically active marrow cells, and the incorporation of ^{32}P into bone.

Dose. ^{32}P is administered intravenously in the form of an isotonic solution of sodium phosphate. The initial dose varies from 111 to 185 MBq (3–5 mCi), depending on the severity of the disorder and the size of the patient; the higher the counts and the heavier the patient, the greater the dose required.

Toxic effects. The injection is free from side-effects or radiation sickness. Pancytopenia is a possible complication, but is rare with usual therapeutic doses. Platelet production is most sensitive to ^{32}P, and treatment is occasionally followed by thrombocytopenia. After repeated courses, there is occasionally a gradual, persistent fall in platelets or white cells, in which case further ^{32}P should be withheld and the patient managed by venesection.

Leukaemia. Modan (1971) reviewed the question of leukaemia as a complication of polycythaemia vera, and concluded that acute leukaemia occurring as a terminal event is largely the result of radiation from ^{32}P. The incidence is dose related, i.e. the risk of developing acute leukaemia increases with the total dose of ^{32}P. The incidence of acute leukaemia in patients treated with radiation is up to 10 per cent, contrasted with about one per cent in patients treated by venesection. Reports from the Polycythaemia Vera Study Group confirm these findings (Berk *et al.* 1986). However, it must be emphasized that vascular complications are readily controlled with this treatment, and for older patients the ease of administration and low intensity of post-treatment supervision means that it remains an attractive choice, especially as earlier studies indicate the overall survival in this group is greater with ^{32}P treatment than with venesection alone.

Response and follow-up. Response to therapy is assessed by regular clinical and haematological follow-up examinations. For practical purposes, it is sufficient to perform blood counts, 6, 12, and 16 weeks after the administration of ^{32}P. The rate of response of the three formed elements of the blood depends in part on their lifespan. Fall in the relatively short-lived platelets and white cells occurs well before that of the red cells, with their lifespan of 120 days. Platelet reduction usually occurs at the end of the third week; the count reaches its minimum in 4–6 weeks (usually about $100 \times 10^9/l$), after which a rise occurs to normal values. The white cell count usually falls along with the platelet count, and tends to rise more slowly. Significant fall in the PCV and red cell count is usually obvious by the sixth week, and is maximal in 3–4 months. An earlier fall occurs, of course, if

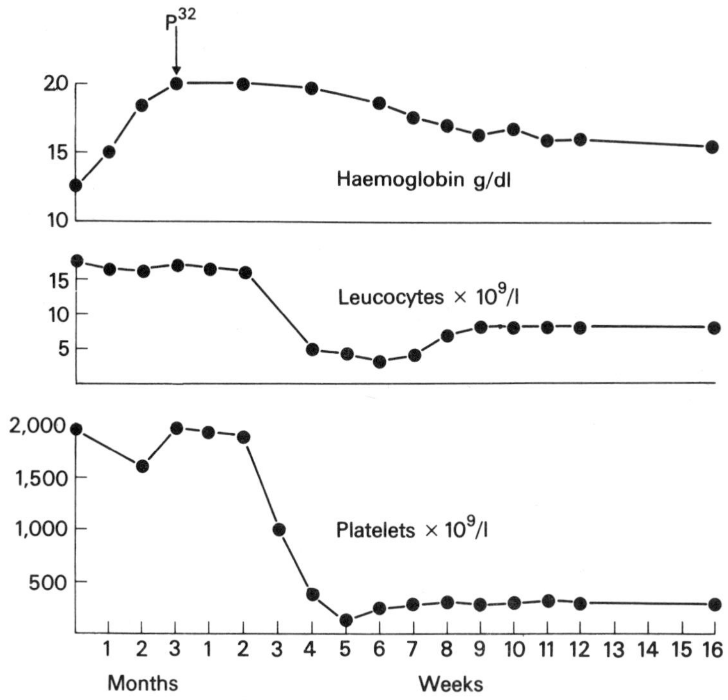

Fig. 12.1. *Polycythaemia vera presenting with anaemia due to occult intestinal bleeding: response to ^{32}P therapy. M.D., a male aged 59 years, presented with priapism, due to thrombosis of the corpora cavernosa. The haemoglobin was 12.3 g/dl, but polycythaemia vera was suspected because of the numerous platelets in the blood film and because the spleen was palpable. Benzidine test for faecal occult blood was positive. Priapism persisted for several weeks. Serial blood examinations over the next three months showed a progressive rise in the haemoglobin to 20 g/dl. ^{32}P (5 millicuries) was administered without preliminary venesection, although venesection should have been performed because of the previous history of thrombosis and the high platelet count. The response of the three cell types is shown. The white cells and platelets started to fall at the end of two weeks; the haemoglobin fall commenced at six weeks, and was maximum after four months. The disease remained under control for 15 months, when a further dose of ^{32}P was necessary. Since then he has had a further seven doses of ^{32}P, and is well and symptom free 16 years after the onset.*

venesection is also used. The response in a typical case is shown in Fig. 12.1.

After 3–4 months, the haematological and clinical responses are assessed. The vast majority of patients have a satisfactory response, with relief of symptoms, reduction in size of the spleen, which may become impalpable, and reversion of the blood picture to normal or near normal. Most symptoms, including headache, fullness in the head, dizziness, weakness, dyspnoea on exertion, and pruritus, are usually relieved. Dyspepsia, when due to peptic ulcer, may persist, and persistent pruritus can be a problem. Hypertension, when present, is usually not eliminated. If a satisfactory remission has not occurred, further treatment is given, and the response followed as before. Patients who have a satisfactory response should be seen at intervals of three months, and assessed for signs of recurrent disease activity. Blood examination should always include a platelet count. Remissions last from six months to more than five years, the average being about 18–24 months. It is quite common for the duration of remission in an individual patient to remain fairly constant after each successive treatment.

A further course of therapy is indicated when there is a rise in platelet count above normal, or a rise in PCV that is not readily controlled by venesection. With an adequate follow-up, relapse is detected early, and the further doses required, especially for the control of thrombocytosis alone, are often relatively small.

Resistance to ^{32}P. In some patients, the response of the red cell count to the usual doses of ^{32}P is unsatisfactory; about 10 per cent show only partial improvement, and five per cent no improvement. In such patients, the larger doses of ^{32}P required to control red cell production predispose to thrombocytopenia, so that it is preferable to control the excess red cell mass by venesection and the thrombocytosis with appropriate doses of ^{32}P. Sometimes, chemotherapy may provide more satisfactory control of the disorder in this setting than ^{32}P.

CHEMOTHERAPY

Cytotoxic agents which have been used in the treatment of polycythaemia vera include *busulphan, chlorambucil, melphalan,* and *hydroxyurea.* A piperazine derivative *pipobroman* has also been successfully employed.

Chlorambucil has now been shown to give rise to a greater incidence of leukaemia than ^{32}P (Berk *et al.* 1981), and hence should not be used. The same is reported to be the case with *melphalan. Busulphan* has a better record in this respect in most published trials (EORTC 1981, Brodsky 1982) but it is too early to be certain of the degree of risk. *Hydroxyurea* has the advantage that it is not an alkylating agent, and preliminary trials show promise (Donovan *et al.* 1984, Kaplan *et al.* 1986). *Pipobroman* is an effective drug, but it is too early to be certain of its oncogenic potential (Najman *et al.* 1982).

Polycythaemia vera is more sensitive to *busulphan* than is chronic myelocytic leukaemia. The usual maximum regular daily dose recommended for the latter disorder is 6 mg (p. 264), and therefore the safest regimens for polycythaemia are those of 4 mg or less per day. Thus a dose of 4 mg/day may be given for a period of 4–12 weeks, depending on the observed response, and after normal blood indices are obtained, the counts are monitored and maintenance therapy should not be given. During treatment, the rate of fall of all three blood cell series should be carefully noted, and Brodsky *et al.* (1968) recommend that busulphan be stopped when the platelet count reaches $300 \times 10^9/l$, as the count may fall considerably after the drug is discontinued. Busulphan has a marked effect on production of platelets and is thus of value in patients with marked thrombocytosis. The marrow suppression produced by *hydroxyurea* is more rapidly reversible than that produced by busulphan, so that hydroxyurea is preferred in patients with normal or low platelet and white cell counts. It is given initially in a dose of 1.5 g daily to an adult of normal size, and the dosage adjusted according to tolerance. As its effects are relatively transient, ongoing therapy is usually required, and prolonged untreated remissions are less common than with busulphan. *Pipobroman* is used in a dose of 50 or 75 mg daily over 5–10 weeks.

VENESECTION

Venesection is the most direct and simple method of treatment. It is especially efficacious in producing rapid relief of symptoms caused by increased blood volume or viscosity. However, it does not reduce the platelet count or have any effect on the underlying disorder, and thus rarely proves adequate as the sole method of treatment throughout the entire course of the disorder. The high incidence of vascular complications in patients treated by this means alone is not reduced by platelet anti-aggregating therapy (Tartaglia *et al.* 1986), but venesection alone is often appropriate treatment for disease that is relatively indolent in activity.

Venesection preliminary to myelosuppressive therapy. The maximum effect of myelosuppressive therapy on the red cell count is not manifested for about three months. Thus, it is advisable in most patients to reduce the total red cell volume by venesection to lessen the possibility of thrombosis, and relieve symptoms over this initial period. Venesection is indicated: (a) when symptoms are distressing. Cerebral symptoms, e.g. headache, dizziness, and fullness in the head, respond particularly well to venesection; (b) in patients with a markedly increased PCV; and (c) in patients with a history of a previous thrombotic episode. In other patients, venesection is optional, although advisable. Venesection of 300–500 ml is carried out either daily or on alternate days, until the PCV is about 0.55; this is usually achieved in 1–2 weeks. In patients with critical ischaemia, it is advisable to replace each unit of blood removed with a high molecular weight dextran preparation to reduce blood viscosity by maintaining the plasma volume. Most patients suffer no ill-effects from rapid venesection, but caution should be exercised with patients in whom cardiovascular symptoms are prominent. Particular caution is necessary in elderly subjects with a previous history of thrombosis, as hypotension which occasionally results from venesection may predispose to thrombosis or ischaemia; these hazards are largely obviated by replacement of blood with a dextran preparation. Following repeated venesections, red cell hypochromia often develops as a result of induction of iron deficiency. *Administration of iron to subjects in whom iron deficiency has contributed to maintaining a low haemoglobin level and PCV can cause an increase in the frequency with which venesections are required to maintain an appropriate PCV.*

SYMPTOMATIC MEASURES

Patients with *hyperuricaemia* may develop gout, renal colic, or even oliguria from urate nephropathy; this is especially so in warmer climates. Thus they should have a high fluid intake with measures to alkalinize the urine, and be given the xanthine oxidase inhibitor allopurinol, in doses of 300 mg daily. After treatment has finished, in patients with hyperuricaemia, allopurinol should be given in a continuous daily dose of 100 or 200 mg. Some authorities recommend its use in all patients with polycythaemia, on the grounds that it may prevent the development of gout or renal calculi. *Pruritus*, which is thought to be due to histamine release, may be controlled by antihistamines, particularly cyproheptidine (Gilbert *et al.* 1966).

Both haemorrhage and thrombosis occur frequently following surgery. Haemorrhage may be persistent, difficult to control, and is sometimes fatal; extensive wound haematomas are common. Wasserman & Gilbert (1966), in their review of surgical bleeding, found the incidence of these complications to be 46 per cent. Comparison of cases controlled by treatment before surgery with uncontrolled cases revealed a three-fold reduction in morbidity, and a seven-fold reduction in mortality in the treated group. Furthermore, they found that patients with a long period of control (four months or more) prior to surgery had a markedly decreased incidence of complications in comparison with patients treated for a shorter period. Thus *elective surgery should be approached with extreme caution*, and *if possible* the patient should be brought under full haematological control for several months before surgery. For emergency surgery, repeated venesections should be performed to bring the red cell volume to normal or near normal, with partial replacement by plasma if necessary to prevent circulatory collapse. At operation, special attention should be paid to local haemostasis. When haemorrhage does occur, platelet transfusion may be necessary if bleeding is judged to be due to platelet dysfunction.

Familial polycythaemia (familial erythrocytosis)

Polycythaemia has been reported rarely as a familial condition; there is evidence to suggest transmission as a Mendelian dominant trait, but recessive inheritance has also been described (Adamson *et al.* 1973). The condition presents at a younger age than classical polycythaemia vera, often in childhood. There may be few, if any, symptoms, and leucocytosis and thrombocytosis are absent. The prognosis appears to be relatively good, and for this reason the condition is sometimes called 'benign familial erythrocytosis'. Some of these families have been identified as possessing a high oxygen affinity haemoglobin; in others, a low erythrocyte 2, 3-DPG has been found; and in a third variety with recessive inheritance, inappropriately increased erythropoietin secretion has been identified (Adamson *et al.* 1973). In others, no definite mechanism has been established.

Relative polycythaemia

In relative polycythaemia, the total number of red cells in the body is not increased. The raised red cell count in the peripheral blood is due to contraction of the plasma volume, while the total red cell volume is normal. The diminished plasma volume may result from marked loss of body fluids, e.g. severe burns, dehydration, marked vomiting, persistent diarrhoea, diuretic therapy, and paralytic ileus. It can be due to reduced fluid intake or redistribution of body fluids, which can occur in crush injuries when the plasma passes into damaged tissues, as well as in other situations. Relative polycythaemia due to acute bodily disturbance seldom presents any difficulty in diagnosis, as the cause of the haemoconcentration is usually obvious.

A further important category of relative polycythaemia is now described under the heading of pseudopolycythaemia.

Pseudopolycythaemia

Polycythaemia of 'stress' and *spurious polycythaemia* are synonyms for pseudopolycythaemia, which is a relative polycythaemia of unknown aetiology, first described by Lawrence & Berlin (1952). They called it 'polycythaemia of stress' because about one-half of their patients had an anxiety state or were mildly neurotic, and it was thought that the condition might be related to nervous stress. However, this condition is now known to be of mixed origin, partly relative polycythaemia, and partly mild secondary erythrocytosis in heavy smokers due to inhalation of carbon monoxide (Sagone *et al.* 1973).

Clinical features. Pseudopolycythaemia occurs much more commonly in males than in females, and although it may occur at any age in adult life, it is most frequently seen in middle-aged persons. There is no typical history. Symptoms of an anxiety state, e.g. fatigue, irritability, headache, and nervousness, are common, and some patients complain of dizziness. Hypertension or obesity is present in about 50 per cent of cases. The facial complexion is florid, often being indistinguishable from that of polycythaemia vera, and dilatation of the superficial vessels about the cheeks and nose is frequently present. The liver and spleen are not palpable.

Blood picture. Red cell values are usually at about the upper limit of normal, or are slightly increased. Thus red cell counts of $6.5–7 \times 10^{12}/l$, haemoglobin levels of 18–20 g/dl, and a PCV of 0.54–0.60 are usual, although both lower or higher values occur. The white cell and platelet counts are normal, as is the neutrophil alkaline phosphatase. The arterial oxygen saturation is normal. The aspirated bone marrow is of normal cellularity.

The total red cell volume is normal. The increase in concentration of red cells is due to an abnormally low plasma volume, of unknown cause.

Diagnosis. The condition is of importance because it may be confused with polycythaemia vera and wrongly treated with myelosuppressive therapy. The main points of differentiation from polycythaemia vera are set out in Table 12.4. It is probable that many cases of Gaisboeck's syndrome are actually examples of pseudopolycythaemia.

Essential thrombocythaemia

Overproduction of platelets is the predominant feature in this myeloproliferative disorder. Defects of platelet function are common, and both thrombosis and haemorrhage can occur (Schafer 1984). Principles of treatment in general resemble those for treatment of polycythaemia vera, although in asymptomatic cases there is usually considerably less emphasis on the extent to which measures should be taken to suppress platelet production (p. 400).

Myelofibrosis

The term myelofibrosis is used to describe fibrosis and collagen formation in the marrow. The terms myelofibrosis and myelosclerosis have both been used to describe cases with collagen deposition and new bone formation, but the term myelofibrosis is now preferred. Myelofibrosis may be classified as primary or secondary.

Primary myelofibrosis. Myelofibrosis developing in polycythaemia vera (p. 328) may be considered as a variant of this disorder. It is probable that in about 25 per cent of cases of primary myelofibrosis there is a preceding history of polycythaemia vera.

Secondary myelofibrosis develops in association with some well-defined disorder of the marrow, or as a result of the toxic action of chemical agents or irradiation. Thus, fibrosis may develop in association with tuberculosis, secondary carcinoma, Hodgkin's disease, leukaemia, and a variety of other haematological disorders.

Primary myelofibrosis is usually accompanied by *myeloid metaplasia* (extramedullary haemopoiesis) in the spleen and liver, and to a much lesser extent in the kidney, lymph nodes, and other organs. The myeloid metaplasia involves the white and red cell precursors and megakaryocytes. In primary myelofibrosis, myeloid metaplasia is consistently found, but in the secondary form it is much less common. Occasionally, myeloid metaplasia is found at post mortem as tumour masses in various organs.

Primary myelofibrosis

Myelosclerosis and agnogenic myeloid metaplasia are synonyms for primary myelofibrosis, which is a proliferative neoplastic disorder related to polycythaemia vera and essential thrombocythaemia. The term *myeloproliferative disorder* is sometimes applied to this group as a whole. Intermediate or transitional forms of these disorders, showing overlapping clinical and pathological features, are seen. Thus, myelofibrosis commonly develops in the terminal phase of polycythaemia vera (p. 328). The blood picture of acute myeloid leukaemia not uncommonly develops in the terminal stages of myelofibrosis. Thrombocythaemia may precede the onset of myelofibrosis, and may become extreme if the spleen is removed. Because of the occurrence of intermediate and transitional forms, the exact classification of the type of myeloproliferative disorder in the individual patient is sometimes difficult.

The myeloproliferative disorders are due to uncontrolled proliferation of abnormal progenitor cells which are capable of producing erythroid, myeloid, and megakaryocytic series. The particular type of disorder is determined by the predominant series into which the cell differentiates, and the extent to which haemopoiesis is 'effective' or 'ineffective'. In polycythaemia vera, the proliferation predominantly involves erythropoiesis and is 'effective', giving rise to increased red cell production and high red cell counts. Similarly, where megakaryocyte proliferation is predominantly involved and thrombopoiesis is 'effective', essential thrombocythaemia results. Some cases with 'panmyelosis' have high blood counts of all three cell forms, as seen in florid polycythaemia vera. As the diseases evolves, haemopoiesis frequently becomes

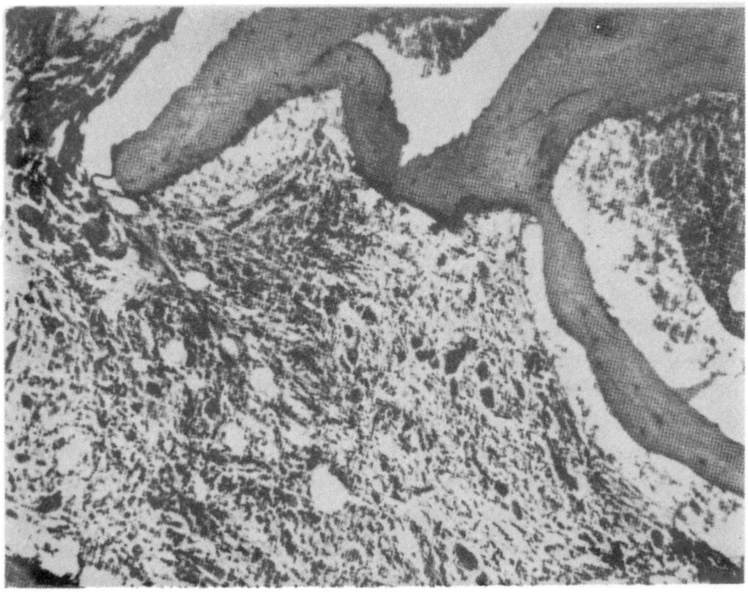

Fig. 12.2. *Bone marrow in myelofibrosis. Section of trephine biopsy of the iliac crest showing replacement of haemopoietic tissue by fibrous tissue, and increased megakaryocytes. Marrow aspiration resulted in a 'dry' tap. From a male, aged 73 years, whose peripheral blood film showed thrombocytopenia, plus anisocytosis with quite marked macrocytosis and poikilocytosis of the red cells.*

'ineffective', and blood cell counts fall. Products of the cells are released in the marrow, including the platelet-derived cell growth factor from megakaryocytes (Castro-Malaspina *et al.* 1981), and stimulate deposition of reticulin and fibrous tissue (McCarthy 1985). Products from other cells may also play a part. This view is supported by evidence that fibroblasts in myelofibrosis are not derived from the same clone as the abnormal haemopoietic cells (Jacobson *et al.* 1978), but are reactive normal cells. Megakaryocytic hyperplasia is often prominent in the marrow in myelofibrosis, even though platelet production may be ineffective (Fig. 12.2).

In the past, the myeloid metaplasia in the spleen, liver, and other organs in myelofibrosis was thought to be a compensatory process to make up for the loss of normal blood-forming marrow. However, it is now considered to represent another manifestation of tissue infiltration by the primary disorder. Support for this theory is derived from the fact that in polycythaemia vera, the histology of the liver and spleen shows that myeloid metaplasia occurs while the bone marrow is still hyperplastic and the blood polycythaemic before the onset of myelofibrosis. Deposition of reticulin and collagen also commences in the marrow at this stage of the disease (Ellis *et al.* 1986).

Clinical features

Myelofibrosis is a disease of adult life, occurring most commonly between the ages of 40 and 70 years; rarely, it occurs in young adults, and even children. It appears to occur equally in both sexes.

The onset is insidious, the condition usually being present for some time before the diagnosis is obvious. The patient most frequently presents with symptoms of anaemia, especially weakness, or with symptoms due to splenomegaly. The accidental finding of an enlarged spleen, either by the patient or doctor, is sometimes the first indication of the disease. Occasionally, weight loss, anorexia, bleeding manifestations, acute abdominal pain, gout, bone pain, leg cramps, or jaundice are presenting manifestations. The development of myelofibrosis in patients with polycythaemia vera is accompanied by a fall in the haemoglobin level, together with relatively rapid enlargement of the spleen.

The symptoms of the *anaemia* are those common to all anaemias, namely weakness, lassitude, fatigue, dyspnoea on exertion, and palpitation. With severe anaemia, signs of congestive cardiac failure may develop.

Splenomegaly is the outstanding physical sign; the spleen usually extends below the umbilicus, and in the later stages may be grossly enlarged, extending into the left iliac fossa, and sometimes appearing to fill the whole abdomen. Slow progressive enlargement of the spleen over many years can often be observed, although in acute myelofibrosis the spleen may not be greatly enlarged (p. 342). Symptoms due to splenomegaly are common, e.g. abdominal fullness, or a dragging, aching sensation, or pain in the left hypochondrium. When the spleen is very large, epigastric discomfort after meals, flatulence, dyspepsia, nausea, and frequency of micturition may occur. Splenic infarction is common, causing acute pain and sometimes a splenic friction rub.

Hepatomegaly is common. Enlargement is usually slight to moderate, although occasionally the liver extends below the umbilicus. The liver is firm, smooth, and non-tender. Following splenectomy, the liver may rapidly increase in size due to an increase in myeloid metaplasia. Mild *jaundice* is common, especially in the later stages, and is mostly unconjugated bilirubin produced by ineffective erythropoiesis. *Portal hypertension* with associated features such as oesophageal varices occurs in up to about one-quarter of cases of myelofibrosis.

Lymph node enlargement is unusual in the typical disorder, and when present is only slight.

Constitutional symptoms. Weight loss, wasting, weakness, and lassitude out of proportion to the degree of anaemia commonly develop in the later stages of the disease, and are sometimes present early. Less commonly, night sweats occur, and pruritus is occasionally present, especially in cases evolving from polycythaemia vera.

Bleeding manifestations are common, especially in the later stages. Bleeding is usually due to thrombocytopenia, purpura and epistaxis being particularly prominent. However, bleeding, especially from the gastrointestinal tract may occur in patients with normal platelet counts. The gastrointestinal bleeding is sometimes due to *peptic ulceration* which is more common than in the general population, and sometimes from oesophageal varices.

The serum uric acid is commonly raised, and *gout* occurs; it may be exacerbated by splenic irradiation or myelosuppressive therapy. Vague *bone pains,* particularly in the legs, are not uncommon, and occasionally *bone tenderness,* especially of the sternum, is present. However, in general, the presence of marked bone pain or tenderness in a patient with leuco-erythroblastic anaemia suggests a cause other than myelosclerosis, such as secondary carcinoma in bone or acute leukaemia.

Radiological bone changes occur in about 30 per cent of cases, and are seen especially in the later stages. The changes are usually not marked, and are best demonstrated by comparison with X-rays of normal persons of similar age. The typical picture is one of patchy sclerosis of the medullary cavity, often with coarsening of trabeculation and rarefaction, sometimes giving a mottled appearance. The bones most commonly involved are the pelvis, spine, and upper ends of the femora and humeri.

Blood picture

The *typical blood picture* is that of a *leuco-erythroblastic anaemia with marked anisocytosis* and *poikilocytosis*. The white cell and platelet counts vary; they may be normal, raised, or reduced. Thus, occasionally, the blood picture is of pancytopenia.

Anaemia is almost invariable at some stage in the course of the disorder, but its severity and rate of progress vary considerably. In many cases, it is of slight to moderate degree at the time of diagnosis, and remains relatively constant over a number of years. However, in the later stages of the disorder anaemia usually becomes more severe. Sometimes the haemoglobin level is within normal range at the time of diagnosis, particularly when the disorder has evolved from polycythaemia vera. Three main factors contribute to the anaemia, namely impairment of red cell production, pooling of red cells in the spleen, and haemolysis. Defective erythropoiesis is usually the major factor, but increased plasma volume associated with the splenomegaly (p. 348) may also contribute to the anaemia.

The red cells are usually normocytic and normochromic, but anisocytosis is often marked. Iron deficiency may develop, in which case microcytosis and hypochromia are found. If macrocytosis is present, it may indicate complicating folate deficiency. Moderate to marked poikilocytosis is usual, pear- or tear-shaped poikilocytes being especially characteristic of the disease; oval or elliptical cells

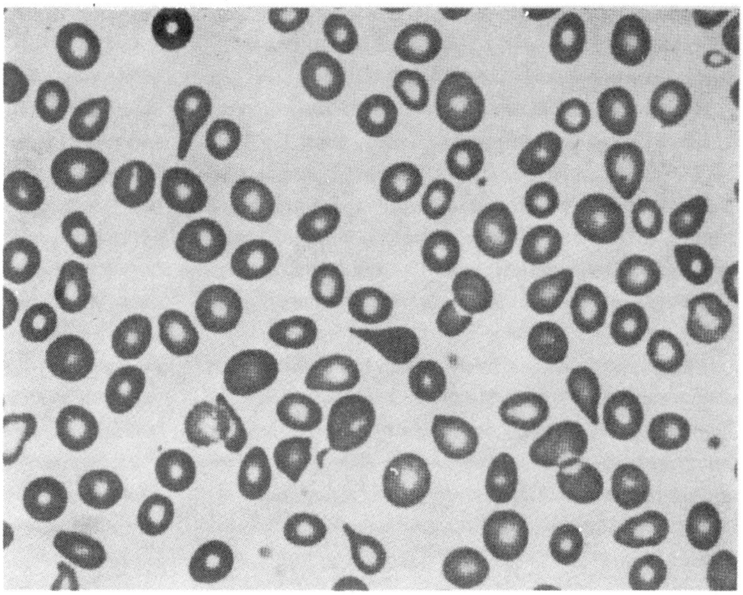

Fig. 12.3. *Myelofibrosis. Blood film. Photomicrograph showing marked anisocytosis and poikilocytosis, with tear-shaped poikilocytes (× 710). From a male, aged 60 years, in whom myelofibrosis developed 10 years after the diagnosis of polycythaemia vera.*

are also common (Fig. 12.3). Polychromasia and basophilia are often prominent, and the reticulocyte count may be moderately raised. Some fragmented and spherocytic cells may be present, especially in the later stages. Nucleated red cells are almost invariably present, usually in small, but sometimes in large, numbers, when they constitute a striking feature of the blood film; they are orthochromatic or late polychromatic, although earlier forms are sometimes seen. Commonly there are up to 10 normoblasts per 100 white cells, but occasionally they form a higher percentage, especially when the total white cell count is low. The number of normoblasts does not parallel the degree of anaemia, and they may be numerous even when anaemia is slight.

The total *white cell count* is usually normal or moderately raised, but it is sometimes reduced. When raised, the count is usually not more than $50 \times 10^9/l$, but occasionally it is higher, and rarely it exceeds $100 \times 10^9/l$, mostly after splenectomy. When reduced, counts range from about 2 to $4 \times 10^9/l$. Myelocytes and metamyelocytes are usually present, but are rarely very numerous, and together commonly comprise 10–20 per cent of the total white cells, although higher proportions may occur. A small number of promyelocytes and myeloblasts may also be seen. There is sometimes a slight increase in the proportion of eosinophils and basophils. The alkaline phosphatase content of the granulocytes is usually increased, but may be normal or rarely decreased.

The *platelet count* is usually normal or reduced, but may be raised, sometimes to more than $1000 \times 10^9/l$. Thrombocytopenia most commonly occurs in the later stages, when it may be severe. Large and abnormal platelets may be seen, and megakaryocytic fragments are sometimes present. A number of abnormalities of platelet function occur (Schafer 1984).

A moderate increase in the sedimentation rate is common. A moderate rise in serum bilirubin, e.g. 30–50 mmol/l, is not uncommon; this is mostly unconjugated. The serum lactate dehydrogenase and lysozyme levels are elevated, reflecting the increased but ineffective haemopoiesis that is taking place.

Serum folate values are commonly reduced because of the increase in folate requirements produced by the utilization of folate by the abnormal tissue. Often, red cell folate values are reduced; in one series, megaloblastic haemopoiesis due to folate deficiency occurred at some time during the course of the disease in one-third of patients with myelofibrosis (Hoffbrand *et al.* 1966). This point is of therapeutic importance in the management of anaemia in this condition (p. 341). Folate deficiency sometimes becomes obvious after an infection. The serum vitamin B_{12} is normal or elevated.

Bone marrow

The essential pathological feature is proliferation of fibroblasts, resulting in a diffuse increase of reticulin fibres and deposition of collagen in the marrow, often with thickening of the bony trabeculae which encroach on the marrow cavity. The degree of fibrosis varies from patient to patient, and often in the same patient at different sites. The increase in reticulin fibres is shown by the reticulin stain (Fig. 12.4), and in the early stages this may be the only significant evidence of fibrosis, with little or no collagen formation. Areas of active haemopoietic tissue are found scattered in the fibrotic tissue. Megakaryocytes are often present in markedly increased numbers; however, there is no correlation between their number and the peripheral platelet count.

Marrow *aspiration* is typically unsatisfactory, usually resulting in a 'dry' tap. Less commonly, aspiration yields a small amount of blood with a few marrow cells, a number of which are megakaryocytes or megakaryocytic nuclei. A gritty sensation is sometimes felt when the needle enters the marrow cavity. Occasionally, the needle enters one of the areas of active marrow interspersed in the fibrotic tissue, and marrow fragments of either normal or increased cellularity are aspirated.

Marrow *trephine biopsy*, preferably of the iliac crest, usually yields a satisfactory sample containing the characteristic histological features (Figs 12.2 & 12.4), which establish the diagnosis. The histological findings on biopsy are well described by Wolf & Neiman (1985), who emphasize the variability of

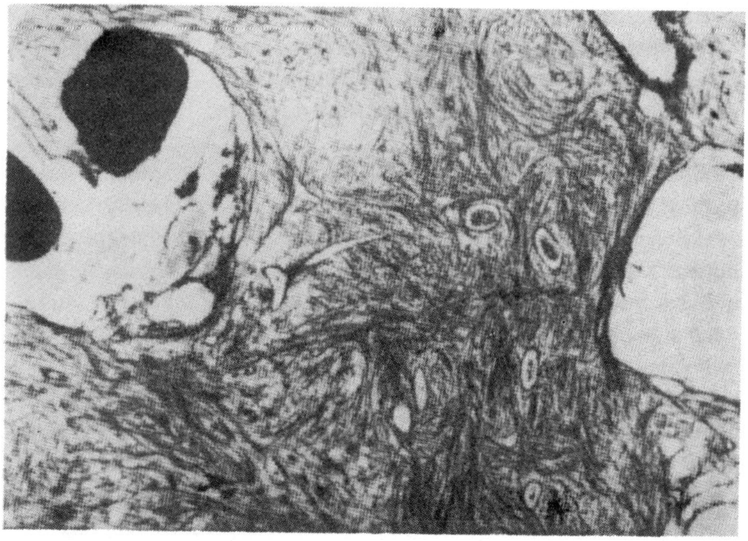

Fig. 12.4. *Myelofibrosis. Reticulin stain of bone marrow.*

the degree of fibrosis and the extent of splenomegaly. An increase in reticulin fibres alone is not in itself diagnostic of primary myelofibrosis, as this may occur in other marrow disorders such as chronic granulocytic leukaemia and other neoplastic diseases.

Diagnosis

The diagnosis is suggested by the occurrence of *marked splenomegaly with leuco-erythroblastic anaemia*, often with relatively little deterioration in general health, in a middle-aged or elderly person. Sometimes, the spleen is known to have been enlarged for a number of years. Cases evolving from polycythaemia vera often have a previous history of symptoms suggesting antecedent polycythaemia, e.g. a plethoric appearance, bloodshot eyes, or pruritus. Failure of marrow aspiration at more than one site further suggests, but does not confirm, the diagnosis. Marrow trephine biopsy is necessary for diagnosis.

Diagnostic difficulty may occur when, on marrow aspiration or trephine, the needle enters one of the areas of active marrow interspersed in the fibrotic tissue, and marrow of either normal or increased cellularity is obtained. In such cases, marrow examination at another site usually reveals the typical findings.

Myelofibrosis associated with tuberculosis. Rare cases of myelofibrosis have been described in association with, and thought to be due to, disseminated tuberculosis. Although the peripheral blood picture may resemble that of myelofibrosis, the clinical picture shows certain general differences—it can occur in younger patients; fever, malaise, and other manifestations of tuberculous toxaemia are present; splenomegaly is less marked; moderate generalized lymph node enlargement is usual; and the course is shorter. The diagnosis is established with certainty only if the marrow biopsy specimen includes a tuberculous focus. The subject is reviewed by Andre *et al.* (1961).

Differential diagnosis

Other causes of splenomegaly (p. 351). The major problem in the diagnosis of primary myelofibrosis is differentiation from *chronic granulocytic leukaemia*, with which it is commonly confused, as patients with both conditions can possess marked splenomegaly and immature granulocytes in the peripheral blood. Fibrosis can occur in the marrow in chronic granulocytic leukaemia, and the main differential points are listed in Table 10.8, p. 263.

Disorders with a similar blood picture. In most cases, careful consideration of the clinical and haematological features and special investigations will distinguish these disorders:

1 *Other causes of leuco-erythroblastic anaemia* (p. 274).

2 *Macrocytic anaemias.* When macrocytosis is prominent, the association of macrocytosis with marked anisocytosis and poikilocytosis, especially when the white count is low, may suggest megaloblastic anaemia. In most cases, the spleen is much larger and firmer than ever occurs in pernicious anaemia or other megaloblastic anaemias; further, the presence of more than occasional myelocytes suggests myelofibrosis.

3 *Haemolytic anaemias.* The occurrence of polychromasia, reticulocytosis, normoblastaemia, and splenomegaly, especially when jaundice is present, may suggest a diagnosis of haemolytic anaemia. In haemolytic anaemia, however, the evidence of dyshaemopoiesis, namely anisocytosis and poikilocytosis, is seldom so great.

Other causes of bone marrow fibrosis. It has been pointed out that bone marrow involvement occurring in certain disorders may be accompanied by fibrosis. These include *secondary carcinoma,* tuberculosis, *malignant lymphomas,* and *leukaemia.* Usually, diagnosis of these disorders is obvious from the clinical features and special investigations, and the marrow fibrosis is simply an incidental finding. In particular, the rate of development of anaemia is usually more rapid in these disorders than in myelofibrosis. As marrow aspiration may result in a 'dry' tap under a variety of circumstances, trephine biopsy is essential. The demonstration of fibrosis does not, on its own, make the diagnosis, and if the other expected clinical and haematological features are not present, other causes of marrow fibrosis must be carefully considered.

Course and prognosis

The course of primary myelofibrosis is usually chronic, but is occasionally relatively rapid. The average duration of life is 5–7 years from diagnosis, but individual survival times vary from 1 to more than 20 years. Survival for 10 years or longer is not uncommon. The anaemia is often only slight to moderate and remains relatively constant for a number of years, with the result that there is little interference with general health even though splenic enlargement may be considerable. Eventually, anaemia becomes severe enough to require transfusion. After repeated transfusions, the increase in haemoglobin level becomes less and is of shorter duration, until it is often impossible to control the anaemia by transfusion. In other cases, the anaemia initially is more severe and progresses more rapidly, with the result that the disorder can be fatal within one year of diagnosis. Unfavourable prognostic signs are severe anaemia responding poorly to transfusion, severe leucopenia, spontaneous bleeding, especially when due to thrombocytopenia, and marked weight loss. Ineffective haemopoiesis may be associated with severe hyperuricaemia, which may prove difficult to control. Death commonly occurs from anaemia, cardiac failure, bleeding, or intercurrent infection. About one-quarter of cases terminate as acute myeloid leukaemia.

Treatment

There is no specific therapy, treatment being primarily symptomatic. However, many patients initially have only mild symptoms and require little or no treatment for years following diagnosis. Anaemia and the discomfort due to splenomegaly are the main symptoms requiring treatment, but treatment of haemorrhage may be necessary. Folic acid, androgens and, in the later stages, blood transfusion are the main forms of treatment for *anaemia.* Iron deficiency should be watched for and treated when present.

Discomfort due to splenic enlargement can sometimes be lessened by the wearing of a supportive abdominal belt. Busulphan may be helpful in reducing splenomegaly, and is particularly useful when the granulocyte count is high. In selected cases, splenic irradiation gives temporary relief, but the reduction in spleen size with radiation in this disease is less than in chronic granulocytic anaemia.

When *haemorrhage* is due to thrombocytopenia,

splenectomy may be considered as an approach to elevating the platelet count. However, in general, severe thrombocytopenic bleeding is difficult to control and carries a poor prognosis. When gastrointestinal bleeding occurs in patients with peptic ulceration and a high platelet count, reduction of the count to normal by the use of busulphan may lessen the liability to bleed (Brody *et al.* 1963). In some patients, on the other hand, a high platelet count may persist for many years without complications (Schafer 1984).

Hyperuricaemia, with its sequelae of gout, nephrolithiasis, and urate nephropathy, usually responds to allopurinol, which is especially important in preventing a further rise in the serum uric acid following treatment with busulphan or splenic irradiation.

Folic acid. Because of the relatively high incidence of folate deficiency in this disorder, folate deficiency must be excluded as a contributing factor in the development of anaemia or thrombocytopenia. Folate deficiency should be especially suspected when there is rapidly developing anaemia associated with thrombocytopenia. Before any other treatment is given, a serum folate (and red cell folate) estimation should be performed. If values are low, a therapeutic trial of folic acid should be given, and this sometimes eliminates the need for transfusion.

Androgens. Administration of androgens such as oxymetholone should be considered for patients with symptoms of anaemia, as a significant minority undergo a degree of improvement. Doses of 100–200 mg daily are usually employed, and responses tend to be delayed for at least six weeks; if no response occurs after 12–16 weeks, treatment should be ceased, as it is unlikely to be beneficial. When response does occur, continued administration is usually necessary to maintain the increased haemoglobin level, but sometimes improvement is sustained after cessation of treatment. Less than one-half of patients obtain some benefit, and those with chromosomal abnormalities are reported to be less likely to respond (Besa *et al.* 1982).

Gardner & Pringle (1961) recommended an initial trial of testosterone enanthate, 600 mg *im* weekly for six weeks; this can then be slowly reduced to a dose necessary to maintain a satisfactory haemoglobin level. This approach remains useful for male patients who do not bruise. Oxymetholone, the anabolic agent most widely used for treatment of aplastic anaemia (p. 132), is now probably the agent of choice.

Blood transfusion. In patients with slight anaemia, transfusion may not be required for many years. When anaemia is sufficiently marked to require transfusion, transfusions should be kept to the minimum necessary to maintain the haemoglobin at a level consistent with a comfortable active life; this is usually about 9 g/dl. Even with the initial transfusion, the rise in haemoglobin is often less than expected for the amount of blood given, but nevertheless a significant rise, followed by a slow fall over a period of weeks or months, is usual. With repeated transfusions, the rise in haemoglobin usually becomes less and of shorter duration, until ultimately a point is reached when even large transfusions may give a response lasting only a week or two, or even less. The cause for this progressive ineffectiveness of transfusion is variable. In some cases, the development of immune isoantibodies plays a part, but in many cases sequestration of the transfused cells in the spleen is the major problem. When transfusion is no longer able adequately to control the anaemia, the administration of corticosteroids should be tried, and if this does not result in a significant lessening of transfusion requirements, splenectomy should be considered. The usual precautions essential in the transfusion of patients with chronic anaemia must be carefully observed (p. 480).

Busulphan, hydroxyurea, or other myelosuppressive therapy can be considered in patients with high leucocyte or platelet counts, relatively cellular marrow, and a large spleen when there are overt problems related to progressive disease. The dosages used are as for the treatment of polycythaemia vera (p. 330), and the response must be carefully monitored and the drug withdrawn if leucopenia is produced.

Corticosteroids in general have little to offer, but in patients with increasing transfusion requirements in whom it is difficult to maintain the haemoglobin level, corticosteroid treatment may be tried. Prednisolone is given initially in doses of 25–75 mg daily for 2–3 weeks, followed by progressive dose reduction, and sometimes results in a lessening of transfusion requirements, together with some increase in haemoglobin level and slight reduction in splenic size. However, in general, the response is disappointing, and, if ineffective, treatment should be ceased.

Splenectomy. In most cases, splenectomy has nothing to offer and is associated with perioperative morbidity and mortality. However, in selected cases, especially in the latter stages of the disease, it may be beneficial. It should be considered: (a) when transfusion requirements have increased to such a degree that it is difficult or impossible to maintain the haemoglobin at a comfortable level. In such cases, splenectomy sometimes lessens transfusion requirements; (b) when thrombocytopenia is sufficiently severe to cause troublesome bleeding, as splenectomy is often followed by a rise in platelet count; and (c) when the spleen, because of its massive size, causes pressure symptoms.

However, splenectomy has several disadvantages; it has a relatively high operative mortality and morbidity, because of the bleeding tendency and, in the later stages, the poor general condition of the patient. In addition, marked elevation of the platelet count sometimes follows splenectomy, particularly in patients with normal or raised presplenectomy counts. This predisposes to thrombosis. If significant thrombocytosis persists after splenectomy, alkylating agents or hydroxyurea should be used to reduce the platelet count. In some patients, marked enlargement of the liver occurs rapidly after splenectomy, causing abdominal discomfort and, sometimes, recurrence of anaemia or thrombocytopenia.

Thus the possible benefit of splenectomy must be carefully weighed against the risks. However, it is important that splenectomy, if indicated, should not be left too late, as seriously ill patients often do not survive the operation.

Splenic irradiation does not favourably affect the course of the disease, and in most cases is not used. However, it may be of value in patients with severe pressure symptoms associated with marked splenomegaly. In such cases, irradiation may be followed by reduction in splenic size, with relief of pressure symptoms and of constitutional symptoms, especially when the leucocyte count is raised. The total white count falls, as does the number of immature white and red cells. The dose of X-ray should be the minimum necessary to relieve the symptoms. The complications of hyperuricaemia may occur, and thus allopurinol should be given. The first course is the most effective. Irradiation is relatively dangerous in patients with low white counts. Szur (1972) summarizes the essential aspects of splenic irradiation, and points out that only the lower half of the spleen needs to be irradiated. The benefit is often short lived, a return to previous splenic size within several months being common.

Acute myelofibrosis

A variant of myelofibrosis has been recognized which runs an acute course and which has clinical and haematological features sufficiently distinctive to require separate classification. It occurs most commonly in middle-aged and elderly subjects. It differs in that splenomegaly is often absent or of relatively minor degree.

The blood picture typically is of pancytopenia, often with profound neutropenia and the presence of blast cells and myelocytes. Nucleated red cells may or may not be present. Marrow trephine usually reveals a cellular marrow with an increase in reticulin, often without a marked increase in collagen. These cases represent malignant proliferation of megakaryoblast series and overlap into frank megakaryoblastic (M7) leukaemia (Bennett *et al.* 1985).

Intensive remission–induction therapy, as for acute leukaemia, can be considered (p. 255), but results are generally disappointing, and occasional beneficial responses have been obtained with low-dosage cytarabine. There is a significant pyrexia without demonstrable infection in some cases, and the condition must be distinguished from poorly differentiated non-Hodgkin's lymphoma with bone marrow involvement, which may produce a similar clinical picture (p. 282).

References and further reading

Polycythaemia

Adamson, J.W. (1968) The erythropoietin/hematocrit relationship in normal and polycythemic man: implications of marrow regulation. *Blood*, **32**, 597.

Adamson, J.W. (1975) Familial polycythemia. *Semin. Hematol.* **12**, 383.

Adamson, J.W. Fialkow, P.J., Murphy, S. *et al.* (1976) Polycythemia vera: stem-cell and probable clonal origin of the disease. *New Engl. J. Med.* **295**: 913.

Adamson, J.W. & Finch, C.A. (1968) Erythropoietin and the polycythemias. *Ann. N.Y. Acad. Sci.* **149**, 560.

Adamson, J.W., Stamatogannopoulos, G. & Koutras, S. (1973) Recessive familial erythrocytosis: aspects of marrow regulation in two families. *Blood*, **41**, 641.

Balcerzac, S.I. & Bromberg, P.I. (1975) Secondary polycythemia. *Semin. Hematol.* **12**, 353.

Berk, P.D., Goldberg, J.D., Donovan, P.B. *et al.* (1986) Therapeutic recommendations in polycythemia vera based on polycythemia vera study group protocols. *Semin. Hematol.* **23**, 132.

Berk, P.B., Goldberg, J.D., Silverstein, M.N. *et al.* (1981) Increased incidence of acute leukemia in polycythemia vera associated with chlorambucil therapy. *New Engl. J. Med.* **304**, 441.

Berlin, N.I. (1975) Diagnosis and classification of the polycythemias. *Semin. Hematol.* **12**, 339.

Berlin, N.I. Jaffe, E.R. & Miescher, P.A. (1976) *Polycythemia*, Grune & Stratton, New York.

Binder, R. & Gilbert, H. (1970) Muramidase in polycythemia. *Blood*, **36**, 228.

Brodsky, I., Kahn, S.B. & Brady, L.W. (1968) Polycythaemia vera: differential diagnosis by ferrokinetic studies and treatment with busulphan (myleran). *Brit. J. Haemat.* **14**, 351.

Brodsky, I. (1982) Busulphan treatment of polycythemia vera. *Brit. J. Haemat.* **52**, 1.

Brownstein, M.H. & Ballard, H.S. (1966) Hepatoma associated with erythrocytosis: report of 11 new cases. *Am. J. Med.* **40**, 204.

Castle, W.B. & Jandl, J.H. (1966) Blood viscosity and blood volume: opposing influences on oxygen transport in polycythaemia. *Semin. Haemat.* **3**, 193.

Dacie, J.V. & Lewis, S.M. (1984) *Practical Haematology*, 6th Ed., Churchill Livingstone, London.

Damon, A., Holub, D.A., Melicow, M.M. *et al.* (1958) Polycythemia and renal carcinoma. *Am. J. Med.* **25**, 182.

Dawson, A.A. & Ogston, D. (1970) The influence of the platelet count on the incidence of thrombotic and haemorrhagic complications in polycythaemia vera. *Postgrad. Med. J.* **46**, 76.

Donovan, P.B., Kaplan, M.E., Goldberg, J.D. *et al.* (1984) Treatment of polycythemia vera with hydroxyurea. *Am. J. Hematol.* **17**, 329.

EORTC (1981) Treatment of polycythaemia vera by radiophosphorus or busulphan: a randomized trial. *Brit. J. Cancer*, **44**, 75.

Ellis, J.T., Peterson, P., Geller, S.A. *et al.* (1986) Studies of the bone marrow in polycythemia vera and the evolution of myelofibrosis and second haematologic malignancies. *Semin. Hematol.* **23**, 144.

Epstein, S. (1964) Primary carcinoma of the liver. *Am. J. Med. Sci.* **247**, 137.

Fialkow, P.J. (1980) Clonal and stem cell origin of blood cell neoplasms. *Contemp. Hematol. Oncol.* **1**, 1.

Gilbert, H.S., Warner, R.R.P. & Wasserman, L.R. (1966) A study of histamine in myeloproliferative disease. *Blood*, **28**, 795.

Hall, C.A. (1964) Gaisbock's Disease: Redefinition of an old syndrome. *Arch. Int. Med.* **116**, 4.

Hammond, D.D. & Winnick, S. (1974) Paraneoplastic erythrocytosis and ectopic erythropoietins. *Ann. N.Y. Acad. Sci.* **230**, 219.

Harris, R.E. & Conrad, F.G. (1967) Polycythaemia vera in the childbearing age. *Arch. intern. Med.* **120**, 697.

Hertko, E.J. (1963) Polycythaemia (erythrocytosis) associated with uterine fibroids and apparent surgical cure. *Am. J. Med.* **34**, 288.

International Committee for Standardisation in Haematology (1980) Recommended methods for measurement of red cell and plasma volume. *J. Nuclear Med* . **21**, 793.

Kan, Y.W., McFadzean, A.J.S., Todd, D. *et al.* (1961) Further observations on polycythemia in hepatocellular carcinoma. *Blood*, **18**, 592.

Kaplan, M.E., Mack, K., Goldberg, J.D. *et al.* (1986) Long-term management of polycythemia vera with hydroxyurea: a progress report. *Semin. Hematol.* **23**, 167.

Koeffler, H.P. & Goldwasser, E. (1981) Erythropoietin radioimmunoassay in evaluating patients with polycythemia. *Ann. Int. Med.* **94**, 44.

Lawler, S.D. (1980) Cytogenetic studies in Philadelphia chromosome negative myeloproliferative disorders, particularly polycythaemia rubra vera. *Clin. Haemat.* **9**, 159.

Lawrence, J.H. & Berlin, N.I. (1952) Relative polycythaemia—the polycythaemia of stress. *Yale J. Biol. Med.* **24**, 498.

Lawrence, J.H. (1955) *Polycythemia: Physiology, Diagnosis and Treatment based on 303 cases*, Grune & Stratton, New York.

Ledlie, E.M. (1966) Treatment of polycythaemia by ^{32}P. *Proc. R. Soc. Med.* **59**, 1095.

Lenfant, C. & Sullivan, K. (1971) Adaptation to high altitudes. *New Engl. J. Med.* **284**, 1298.

Mitus, W.J. & Kiossouglou, K.A. (1968) Leukocyte alkaline phosphatase in myeloproliferative syndrome. *Ann. N.Y. Acad. Sci.* **155**, 976.

Modan, B. (1971) *The Polycythemic Disorders*, Charles C. Thomas, Springfield, Illinois.

Najman, A., Stachowiak, J., Parlier, Y. *et al.* (1982)

Pipobroman therapy of polycythemia vera. *Blood*, **59**, 890.

Nakao, K., Kimura, K., Miura, Y. *et al.* (1966) Erythrocytosis associated with carcinoma of the liver (with erythropoietin assay of tumour extract). *Am. J. Med. Sci.* **251**, 161.

Nies, B.A., Cohn, R. & Schrier, S.L. (1965) Erythraemia after renal transplantation. *New Engl. J. Med.* **273**, 785.

Noble, J.A. (1967) Hepatic vein thrombosis complicating polycythemia vera. *Arch. Int. Med.* **120**, 105.

Osgood, E.E. (1968) The case for ^{32}P in treatment of polycythemia vera. *Blood*, **32**, 492.

Penington, D.G (1974) The myeloproliferate syndromes. *Med. J. Aust.* **2**, 56.

Pollycove, M., Winchell, H.S. & Lawrence, J.G. (1966) Classification and evolution of patterns of erythropoiesis in polycythaemia vera as studied by iron kinetics. *Blood*, **28**, 807.

Prchal, J.F., Adamson, J.W., Murphy, S. *et al.* (1978) Polycythemia vera. The *in vitro* response of normal and abnormal stem cell lines to erythropoietin. *J. Clin. Invest.* **61**, 1044.

Rosenthal, A., Nathan, D.G., Marty, A.T. *el al.* (1970) Acute haemodynamic effects of red cell volume reduction in polycythemia of cyanotic congenital heart disease. *Circulation*, **42**, 297.

Rosse, W.F., Waldmann, T.A. & Cohen, P. (1963) Renal cysts, erythropoietin and polycythaemia. *Am. J. Med.* **34**, 76.

Russell, R.P. & Conley, C.L. (1964) Benign polycythaemia: Gaisbock's syndrome. *Arch. Int. Med.* **114**, 534.

Sagone, A.L., Jr, Lawrence, T. & Balcerzak, S.P. (1973) Effect of smoking on tissue oxygen supply. *Blood*, **41**, 845.

Shield, L.K. & Pearn, J.H. (1969) Platelet adhesiveness in polycythaemia rubra vera. *Med. J. Aust.* **1**, 711.

Silverstein, M.N. (1976) The evolution into and treatment of late stage polycythemia vera. *Semin. Hematol.* **13**, 79.

Smith, J.R. & Landaw, S.A. (1978) Smokers polycythemia. *New Engl. J. Med.* **298**, 6.

Starr, G.F., Stroebel, C.F. & Kearns, T.P. (1958) Polycythemia with papilledema and infratentorial vascular tumors. *Ann. Int. Med.* **48**, 978.

Tartaglia, A.P. Goldberg, B.D., Berk, P.D. *et al.* (1986) Adverse effects of antiaggregating platelet therapy with treatment of polycythemia vera. *Semin. Hematol.* **23**, 172.

Thorling, E.B. (1972) Paraneoplastic erythrocytosis and inappropriate erythropoietin production. A review. *Scand. J. Haemat.* Suppl. No. 17.

Wasserman, L.R. & Gilbert, H.S. (1966) Surgical bleeding in polycythaemia vera. *Ann. N.Y. Acad. Sci.* **115**, 122.

Wasserman, L.R. (1976) The treatment of polycythaemia vera. *Semin. Hematol.* **13**, 57.

Wasserman, L.R. (1986) Polycythemia Vera Study Group: a historical perspective. *Semin. Hematol.* **23**, 183.

Weatherall, D.J. (1969) Polycythaemia resulting from abnormal haemoglobin. *New Engl. J. Med.* **280**, 604.

Weinreb, N.J. & Shih, C-F. (1975) Spurious polycythemia. *Semin. Hematol.* **12**, 397.

Weiss, E.A.B., Mosehos, C.B., Frank, M.J. *et al.* (1975) Haemodynamic effects of staged hematocrit reduction in patients with stable cor pulmonale and severely elevated hematocrit levels. *Am. J. Med.* **58**, 92.

York, E.L., Jones, R.L., Menon, D. *et al.* (1980) Effects of secondary polycythemia on cerebral blood flow in chronic obstructive pulmonary disease. *Am. Rev. Resp. Dis.* **121**, 813.

Myelofibrosis and thrombocythaemia

Adamson, J.W. & Fialkow, P.J. (1978) The pathogenesis of myeloproliferative syndromes. *Brit. J. Haemat.* **38**, 299.

Andre, J. Schwartz, R. & Dameshek, W. (1961) Tuberculosis and myelosclerosis with myeloid metaplasia. *J. Am. Med. Ass.* **178**, 1169.

Bennett, J.M., Catovsky, D., Daniel, M-T. *et al.* (1985) Criteria for the diagnosis of acute leukemia in megakaryocyte lineage (MT). *Ann. Int. Med.* **103**, 460.

Besa, E.C., Nowell, P.C., Geller, N.L. *et al.* (1982) Analysis of androgen response of 23 patients with agnogenic myeloid metaplasia. *Cancer*, **49**, 308.

Brody, J.I., McKenzie, D. & Kimball, S.G. (1963) Myleran as a therapeutic adjunct in gastrointestinal bleeding complicating myeloproliferative disorders. *Gastroenterology*, **45**, 499.

Castro-Malaspina, M., Rabellino, E.M., Yen, A. *et al.* (1981) Human megakaryocyte stimulation of proliferation of bone marrow fibroblasts. *Blood*, **57**, 781.

Failkow, P.J., Faguet, G.B., Jacobson, R.J. *et al.* (1981) Evidence that essential thrombocythemia is a clonal disorder with origin in a multipotential stem cell. *Blood*, **58**, 916.

Gardner, F.H. & Pringle, J.C., Jr. (1961) Androgens and erythropoiesis. II. Treatment of myeloid metaplasia. *New Engl. J. Med.* **264**, 103.

Gardner, F. H. & Nathan, D.G. (1966) Androgens and erythropoiesis. III. Further evaluation of testosterone treatment of myelofibrosis. *New Engl. J. Med.* **274**, 420.

Gunz, F.W. (1960) Haemorrhagic thrombocythemia: a critical review. *Blood*, **15**, 706.

Hickling, R.A. (1968) The natural history of chronic non-leukaemic myelosis. *Quart. J. Med.* **37**, 267.

Hoffbrand, A.V., Kremenchuzky, S., Butterworth, P.J. *et al.* (1966) Serum lactate dehydrogenase activity and folate deficiency in myelosclerosis and haematological diseases. *Brit. Med. J.* **1**, 577.

Jacobson, R.J., Salo, A. & Kialkow, P.J. (1978) Agnogenic myeloid metaplasia: a clonal proliferation of hemopoietic cells with secondary myelofibrosis. *Blood*, **51**, 189.

Laszlo, J. (1975) Myeloproliferative disorders (MPD):

myelofibrosis, myelosclerosis extramedullary haematopoiesis, undifferentiated MPD and hemorrhagic thrombocythemia. *Semin. Hematol.* **12**, 409.

Lau, S. & White, J.C. (1969) Myelosclerosis associated with systemic lupus erythematosus in patients in West Malaysia. *J. Clin. Path.* **22**, 433.

Lewis, S.M. & Szur, L. (1963) Malignant myelosclerosis. *Brit. Med. J.* **2**, 472.

McCarthy, D.M. (1985) Fibrosis of the bone marrow: content and causes *Brit. J. Haemat.* **59**, 1.

Murphy, S. (1983) Thrombocytosis and thrombocythaemia. *Clin. Haemat.* **12**, 89.

Murphy, S., Iland, H., Rosenthal, D. *et al.* (1986) Essential thrombocythemia: an interim report from the polycythemia vera study group. *Semin. Hematol.* **23**, 177.

Pegrum, G.D. & Ridson, R.A. (1970) The haematological and histological findings in 18 patients with clinical features resembling those of myelofibrosis. *Brit. J. Haemat.* **18**, 475.

Schafer, A. (1984) Bleeding and thrombosis in the myeloproliferative disorders. *Blood*, **64**, 1.

Szur, L. (1972) The non-leukaemic myeloproliferative disorders. *In* Hoffbrand, A.V. & Lewis, S.M. (eds) *Haematology Tutorials in Postgraduate Medicine*, Vol. 2, p. 257. Heinemann, London.

Wolf, B.C. & Neiman, R.S. (1985) Myelofibrosis with myeloid metaplasia: Pathophysiologic implications of the correlation between bone marrow changes and progression of splenomegaly. *Blood*, **65**, 803.

Chapter 13
The Spleen:
Hypersplenism and Splenomegaly

Functions of the spleen

The spleen may be regarded as a large mass of lymphatic tissue with special anatomical features which enable it to serve as a filter of cellular components of the blood. Like other lymphatic tissues it consists predominantly of cells of the lymphatic and reticulo-endothelial systems. The histological structure of the spleen, and the relationship between the elaborate structure of the red pulp, with its cords and sinusoids, and its effects on the formed elements of the blood is discussed by Weiss (1983). The role of the spleen in defence against infection and in other immunological functions involves both the red and the white pulp, the latter characterized by the Malpighian follicles containing both B and T lymphocytes (Weissman *et al.* 1978). Although the normal processes of the spleen are not entirely clarified, the following are recognized.

Antibody formation

The spleen shares with the lymphatic tissues in other parts of the body the function of producing antibodies. It appears to be concerned especially with the immune response to circulating particulate antigens.

Erythrocyte removal and phagocytosis

Red cells at the end of their lifespan are normally removed from the circulation by phagocytic cells of the reticulo-endothelial system. The spleen contains a large number of these cells which are in intimate contact with the cells of the blood as they pass slowly through the red pulp. It is consequently an important site of destruction of aged red cells, but red cell lifespan is not prolonged following splenectomy because other tissues of the reticulo-endothelial system take over the role of the spleen under these circumstances. The spleen is particularly effective in removing inflexible or antibody-coated red cells from the circulating blood, and it can also selectively remove inclusions from intact red cells.

Particulate matter and micro-organisms are also removed from the circulation by phagocytosis in the spleen.

Blood storage

Red cells. In some animals, the spleen forms an important reservoir for red cells, and by active contraction supplies red cells in response to physiological demand, e.g. during exercise or following haemorrhage. However, in humans, the amount of blood contained in the normal spleen is small (estimated at 20–60 ml of red cells) compared with the total blood volume. Its function as a reservoir of red cells is thus unimportant. Splenectomy in an otherwise healthy person does not impair exercise tolerance.

In certain disorders where the spleen is greatly enlarged, there may be pooling of red cells in the spleen, and when enlargement is gross, the spleen may contain a significant proportion of the total red cell volume (p. 349).

Platelets. The spleen acts as a significant reservoir

of platelets, in dynamic exchange with platelets in the blood. The exchangeable pool in the normal spleen is approximately 30 per cent of the total mass of platelets in the circulation, and increases with increasing splenic size (Penny *et al.* 1966). An increase in this platelet pool is a major factor in the thrombocytopenia of hypersplenism.

White cells. Lymphocytes occur naturally in the spleen and constitute about one-half of the normal spleen cell population. Granulocytopenia of mild to moderate degree is relatively common in patients with splenomegaly, due to an increase of 'marginated' granulocytes in the spleen.

The degree of pooling, and transit times for particular cell types in the spleen, have been categorized (Peters 1983).

Blood production

In fetal life, the spleen contributes to the formation of all types of blood cells, but after birth it normally forms only lymphocytes. In certain pathological circumstances, the spleen may undergo myeloid metaplasia and produce red cells, granulocytes and platelets (p. 335).

Effects of splenectomy

Haematological effects

The changes described below refer to those that occur in normal subjects after splenectomy. Consequences of splenectomy for pathological conditions on one or more of the cellular elements may be substantially modified by the effect of the underlying disorder on the production of blood cells by the bone marrow. In auto-antibody-mediated haemolysis or thrombocytopenia, for example, the relative increase in the respective cell counts following splenectomy is often significantly increased.

Red cells. Target cells usually appear in the blood film, and the cells have increased resistance to haemolysis in the osmotic fragility test (p. 181). Occasional spherocytes may be detected. Small remnants of nuclear material, Howell–Jolly bodies, characteristically are present in red cells, as they are no longer selectively 'pitted' from circulating red cells by the spleen. Other inclusions, such as aggregates of iron-containing material, may also be observed. Changes of this type often persist indefinitely after splenectomy.

When increased demand for red cells leads to marrow hyperplasia in the splenectomized subject, e.g. after haemorrhage or in haemolysis, the appearance of erythroblasts in the peripheral blood is often more marked, together with occasional myelocytes.

White cells. After splenectomy, there is an increase in the total white cell count within several hours, and it usually reaches a maximum after a day or two. The count then gradually falls over a period of weeks or months in the uncomplicated situation, to normal values. In some cases, a mild increase, e.g. up to 15×10^9/l, persists for many years. The maximum reached by the white cell count is usually about twice normal, although it may be higher. The sharp rise in the count is due mainly to an increase in neutrophils, but after a few weeks to months, the neutrophil count falls to near normal levels, and the count of circulating lymphocytes and monocytes rises, and remains increased, apparently permanently. There may also be a slight increase in eosinophils and basophils. In splenectomized subjects, *leucocytosis in response to infection is characterized by a greater than normal shift to the left,* with the appearance of myelocytes.

Platelets. The platelet count rises sharply, often within a matter of hours, reaches a peak in 1–2 weeks, and then usually falls to normal values over a period of weeks or months. In about one-third of cases, it remains raised indefinitely. This is especially so in patients with continuing haemolysis, and this group has a reported increased risk of thromboembolism (Hirsh & Dacie 1966). The maximum platelet count is usually 3–4 times normal, and on occasion reaches $2000–3000 \times 10^9$/l.

The current view is that changes after splenectomy are a reflection of the capacity of the spleen to sequester cells newly released from the bone marrow. The spleen contributes to the maintenance of normal red cell appearance by its 'pitting' function—the selective removal of particles from the cytoplasm of the red cell without injuring the cell (Crosby 1963).

SPLENIC ATROPHY

Changes similar to those occurring after splenectomy have been described accompanying congenital absence or acquired atrophy of the spleen. Disorders in which acquired atrophy may occur include sickle cell disease, coeliac disease, dermatitis herpetiformis, and essential thrombocythaemia.

Clinical effects

The spleen is not essential for life. In otherwise healthy *adults* it can be removed without apparent alteration of health or longevity.

Susceptibility to infection after splenectomy. Splenectomy does not appear to render normal adults more susceptible to infection. However, there is evidence in *infants* and *young children* of an increased incidence of severe, and sometimes fatal, infections after splenectomy. It appears that children under the age of three years are most frequently affected, particularly infants under one year. The interval between splenectomy and the onset of infection has been less than three years in most reported cases, but may be longer. The *pneumococcus* has been the organism most commonly isolated (over 50 per cent of cases) but infections with Group A *streptococcus, Haemophilus influenzae,* enteric bacteria, and other organisms have also been reported. No increase in incidence of viral infections has been noted. Reported infections include septicaemia, meningitis, pneumonia, pericarditis, and acute endocarditis. A feature of many infections has been their fulminating character. With septicaemia and meningitis, death may occur within 12–24 hours of the onset of symptoms. Whitaker (1969) has shown that some cases of severe infection are associated with acute disseminated intravascular coagulation. Although the incidence of infection in children over the age of three years does not appear to be much increased, when it does occur, infection may be severe and overwhelming. It is recommended that the young splenectomized patient has close supervision for several years postoperatively, so that immediate and energetic treatment can be instituted in the event of sudden and severe infectious illness.

Diamond (1969) has pointed out that the nature of the disorder that led to the splenectomy influences the risk of postoperative infection. Infection is not markedly increased following splenectomy for trauma, hereditary spherocytosis, idiopathic thrombocytopenic purpura, Gaucher's disease, and portal vein thrombosis with congestive splenomegaly, while it is more common in other disorders such as thalassaemia major, lymphoma, leukaemia, hepatitis with portal hypertension, and diseases requiring treatment with corticosteroids in relatively high doses. Septicaemia of an unusually fulminant nature is sometimes encountered in hyposplenism due to sickle-cell disease. Prophylactic immunization with pneumococcal vaccine should be considered in individuals at increased risk. However, even when polyvalent vaccines are employed, septicaemia may still occur (Overturf *et al.* 1979). Long-term prophylaxis with penicillin may therefore be needed in susceptible patients.

Hypersplenism

Definition and pathogenesis

It has been known for many years that certain patients with splenomegaly secondary to a number of disorders develop neutropenia, anaemia, or thrombocytopenia, either singly or in combination, and that splenectomy results in varying degrees of improvement in the peripheral blood picture, even to normal. The fact that the peripheral blood picture is corrected by splenectomy led to the concept of *hypersplenism.* In rare cases of splenic enlargement with hypersplenism, where no histologically identifiable cause of the enlargement of the spleen can be found, the term *primary hypersplenism* is applied. The term *secondary hypersplenism* is applied to the much more common group in which splenomegaly is caused by a well-defined disease. The syndrome of hypersplenism is thus characterized by reduction of one or more of the cellular elements of the blood.

Hypersplenism is generally not a direct cause of death, and a fatal outcome in a patient with hypersplenism is usually due to complications of the condition responsible for enlargement of the spleen. There is, however, no doubt that hypersplenism can cause marked depression of cell counts in the blood, and these can substantially increase the severity of clinical problems produced by the underlying disorder.

Mechanism of hypersplenism. There has been considerable speculation over the mechanism by which enlargement of the spleen causes reduction in the count of cells in the peripheral blood. One of the processes involved in depression of the red cell count is pooling of red cells within the enlarged spleen. The extent to which pooling, or sequestration, of red cells takes place bears a general relationship to the degree of splenomegaly, but the correlation can be poor in some instances. Studies with radio-isotope labelled red cells indicate that passive pooling of red cells in the spleen has a greater impact on lowering the red cell count in the blood than accelerated destruction of entrapped red cells, although the latter can occur to some extent in some instances. The degree of anaemia can be considerably accentuated in some instances by expansion of the plasma volume, but the underlying mechanism responsible for this phenomenon remains to be clarified (Christensen 1973).

The decrease that occurs in the blood platelet and leucocyte count is likewise a reflection of an increase in the pool of platelets, and in the number of marginated leucocytes in the enlarged spleen (Peters 1983).

Aetiology

Causes of enlargement of the spleen associated with hypersplenism are listed in Table 13.1. The most common cause is congestive splenomegaly secondary to portal hypertension. It must be remembered that in a number of the conditions listed, e.g. lymphomas, hypersplenism is uncommon, and that changes in blood count in these disorders are often brought about by some other mechanism. Primary hypersplenism is very rare, and should be diagnosed only by exclusion after complete investigation has failed to reveal any underlying disorder.

In some cases of anaemia associated with abnormal bone marrow and marked splenomegaly, such as thalassaemia major, myelofibrosis, and chronic lymphocytic leukaemia, transfusion requirements increase steadily. *Whilst it may be difficult to define the contribution made by hypersplenism in an individual case, splenectomy in these disorders is often followed by reduction in the severity of anaemia, although sometimes the extent of the bone marrow abnormality can prevent an effective response.*

Table 13.1. *Causes of hypersplenism*

Secondary
Portal hypertension with congestive splenomegaly
Lymphomas
Sarcoidosis
Felty's syndrome
Lipid storage disease—Gaucher's disease
Kala-azar, chronic malaria, 'tropical splenomegaly'
Bacterial infections—tuberculosis, brucellosis, bacterial endocarditis, chronic bacteraemia
Thalassaemia
Chronic lymphatic leukaemia
Myelofibrosis
Hairy cell leukaemia
Primary (idiopathic)

PRIMARY HYPERSPLENISM

A small series of patients has been described in whom marked splenomegaly occurred with the haematological features of hypersplenism, but without an obvious underlying causative disorder (Dacie *et al.* 1969). Splenectomy was usually followed by immediate and often sustained haematological improvement. Histological examination of the spleen revealed hyperplasia, commonly with a disproportionate increase in lymphoid tissue. Some of the patients subsequently developed non-Hodgkin's lymphoma, and the preceding enlargement of the spleen evidently reflected a non-malignant reaction to the disease, or lymphomatous involvement of a type that was difficult to recognize on histological grounds. A diagnosis of primary hypersplenism should thus be made only with considerable reservations.

Diagnosis

There are two problems in diagnosis: (i) to establish that hypersplenism exists; and (ii) to establish the cause of the enlargement of the spleen.

The first question is sometimes clarified by establishing the underlying cause. Thus, if a patient with splenomegaly, neutropenia, and thrombocytopenia has clear-cut evidence of portal hypertension, it is probable that the patient has congestive splenomegaly with secondary hypersplenism.

THE DIAGNOSTIC CRITERIA OF HYPERSPLENISM

The four criteria laid down for the diagnosis of hypersplenism are:

1 a peripheral blood picture of anaemia, neutropenia, and thrombocytopenia, either singly or in combination;

2 a normally cellular or hypercellular bone marrow;

3 splenomegaly;

4 significant improvement in the peripheral blood picture following splenectomy.

Blood picture. There is nothing specifically diagnostic in the peripheral blood picture. In the absence of additional factors, *anaemia* is usually normocytic and normochromic. Marked anisocytosis and poikilocytosis are uncommon in uncomplicated cases. It is not typical to have features of significant haemolysis. *Leucopenia* is due primarily to neutropenia, but in severe cases all white cells are reduced in number. The white cell count is usually not reduced sufficiently to predispose to infection—total counts from 3 to 4×10^9/l, with neutrophil counts of $1–2 \times 10^9$/l being usual. Only occasionally is the total leucocyte count less than 1×10^9/l. Moderate *thrombocytopenia* occurs with a platelet count of about 100×10^9/l being usual, but occasionally values are $50–100 \times 10^9$/l, or lower. The reduction in cell count tends to be slowly progressive, although this may reflect progressive increase in the size of the spleen, and in some cases the counts remain relatively stationary over many years.

The *bone marrow* is either of normal or increased cellularity, and may of course be infiltrated by a disease process that has been responsible for the enlargement of the spleen. Uncommonly, the picture is complicated by reduction in the proportion of neutrophil precursors more mature than the myelocyte.

Splenomegaly is present by definition. It may be either moderate or marked. However, in obese patients a moderately enlarged spleen may not be palpable. Thus, although the diagnosis should be seriously questioned when the spleen is not palpable, the *absence of a clinically palpable spleen does not absolutely exclude the diagnosis in a patient in whom the other features are suggestive*. Under such circumstances, the size of the spleen can be assessed by an isotope scan. When the splenomegaly is first noted, blood changes may be minimal or absent, but may progress over the following months or years. On occasion, neutropenia and thrombocytopenia may be prominent features well before splenomegaly has become marked.

Splenectomy results in a return of the blood picture to normal, provided this is not prevented by interference with the productive capability of the bone marrow by disease, such as marrow infiltration. There can be an immediate rise in neutrophils and platelets to higher than normal values, followed by a gradual fall to normal or near normal values.

It must be realized that in many cases the reduction in cell counts is not sufficient to cause clinical problems, and splenectomy is not indicated.

Distinction from other causes of splenomegaly with a reduction in the formed elements of the blood. In considering hypersplenism as a cause for reduced blood cell counts in a patient with splenomegaly, two facts must be borne in mind: (a) the association of splenomegaly with the reduction of one or more formed elements occurs in a number of disorders which may cause cytopenia by other mechanisms. These include lupus erythematosus and leukaemia; and (b) in diseases known to cause hypersplenism, a similar blood picture may be brought about by a different mechanism, and hence is not corrected by splenectomy. Thus, pancytopenia due to marrow infiltration can occur in advanced stages of lymphoma, and indeed is a more common cause of pancytopenia than hypersplenism. Presence of marked anisocytosis and poikilocytosis is more suggestive of marrow infiltration than hypersplenism under these circumstances. Neutropenia may be caused predominantly by mechanisms other than hypersplenism in some cases of Felty's syndrome, when it is unlikely to recover after splenectomy. Careful consideration should thus be given to the cellularity and composition of the bone marrow, and this requires examination of a trephine biopsy.

DIAGNOSIS OF THE CAUSE OF HYPERSPLENISM

In many cases of hypersplenism, the cause of the splenomegaly is suggested by the presence of manifestations of the underlying disease, e.g. portal hypertension or lymphoma, and is confirmed by appropriate investigations. Occasionally, however, there are no obvious clinical features of an underlying disorder, and investigations are not conclusive. Such cases may be examples of primary (idiopathic) hypersplenism, but it must be realized that with adequate follow-up the majority subsequently develop evidence of an underlying disease which was not obvious at the time of presentation. Splenectomy should be carried out, as the histology of the spleen may reveal the first evidence of an underlying disease, e.g. sarcoidosis, Hodgkin's disease, or non-Hodgkin's lymphoma. In apparently idiopathic cases in which the histological picture is one of non-specific hyperplasia, clinical features of the underlying disease, such as lymphoma, may appear subsequently.

Treatment

Splenectomy produces partial or complete recovery of the abnormal blood picture in otherwise uncomplicated cases. When the effect of the hypersplenism is not sufficient to cause symptoms, splenectomy offers no benefit to the patient. Splenectomy is indicated when significant problems are caused by the sole or the additional effect of hypersplenism in reducing the count of blood cells, usually anaemia of sufficient severity to cause symptoms, neutropenia predisposing to infections, or thrombocytopenia causing spontaneous bleeding.

Disorders causing splenomegaly

Splenomegaly is a relatively common clinical finding, which may occur in a wide variety of disorders (Table 13.2). In one series of nearly 6000 unselected adult outpatients, two per cent had palpable spleens (Schloesser 1963). In the majority of cases, clinical examination and appropriate investigations reveal the cause of the splenomegaly. Nevertheless, occasionally a slight to moderate degree of splenomegaly is present in apparently normal persons without any obvious cause. Such splenomegaly may be found accidentally on routine medical examination, and in Schloesser's series accounted for one-quarter of cases; McIntyre & Ebaugh (1967)

Table 13.2. *Causes of splenomegaly*

Slight enlargement (just palpable or to about 5 cm)
Acute, subacute, and chronic infections (Table 13.3)
Disorders in which splenomegaly is occasionally present—megaloblastic anaemias, rheumatoid arthritis, systemic lupus erythematosus*, sarcoidosis*, amyloidosis*
Disorders listed below which cause moderate or marked enlargement in the early stage or following treatment
No demonstrable cause
Moderate enlargement (to umbilicus)
Lymphomas
Chronic granulocytic leukaemia
Chronic lymphatic leukaemia
Acute leukaemia
Portal hypertension with congestive splenomegaly
Chronic haemolytic anaemias
Polycythaemia vera
Essential thrombocythaemia
Myelodysplastic disorders
Marked enlargement (below umbilicus)
USUAL OR COMMON
Myelofibrosis
Hairy cell leukaemia
'Tropical splenomegaly', kala–azar, bilharzia, chronic malaria
Thalassaemia major
Splenic cysts and tumours
Gaucher's disease
LESS COMMON
Disorders which more usually cause moderate enlargement, especially lymphomas and portal hypertension

*Moderate enlargement can also occur.

Table 13.3. *Infective causes of splenomegaly*

Acute
Infectious mononucleosis
Typhoid
Brucellosis
Infectious hepatitis
Toxoplasmosis
Typhus
Septicaemia
Subacute and chronic
Bacterial endocarditis
Tuberculosis
Brucellosis
Syphilis
Histoplasmosis
Chronic bacteraemia
Parasitic
Malaria
Kala–azar
Hydatid
Trypanosomiasis

found that about 2.5 per cent of 2200 students entering college had a palpable spleen with no obvious cause. Englargement of the spleen sometimes persists for a long time after recovery from the causative disorder, and a number of cases of unknown cause are probably due to a previous illness not recognized at the time as causing splenomegaly, e.g. infectious mononucleosis or hepatitis. In other cases, after observation over a period of time, an underlying causative disorder may become obvious, but sometimes the splenomegaly persists indefinitely without any obvious cause. While the spleen is usually palpable only when it is enlarged, in a small proportion of individuals their physique is such that a normal spleen can be tipped on inspiration. Conversely, the physique in other individuals can be such as to prevent palpation of a moderately enlarged spleen.

The *size* of the spleen varies with the nature and duration of the causative disorder. Splenomegaly is usually classified as slight (when the spleen is just palpable or palpable up to about 5 cm below the costal margin), moderate (when the spleen extends up to, but not beyond, the umbilicus), and marked (when the spleen extends below the umbilicus). With massive enlargement, the spleen can extend into the right iliac fossa. Table 13.2 summarizes the usual maximum size attained by the spleen in disorders causing splenomegaly. Clearly, in any disorder, the enlarging spleen can progress along a course of increasing size, and it should be realized that there is considerable overlap between the groups, particularly in disorders causing slight and moderate splenomegaly.

Clinical features of splenomegaly

In many cases, splenomegaly itself is symptomless, especially when the enlargement is only slight to moderate in degree. However, it may cause a dull ache in the left hypochondrium, and when the spleen is particularly large, a heavy dragging sensation. Sometimes there is actual pain over the spleen. In disorders characterized by splenic infarction, the perisplenitis due to the infarct may cause acute pain, sometimes worse on breathing. This may be accompanied by an audible friction rub, which is occasionally also palpable.

With *marked enlargement*, especially in children, there may be symptoms due to pressure on adjacent organs; these include a feeling of fullness after meals, flatulence, dyspepsia, epigastric pain, nausea, and vomiting due to pressure on the stomach, and frequency of micturition due to pressure on the bladder.

Most of the disorders causing splenomegaly associated with haematological manifestations are described elsewhere. In the following section, several other disorders in which splenomegaly is an important feature are discussed. These are congestive splenomegaly, Gaucher's and Niemann–Pick disease, and tropical splenomegaly.

Portal hypertension with congestive splenomegaly

In 1898, Banti described a disorder characterized by splenomegaly, anaemia, leucopenia, gastric haemorrhage, cirrhosis of the liver, and ascites. He considered the splenic enlargement was the primary lesion, and that the enlarged spleen produced a toxin which was carried by the bloodstream to the liver to cause cirrhosis. He described an initial stage of splenic enlargement with anaemia and leucopenia, the development of hepatic cirrhosis, and a terminal stage in which the liver becomes atrophic and impalpable, and severe haemorrhage, ascites, and cachexia develop. Since the original description, there has been much confusion about both the pathology and the terminology of the condition which Banti described. It is now recognized that the splenomegaly is produced primarily by congestion of the spleen resulting from increased pressure in the portal venous system, i.e. from portal hypertension, but lymphoid hyperplasia may also contribute in certain types of liver disease as part of the immune reaction associated with chronic active hepatitis. Cirrhosis is the most common, but not the only, cause of portal hypertension. Splenic venous obstruction and extrahepatic portal vein obstruction must also be considered.

Aetiology

Cirrhosis with *intrahepatic obstruction* of the portal vein is responsible for at least 80 per cent of cases of portal hypertension with congestive splenomegaly. The remaining 20 per cent are due either to obstruction of the portal vein outside the liver, or to obstruction of the splenic vein. Only rarely is there no obvious obstruction to the portal venous system.

Extrahepatic obstruction with a normal liver is most frequently due to congenital stenosis, atresia, angiomatous malformation, or extension of umbilical vein thrombosis into the portal vein. In such cases, clinical manifestations usually occur before the age of 20 years. Thrombosis of either portal or splenic vein in adult life occurs most frequently as a complication of hepatic cirrhosis, but occasionally follows trauma, intra-abdominal inflammation, or occurs in disorders with a thrombotic tendency, such as polycythaemia vera.

No discernible venous obstruction. Rarely, portal hypertension develops in the absence of definite intrahepatic or extrahepatic obstruction, presumably due to increased flow through the splenoportal system.

Pathophysiology

Portal hypertension. The normal pressure in the portal venous system, as measured at operation, is 100–150 mm water. In portal hypertension with congestive splenomegaly, readings usually range from 250 to 400 mm water, and are sometimes higher. Because of the increased pressure in the portal venous system, a collateral circulation between the portal and systemic veins develops in the region of the lower end of the oesophagus and upper end of the stomach, the diaphragm, retroperitoneal tissues, umbilicus, and rectum. The collaterals in the rectum and umbilicus may manifest themselves clinically as haemorrhoids and dilated veins on the abdominal wall, respectively. In general, the collateral circulation is beneficial to the patient as it tends to lower the pressure in the portal system, but the submucous oesophageal and gastric veins in the region of the cardia are poorly supported, subject to trauma, and hence are frequently the site of massive and often fatal haemorrhage.

In cirrhosis, the increased portal pressure is in part due to obstruction to flow in the intrahepatic vascular bed, and in part due to anastomosis between the small branches of the hepatic artery and portal vein in the disorganized fibrotic liver, with the result that pressure in arterioles is transmitted to the portal vein.

Haematological changes. Anaemia is not uncommon, and is usually due to bleeding and hypersplenism, but in some cases the liver disease itself contributes (p. 111). Leucopenia and thrombocytopenia are usually manifestations of hypersplenism. Bleeding and bruising may occur, due predominantly to deficiency of coagulation factors normally produced by the liver. Chronic mild disseminated intravascular coagulation may contribute in some cases. These coagulopathies may predispose to bleeding from oesophageal and gastric veins, but the major element in such bleeding is the high pressure in poorly supported large varices.

Liver damage. Jaundice and ascites, when present, are manifestations of the underlying liver disease. It is probable that portal hypertension alone does not cause ascites, although it may contribute in the presence of other factors, e.g. the lowering of the serum albumin level, and the sodium retention that occur in cirrhosis.

Clinical features

Portal hypertension may occur at any age. A small proportion of cases occur in children, mostly due to a developmental anomaly or perinatal thrombosis of the portal vein. The history sometimes suggests the cause, e.g. a history of umbilical stump infection, alcoholism, or chronic hepatitis, but in many cases there is no such history.

Massive gastrointestinal bleeding eventually occurs in about 50 per cent of all cases of portal hypertension. The bleeding tends to be repeated, and can be fatal. The splenic enlargement may cause a dragging sensation under the left costal margin or, when more marked, flatulent dyspepsia. Occasionally, the first manifestation is the accidental discovery of an enlarged spleen. The splenomegaly may precede the onset of clinical manifestations by years, and apart from the progressive development of a moderate anaemia and leucopenia, the patient may be in relatively good general health.

Examination. Splenomegaly is nearly always present in portal hypertension. It is usually moderate in degree, but occasionally it is marked, and rarely the spleen extends into the left iliac fossa. The spleen is firm. The liver is commonly palpable, but in some cases the liver is small and impalpable. Sometimes, progressive shrinking of the liver can be observed over a period of time. Evidence of collateral circulation may be present. When liver failure is extensive there may be jaundice, oedema, ascites, wasting of muscle mass, spider naevi, and palmar erythema. These are late manifestations and relate to the severity of liver cell disease rather than to the severity of portal hypertension. Features of hepatic encephalopathy may also be found, such as flapping tremor and impairment of cerebral function.

Blood picture

The blood picture is not diagnostic. In the absence of bleeding, the typical picture is of mild normochromic normocytic anaemia and leucopenia, with or without thrombocytopenia. In the early stages, the blood picture may be normal. The picture is complicated by associated bleeding in which the hypochromic microcytic anaemia of iron deficiency supervenes. The white cell count is usually less than 5×10^9/l, and commonly ranges from 2 to 4×10^9/l. It may be the only abnormality, but it is rare for the neutrophil count to fall to a level that predisposes to infection. The white cell count may be elevated in response to associated problems, e.g. acute haemorrhage, infection, or thrombosis. A moderate, symptomless thrombocytopenia is common, but sometimes the platelet count can be less than 50×10^9/l. The lowering of the platelet count may be exaggerated in alcoholic subjects who have recently ingested large amounts of alcohol.

The *bone marrow* findings vary. In the early phases, the marrow picture may be normal, but later there may be hyperplasia of red cell and white cell precursors.

Diagnosis

The diagnosis of portal hypertension with congestive splenomegaly is suggested by the occurrence of splenomegaly, hepatomegaly, together with distension of the veins of the abdominal wall, either with or without clinical evidence of liver failure. A history of haematemesis supports the diagnosis.

The major diagnostic difficulty is when the patient with splenomegaly and neutropenia or pancytopenia has no clinical evidence of liver damage or portal hypertension. In such patients, the demonstration of oesophageal varices by barium swallow, as shown in Fig. 13.1 establishes the diagnosis, but these varices are demonstrable in only about 40 per cent of cases. Aspiration liver biopsy and portal venography may establish the diagnosis and are discussed in detail by Sherlock (1985).

Course and prognosis

The course of portal hypertension displays marked individual variation, which is determined chiefly by two factors: the degree of pressure elevation, and the degree of liver damage. In patients presenting with splenomegaly without haematemesis, the condition may run a chronic course for many years with few clinical problems. Onset of massive haemorrhage is a serious prognostic factor, as massive bleeds are usually repeated and ultimately fatal. In a few cases, there are intervals of several years between bleeds, possibly due to the development of better collateral circulation at other sites of anastomosis with systemic veins, or other causes of lowered pressure in the oesophageal varices. The severity of associated liver disease is a major factor in prognosis. In patients whose liver function is not markedly impaired and remains relatively unchanged over a period of years, survival may be long. Prognosis is poor in patients with progressive development of features of hepatic insufficiency such as jaundice, ascites, and cachexia. Prognosis is best in patients with a normal liver and no other disease apart from isolated obstruction of the splenic vein.

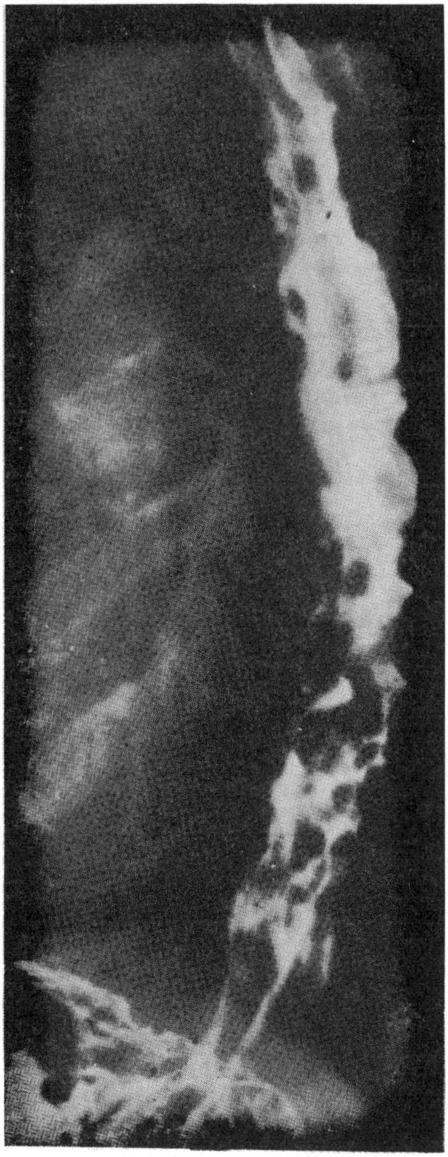

Fig. 13.1. *Oesophageal varices displayed by barium swallow. Oesophageal varices can be demonstrated radiologically in about 40 per cent of cases of portal hypertension, and thus the absence of demonstrable varices does not exclude portal hypertension. The varices in this case are more extensive than usual.*

Treatment

The relief of symptoms due to hypersplenism. In most cases of congestive splenomegaly, the reduction in the cell counts is not sufficient to cause significant symptoms and thus splenectomy is not indicated. If, however, splenectomy is indicated because of hypersplenism, the question of performing a lienorenal shunt at the same time must be considered. If this is not done at the time of splenectomy, the splenic vein cannot be used for a lienorenal anastomosis should this subsequently become necessary for the relief of portal hypertension. Splenectomy alone is of no lasting value in the relief of portal hypertension, except in the occasional case in which venous obstruction is confined to the splenic vein.

Gaucher's disease

Gaucher's disease is an inherited disorder of metabolism characterized by the accumulation of lipid in the form of glucocerebroside in the cells of the reticulo-endothelial system. The organs most commonly involved are the spleen, liver, and bone marrow, but the lymph nodes, nervous system, and lungs can also be involved. It is relatively common in Jewish communities, but much less common in others. The majority of cases appear to be inherited as an autosomal recessive trait. The nature of the biochemical defect is a deficiency of the enzyme involved in the hydrolysis of glucocerebroside, causing this material to accumulate in grossly excessive amounts in cells of the reticulo-endothelial system. Detection of low levels of enzyme activity in leucocytes is of diagnostic value (Kampine *et al.* 1967).

Two forms distinguished on the basis of age of onset are recognized—an infantile type, and an adult type. The former can run an acute course, and the latter a chronic course.

Adult Gaucher's disease

This is the more common type, and it may be first detected in childhood, in young adults, or even in patients over the age of 30 years. A particularly common presenting feature is splenic enlargement. Less common presenting manifestations are pain secondary to bone infiltration, anaemia, thrombocytopenia, and pigmentation. Splenic enlargement, which is often extreme, is the outstanding feature on examination. Moderate to marked smooth non-tender hepatomegaly is usual. The superficial lymph nodes may be enlarged in children, but are seldom palpable in adults. Brownish pigmentation of the skin, affecting the face and other exposed areas, and sometimes the legs, is common. In some older patients, yellow-brown wedge-shaped thickenings—pingueculae—are present in the conjunctivae on both sides of the cornea. There may be either a generalized rarefaction with cortical thinning, or localized osteolytic lesions in bone on X-ray. The most typical abnormality in the early stages is a club-shaped widening of the lower end of the femur, and pathological fractures can develop at a later stage. Changes in the spine may result in vertebral collapse.

Blood picture. Changes in the blood count are due to two factors: marrow replacement by Gaucher's cells, and hypersplenism. Moderate normochromic normocytic anaemia is usual, and in some cases anaemia is severe. Mild to moderate leucopenia and thrombocytopenia are common. and occasionally thrombocytopenia is sufficiently marked to cause bleeding.

Bone marrow. The typical and diagnostic feature on marrow aspiration is the presence of Gaucher's cells. These cells are large, pale, round or polyhedral, and range in diameter from 20 to 40 microns or more. The nuclei are relatively small, eccentric, and vary in chromatin content. The cytoplasm is pale, and has a pattern of fine wavy fibrils. It is strongly positive to the acid phosphatase and the periodic acid–Schiff (PAS) stains. Effects of hypersplenism increase the cellularity of haemopoietic tissue, but in some regions the marrow can be extensively replaced by sheets of Gaucher's cells.

Course and treatment. The disorder runs a chronic course, and often the patient dies of some other disorder. When death results from the disease itself, it is usually due to pathological fracture, especially of the spine, thrombocytopenia, anaemia, or intercurrent infection. Splenectomy is indicated in patients in whom hypersplenism causes symptoms, especially thrombocytopenia, and when the massive size causes severe discomfort. Pain due to local bone destruction may be relieved by irradiation.

Infantile Gaucher's disease

Less commonly, some cases of Gaucher's disease present in infancy, usually during the first six months of life, and deterioration is rapid. Infiltration of the liver and spleen occurs, but there is also widespread neurone degeneration. Death from intercurrent infection or cachexia usually occurs in the first two years of life, although in some instances the rate of clinical deterioration is less rapid.

Niemann–Pick disease

Niemann–Pick disease is a rare disorder of lipid metabolism characterized by the accumulation of sphingomyelin in the cells of the reticulo-endothelial system and other tissues. It occurs most commonly in Jews, and is often familial. The basic defect is a marked reduction in the tissues of the enzyme sphingomyelinase, which catalyses the first step in the catabolism of sphingomyelin (Brady 1969). Assay of the enzyme in leucocytes is of diagnostic value.

Onset is in the first year of life, with loss of weight, vomiting, and abdominal enlargement due to marked enlargement of the liver and spleen. The nervous system then becomes involved, with muscular weakness, spasticity, blindness, and deafness; fundal examination commonly shows a cherry-red spot in the macula. A moderate anaemia is usual, often with leucocytosis. Diagnosis is established by demonstration of Niemann–Pick cells, which in general resemble those of Gaucher's disease but are filled with small hyaline droplets giving a honeycomb appearance; the droplets stain positively with fat stains. The disorder is usually, but not invariably, fatal in the first few years of life, and no effective treatment has yet been devised.

Splenomegaly in tropical diseases

Splenomegaly is common is tropical diseases, especially malaria, kala-azar, and bilharzia. Thus a history of residence in, or passage through, a tropical or subtropical area, or of malarial or other tropical infections, should be sought in any patient with splenomegaly.

Tropical splenomegaly

In tropical areas, in addition to splenomegaly for which a definite cause can be demonstrated, cases of marked and often massive splenic enlargement are seen in which the aetiology cannot be established. The term 'tropical splenomegaly' is sometimes used to describe such cases, which are associated with anaemia and varying degrees of neutropenia and thrombocytopenia.

Cases of 'tropical splenomegaly' do not form a homogeneous group, and it appears that the cause varies in different parts of the world. Two main types have been described.

The first is associated with hepatic cirrhosis, often with portal hypertension, although there is not necessarily a correlation between the degree of portal hypertension and the size of the spleen. This type of disorder has been described in many countries, including Africa, India, and South-East Asia, and is generally associated with chronic infection of the liver with hepatitis B.

The second type, now termed the *tropical splenomegaly syndrome*, is not associated with cirrhosis but with a liver biopsy appearance in which there is lymphocytic infiltration of the hepatic sinusoids, and Kupffer cell hyperplasia. It has been reported in Uganda, Nigeria and other parts of Africa, and also New Guinea. There is evidence to suggest a relationship with malaria, as it occurs in areas where malaria is endemic, and rarely occurs in malaria-free regions. Malarial parasites in general are not seen on routine examination of the blood film, but in Uganda small numbers of *Plasmodium malariae* trophozoites were found after a *prolonged search* of the peripheral blood of nearly 50 per cent of the patients. Striking evidence of a causal relationship with malaria is the fact that continuous antimalarial therapy resulted in progressive diminution of splenic size in a high proportion of patients.

The disorder usually presents in adult life, most commonly in young adults, but it may occur in children. The patient complains of abdominal discomfort, occasional fever, and general debility. Marked hepatosplenomegaly can be an outstanding feature. Portal hypertension is sometimes present in the absence of cirrhosis, and is considered to be due to an increase in portal blood flow or, less commonly, to presinusoidal obstruction to blood flow (Williams *et al.* 1966). Anaemia, leucopenia, and thrombocytopenia are common, but spontaneous bleeding is unusual. Acute self-limiting episodes of haemolytic anaemia may occur, especially in pregnancy. The bone marrow is commonly hyperplastic. There may be up to a ten-fold increase in polyclonal IgM concentration in the serum, of which only a small proportion represents malaria antibody (Fakunle 1981).

Diagnosis. There is no specific diagnostic test, and the diagnosis is usually made by exclusion of other causes of splenomegaly in an area where the disease is endemic. In areas where thalassaemias, haemoglobinopathies, malaria, leishmaniasis, and schistosomiasis are present, these disorders must be excluded by appropriate investigation. The liver biopsy appearance of lymphocytic infiltration associated with Kupffer cell hyperplasia, but with no alteration of liver architecture, is suggestive although not specifically diagnostic.

Treatment. Both splenectomy and antimalarial chemotherapy have been used. While splenectomy may relieve symptoms and improve the blood picture, there is evidence that it is followed by an increased risk of serious malarial infection (Fakunle 1981). Malarial chemotherapy appears to be the initial treatment of choice, and Stuvier *et al.* (1971) consider prolonged therapy with antimalarial drugs appropriate for the sensitivity of the organism in that region is the most reasonable and effective treatment for umcomplicated cases.

Kala–azar. Marked splenomegaly is common in kala–azar (leishmaniasis). Kala–azar is characterized by irregular pyrexia, and normocytic anaemia with leucopenia. Lymph node enlargement is sometimes present. Diagnosis is established by demonstration of the parasite, *Leishmania donovani,* by bone marrow aspiration or by splenic puncture. In marrow films stained by Romanovsky stains, the organisms are present in phagocytic cells, but may also be found free. They are about the same size as platelets, from which they have to be differentiated. The Leishmania are oval with two deeply staining bodies, the larger the trophonucleus, and the smaller the kinetoplast. The marrow is hyperplastic, the hyperplasia involving the myeloid and erythroid series, as well as monocytes and macrophages. However, the differential count reveals a decrease in the proportion of mature granulocytes, as can be seen in other types of hypersplenism. Occasionally, the parasite can be observed in monocytes in the peripheral blood.

The disease is endemic in many parts of the world, especially Africa and the Indian subcontinent. It is usually a progressive, debilitating infection which is ultimately fatal in most cases, unless treated. Organic antimony drugs such as stibogluconate are the most effective.

Table 13.4. *Indications for splenectomy*

Disorders in which splenectomy is usually indicated
Hereditary spherocytosis (p. 182)
Chronic idiopathic thrombocytopenic purpura (p. 377)
Hypersplenism responsible for clinical problems
Portal hypertension due to splenic vein thrombosis (p. 352)
'Hairy cell' leukaemia (p. 271)
Disorders in which splenectomy is sometimes indicated
Lymphomas (p. 278)
Auto-immune acquired haemolytic anaemia (p. 192)
Acute idiopathic thrombocytopenic purpura
Hereditary elliptocytosis (p. 184)
Thalassaemia major (p. 157)
Felty's syndrome (p. 229)
Disorders in which splenectomy is occasionally indicated
Myelofibrosis (p. 334)
Chronic lymphocytic leukaemia (p. 265)

Indications for splenectomy

The role of splenectomy in the management of individual disorders is considered in the discussion of each disorder, but for convenience, the indications for splenectomy are summarized in Table 13.4.

References and further reading

Banti, G. (1898) Splenomegalie mit Lebercirrhose. *Beitr. path. Anat.* **24**, 21.

Bowdler, A.J. (1983) Splenomegaly and hypersplenism. *Clin. Haemat.* **12**, 467.

Brady, R.O. (1969) Genetics and the sphingolipidoses. *Med. Clin. N. Amer.* **53**, 827.

Cartwright, G.E., Chung, H-L. & Chang, A. (1948) Studies on the pancytopenia of kala–azar. *Blood,* **3**, 249.

Christensen, B.E. (1973) Erythrocyte pooling and sequestration in enlarged spleens. Estimation of splenic erythrocyte and plasma volume in splenomegalic patients. *Scand. J. Haemat.* **10**, 106.

Christensen, B.E. (1975) Quantitative determination of splenic red blood cell destruction in patients with splenomegaly. *Scand. J. Haemat.* **14**, 295.

Crosby, W.H. (1963) Hyposplenism: an inquiry into normal functions of the spleen. *Ann. Rev. Med.* **14**, 349.

Dacie, J.V., Brain, M.C., Harrison, C.V. *et al.* (1969) Non-tropical idiopathic splenomegaly ('primary hypersplenism'): a review of ten cases and their relationship to malignant lymphomas. *Brit. J. Haemat.* **17**, 317.

Diamond, L.K. (1969) Splenectomy in childhood and the hazard of overwhelming infection. *Pediatrics,* **43**, 886.

Eraklis, A.J., Kevy, S.V., Diamond, L.K. *et al.* (1967) Hazard of overwhelming infection after splenectomy in childhood. *New Engl. J. Med.* **276**, 1225.

Erickson, W.D., Burgert, E.O., Jr & Lynn, H.B. (1968) The hazard of infection following splenectomy in children. *Am. J. Dis. Child.* **116**, 1.

Fakunle, Y.M. (1981) Tropical splenomegaly. *Clin. Haemat.* **10**, 963.

Gupta, P.S., Gupta, G.D. & Sharma, M.L. (1963) Veno-occlusive disease of the liver. *Brit. Med. J.* **1**, 1184.

Hirsh, J. & Dacie, J.V. (1966) Persistent post-splenectomy thrombocytosis and thrombo-embolism. *Brit. J. Haemat.* **12**, 44.

Islam, N. (1965) Splenic cysts. *Postgrad. Med. J.* **41**, 139.

Jandl, J.H., Files, N.M., Barnett, S.B. *et al.* (1965) Proliferative response of the spleen and liver to hemolysis. *J. Exp. Med.* **122**, 299.

Jandl, J.H. & Aster, R.H. (1967) Increased splenic pooling and pathogenesis of hypersplenism. *Am. J. Med. Sci.* **253**, 383.

Kampine, J.P., Brady, R.O., Kanfer, J.N. *et al.* (1967) Diagnosis of Gaucher's disease and Niemann–Pick disease with small samples of venous blood. *Science,* **155**, 86.

Lipson, R.L. Bayrd, E.D. & Watkins, C.H. (1959) The post-splenectomy blood picture. *Am. J. Clin. Path.* **32**, 526.

Lowdon, A.G.R., Stewart, R.H.M. & Walker, W. (1966) Risk of serious infection following splenectomy. *Brit. Med. J.* **1**, 446.

McBride, J.A., Dacie, J.V. & Shapley, R. (1968) The effect of splenectomy on the leucocyte count. *Brit. J. Haemat.* **14**, 225.

McFadzean, A.J.S. Todd, D. & Tsang, K.D. (1958) Observations on the anaemia of cryptogenic splenomegaly. II. Expansion of the plasma volume. *Blood,* **13**, 524.

McIntyre, O.R. & Ebaugh, F.G. (1967) Palpable spleens in college freshmen. *Ann. Int. Med.* **66**, 301.

Marsden, P.D. & Hamilton, P.J.S. (1969) Splenomegaly in the tropics. *Brit. Med. J.* **1**, 99.

Marsh, G.W. & Stewart, J.S. (1970) Splenic function in adult coeliac disease. *Brit. J. Haemat.* **19**, 445.

Overturf, G.D., Field, R. & Edmonds, R. (1979) Death from type 6 pneumococcal septicemia in a vaccinated child with sickle-cell disease. *New Engl. J. Med.* **300**, 143.

Penny, R., Rozenberg, M.G. & Firkin, B.G. (1966) The splenic platelet pool. *Blood,* **27**, 1.

Peters, A.M. (1983) Splenic blood flow and blood cell kinetics. *Clin. Haemat.* **12**, 421.

Pettit, J.E. (1977) Spleen function. *Clin. Haemat.* **6**, 639.

Pitney, W.R. (1968) The tropical splenomegaly syndrome. *Trans. R. Soc. Trop. Med. Hygiene,* **62**, 717.

Pitney, W.R., Pryor, D.S. & Tait Smith, A. (1968) Morphological observations on livers and spleens of patients with tropical splenomegaly in New Guinea. *J. Path. Bact.* **95**, 417.

Pryor, D.S. (1967a) Tropical splenomegaly in New Guinea. *Quart. J. Med.* **36**, 321.

Pryor, D.S. (1967b) The mechanism of anaemia in tropical splenomegaly. *Quart. J. Med.* **36**, 337.

Richmond, J., Donaldson, G.W.K., Williams, R. *et al.* (1967) Haematological effects of the idiopathic splenomegaly seen in Uganda. *Brit. J. Haemat.* **13**, 348.

Rivero, S.J., Alber, M. & Alcarcon-Segovia, D. (1979) Splenectomy for hemocytopenia in systemic lupus erythematosus. *Arch. Int. Med.* **139**, 773.

Rosenbaum, D.L., Murphy, G.W. & Swisher, S.N. (1966) Haemodynamic studies of the portal circulation in myeloid metaplasia. *Am. J. Med.* **41**, 360.

Shaldon, S. & Sherlock, S. (1962) Portal hypertension in the myeloproliferative syndrome and the reticuloses. *Am. J. Med.* **32**, 758.

Sherlock, S. (1985) *Diseases of the Liver and Biliary System,* 7th Ed., Blackwell Scientific Publications, Oxford.

Spivak, J.L. (1977) Felty's syndrome: an analytic review. *Johns Hopk. Med. J.* **141**, 156.

Stuvier, P.C., Ziegler, J.L., Wood, J.B. *et al.* (1971) Clinical trial of malaria prophylaxis in tropical splenomegaly syndrome. *Brit. Med. J.* **1**, 426.

Szur, L., Marsh, G.W. & Pettit, J.E. (1972) Studies of splenic function by means of radioisotope-labelled red cells. *Brit. J. Haemat.* **23**, Suppl., 183.

Weiss, L. (1983) The red pulp of the spleen: structural basis of blood flow. *Clin. Haemat.* **12**, 375.

Weissman, I.L., Warnke, R., Butcher, E.C. *et al.* (1978) The lymphoid system. Its normal architecture and potential for understanding the system through the study of the lymphoproliferative diseases. *Human Pathol.* **9**, 25.

Wennberg, E. & Weiss, L. (1969) The structure of the spleen and hemolysis. *Ann. Rev. Med.* **20**, 29.

Whitaker, A.N. (1969) Infection and the spleen: association between hyposplenism, pneumococcal sepsis and disseminated intravascular coagulation. *Med. J. Austr.* **1**, 1213.

Williams, R., Parsonson, A, Somers, K. *et al.* (1966) Portal hypertension in tropical splenomegaly. *Lancet,* **i**, 329.

Chapter 14
The Haemorrhagic Disorders: Capillary and Platelet Defects

The haemorrhagic disorders are a group of disorders of widely differing aetiology, which have in common an abnormal tendency to bleed due to a defect in the mechanism of haemostasis.

Clinical features. Clinically, the haemorrhagic disorders are characterized by: (a) spontaneous bleeding into the skin, mucous membranes and internal tissues; (b) excessive or prolonged bleeding following trauma or surgery; and (c) bleeding from more than one site. The bleeding varies in severity. In some disorders, it is mild and limited to the skin and is therefore of nuisance value only; in other disorders, uncontrollable bleeding from mucous membranes or bleeding into internal organs may threaten life.

Pathogenesis. There are three major components of the normal haemostatic mechanism—the *vascular, platelet,* and *coagulation components*—which act together in a co-ordinated fashion to arrest bleeding. A breakdown in the normal haemostatic mechanism, and thus an abnormal tendency to bleed, may result from a defect in any one of these three components. Bleeding is especially liable to occur when more than one component is defective. It should be noted that bleeding may arise from either quantitative (deficiency) or qualitative (functional) defects.

In this chapter, haemorrhagic disorders due to vascular and platelet abnormalities are discussed. Coagulation defects are discussed in the next chapter.

The normal haemostatic mechanism

The functions of the normal haemostatic process are to prevent blood loss from intact vessels and to arrest bleeding from injured vessels. Relatively little is known about the mechanism by which blood loss is prevented from intact vessels; however, both the structural integrity of the vessels and the presence of adequate numbers of normal viable platelets are necessary for this function. The precise nature of the functional support of the endothelium provided by platelets is not known, but there is evidence for structural changes in the vessel wall as a consequence of thrombocytopenia both in experimental animals (Kitchens & Weiss 1975), and in humans (Kitchens & Pendergast 1986). Although there has been controversy surrounding the question, there appear to be growth factors within platelets which

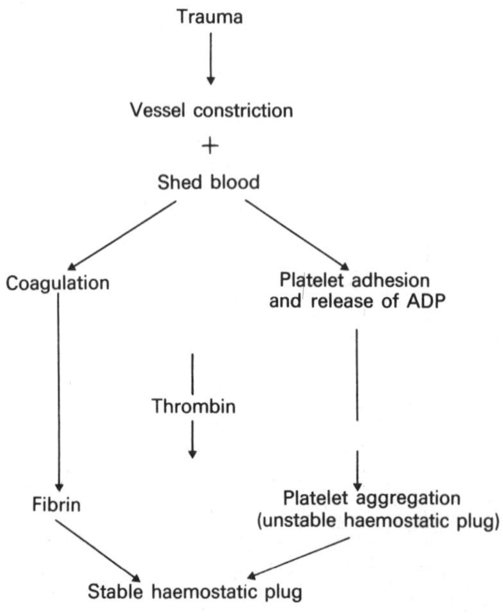

Fig. 14.1. *Normal haemostasis.*

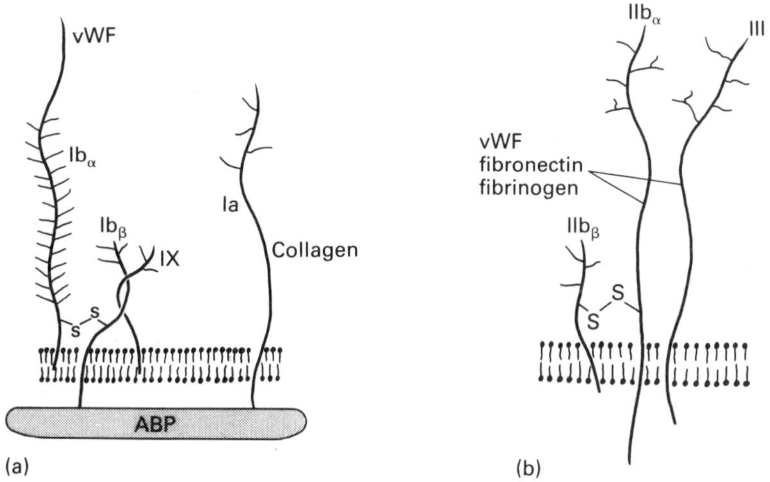

Fig. 14.2. *Diagrammatic representation of the structures of the human platelet glycoprotein: (a) Ib complex and Ia; and (b) IIb/IIIa complex. vWF = von Willebrand factor; ABP = actin-binding protein (from Chesterman & Berndt 1986, with permission of the authors and publishers).*

may be involved in stimulating endothelial repair processes (Miyazono *et al.* 1987).

A simplified scheme of normal haemostasis is shown in Fig. 14.1. Immediately after injury the damaged blood vessel undergoes a temporary reflex nervous vasoconstriction, resulting in slowing of blood flow. Blood escapes into the tissues and so increases the tissue tension, with further narrowing of the vessels (see extravascular factors below). The escaping blood comes in contact with the damaged vessel wall and the extravascular tissues, and the processes of platelet adhesion, platelet aggregation, and blood coagulation are initiated. The response to an endothelial breach is extremely rapid; the time available for a platelet to leave the blood flow and react to the subendothelium may be measured in milliseconds.

Platelet adhesion to subendothelium has two definable components, each with its own functional determinants (reviewed by Chesterman & Berndt 1986). The initial *contact adhesion* is to types I and III collagen fibrils and to the elastin-associated collagenous microfibrils in subendothelium. At high shear flow (> 800 sec^{-1}) in the capillary bed, platelet adhesion to these subendothelial components depends on the plasma protein, von Willebrand factor (factor VIII-related antigen) which forms a bridge to the platelet membrane receptor, glycoprotein Ib complex (Fig. 14.2). In larger vessels, e.g. the aorta, platelet adhesion is independent of von Willebrand factor and probably involves the direct adhesion of platelets to collagen fibrils. This may be via the platelet membrane glycoprotein IIb/IIIa complex and glycoprotein Ia (see Fig. 14.2).

Platelet contact is closely followed by a process of *spreading adhesion* dependent on at least three components: (a) adhesive proteins such as von Willebrand factor and/or fibronectin incorporated in the subendothelial matrix; (b) divalent cations, calcium or magnesium; and (c) the glycoprotein IIb/IIIa complex in the platelet membrane.

Release of platelet components (Fig. 14.3) and the recruitment of further platelets occur simultaneously, but can be conveniently considered as two distinct events. Both are stimulated by the

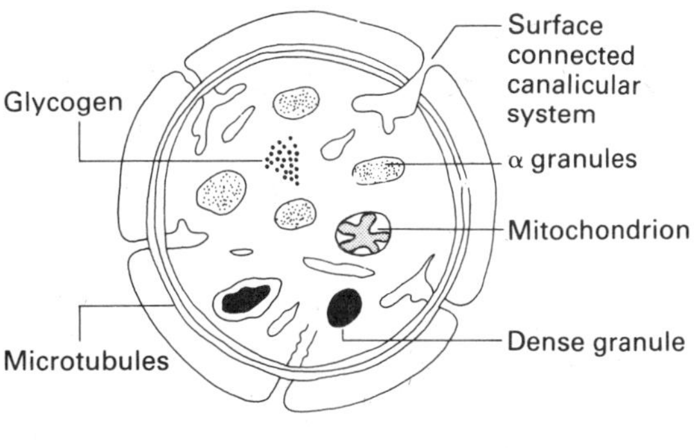

Fig. 14.3. *Ultrastructural features of the platelet. Granule contents either fuse with the membrane or with the surface-connected open canalicular system before being extruded from the cell.*

adhesion process to collagen and by a number of other agonists made available in the vicinity of tissue injury, particularly adenosine diphosphate (ADP) and thrombin, and, in some situations, platelet activating factor (PAF) derived from inflammatory cells. There are also common internal pathways within the platelet which initiate the processes of release and aggregation. The *signal transduction* of receptor occupation involves the hydrolysis of phospho-inositol by phospholipase C; hydrolysis of phosphatidylcholine and phosphatidylethanolamine by phospholipase A, with release of arachidonic acid; the activation of protein kinase C; and the ultimate increase of cytosol [Ca^{++}] released from the dense tubular system and by influx from the outside (reviewed by Haslam 1987).

Aggregation is dependent, firstly, on shape change involving the loss of the platelet discoid configuration and the formation of pseudopods to increase the surface area and the likelihood of contact. (Fig. 14.4). Shape change and the later release process depend on contraction of actin–myosin in the periphery of the platelet. Associated conformational changes to the membrane glycoprotein IIb/IIIa complex expose fibrinogen receptors on the platelet surface, enabling platelet bridging to take place via fibrinogen molecules, probably being enchanced by von Willebrand factor and fibronectin. The *release* of dense granule components, ADP, calcium, and serotonin, combined with the synthesis and release (see Fig. 14.5) of thromboxane A_2 (TXA_2) from arachidonic acid, provides a powerful amplification feedback to aggregate platelets in the vicinity. The release is achieved by a combination of fusion and extrusion of granules.

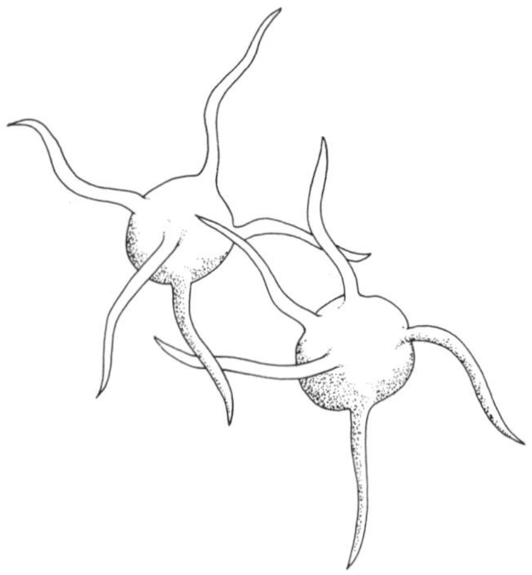

Fig. 14.4. *Shape change and aggregation of platelets. Features of activation include the change to spherical shape, formation of pseudopodia, centralization of granules, and close contact with contiguous platelets.*

Alpha granule proteins, factor V, fibrinogen, von Willebrand factor, and thrombospondin, released simultaneously, may contribute further to the

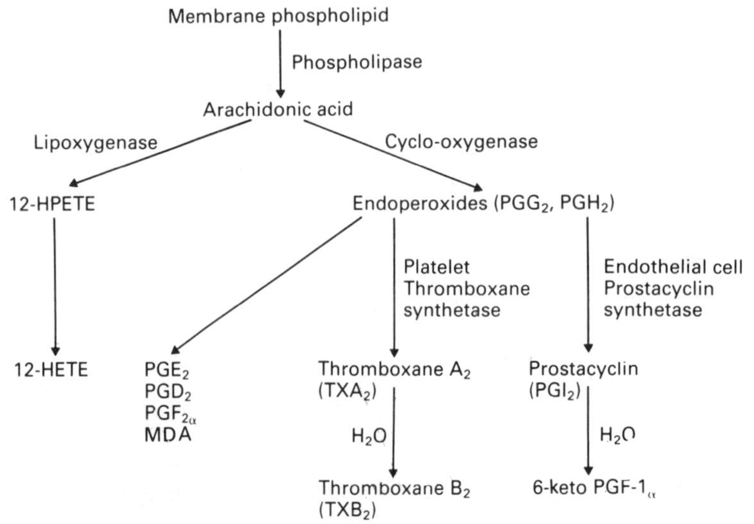

Fig. 14.5. *Arachidonic acid metabolism in platelets and vascular endothelium. Thromboxane A_2 and prostacyclin are short-lived intermediates whose end-products, thromboxane B_2 and 6-keto-prostaglandin $F_{1\alpha}$, are stable and may be measured by radio-immunoassay. HPETE = hydroperoxyeicosatetranoic acid; HETE = hydroxyeicosatetranoic acid; MDA = malondialdehyde.*

process by raising their local concentration. Other alpha granule proteins and arachidonate products produced simultaneously are involved in repair processes following injury. Many alpha granule components are well characterized and include polypeptides such as the beta-thromboglobulin family (chemotaxis and possibly mitogenesis), platelet factor 4 (antiheparin, chemotaxis) and platelet-derived growth factor (chemotaxis, mitogenesis, and vaso-activity). Lipid-derived mediators such as 12-hydroxyeicosatetranoic acid (12-HETE), a lipoxgenase product of released membrane arachidonic acid have powerful chemotactic activity for neutrophils (reviewed by Chesterman & Berndt 1986). Lyzosomal enzymes, released separately, include glucuronidase, *n*-acetyl glucosaminidase, elastase, heparinitase, and collagenase. These enzymes may reach local concentrations high enough to disrupt subendothelial basement membrane and internal elastic lamina.

In addition, in the process of aggregation, the platelet membrane exposes a number of receptor sites for coagulation components making a 'solid phase' system for the coagulation mechanism, in part protected from inhibitors. The negatively charged phospholipid component that enhances coagulation enzyme systems, previously termed 'platelet factor 3', lies on the inner aspect of the platelet membrane but is exposed during activation, providing a surface for calcium and activated coagulation factor complexes. Factor V is released from alpha granules, activated by protease, and binds to specific sites on the platelet membrane. Membrane-bound factor Va becomes a receptor for activated factor X, accelerating the activation of prothrombin to thrombin some 300 000-fold.

The relative importance of various factors concerned with haemostasis varies with the size of the vessel involved. In small arterioles and venules, haemostasis depends mainly on vessel constriction and on a platelet plug. In larger vessels, although constriction is important in limiting the initial loss of blood, the formation of the haemostatic plug to seal the defect in the vessel plays the major role.

Finally, *limitation* of the processes of platelet adhesion and activation is obviously of importance in maintaining blood fluidity and vascular patency. The aggregating compounds have extremely short survival times due to hydrolysis (TXA_2), enzymatic degradation (ATP and ADP), cellular uptake (serotonin), and specific inhibitors (antithrombin). In addition, vascular endothelial responses to local platelet activation include the release of specific platelet inhibitory substances, in particular prostacyclin, a cyclo-oxygenase product of arachidonic acid (Fig. 14.5). These interactions are discussed in more detail in Chapter 16 (p. 457). The *plasma coagulation* system is described in Chapter 15.

Fate of the haemostatic plug

The platelets in the haemostatic plug gradually undergo autolysis and are replaced by fibrin, so that after 24–48 hours the haemostatic plug has been transformed into a dense fibrin mass. This is then gradually digested by the *fibrinolytic enzyme system* (see Chapter 15), and the defect in the vessel wall then becomes covered with endothelial cells.

Extravascular factors

Haemostasis is also influenced by extravascular factors, namely tissue tension and the support of the vessels, which play an important subsidiary role, particularly in venous bleeding. In tissues with a relatively high tissue tension, the natural tension, together with the increased tension caused by the mass of escaped blood, compresses these damaged vessels and lessens blood loss. When vessels are contained in loose tissue and are poorly supported, bleeding tends to continue. Thus, vessels in the nasal septum, which have a rigid unyielding septum on one side and no support on the other, are particularly liable to bleed. Vessels in the gastro-intestinal mucosa, in the bladder, and in the pelvis of the kidney are not well supported; bleeding from these sites occurs relatively easily after slight trauma and in disorders of the haemostatic mechanism, and can be difficult to control. In other areas where the tissue tension is low, e.g. in the subcutaneous tissues of the scrotum and about the orbit, mild trauma may result in extensive haematoma formation.

Haemorrhagic disorders due to capillary defects: non-thrombocytopenic purpura

Vascular defects are a common cause of bleeding disorders seen in clinical practice. However, it is now recognized that in a number of the acquired vascular haemorrhagic disorders qualitative platelet defects may co-exist and contribute.

Most cases of bleeding due to a vascular defect alone are not severe, and frequently the bleeding is mainly or wholly into the skin, causing petechiae or ecchymoses, or both. Petechiae may be rather pale and tend to be confluent; ecchymoses are usually small. In some disorders there is bleeding from mucous membranes, but only rarely is there bleeding into muscles and internal organs. Excess bleeding from wounds tends to occur at once, usually persists for less than 48 hours, and rarely recurs.

In many of these conditions, the standard screening tests used in the investigation of patients with a bleeding disorder show little or no abnormality. The bleeding time is sometimes prolonged, and the tourniquet test may be positive (for a description of these tests see pp. 376–7). However, in many cases either one or both are normal. When they are abnormal, and especially when the bleeding time is prolonged, bleeding is likely to be more severe, particularly following trauma and with surgery. The platelet count, the one-stage prothrombin time, and the activated partial thromboplastin time are typically normal. However, in certain disorders, e.g. infection and uraemia, associated thrombocytopenia may contribute to bleeding. In addition, in those disorders with platelet functional defects (Table 14.1), especially uraemia and dysproteinaemia, there are abnormalities in the tests of platelet adhesion or aggregation.

The causes of haemorrhagic disorders due to vascular defects are listed in Table 14.1.

Table 14.1. *Haemorrhagic disorders due to vascular defects*

Acquired
Simple easy bruising ('devil's pinches')*
Senile purpura
The symptomatic vascular (non-thrombocytopenic) purpuras
Infections
Drugs
Uraemia*
Cushing's disease and adrenocorticosteroid administration
Scurvy*
Dysproteinaemias*—cryoglobulinaemia, benign purpura hyperglobulinaemia, macroglobulinaemia, multiple myeloma
Henoch–Schöenlein syndrome (anaphylactoid purpura)
Miscellaneous disorders
Orthostatic purpuras
Mechanical purpura
Fat embolism
Auto-erythrocyte sensitization
Systemic disorders—collagen disease, especially polyarteritis nodosa, amyloidosis, allergy
Congenital
Hereditary haemorrhagic telangiectasis (Osler–Rendu–Weber disease)
Ehlers–Danlos disease

*Abnormalities of platelet function may contribute to the bleeding tendency in these disorders.

Acquired haemorrhagic vascular disorders

Simple easy bruising (purpura simplex)

Simple easy bruising is a benign disorder which occurs predominantly in otherwise healthy women. Onset is often during adolescence or early adult life.

The disorder is relatively common. It is characterized by the occurrence of circumscribed bruises, either on minor trauma or without obvious cause ('devil's pinches'). They are most often seen on the legs and trunk. The bruises are occasionally preceded by pain due to the rupture of a small blood vessel. Although abnormalities are not found in tests of blood coagulation and the bleeding time is usually normal, the tourniquet test occasionally gives a weakly positive result. More extensive investigations of platelet function by one group revealed mild abnormalities in a proportion of these patients. Lackner & Karpatkin (1975) found a high incidence of impaired platelet aggregation with adrenaline and some impairment with ADP and connective tissue. They also detected platelet antibodies in a proportion of the patients and suggested that the 'easy bruising' syndrome may include a proportion of patients with abnormal platelet function on an immune basis. This concept is not generally held, but has not been disproven.

Simple easy bruising is of importance only because of its cosmetic significance and because it may give rise to suspicion of a serious blood disorder. It is probably the most common cause of referral of patients for diagnosis and assessment of unexplained skin bruising. Diagnosis is made on the clinical features and by the exclusion of other causes of purpura. A history of aspirin ingestion should be sought, as it may cause similar bruising. There is no effective treatment; in particular, corticosteroids and other hormones are of no benefit and should be avoided. The patient should be reassured and advised to avoid aspirin when possible. The disorder does not cause excessive bleeding at operation.

Senile purpura (involutional purpura)

Senile (involutional) purpura is a form of purpura that occurs commonly in elderly subjects, mainly on the extensor aspect of the forearms and hands. It occurs equally in males and females over the age of 60 years. Tattersall & Seville (1950) found an incidence of 2 per cent in the seventh decade, increasing progressively to 25 per cent in the tenth decade. The lesions occur on the extensor surface and radial border of the forearm and on the back of the hand, but they do not extend onto the fingers. They do not occur on any other parts of the body, although they are occasionally seen on the face in relation to spectacle frames, either across the bridge of the nose or along the side pieces. The purpuric areas are large (1–4 cm in diameter), irregular, dark purple, and have a clear-cut margin. The skin in the affected areas is inelastic, thin, smooth, pigmented, and may show non-pigmented scars; hair is scanty or absent. The purpuric lesions last for varying periods, ranging from a few days to many weeks. The tourniquet test is negative. The lesions are commonly due to minor trauma. There is no effective treatment; in particular, corticosteroids are of no value and indeed may aggravate the disorder and retard resolution of the lesions.

Pathogenesis. Histological section of the skin in affected areas shows marked atrophy of collagen; this results in the skin being freely moveable over the deeper tissues. The purpuric lesions are easily induced by a shearing strain to the skin, which tears the vessels passing to the skin because of the excessive mobility of the skin on the subcutaneous tissues. Once the vessels are ruptured, abnormal spread of the blood is permitted by the atrophied collagen fibres. The long persistence of the lesion is due to slow resorption of the blood because of impairment of the normal phagocytic response to extravasated blood (Schuster & Scarborough 1961).

Purpura similar in distribution and type to that of involutional purpura may occur in patients with *rheumatoid arthritis*. The assciation may be related to the duration of rheumatoid disease. Corticosteroid therapy, however, is likely to contribute in some patients.

The symptomatic vascular (non-thrombocytopenic) purpuras

The term symptomatic vascular purpura is used to describe the purpura occurring in association with a number of disorders, in which the essential lesion is damage to the capillary endothelium resulting in increased capillary fragility or permeability.

Diagnosis is, in general, made on clinical features, especially the presence of the causative disorder. The platelet count is typically normal, although in some disorders an associated thrombocytopenia may occur. The tourniquet test is commonly, but by no means constantly, positive. The bleeding time is usually normal, but is occasionally prolonged. Symptomatic purpura is a common cause of purpura seen in clinical practice.

INFECTIONS

Purpura may occur with many infections, especially severe infections, but it occurs more constantly in some. These include *typhoid fever, subacute bacterial endocarditis, meningococcal septicaemia, Gram-negative septicaemia,* and *smallpox*. The purpura is generally considered to be due to toxic damage to the capillary endothelium. However, associated thrombocytopenia, sometimes severe, may be present, especially in septicaemia (p. 386). Intravascular coagulation with a resulting haemostatic defect may also occasionally be a contributing factor (p. 442). Purpura also occurs as an occasional or rare complication of certain other infections; these include *scarlet fever, chickenpox, rubella, measles, tuberculosis,* and *infectious mononucleosis*. In these disorders, thrombocytopenia is an occasional finding, although the purpura usually represents an allergic response to the infection, not related to its severity. The purpura may occur either in the acute stage of the infection or during the period of convalescence.

Occasionally, purpura is the first manifestation of an occult infection in which neither fever nor local signs of infection are present. This is particularly so in children, in whom search for infection, e.g. of the renal tract, should always be carried out in any case of unexplained non-thrombocytopenic pupura.

DRUGS

Petechiae and ecchymoses are relatively uncommon manifestations of drug and chemical toxicity, other types of skin rash, particularly erythematous, urticarial, and morbilliform rashes, being more common. However, a number of drugs have been recorded as causing purpura, occasionally with mucous membrane bleeding; they include chlorothiazide, frusemide, penicillin, streptomycin, sulphonamides, carbromal, phenacetin, aspirin, salicylates, amidopyrine, phenylbutazone, hydantoin, barbiturates, chloral hydrate, iodides, gold, arsenic, bismuth, mercury, antihistamines, quinine, quinidine, thiouracils, oestrogens, insulin, isoniazid, chlorpromazine, and trinitrin. The development of purpura is due to idiosyncrasy of the patient to the drug, and may be a consequence of specific antibodies to vascular components or of the formation of immune complexes with secondary endothelial damage. The purpura usually clears within a few days to a week of stopping the drug, but pigmentation, when associated, may last up to a month or more. The purpura commonly recurs if the drug is re-administered. Some of the drugs listed above may also cause thrombocytopenic purpura (see Table 14.4, p. 388).

URAEMIA

A bleeding tendency is not uncommon in uraemia and is occasionally the first clinical manifestation; in general bleeding occurs only with marked nitrogen retention. Epistaxis is the most frequent symptom, but bleeding into the skin, from the gastrointestinal tract and renal tract, may also occur. In the past, the primary defect was thought to be mainly in the capillary endothelium, but recent studies have shown that a number of abnormalities in platelet function are commonly present. Further, the low haematocrit associated with chronic renal failure appears to play a significant role. Thrombocytopenia may contribute in some cases.

Abnormalities in platelet function include defective aggregation to adenosine disphosphate (ADP), collagen, and adrenaline; decreased platelet retention in glass bead columns; reduction in thromboxane A_2 synthesis; and decreased availability of platelet factor III. In some cases, these abnormalities are improved by dialysis (Stewart & Castaldi 1967). The responsible factor is not urea but guanidinosuccinic acid (Horowitz *et al.* 1970) and phenol acetic acid (Rabiner & Molinas 1970) have both been implicated. Associated increase in prostacyclin production by the vascular endothelium may compound platelet dysfunction (Remuzzi *et al.* 1978), and this may be due to a circulating factor (Defreyn *et al.* 1980).

Von Willebrand factor activity and factor VIII have been reported to be abnormal in chronic renal failure, but the results have been inconsistent and, for the most part, functional defects have not been demonstrated. Finally, two studies (Livio *et al.* 1982, Fernandez *et al.* 1985) have shown a striking relationship between severity of the anaemia and degree of haemostatic defect in these patients. The mechanism is not clear.

Bleeding in uraemia is of particular clinical importance in patients in whom renal biopsy or surgery is contemplated. Before these procedures are performed in a patient with raised serum creatinine, skin bleeding time and platelet count should be performed. A prolonged bleeding time is the best clinical correlate, and the following measures should be undertaken if an abnormality is detected. Thrombocytopenia should be corrected by a platelet transfusion. The haematocrit should be increased to greater than 26 per cent by red cell transfusion (Fernandez *et al.* 1985). Dialysis may also improve the haemostatic defect.

Two somewhat empirical approaches have been reported to shorten transiently the bleeding time. These are infusion of 10 units cryoprecipitate (Janson *et al.* 1980) and intravenous infusion of desamino arginine vasopressin (DDAVP) (Mannucci *et al.* 1983). Subsequently, a conjugated oestrogen preparation, Premarin (10 mg daily), was shown to reduce the bleeding time in six uraemic patients (Liu *et al.* 1984). There was no improvement in platelet aggregation tests, nor increase in plasma von Willebrand factor activity in these patients. These treatment options are successful in some patients and not in others, suggesting a multifactorial defect; in practice, it may be necessary to combine therapy, monitoring the skin bleeding time meanwhile.

CUSHING'S DISEASE AND CORTICOSTEROID ADMINISTRATION

Ecchymoses are not uncommon in Cushing's disease, and are sometimes the presenting manifestation; they may be slow to disappear. The administration of adrenocortical steroids may be accompanied by ecchymoses, easy bruising on minor trauma, and sometimes petechiae. These haemorrhagic skin phenomena occur particularly in women about the menopause. The disorder appears to be due to a vascular defect and is associated with atrophy of collagen; the platelet count and the tests of coagulation are normal. The tourniquet test is positive in some cases. Cessation of steroid administration results in disappearance of the haemorrhagic skin manifestations.

SCURVY

Haemorrhage is usual in scurvy, and is the major feature of adult scurvy. It is primarily due to the increased capillary fragility which results from defective formation of the intercellular substance of the capillary wall. In addition, a defect of platelet function may be a contributing factor. The skin is the most common site of haemorrhage, which occurs as both petechiae and ecchymoses of varying size. Haemorrhages may occur anywhere in the skin, but are particularly common in the legs and at the site of trauma; petechiae are commonly perifollicular. Haemorrhage into muscle also occurs, resulting in areas of brawny induration and tenderness. Less common manifestations are epistaxis and conjunctival and retinal haemorrhage; in severe cases, haematemesis, melaena, haematuria, and cerebral haemorrhage may occur. The tourniquet test is usually, but not invariably, positive. The anaemia of survey is described elsewhere (p. 113).

The diagnosis is suggested by a history of inadequate dietary intake and by the other manifestations of scurvy when present; it is confirmed by the rapid relief of symptoms following adequate vitamin C administration, the purpura commencing to fade within 24–48 hours. Estimation of the ascorbic acid content of white cells and the ascorbic acid saturation test may be used to confirm the diagnosis. Other manifestations of scurvy include follicular hyperkeratosis, particularly on the anterior aspects of the thighs and the ulnar border of the forearms, swelling and congestion of the gums, especially at the site of dental caries, and, in children, bone tenderness and swelling of the extremities. However, the absence of these signs does not exclude the diagnosis of scurvy in the patient who presents with skin haemorrhage.

In adults, scurvy is most often seen in elderly people, particularly men, who live alone and eat inadequate meals, and in chronic alcoholics. In children, it is most often seen in infants on artificial feeding which is not supplemented by vitamin C; thus it may occur in all social groups.

DYSPROTEINAEMIA

Bleeding may be present in certain disorders characterized by an abnormality of the plasma proteins—the dysproteinaemias. These are cryoglobulinaemia, hyperglobulinaemia, macroglobulinaemia (p. 310), and multiple myeloma (p. 299). The pathogenesis of the bleeding is not completely understood; in some cases, interference with platelet function is the result of coating of the platelet outer membrane by protein. In many cases, the abnormal protein results in coagulation defects. Increased blood viscosity may cause sludging and increased intracapillary pressure. Thus, troublesome bleeding may be controlled, at least in part, by a reduction in the level of plasma proteins, either by plasmapheresis or specific chemotherapy.

Cryoglobulinaemia. Cryoglobulins are abnormal globulins which have the property of precipitating or gelling in the cold. Cryoglobulinaemia is of rare occurrence and is nearly always secondary to some underlying disorder, the most common being multiple myeloma or macroglobulinaemia; others include malignant lymphomas and leukaemia. In rheumatoid arthritis and systemic lupus erythematosus, immune complexes may behave as cryoglobulins. The purpura of cryoglobulinaemia occurs after exposure to cold and may be accompanied by Raynaud's phenomenon. There is sometimes associated urticaria and pruritus. In some cases, the diagnosis is suggested by 'clotting' of the blood in the syringe. In suspected cases, blood should be taken into a warmed syringe and allowed to clot in a water bath at 37°C. The separated serum is then cooled to 4°C; serum containing cryoglobulin forms a gel at 4°C but liquefies again when heated to 37°C.

Benign purpura hyperglobulinaemia. This is a rare disorder, described by Waldenström (1952) and characterized clinically by the appearance at irregular intervals of petechiae, which occur most commonly on the legs, and sometimes follow exertion or an infection. Purpura also tends to occur under areas of pressure. The attacks may be preceded by a feeling of tenderness or swelling in the legs. The disorder is seen mainly in women. Pigmentation commonly develops after a number of attacks. There are usually no positive physical findings other than the purpura and pigmentation, but in some cases there is moderate lymph node enlargement and hepatosplenomegaly, or associated collagen disorders (Lee & Miotti 1975). The tourniquet test is usually strongly positive. A moderate normochromic normocytic anaemia is usual, and the sedimentation rate is markedly increased. There is a polyclonal increase in serum immunoglobulins, predominantly IgG, and the histology of the lesions shows evidence of vasculitis. While plasmapheresis may be of value in the acute event, there is no satisfactory long-term therapy.

THE HENOCH-SCHÖNLEIN SYNDROME (ANAPHYLACTOID PURPURA)

This disorder is thought to be a hypersensitivity reaction, allied to acute glomerulonephritis and rheumatic fever. The fundamental disturbance is a widespread acute inflammatory reaction of the capillaries and small arterioles, resulting in increased vascular permeability and thus in exudation and haemorrhage into the tissues. Bacterial hypersensitivity is the most common cause, but occasional cases result from food and drug hypersensitivity. Foods that have caused anaphylactoid purpura include milk, eggs, tomatoes, strawberries, plums, crab, fish, pork, beans, and peaches. Rare cases following insect bites and smallpox vaccination have been recorded. In some cases, there is no obvious cause. The aetiology is not established, although antigenic stimulus by bacteria or food may produce an IgA immune complex-mediated disease. IgA and fibrin deposition can be demonstrated in biopsy specimens from the kidney, and IgA and C3 have been demonstrated in blood vessels from both involved and adjacent normal skin.

Clinical features

The disorder may occur at all ages, but most cases are seen in childhood and adolescence. Males are affected more often than females. There is commonly a history of an upper respiratory tract infection with a sore throat 1–3 weeks before the onset, and in such cases a group A beta-haemolytic streptococcus may be isolated from the throat and the antistreptolysin O titre may be raised; occasionally, there is an infective focus at some other site, e.g. skin.

There are four main clinical features—a purpuric rash, joint, abdominal, and renal manifestations; these usually occur in combination, but occasionally only one is present. Most cases present with purpura which is followed shortly by joint and abdominal symptoms. However, sometimes joint or abdominal symptoms first bring the disorder to notice, which may result in diagnostic difficulty, especially in the occasional case in which skin lesions do not develop.

Purpuric rash. The rash is typically of large and often confluent haemorrhagic macules, but smaller petechial purpuric spots also occur (Fig. 14.6). Initially, the lesions may appear as raised urticarial areas, but within hours they alter to the typical purpuric lesions. They occur most commonly on the buttocks, on the backs of the elbows and extensor surfaces of the arms, and on the extensor surfaces of the lower leg, the ankle, and foot; they are usually bilateral. They may also appear on the face, but the trunk is generally spared. They occur in recurrent crops which progressively fade over about two weeks. Occasionally, frankly haemorrhagic lesions become bullous and may progress to local necrosis.

The *abdominal manifestations* are due to mural vasculitis and the extravasation of serosanguinous fluid into the wall of the intestine. Colicky abdominal pain is common; it may be accompanied by vomiting, diarrhoea, and the passage of bright red blood. The pain varies in severity from mild cramps to severe pain simulating an acute abdominal emergency; most often it is central. Rarely, perforation or intussusception occurs.

Joint involvement with polyarthritis is common; occasionally only one joint is affected. The involvement ranges from mild pain without objective findings to painful swelling of the joints with limitation of movement. The swelling is mainly peri-articular, effusion into the joint being unusual; it lasts only a few days, and resolves without damage. The joints most often affected are the knees and ankles, less commonly the wrists, elbows, and hips. It is not uncommon for swelling to recur, either in the same or other joints. A mild *pyrexia* is sometimes present, but usually lasts only a few days and seldom longer than a week.

Renal manifestations. Haematuria, either macroscopic or microscopic, is common and is frequently accompanied by albuminuria and the presence of casts. Recovery of the renal lesion is usual, but signs not infrequently persist for many months or years; follow-up shows the development of chronic glomerulonephritis in some cases (probably 5–10 per cent). Rarely, an acute rapidly fatal renal insufficiency develops.

Other manifestations. Localized areas of oedema, most commonly seen on the scalp, the dorsum of the hand, and around the eyes, sometimes unilaterally, are relatively common. Pleurisy, pericarditis,

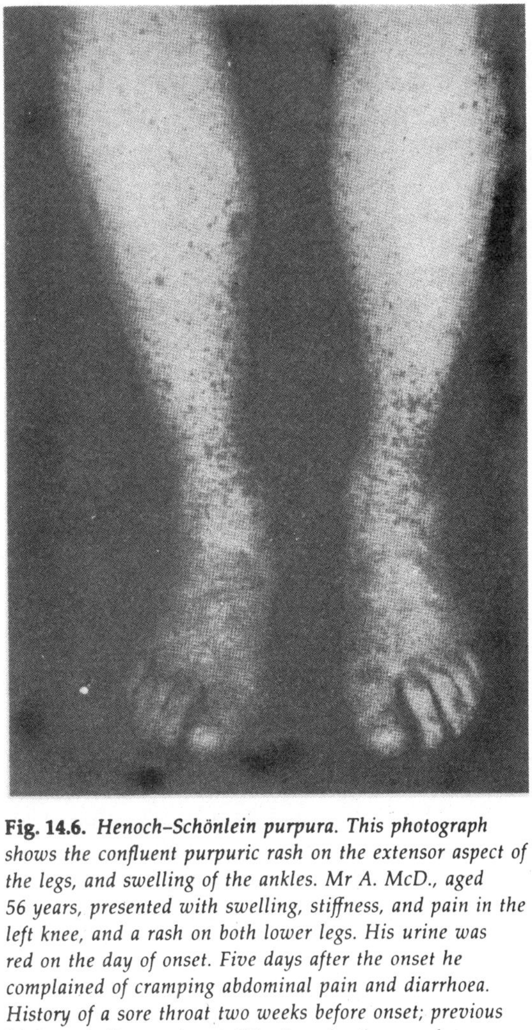

Fig. 14.6. *Henoch–Schönlein purpura. This photograph shows the confluent purpuric rash on the extensor aspect of the legs, and swelling of the ankles. Mr A. McD., aged 56 years, presented with swelling, stiffness, and pain in the left knee, and a rash on both lower legs. His urine was red on the day of onset. Five days after the onset he complained of cramping abdominal pain and diarrhoea. History of a sore throat two weeks before onset; previous history of allergy to penicillin. Examination—rash on exterior surfaces of both legs and buttocks, swelling of both ankles. Tourniquet test negative. Urine—moderate number of red cells, no casts, no albumin. Throat swab produced on culture a group A beta-haemolytic streptococcus. Antistreptolysin titre 1/625.*

and iritis occur occasionally. Cerebral haemorrhage is a rare complication.

Blood picture

There are no significant abnormalities other than a moderate polymorph leucocytosis and occasionally a mild eosinophilia. The sedimentation rate is usually moderately increased, but it may be normal. The platelet count, bleeding time, and coagulation screening tests are normal. The tourniquet test is moderately positive in about 25 per cent of cases. As indicated above, biopsy specimens from kidney or clinically involved skin show IgA, fibrin and C3 deposition.

Course and prognosis

The immediate prognosis is excellent, except for those rare cases with intestinal perforation, intussusception, acute renal failure, or cerebral haemorrhage. Typically, recurrences of the clinical manifestations occur over a varying period lasting from a week to several months, with an average of about one month; occasionally, they recur for many months or even a year or longer. In the 5–10 per cent of cases that develop chronic glomerulonephritis, the prognosis is that of the renal lesion.

Treatment

The disease is usually self-limiting, and treatment is therefore mainly symptomatic to control the joint manifestations and abdominal pain. The administration of antihistamines may lessen exudation.

Allen *et al.* (1960) gave an excellent account of the results of corticosteroid treatment. They found that corticosteroids were not useful in the management of the skin manifestations, although they improved painful joint involvement or soft tissue swelling and provided uniform relief of scalp oedema. They found that corticosteroids in adequate dosage usually relieved abdominal pain within 24 hours; if this does not occur, a fixed lesion of the bowel should be suspected. Gastrointestinal bleeding may be well controlled by the drug, but the effect is less dramatic than with other symptoms.

In the event of progressive renal involvement, a trial of corticosteroid therapy or even cytotoxic therapy is warranted (Cupps & Fauci 1981). In the occasional case due to food or drug allergy, the offending agent, when identified, should obviously be eliminated.

Miscellaneous disorders

ORTHOSTATIC PURPURA

The term 'orthostatic purpura' is used to describe the occurrence of purpura on the legs after prolonged standing. It is seen most often in persons with varicose veins and in elderly subjects. There is no demonstrable disorder of the haemostatic mechanism, and the purpura is thought to be due to orthostatic pressure resulting from standing. The effect of this high local orthostatic pressure is also seen in persons with generalized purpuric disorders, as the purpura is often most prominent on the legs.

MECHANICAL PURPURA

Mechanical purpura is due to a local increase in intracapillary pressure. It is most often seen about the head and neck as a result of violent coughing, crush injuries to the chest, or epileptiform seizures. It may also occur on the legs as a result of venous obstruction due to thrombosis, compression by tumour, or the wearing of tight garters.

FAT EMBOLISM

Petechial haemorrhages may be seen in the skin and mucous membranes of patients with fat embolism at the time of onset of stupor, and when present in a suspected case are an important aid to diagnosis. They are most often seen in the skin of the upper part of the chest, the shoulders, and the anterior part of the neck, and less commonly in the conjunctivae and soft palate.

AUTO-ERYTHROCYTE SENSITIZATION

This rare disorder was first described by Gardner & Diamond in 1955. It usually occurs in adult women,

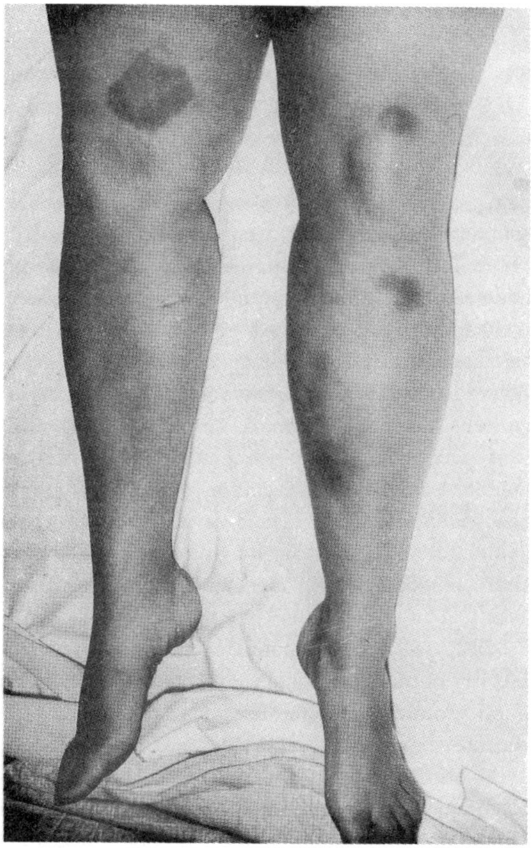

Fig. 14.7. *Auto-erythrocyte sensitization in a young female. At the age of 23 years, the patient was involved in a motor vehicle accident. Two months later she developed crops of painful, raised bruises, mainly on the anterior surfaces of the lower limbs. It was possible to prevent the development of lesions by encasing the limb in plaster of Paris. Personality traits were as described in the text.*

and often follows an injury. The main clinical feature is the appearance of repeated crops of large painful ecchymoses (Fig. 14.7). The ecchymoses are preceded by the sudden onset of localized sharp pain or a stinging or burning sensation, and a feeling that a lump is present at the affected site. The area then gradually becomes erythematous, and within an hour or so the ecchymosis appears, which seems to spread from the margin of the erythematous area. The ecchymoses are usually tender and painful for at least several days, and they persist for a week or longer. They tend to occur in crops over several weeks or longer, followed by a period of weeks or months with few or no ecchymoses. They occur on the extremities, especially the legs, on the trunk and, rarely, on the face. Other manifestations that sometimes occur are menorrhagia, abdominal pain, headache, gastrointestinal bleeding, epistaxis, haematuria, and syncope.

The pathogenesis is poorly understood. The first attack commonly occurs within a few months of an injury or surgical procedure. It is postulated that the patients become sensitive to the red cell stroma of their own extravasated blood. Thus it has been demonstrated that typical lesions can be produced by the intracutaneous injection of the patient's own blood, and in particular by the erythrocyte stroma; a positive reaction to this test, however, is not invariable, and its absence does not exclude the diagnosis. The technique is described by Ratnoff & Agle (1968). A high incidence of emotional disturbance has been recorded in these patients, and in some cases the onset or exacerbation of the symptoms has been preceded by emotional stress. Ratnoff & Agle (1968) found that five psychological components were almost always present in their patients, namely hysterical and masochistic character traits, problems in dealing with their own hostility, and overt symptoms of depression and anxiety. They suggest that the term 'psychogenic purpura' may be more appropriate than auto-erythrocyte sensitization. In a proportion of cases the lesions are factitious, but considerable ingenuity is required to prove that this is so.

Blood examination is normal. Treatment is unsatisfactory, but a short course of corticosteroids may give temporary symptomatic relief. Psychotherapy should be directed toward treatment of the main emotional disturbances.

DNA autosensitivity. A somewhat similar clinical disorder in which acute and painful ecchymoses are confined to the legs has been described; the lesions can be reproduced by the intradermal injection of a solution of the patient's white cells or a solution of deoxyribonucleic acid (DNA) (Chandler & Nalbandian 1966). Treatment with chloroquine causes prompt clinical improvement, but relapse follows cessation of the drug.

SYSTEMIC DISORDERS

Systemic vascular disorders may be accompanied by an increased capillary fragility, with a positive tourniquet test; these include some cases of *collagen disease* and *amyloid*. In the latter disease, coagulation factor deficiencies, thought to be due to absorption of the factor to the amyloid protein, may contribute to the tendency to bleed. Factor X and sometimes factor IX are particularly susceptible (McPherson *et al.* 1977). Bleeding is also common in *polyarteritis nodosa*, presumably as a result of the vascular lesions.

Allergy. Rare cases of non-thrombocytopenic purpura have been described due to *food allergy* and *cold allergy*.

Congenital haemorrhagic vascular disorders

Hereditary haemorrhagic telangiectasia

Osler–Rendu–Weber disease is a synonym for this condition, which is an uncommon disorder transmitted as a simple dominant trait and affecting both sexes equally. The basic lesion is the presence in the skin and mucous membranes of telangiectases due to multiple dilatations of capillaries and arterioles. The telangiectases are lined by a thin layer of endothelial cells; because of their thinness they bleed easily, and because they contract poorly the bleeding is often prolonged.

Clinical features. The most common sites of lesions are the skin and mucous membranes of the nose and mouth; however, they may also occur in the conjunctivae, bronchi, gastrointestinal and renal tracts, and in the vagina. Lesions in the skin are seen mainly on the face, particularly the ears and cheeks, on the hands, especially the tips of the fingers, and on the feet; in the mouth, they occur on the lips, tongue, cheeks, and palate. The telangiectatic spots range in size from a pin-point to lesions up to several millimetres in diameter; they vary in colour from purple to bright red, and they blanch on pressure. They are usually raised, but may be flat. Spider-like telangiectases may also occur. The lesions tend to become more numerous and larger with advancing age.

Although the lesions may be present in childhood, bleeding often does not occur until early adult life. It may occur either spontaneously or following mild trauma. Epistaxis is the most common symptom, and is usually the presenting manifestation. It may occur every day, sometimes several times a day, and it lasts from minutes to hours. Bleeding sometimes lessens or ceases during pregnancy. Much less common manifestations are melaena, haematemesis, haemoptysis, haematuria, and menorrhagia. Retinal and cerebral haemorrhages have also been reported. Bleeding from the skin is not as severe as from mucous membranes, and it may be entirely absent. Pulmonary arteriovenous aneurysm is occasionally present, and splenic enlargement associated with aneurysm of the splenic artery has been described. The liver is sometimes palpable, due to hepatic cirrhosis, a recognized association, or occasionally due to telangiectasis of the liver.

Blood picture. Anaemia proportional to the severity of the bleeding is usual. It is commonly the hypochromic microcytic anaemia of iron deficiency, because the chronic blood loss leads to exhaustion of the body's iron stores; however, with less severe bleeding, it may be normochromic and normocytic. The platelet count and tests of coagulation are usually normal, but some have discovered mild abnormalities in coagulation and fibrinolysis, suggestive of low-grade disseminated intravascular coagulation (Bick 1979). The tourniquet test and bleeding time are also usually normal, but rare cases have been described in which the former is positive and the latter prolonged.

Diagnosis. The diagnostic triad consists of repeated haemorrhages from one, or mainly one, site (particularly epistaxis), the presence of typical lesions in the skin and the mouth, and the family history. As lesions are not always very obvious in the skin, the diagnosis may be overlooked if the mouth is not examined (Fig. 14.8). A family history is usual, but occasionally neither parent gives a history of bleeding; nevertheless, careful examination usually reveals the presence of typical lesions. Diagnostic difficulty may occur when bleeding is predominantly gastrointestinal or renal.

Course and prognosis. The severity of the disorder

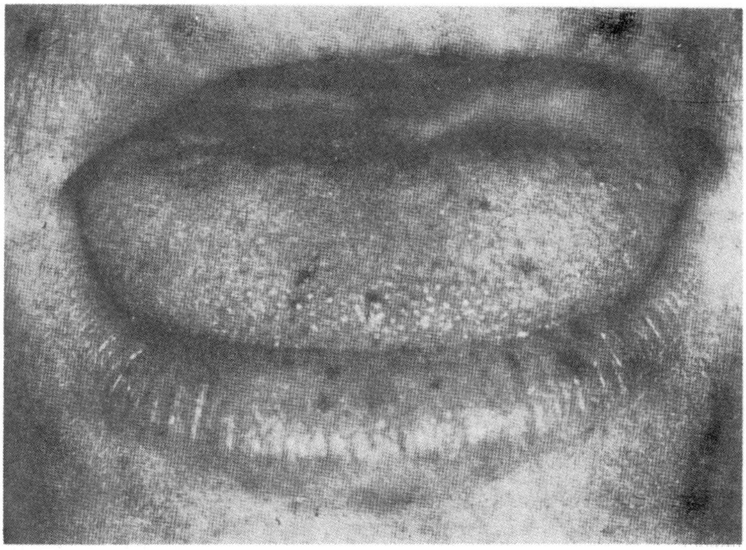

Fig. 14.8. *Hereditary haemorrhagic telangiectasia. This photograph shows typical telangiectatic spots on the tongue and lip. Mrs J.K., aged 25 years, presented with severe epistaxis requiring transfusion; history revealed mild intermittent epistaxis since the age of two years. There were no telangiectatic spots on the face; diagnosis was established by examination of the mouth, which revealed the typical lesions on the tongue. During the next few years, lesions appeared on the cheeks and lip, and those on the tongue became larger.*

varies; in mild cases, bleeding is slight and is only of nuisance value, while in severe cases it may cause death. The bleeding often becomes more frequent and severe with advancing years. The chronic anaemia associated with frequent and persistent bleeding causes varying degrees of invalidism.

Local treatment. Epistaxis is usually the most common problem requiring treatment. Short-term measures include digital pressure, nasal packing, and the local application of topical haemostatic agents. The main long-term treatment is the administration of large doses of oestrogen which significantly lessens epistaxis in many, but not all, patients; it acts by causing squamous metaplasia of the nasal mucous. The usual dose is 0.25 mg/day ethinyl oestradiol; this can be increased to 0.5 mg/day at the end of four weeks if the epistaxis is not well controlled. The daily dose is then varied, either up or down, until a level is reached that keeps the patient epistaxis free. In males, testosterone (2.5–5.0 mg daily) is also given to lessen undesirable feminizing effects. Because of the possible side-effects of large doses of long-term oestrogen therapy (particularly jaundice), it should be used only in patients with troublesome epistaxis. Furthermore, the question of these side-effects must be carefully explained to the patient. In patients with undesirable side-effects, a concentrated oestrogen cream applied locally may be a successful substitute. Cautery may be of value, but new lesions often develop about the treated site, and bleeding may recur. The operation of septal dermatoplasty i.e. resection of the mucosa of the anterior part of the nasal septum and its replacement by a skin graft, may result in permanent control of nose bleeds and should be considered in patients with severe refractory bleeding. With severe recurrent epistaxis which threatens life, ligation of the external carotid artery or the anterior ethmoidal artery, or both, may be necessary. Intestinal resection may be necessary in patients with severe gastrointestinal bleeding; however, fresh lesions develop and bleeding usually recurs.

General treatment. Chronic iron deficiency is common, and thus iron therapy is often indicated. In more severe cases, parenteral iron is preferred as it enables iron stores to be replenished (p. 54). Transfusion is sometimes required in patients with severe blood loss.

Ehlers–Danlos disease

This is a very rare familial disorder, transmitted as a Mendelian dominant trait. The basic lesion is a developmental abnormality of the mesenchyme which results in increased fragility of the blood vessels of the skin, together with increased elasticity of the skin and hyperextensibility of joints. A defect of platelet interaction with the abnormal collagen in the vessel wall has also been suggested. The haemostatic defect results in the occurrence of large haematomas following slight trauma or excessive torsion of the skin. There is no effective treatment other than avoidance of trauma.

Haemorrhagic disorders due to platelet abnormalities

The function of the platelet and its essential role in normal haemostasis has been described earlier in the chapter (p. 360). A brief comment regarding platelet production and kinetics is relevant to the following section describing the haemorrhagic disorders due to platelet abnormalities.

Platelet production (p. 9)

Mature megakaryocytes are unique cells in the body in that they can increase their nuclear DNA content within the same nucleus, allowing them to increase protein-producing capacity without undergoing mitosis. Platelets share common antigens with bone marrow megakaryocytes, and the ultrastructural features of platelets are clearly demonstrable in maturing megakaryocytes. Each megakaryocyte produces about 1000 platelets. Any increase in platelet destruction is followed by a change to a higher mean nuclear DNA content of bone marrow megakaryocytes with the production of more active and larger platelets. This is probably a basic mechanism of haemostasis, and is likely to be under hormonal control.

The platelet count is related to red and white cell counts under normal resting conditions, indicating that the basal platelet count is probably fixed by the hormone acting on the pluripotential stem cell in the bone marrow. The proposed hormone 'thrombopoietin' has not been characterized. However, such a factor exists, since thrombocytopenic serum can cause an increase in protein synthesis in megakaryocytes. The control mechanism of platelet production is likely to be complex and to involve more than one chemical messenger.

The formation of platelets from megakaryocyte cytoplasm is also poorly understood. Budding of cytoplasmic processes from the surface of the megakaryocyte within the bone marrow has been accepted, but the evidence for such a mechanism is subjective. Two alternative processes have been proposed. These proposals seek to explain the unique platelet volume distribution, which is log-Gaussian as opposed to the Gaussian distribution for all other cells. It should be pointed out that platelet formation without mitosis is a unique process.

The first proposal is that platelets are preformed within the megakaryocyte by the demarcation membrane system, a series of membranes extending throughout the cytoplasm over the mature megakaryocyte. The second theory proposes that megakaryocyte cytoplasm undergoes sequential binary division, an idea supported by computer model for such a mechanism. Platelets might be formed and released by either mechanism without the bone marrow or within the lungs, or at both sites. There is no doubt that megakaryocytes leave the bone marrow and circulate. Their relatively large size would prevent passage through the pulmonary capillaries. Megakaryocyte nuclei in the pulmonary capillaries, naked megakaryocyte nuclei on the left side of the circulation but not on the right, all suggest that these circulating megakaryocytes lose their cytoplasm in the lungs, giving rise to platelets. The proponents of sequential binary division of megakaryocytes suggest that this might be achieved by physical fragmentation of the cytoplasm within the pulmonary capillary network.

Since platelets are involved in both thrombotic and bleeding disorders, abnormalities of platelet production might lead to either dysfunction. Resolution of our knowledge concerning the site and mechanism of platelet production is a prerequisite for a full understanding of platelet disorders.

The lifespan of platelets once they enter the circulation is about 8–10 days. About 10 per cent of the population of platelets in the blood is destroyed each day. It seems probable that there is a small random loss of platelets each day due to the use of platelets in normal maintenance of haemostasis. Measurement of platelet lifespan is best done by labelling the platelet with radioactive chromium (^{51}Cr) or indium (^{111}In), *ex vivo*, and returning them to the circulation. The disappearance of radioactivity from the blood on succeeding days provides a measure of the platelet survival. An approach to methodology was published by the International Committee for Standardisation in Haematology (ICSH Panel 1977). The topic was reviewed by Harker (1978).

Platelet antigens and antibodies. Platelets contain specific antigens, and thus platelet antibodies of several types may occur in the plasma. These antibodies are of significance in platelet transfusion and in the pathogenesis of some cases of thrombocytopenia, especially idiopathic (or immune), neonatal, and drug-induced. Platelet antibodies can be classified as follows:

1 *Allo-antibodies* (usually anti-$P1^{A1}$ or anti-Bak^a (Lek^a) induced by transfusion and pregnancy. $P1^{A1}$ antigen is probably located on glycoprotein IIIa, and Bak^a on the glycoprotein IIb subunit (reviewed by Kunicki & Newman 1986). Platelets also contain histocompatibility antigens which may induce antibody formation.

2 *Auto-antibodies*, in idiopathic or immune thrombocytopenia (p. 377), and in certain symptomatic thrombocytopenias (p. 380).

Details of the identification and significance of these antibodies are given in references at the end of the chapter, in particular those of Hegde *et al.* (1977), Cines & Schreiber (1979), McMillan (1983), and Court *et al.* (1987). It is interesting to note that antibodies to glycoprotein IIb–IIIa are detected in a proportion of patients with chronic ITP.

NORMAL VALUES

The normal values for *platelet numbers* in peripheral blood vary with the method used for their estimation. The platelet count under phase-contrast described by Brecher & Cronkite (1950) is still the preferred visual method (Dacie & Lewis 1984). The normal range in health is approximately 150–400 $10^9/l$, average values being about $250 \times 10^9/l$. Platelet counts tend to be subject to error, both because clumping of platelets occurs (particularly with some individuals whose platelets clump in the presence of EDTA anticoagulant used for routine blood specimens) and also because small extraneous particles in the preparation may be mistaken for platelets. However, a careful and experienced worker can produce results that are sufficiently accurate for clinical purposes. The electronic particle counters now widely employed give accurate results, provided that they are calibrated and regularly checked. In the Technicon system, sampling is done from whole blood and, like the Coulter system, gives good correlation with visual counting (Bull *et al.* 1965, Rowan *et al.* 1972). References to sources of error in platelet counting are given by Dacie & Lewis (1984).

The *mean platelet volume* is about 9 femtolitre (fl), and the 'plateletcrit' (PCT) about 0.15–0.3 per cent. These measurements are frequently included in automated systems. Both their accuracy and their clinical value are questionable, although the platelet volume is usually greater in immune than in the other causes of thrombocytopenia.

Physiological variation. There are no sex differences in counts, and the count in an individual patient tends to remain relatively constant. However, in some normal subjects there is a platelet cycle, with periods of oscillation of 21–35 days (Morley 1969). A fall in platelet count may occur in normal women about the time of menstruation. There may also be racial differences, and Mediterranean migrants in Australia have been reported to have significantly lower platelet counts than their northern European counterparts (von Behrens 1975). The platelet volume was greater in the Mediterranean subjects, suggesting that the circulating platelet mass is the critical parameter in homeostasis.

Thrombocytopenia

Thrombocytopenia is defined as a reduction in the peripheral blood platelet count below the lower normal limit of $150 \times 10^9/l$. Because platelet counts are prone to error, a single platelet count that is lower than normal should always be confirmed by a second count. Further, the *thrombocytopenia should also be confirmed by inspection of the blood film.*

General considerations

Relation of the platelet count to bleeding. Haemorrhage is common in thrombocytopenia; nevertheless, many patients with mild to moderate thrombocytopenia, and some with severe thrombocytopenia, go for months or even years without spontaneous bleeding. There is no absolute relationship between the platelet count and the occurrence and severity of bleeding. However, certain broad generalizations can be made. Bleeding is common when the count is less than 30–40 × 10^9/l, but is by no mean invariable; with counts of less than 10 × 10^9/l, bleeding is usual and is often severe. With values of 40–80 × 10^9/l, bleeding is usually absent, although it occurs occasionally. The skin bleeding time, however, has been shown to have a close relationship to platelet count (Fig. 14.9) when platelet function is unimpaired (Harker & Slichter 1972).

The conditions under which thrombocytopenia has developed have an important influence on the occurrence of bleeding. When there is associated infection, vascular disease, or metabolic disorder such as the uraemic state, bleeding may occur with relatively mild thrombocytopenia, functional defects contributing to bleeding.

A detailed description of the pattern of bleeding in thrombocytopenia is given on page 378. Thrombocytopenia is accompanied by a positive tourniquet test and a prolonged bleeding time.

Positive tourniquet test. There is an incompletely understood relationship between the number of platelets and capillary integrity; thrombocytopenia is accompanied by an increased capillary fragility. This is most conveniently demonstrated by the tourniquet test (capillary resistance test of Hess), which, although crude, is a useful part of the examination of any patient with a bleeding tendency.

The tourniquet test is performed by placing a sphygmomanometer cuff around the upper arm and raising the pressure to 100 mmHg for 5–7 minutes. If systolic blood pressure is less than 100 mmHg, the pressure is raised to half way between the systolic and diastolic pressure. Two to three minutes after the cuff has been deflated and the congestion has disappeared, the number of petechiae in an area

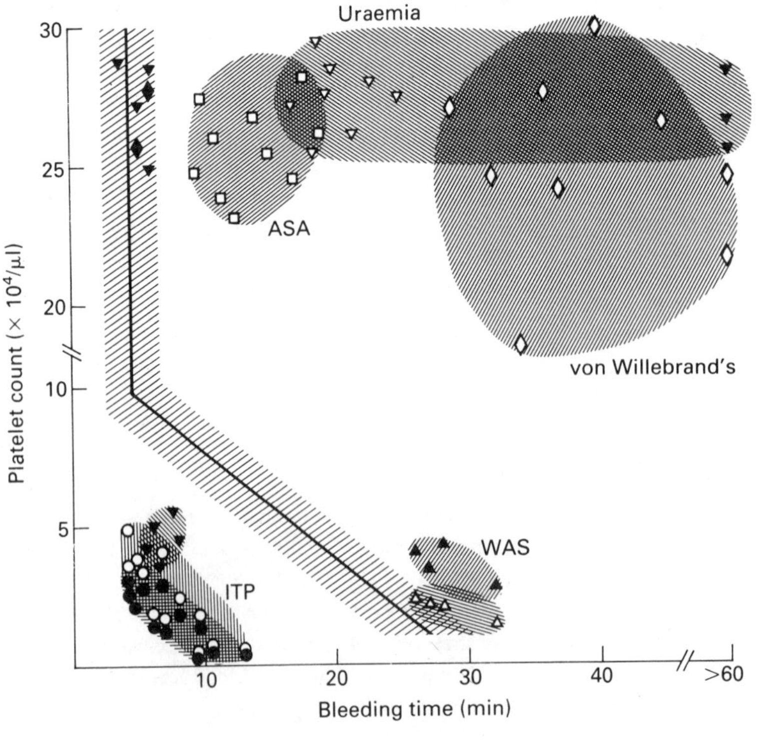

Fig. 14.9. *The inverse relationship between the skin bleeding time and the peripheral blood platelet count. The hatched area represents the relationships in normal individuals and in thrombocytopenia caused by impaired platelet production. In the case of platelet dysfunction, the bleeding time is relatively prolonged, whereas in idiopathic thrombocytopenic purpura the bleeding time is shorter than might be expected. ASA = aspirin; WAS = Wiskott–Aldrich Syndrome; ITP = idiopathic thrombocytopenic purpura. (Reproduced from Harker & Slichter 1972, with the permission of the authors and publishers.)*

with a 3 cm diameter, 1 cm below the cubital fossa, is counted. In most normal subjects, the number of petechiae is up to 10, although up to 20 may be present. More than 20 is abnormal. In severe thrombocytopenia, the count is increased up to 100 or more. The petechiae vary in size from pin-point to pin-head or larger. The tourniquet test is positive in most cases of reasonably significant thrombocytopenia, but is occasionally negative in patients with mild or moderate thrombocytopenia. In patients with widespread purpura, the test is redundant and inappropriate.

Prolonged bleeding time. The bleeding time is the time required for the cessation of haemorrhage from a small puncture wound of the skin made under standard conditions. There are two techniques commonly used, the template method and Ivy's method. In both, a standardized incision is made on the volar aspect of the forearm, while the venous and capillary tension is raised by a sphygmomanometer cuff around the upper arm inflated to 40 mmHg throughout. Variation in the methods relate to the cutting instrument which may consist of a scalpel blade, with guard, protruding through a slit in a template or, simply, a disposable lancet. The bleeding time does correlate to the circulating platelet count when platelet function is normal (Fig. 14.9), particularly when there is imparied platelet production. An inappropriately short bleeding time may be encountered if there is peripheral platelet destruction because of larger and more reactive platelets produced by the 'stressed' bone marrow. Conversely, an unexpected, prolonged bleeding time suggests platelet dysfunction either due to an intrinsic platelet defect or to plasma protein abnormalities, e.g. von Willebrand's disease, or to the presence of certain types of paraproteins. It is essential that drugs affecting platelet function are omitted for an appropriate period (ideally 6–7 days) before bleeding time estimation, and this applies especially to aspirin. The techniques are described by Dacie & Lewis (1984).

Aetiology. Thrombocytopenia may result from impaired platelet production, accelerated platelet destruction, or dilution and/or splenic sequestration.

Thrombocytopenia is associated with a number of disorders, and other causes should be excluded before assuming a diagnosis of immune (idiopathic) thrombocytopenia. A classification of thrombocytopenia, giving prominence to the more common causes, is listed in Table 14.2.

Table 14.2. *Classification of thrombocytopenia*

Acquired
More common causes (especially of moderate to severe thrombocytopenia)
Idiopathic (immune) thrombocytopenic purpura
acute
chronic
Drugs and chemicals
Leukaemias
Aplastic anaemia
Bone marrow infiltration—secondary carcinoma, multiple myeloma, malignant lymphomas, myelofibrosis
Hypersplenism
Disseminated lupus erythematosus
Less common causes
Infection including HIV
Megaloblastic macrocytic anaemia
Liver disease
Alcoholism
Massive blood transfusion
Disseminated intravascular coagulation
Rare causes
Thrombotic thrombocytopenic purpura
Post-partum thrombocytopenia
Post-transfusion thrombocytopenia
Haemangiomas
Food allergy
Idiopathic cryoglobulinaemia
Neonatal and congenital (see Table 14.5)

Idiopathic thrombocytopenic purpura

Primary or essential thrombocytopenic purpura, purpura haemorrhagica, Werlhof's disease, and auto-immune thrombocytopenia are synonyms for *idiopathic (immune) thrombocytopenic purpura.* This is a disorder characterized by thrombocytopenia in almost all cases due to antibody formation. It is not hereditary or familial, although in occasional cases there is a family history of easy bruising or even of frank bleeding such as expistaxis.

Clinical features

The disorder may occur at any age, but is most common in children and young adults. Until the age of about 12 years, the sex incidence is approximately equal, but thereafter females are affected 3–4 times more commonly than males.

Broadly, two clinical types are recognized—an acute self-limiting type, and a chronic type characterized by chronic recurring bleeding over months or years. Although the majority of cases fit into one or other of these groups, there is considerable clinical overlap between them.

TYPE AND SITE OF BLEEDING

The bleeding, as with all bleeding due to thrombocytopenia, commonly occurs spontaneously. It also occurs following trauma, surgery, and dental procedures. Bleeding from wounds tends to occur at once, ceases within 48 hours, and does not recur. The skin is the most common site of haemorrhage, and in mild cases it may be the only site. The haemorrhage may take the form of multiple petechiae or ecchymoses, or both. Although petechiae are usually present, ecchymoses may occur in their absence. The petechial spots vary from the size of a pin-point to a pin-head or somewhat larger; they are not raised and do not blanch on pressure. When fresh, they are red in colour, but with time they pass through the colour changes of absorbing blood. They characteristically occur in groups or crops, and although they may occur in any part of the body, they are seen especially on the arms and legs, the neck, and the upper part of the chest. They may vary in number from a few scattered crops to innumerable spots covering almost the whole of the body. Ecchymoses vary in size and are initially purple; occasionally, larger haematomas form in the subcutaneous tissue. Haemorrhages are not accompanied by urticaria or erythema.

Bleeding from the *mucous membranes* is common, although less so than skin bleeding; occasionally, it occurs in the absence of skin bleeding. Epistaxis and bleeding from the gums are the most common forms of haemorrhage, but haematuria, menorrhagia and metrorrhagia, and melaena are not infrequent. Petechiae similar to those of the skin may be seen in the mouth and nose. Less commonly, haematemesis or haemoptysis occurs. Rarely, there is haemorrhage into the peritoneal or pleural cavities.

Bleeding into *internal organs* is relatively uncommon, but may be serious. The most important site is the nervous system, especially the brain. Cerebral haemorrhage is the most common cause of death in severe thrombocytopenia. Haemorrhage into the spinal cord and into the meninges may also occur. Rarely, haemorrhage occurs in the tongue, larynx, muscles, fallopian tubes, or ear. Bleeding into joints is very rare.

On *examination,* the outstanding feature is the absence of physical findings other than those due to the haemorrhage and, when blood loss is severe, to anaemia. Subconjunctival and retinal haemorrhages are relatively common. The spleen in enlarged in less than 10 per cent of cases, and when enlarged is only slightly so. The lymph nodes and liver are not palpable, and there is no sternal tenderness. Jaundice is absent except when there is extensive tissue haemorrhage, e.g. large haematomas, which results in the absorption of large amounts of bile pigment from the broken-down blood. Fever is usually absent, but there may be a moderate rise in temperature with extensive haemorrhage into the tissues or gastrointestinal tract. Rarely, there is chronic ulceration of the legs.

COURSE OF THE BLEEDING

There are two clinical types, namely acute and chronic, but not uncommonly these overlap.

The acute variety occurs most commonly in children aged from 2 to 6 years, and accounts for most cases seen in children. It is characterized by a relatively acute onset with haemorrhage into the skin or mucous membranes, or both; the haemorrhage is often severe. Epistaxis is particularly common. There is frequently a history of a viral infection in the preceding several weeks before the onset. In most cases, bleeding ceases spontaneously after a period varying from a few days to 12 weeks; in the remainder it usually ceases within six months, but in about 10 per cent of cases it persists and the disorder runs the course of chronic idiopathic thrombocytopenia. In general, bleeding is most severe at the onset, and tends to lessen in severity as time passes. Death is uncommon (less than one per cent); it occurs usually within the first four weeks of onset.

Chronic idiopathic thrombocytopenic purpura is most commonly a disease of young to middle-aged females (F,3:M,1). The onset is usually less abrupt. The severity of the symptoms varies; in some cases it is mild and there may be only recurrent crops of petechiae or 'easy' bruising, while in other cases there may be relatively severe bleeding from mucous membranes, sometimes localized to one site. Occasionally, the first manifestation is menorrhagia occurring at the menarche. In the chronic disease, symptoms are often intermittent, with remissions lasting weeks, months, or even years. In other cases, symptoms persist but fluctuate in severity.

Blood picture

The outstanding feature is the reduction in platelet count; it occurs in all degrees, values ranging from just below normal to less than 10×10^9/l, lower counts tending to be associated with the acute disease. The platelets sometimes appear to be morphologically abnormal, with large, small, and atypical forms. The usual associations of thrombocytopenia—a prolonged bleeding time and a positive tourniquet test—are present. The bleeding time is prolonged up to 30 minutes or longer. Coagulation studies (see Chapter 15) are normal. Anaemia proportional to the degree of blood loss may be present when bleeding is severe; in the early stages, it is normocytic and normochromic, but with prolonged bleeding (e.g. menorrhagia) the iron stores are diminished and the hypochromic microcytic anaemia of iron deficiency develops. Rarely, there is an associated auto-immune haemolytic anaemia with spherocytosis and other typical features (p. 192); this is termed Evans' syndrome (Evans *et al.* 1951). The leucocyte count is normal or moderately increased during bleeding episodes. The sedimentation rate is usually normal. About 30 per cent of cases have positive anticardiolipin antibodies in the serum (Harris *et al.* 1985). The test is by no means specific, and these antibodies are also commonly present in SLE.

Bone marrow

Megakaryocytes and their precursors are present in normal, and often in increased, numbers (Fig. 14.10). There is an increase in the percentage of immature cells; these cells have a lesser degree of

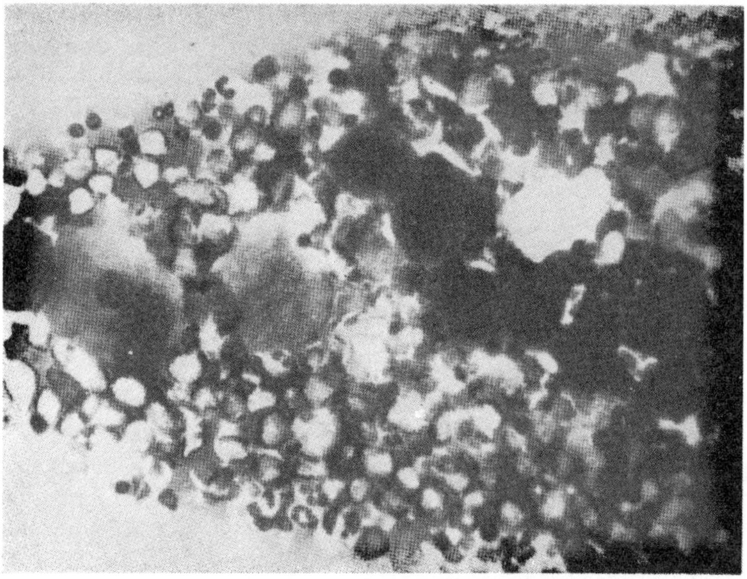

Fig. 14.10. *Bone marrow in idiopathic thrombocytopenic purpura. Photomicrograph of a bone marrow film from a boy aged 15 years, showing an increased number of megakaryocytes (× 260).*

cytoplasmic granularity. Vacuolization may be present in some cells. In a few cases, there is a moderate increase in mature lymphocytes or in eosinophils. Otherwise, the marrow is normal. When haemorrhage is severe enough to cause anaemia there is an associated erythroid hyperplasia, and iron stores may be absent if bleeding has been prolonged.

Diagnosis

Idiopathic thrombocytopenic purpura is characterized by thrombocytopenia with a normal or increased number of megakaryocytes in the bone marrow; the white cell count is normal or slightly increased, and anaemia (when present) is proportional to the amount of blood loss. There are usually no positive physical findings other than those due to thrombocytopenia and anaemia. As the spleen is enlarged in less than 10 per cent of cases, the presence of splenomegaly in a patient with thrombocytopenia suggests another cause.

The laboratory demonstration of antiplatelet antibodies is a potentially useful diagnostic tool. Recently introduced tests for detecting platelet-associated immunoglobulin are standard procedures. Unfortunately, in other conditions frequently associated with thrombocytopenia, e.g. acute leukaemia and septicaemia, there is increased platelet associated immunoglobulin with considerable overlap with ITP. In spite of these problems of specificity, the tests are clearly superior to the previously available rather insensitive techniques which used indirect measures such as platelet 'injury' to detect antibodies.

EXCLUSION OF OTHER CAUSES

The majority of cases of thrombocytopenia seen in clinical practice are secondary to other disorders, and thus the diagnosis of idiopathic thrombocytopenia can be made only after careful clinical and haematological investigations.

The presence of lymph node enlargement, marked splenomegaly, bone tenderness, fever, anaemia out of proportion to the degree of bleeding, or a markedly increased sedimentation rate suggest that the thrombocytopenia is not idiopathic. However, it is not uncommon for none of the above features to be present in other disorders, and their absence does not exclude secondary thrombocytopenia. Bone marrow aspiration is always essential, to exclude leukaemia, aplasia, and marrow infiltration, and to demonstrate the typical features of idiopathic thrombocytopenia.

Table 14.3 lists the main points in differential diagnosis of the disorders most likely to be confused with idiopathic thrombocytopenia. *Drug-induced thrombocytopenia is particularly important as it gives a clinical and haematological picture indistinguishable from that of idiopathic thrombocytopenia;* thus a careful history about drug ingestion or exposure to chemical agents must always be taken. Appropriate tests such as those for antinuclear factor, anti-DNA antibodies, and the LE cell test should be performed, as thrombocytopenia may be the first manifestation of *disseminated lupus erythematosus.* In the appropriate setting, testing for antibodies to *human immunodeficiency virus* should be carried out (p. 488).

In cases that come to splenectomy, the spleen should always be examined histologically, as occasionally it gives the first evidence of an unsuspected causative disorder, e.g. *lupus erythematosus, tuberculosis,* or *sarcoidosis.*

Bleeding localized to one site. Occasionally, bleeding occurs wholly or mainly from one organ, e.g. in menorrhagia, haematuria, or epistaxis. In such cases, a local cause for the abnormal bleeding may be suspected; this is especially so in patients presenting with menorrhagia.

Pathogenesis

It is believed that idiopathic thrombocytopenic purpura is virtually always due to antiplatelet antibodies. IgG antibodies may be identified in the majority of cases, and bound complement in a proportion. These antibodies are often not demonstrable by the standard serological techniques of agglutination and complement fixation, and other evidence for their existence has been sought.

1 They are often shown by tests that reflect platelet

damage induced by antibodies, such as platelet factor 3 availability or platelet serotonin release. However, detection of platelet-associated immunoglobulin or 'bindable' immunoglobulin in the serum is the most useful approach, with greater sensitivity (Hegde *et al.* 1977, Cines & Schreiber 1979, McMillan 1983, Court *et al.* 1987).

2 The transfusion of plasma from a patient with idiopathic thrombocytopenic purpura has been shown to cause thrombocytopenia with clinical purpura in recipients.

3 A transient thrombocytopenia may occur in newborn infants born to mothers with idiopathic thrombocytopenic purpura, suggesting the transplacental passage of an antiplatelet factor from the mother to the fetus.

4 It has been shown that normal platelets can adsorb the factor from the plasma of patients with the disorder; furthermore, the factor reacts with autologous as well as homologous platelets, and is species specific. Even in remission with normal platelet counts, persisting abnormalities in tests of platelet function may result from the subclinical effects of antibodies (Clancy *et al.* 1972).

5 Platelets with bound antibody are removed by the reticulo-endothelial system (Aster & Keene 1969), in particular the spleen, but with the tendency that increasing platelet antibody load increases hepatic sequestration. Little intravascular platelet lysis occurs. The mechanism of acute idiopathic thrombocytopenia is less well understood. In about 75 per cent of cases, there is a preceding infection and antibody formation resulting from some reaction between virus and platelets. It may be that the thrombocytopenia represents a hypersensitivity reaction to the infection. Basic aspects of immunological reactions of platelets are reviewed by Hanson & Ginsberg (1981), and clinical laboratory techniques by McMillan (1983).

Treatment

Patients should be in hospital for diagnosis and initiating treatment if there is a significant bleeding tendency. Trauma and agents likely to interfere with platelet function, e.g. aspirin, alcohol, must be forbidden. Cough and constipation should be treated to lessen sudden elevations in intracranial pressure.

The main therapeutic measures are the administration of *corticosteroids* and *splenectomy*. *Immunosuppressive* therapy and intravenous administration of *immunoglobulin* are indicated in selected cases.

The age of the patient is an important factor in determining the therapeutic approach. Thus, although it is not possible to predict from either the clinical or haematological features whether a particular case will be acute or chronic, it is known that most cases in children run an acute self-limiting course, while most cases in adults run a chronic course with recurring attacks. Splenectomy is therefore only rarely necessary in children, while it is commonly performed in adults.

Children. In general, the trend is conservative. In mild cases with bleeding only into the skin or slight bleeding from the mucous membranes, no active treatment may be necessary, although the patient must be closely observed. With more severe bleeding, a course of corticosteroid is given as outlined below. This is usually followed by either a clinical remission or at least sufficient improvement to allow an expectant policy to be followed until the natural remission occurs. If, however, the thrombocytopenia persists for longer than six months, the case can be classified as chronic, and splenectomy should be considered if the bleeding tendency is causing more than minor disability. Keep in mind, however, the increased risk of infection after splenectomy, particularly in younger children, and pneumococcal prophylaxis should be instituted (p. 348). Emergency splenectomy is indicated when, despite corticosteroid therapy, the bleeding is sufficiently severe to endanger life; however, with adequate steroid therapy it is seldom necessary. A further option is the intravenous infusion of high-dosage immunoglobulin (p. 384). Because of the comparatively rapid response to this mode of therapy it may be of great value in the emergency situation or when splenectomy is contemplated due to a poor response to corticosteriod.

Adults. The principles are the same as for children, but as the majority of cases tend to run a chronic rather than acute course, splenectomy should be considered earlier, e.g. if after 2–3 months bleeding is troublesome despite corticosteroid therapy. When a chronic case with a long history is seen for the first time, a course of corticosteroids should be tried, but if this fails then splenectomy is indicated. The results of treatment with corticosteroids, splenectomy, and immunosuppressive treatment in 934 adults have recently been reviewed (Pizzuto & Ambriz 1984).

CORTICOSTEROID HORMONES

The dose is determined by the age of the patient and the severity of the bleeding. The initial dose for adults is 1–2 mg/kg prednisolone, higher doses being used if bleeding is severe. The dosage for children is 0.5–1 mg/kg prednisolone. Treatment is usually followed promptly by an improvement in the capillary fragility as shown by the tourniquet test, a shortening of the bleeding time, and a lessening or cessation of haemorrhage; this is followed by an increase in the platelet count, which is usually obvious within 2–4 days but sometimes does not occur for 10–14 days, and occasionally for 3–4 weeks. In about 25 per cent of cases, there is no improvement. Treatment with full doses is continued for at least two weeks, and for 3–4 weeks if necessary, when the dose is gradually reduced. Cessation of therapy may be followed by a permanent clinical and haematological remission, particularly in children. However, in adults it is more common for a partial or complete relapse to occur as dosage is reduced, and if an unacceptably high maintenance dosage is required to control thrombocytopenia, splenectomy should be considered. As it is uncommon for such relapsed cases to remit subsequently, there is a strong case for splenectomy to be performed within a few weeks rather than waiting for three months or more, a commonly recommended procedure.

In summary, the principal aims of treatment with steroids are to protect the patient from the haemorrhagic consequences of severe thrombocytopenia, to reduce the levels of antiplatelet antibodies, and to suppress macrophage function. In chronic cases, the use of steroids is determined by the severity of the bleeding tendency. Prednisolone may be used in the attempt to induce a remission, and a significant proportion of patients respond favourably. Other uses are as a postoperative measure in cases of failed splenectomy and in pregnant women after the fifth month of pregnancy.

SPLENECTOMY

Indications. The main indications for splenectomy are chronic cases, particularly in adults, which have not had a sustained response to steroids, and in which troublesome bleeding persists after several weeks. Less common indications are as an emergency measure in both adults and children when, despite adequate steroid therapy, the bleeding is sufficiently severe to endanger life or when cerebral haemorrhage threatens, and in the first 4–5 months of pregnancy, if steroids have not induced a full remission.

Results. Splenectomy results in a sustained clinical remission in approximately 75 per cent of cases. In patients who respond, splenectomy is followed by an improvement in capillary fragility and a shortening of bleeding time, together with lessening or cessation of bleeding, commencing within a matter of minutes, sometimes as soon as the splenic pedicle is clamped. The platelet count starts to rise within a few hours to a few days. The maximum value is reached within three weeks, with an average of about ten days; it usually exceeds normal values, commonly ranging from 500 to 1000 $\times 10^9$/l (Fig. 14.11). The count slowly returns to normal; occasionally it falls to presplenectomy levels, but the clinical cure persists.

Prediction of results. At present, it is not possible to predict accurately the response of the individual patient to splenectomy. Studies with radioactively labelled platelets estimating platelet survival time and the site of platelet destruction as indicated by surface scanning are probably not of help in the decision for or against splenectomy (Aster & Keene 1969). There is evidence for a relationship between *age* and *response to corticosteroids* and response to splenectomy (Harrington & Arimura 1961):

1 Under the age of 45 years, there were 80 per cent good responses, but only about 50 per cent in the older age group.

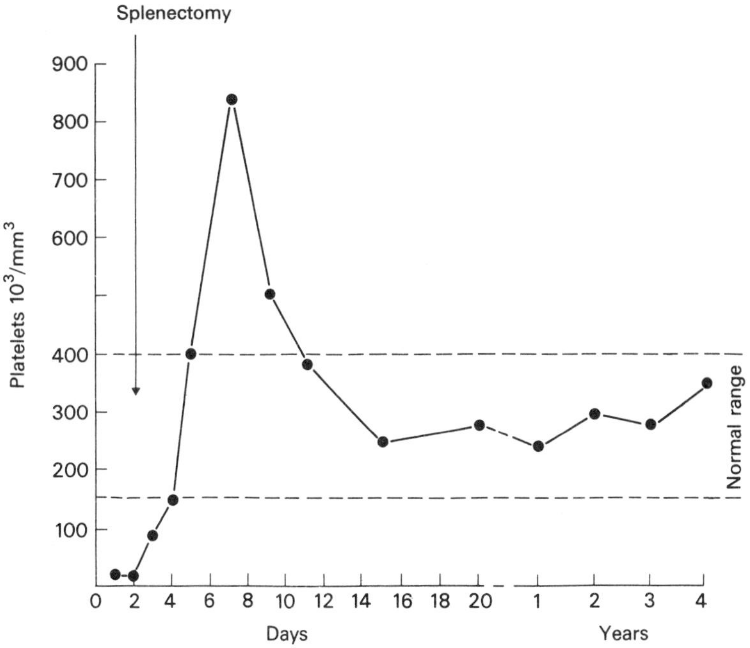

Fig. 14.11. *Idiopathic thrombocytopenic purpura. Response to splenectomy. Mrs J.D., aged 62 years, presented with spontaneous bruising. Platelet count, 40 × 10⁹/l. Clinical picture, blood picture, and bone marrow consistent with idiopathic thrombocytopenic purpura. No history of drug ingestion or exposure to chemicals. Because of the mild nature of the symptoms, no active treatment was given. Bruising occurred intermittently for three years. When a 14-day course of corticosteroid was given, the tourniquet test became temporarily negative, but there was no increase in platelets and the bruising continued. She suddenly developed severe headache, followed shortly by aphasia and weakness of the right arm. Splenectomy was performed as an emergency measure and resulted in a prompt rise in the platelet count. The cerebral signs recovered in several months, and the patient has remained symptom-free with a normal platelet count for 11 years.*

2 The vast majority of cases that respond to steroids will respond to splenectomy; however, failure to respond to steroids does not imply that splenectomy will be similarly ineffective, since about 50 per cent of patients who do not respond to steroids have a good response to splenectomy.

3 A high concentration of *platelet-associated antibody* is likely to be associated with a poor result.

Failed splenectomy. About 25 per cent of cases do not respond or do so only temporarily, the platelet count relapsing to presplenectomy values in weeks or months. Rarely, relapse occurs several years later. Occasionally, the count increases slowly over a period of months to years. Continuation or recurrence of troublesome bleeding after splenectomy may be lessened or abolished by steroids or by other forms of therapy (see below). The development of an accessory spleen is reported as a cause of recurrent thrombocytopenia after a successful splenectomy, and should be excluded by splenic scan using heat-treated isotopically labelled red blood cells. However, an exacerbation of the underlying immune disorder is more likely to be responsible.

Mechanism of response to splenectomy. The available evidence suggests that in idiopathic thrombocytopenic purpura platelets sensitized by reaction with plasma antiplatelet antibodies are removed from the circulation by the spleen and the liver. Thus, splenectomy works by removing a major site of platelet destruction; there is also evidence that the concentration of circulating antiplatelet antibodies decreases after splenectomy at least in some patients (Cines & Schreiber 1979).

Histology. Histological section of the spleen does not show any characteristic or constant features.

The most common change is an increase in the size of the germinal centres of the lymphoid follicles; other changes observed include an increase in neutrophils and eosinophils in the splenic pulp, and the presence of megakaryocytes in the splenic pulp. Examination of spleen by electron microscopy has shown platelet phagocytosis in splenic macrophages, supporting the belief that this is the major site of removal of antibody-damaged platelets (Firkin *et al.* 1969). The importance of careful histological examination of the spleen for evidence of an occult underlying disease in every apparent case of ITP has been emphasized (p. 380).

SUPPORTIVE THERAPY

Blood transfusion may be necessary when haemorrhage causes severe anaemia. Because transfused platelets are rapidly destroyed by the patient's immune system, platelet transfusion is generally of little value. However, it may be employed in patients with severe bleeding uncontrolled by steroids, when they require splenectomy. The transfusion is probably best commenced just before the first surgical incision is made, a second transfusion being administered after the clamping of the splenic pedicle. Despite its limitation, transfusion may also be used when surgery is needed for bleeding complications or for an unrelated disorder.

IMMUNOSUPPRESSIVE THERAPY

There are reports of good results of treatment with immunosuppressive agents such as vincristine, azathioprine, or cyclophosphamide. However, the inherent risks of immunosuppression and cytotoxic drugs restrict their use to 'refractory' cases, i.e. those that have failed to respond to corticosteroids and splenectomy, or those in which these methods of treatment are contra-indicated. Details are given by Bouroncle & Doan (1966), Sussman (1967) and Ahn *et al.* (1974, 1984). Of the various modalities, vincristine or vinblastine are probably the best choice, with good responses in more than half of postsplenectomy patients so treated. Responses, however, are usually transient, necessitating further courses of treatment. The vincristine is administered by intravenous push (1 mg/m^2) or by infusion over several hours at a dose of 0.02 mg/kg. Vinblastine has been used at a dosage of 0.1 mg/kg, and is probably less toxic than vincristine. This may be repeated at weekly intervals for 3–4 doses. If there is no response at this stage, success is not likely.

INFUSION OF IMMUNOGLOBULIN

Intravenous infusions of immunoglobulin have been shown to result in remissions in both acute and chronic idiopathic thrombocytopenic purpura. The mechanism of action is uncertain, but evidence suggests interference with phagocyte Fc-receptor-mediated immune clearance (Fehr *et al.* 1982). The therapeutic effect is, however, frequently not transient. In practice, polyvalent intact immunoglobulins are administered in large dosage (0.4 g/kg/day over five days) diluted in normal saline. In children, remissions are achieved in almost 100 per cent and are usually permanent. In adults, not surprisingly, the remission rate is less (perhaps 75 per cent), and in the small series so far reported the permanent remission rate is less than half of these. Sometimes, infusions at intervals of weeks can maintain remission.

The unwanted effects seem to be confined to immediate reactions to the immunoglobulin preparation, for example dyspnoea, chest pain, nausea, vomiting, and abdominal pain, particularly on the first or second days of therapy (Brearley & Rowbotham 1984). The incidence of these side-effects appears to vary with the commercial source of the immunoglobulin preparation (perhaps as a consequence of anticomplementary IgG aggregates), the reported rate varying from 5 to 50 per cent. Viral hepatitis, both hepatitis B and non-A, non-B hepatitis, have been described after use of immunoglobulin fractions, but appear to be rare complications of this therapy.

Details of administration are discussed by Fehr *et al.* (1982), Newland *et al.* (1983), Brearley & Rowbotham (1984), and Bussel & Hilgartner (1984). This form of therapy appears particularly suited to acute situations, prior to surgery or childbirth, and in individuals in whom corticosteroids or splenectomy could be contra-indicated, for example in cases of thrombocytopenia associated with HIV infection.

ANDROGENS

Androgens have been shown to have a steroid-sparing effect in the treatment of idiopathic thrombocytopenic purpura. The mechanism of this activity is unknown, but possible explanations include displacement of steroids from steroid-binding globulin. Certainly, free antiplatelet antibody has been reported to be reduced by several weeks' treatment with danazol, an androgen with reduced virilizing activity (Ahn *et al.* 1983). This was associated with clinical benefit in 15 of 22 patients so treated, 11 with sustained normalization of platelet counts. Unfortunately, there is little subsequent confirmatory information to support this form of treatment, and its place in the overall therapeutic plan is not clear.

Pregnancy

Maternal mortality would appear to have lessened over the years. Territo *et al.* (1973) calculated 5.5 per cent maternal mortality from the literature while Kelton (1983), reviewing more recent literature, reported only one death in 88 patients with immune thrombocytopenia, that death not being due to the low platelet count.

The intra-uterine death rate with thrombocytopenic mothers varies widely, from up to one-third terminating in spontaneous abortion (Territo *et al.* 1973) to five per cent in the review of Kelton (1983). Neonatal mortality is low, but a significant bleeding defect is present in 10–20 per cent, and thrombocytopenia in 50 per cent. Unfortunately, neither the maternal platelet count nor the quantity of platelet-associated Ig appear to be good predictors of fetal platelet count at term, although some authors have found them to be so (Laros & Kagan 1983). A prior history of significant neonatal thrombocytopenia may be a better index.

The management of maternal thrombocytopenia is very much dependent on severity. A platelet count below $50 \times 10^9/l$ or clinical bleeding is an indication for prednisolone in standard dosage (p. 382), reducing as quickly as possible. In the of steroid failure, splenectomy may be indicated, ideally in the second trimester. Intravenous high-dose gamma globulin has been used with effect, and should certainly be given to raise the platelet count to cover surgery if required.

The ideal management of delivery is contentious. In the presence of significant maternal thrombocytopenia, attempts should be made to increase the platelet count by either infusion of high-dose gamma globulin, using the five-day protocol some two weeks before delivery, or by administration of corticosteroids. To lessen the danger to the fetus with potential neonatal thrombocytopenia, several options are available: (a) predelivery attempts to raise the maternal and fetal platelet count either by corticosteroids or infusion of high-dose intravenous gamma globulin started two weeks before delivery; (b) delivery by Caesarian section in the presence of a low maternal platelet count, e.g. below $100 \times 10^9/l$; and (c) delivery by Caesarian section on the basis of a proven low fetal platelet count performed on a scalp blood sample. In any event, the importance of avoiding a prolonged labour and avoiding forceps delivery would seem self-evident. Any indication that these might occur would weight the decision towards Caesarian section.

The infant's platelet count may fall during the first few days after birth, and this should be monitored. In the case of severe thrombocytopenia or haemorrhage intervention with corticosteroids, platelet transfusion or exchange transfusion may be indicated. The topic is reviewed by Colvin (1985).

Idiopathic cyclical thrombocytopenia purpura

This is a rare variant of idiopathic thrombocytopenic purpura in which thrombocytopenia is cyclical, recurring at regular intervals. Most reported cases have occurred in women and have been related to some phase of the menstrual cycle; usually it appears as an exaggeration of the physiological decrease that occurs during menstruation, but cases with the count lowest at the time of ovulation have been described.

Secondary thrombocytopenia

The majority of cases of thrombocytopenia seen in clinical practice are secondary to some underlying disorder. The problem of diagnosis from idiopathic thrombocytopenic purpura is discussed on p. 380.

Aetiology (Table 14.2, p. 372)

MORE COMMON CAUSES

(Differential diagnosis, Table 14.3, p. 380)

Drug-induced thrombocytopenic purpura. Careful questioning about the administration of drugs should be carried out in all patients with thrombocytopenia, especially when no definite cause is obvious. The problem is discussed more fully on p. 388.

Leukaemias. In acute leukaemia, thrombocytopenia is almost invariable and is frequently severe. Bleeding is a common presenting manifestation and a frequent cause of death. In chronic lymphocytic leukaemia, thrombocytopenia is usual; in the early stages it is usually mild and asymptomatic, but in the later stages it may be marked and cause severe bleeding. Efforts should be made to identify the occurrence of auto-immune antiplatelet antibodies if severe thrombocytopenia develops during the course of this disease or *malignant lymphoma* because specific therapy, as for idiopathic thrombocytopenic purpura, may be successful. In chronic granulocytic leukaemia, the platelet count is initially normal or raised, but it falls in the later stages of the disease.

Aplastic anaemia. Thrombocytopenia is common in aplastic anaemia, especially acute drug-induced cases, and bleeding may be the first manifestation (p. 121).

Bone marrow infiltration. Thrombocytopenia may occur as a consequence of *secondary carcinoma, multiple myeloma* (p. 299), *myelofibrosis* (p. 335), and the *malignant lymphomas* (p. 278). Occasionally, thrombocytopenic bleeding is the first manifestation of secondary carcinoma of bone and multiple myeloma.

Hypersplenism is a cause of secondary thrombocytopenia, and is more fully discussed on p. 348.

Disseminated lupus erythematosus. Thrombocytopenia is quite common in this condition. Although the history and clinical examination usually reveal one or more of the other features of the disease, the disorder occasionally presents with thrombocytopenia as the only manifestation.

LESS COMMON CAUSES

Infection. In acute idiopathic thrombocytopenic purpura of children, there is frequently a history of infection, especially of the upper respiratory tract, several weeks before the onset. In addition, thrombocytopenia occurs as an uncommon or rare complication of certain acute and chronic infections; these include scarlet fever, infectious mononucleosis, measles, rubella (both acquired and congenital), chickpenpox, tuberculosis, diphtheria, and subacute bacterial endocarditis. With acute infections, the thrombocytopenia may occur either during the acute phase or during convalescence. The thrombocytopenia probably represents an allergic response to the infection, or a manifestation of bone marrow suppression; there is no relation between the severity of the primary disorder and the occurrence of purpura.

In septicaemia, thrombocytopenia is not uncommon in both adults and children. Thrombocytopenia is particularly common with Gram-negative bacteraemia. Falciparum malaria is complicated by thrombocytopenia in severe cases. Immune complex-mediated platelet injury has been suggested as the mechanism for this association.

Megaloblastic macrocytic anaemia is commonly accompanied by a mild, symptomless thrombocytopenia; rarely, there is a mild bleeding tendency.

Liver disease. Thrombocytopenia associated with liver disease is most often due to hypersplenism caused by congestive splenomegaly associated with cirrhosis of the liver. However, it occasionally occurs in cirrhotic patients in whom the spleen is not palpable and there is no evidence of portal hypertension. Thrombocytopenia may also occur in severe acute infective hepatitis, probably on the basis of disseminated intravascular coagulation.

Alcoholism. Chronic thrombocytopenia is not uncommon in chronic alcoholics, in whom it is usually considered to be due to hypersplenism associated with cirrhosis and congestive splenomegaly, or to nutritional megaloblastic anaemia. However, an acute transient thrombocytopenia may occur in alcoholics without cirrhosis, related to drinking bouts; the platelet count usually rises within a few days of cessation of alcohol. The thrombocytopenia is due to a direct effect of alcohol intoxication on the developing megakaryocytes (Lindenbaum & Hargrave 1968, Sullivan *et al.* 1977).

Disseminated intravascular coagulation (defibrination) may also be associated with thrombocytopenia (p. 442).

Massive blood transfusion. Thrombocytopenia causing severe bleeding may occur in patients transfused with massive amounts of stored whole blood, when the blood is given either to patients undergoing surgery or to patients with massive bleeding (e.g. gastrointestinal) in whom no surgery has been performed. The thrombocytopenia is related to the amount of whole blood transfused and the rate of infusion. Thrombocytopenia can be expected when there is replacement of 50 per cent or more of the patient's blood volume. Dilution of the recipient's platelets, the non-viable state of the platelets in stored blood, or their lack in packed red blood cells, are the causes of the thrombocytopenia. Consumption at the site of haemorrhage and activation of coagulation are often additional factors. The platelet count usually returns to normal levels within 3–5 days. Transfusion of 6–8 platelet concentrates is indicated in the presence of haemorrhage when the platelet count falls to levels of around $50 \times 10^9/l$ in association with massive transfusion.

RARE CAUSES

Thrombotic thrombocytopenic purpura is more fully discussed on pp. 208, 391.

Haemangiomas. Thrombocytopenic purpura has been described in association with congenital haemangiomas in infants; they are usually large and solitary, but are sometimes smaller and multiple. Bleeding often occurs in the first month of life. It is considered to be due to utilization and destruction of platelets in the tumour mass; hypofibrinogenaemia and reduction in factors II, V, and VIII occurs in some cases. Successful treatment of the haemangioma usually results in a rise in platelet count and disappearance of the purpura. Treatment with heparin may correct the coagulation abnormalities prior to surgery.

Post-partum thrombocytopenia. An acute thrombocytopenic purpura occurring about one month after delivery has recently been described; it has also been noted after miscarriage. Most commonly it has occured in multiparous women; the infants have been normal. The disorder is self-limiting and responds well to corticosteroids, and thus splenectomy is not necessary.

Idiopathic cryoglobulinaemia. Thrombocytopenia may be associated with the rare disorder idiopathic cryoglobulinaemia (p. 368). Response to steroids is generally poor.

Food allergy. Rare cases of thrombocytopenic purpura have been described in food allergy.

Post-transfusion thrombocytopenia. This rare syndrome has been described in middle-aged multiparous women in whom severe purpura develops about 5–7 days after their first blood transfusion, and in whom a platelet iso-antibody is found in the plasma. The antibody is directed against either $P1^{A1}$ or Bak^{a} antigens, which these patients lack. The disorder is self-limiting, thrombocytopenia persisting about 3–6 weeks; it is thought to be a result of the development of a platelet iso-antibody which cross-reacts with the subject's own platelets or which produces immune complexes with the transfused platelets, resulting in an 'innocent bystander' destruction of the patient's platelets. High-dose intravenous immunoglobulin has been found effective, and is probably the treatment of choice (Berney *et al.* 1985). Corticosteroids may also be effective.

Thrombocytopenia with acquired immunodeficiency (AIDS) or related syndromes is becoming increasingly recognized (p. 488). The prevalence of thrombocytopenia is about 10 per cent in patients with persistent generalized lymphadenopathy, and 30 per cent in AIDS (Murphy *et al.* 1987). The features are those of immune thrombocytopenia. Corticosteroids may be contra-indicated, depending on the clinical status of the patient, and high-dosage intravenous immunoglobuin may be the best initial treatment (Bussel & Hilgartner 1984). Nevertheless, the response to corticosteroids and splenectomy is similar to that in patients with idiopathic thrombocytopenic purpura (Oksenhendler *et al.* 1987).

Treatment

Treatment of secondary thrombocytopenic purpura consists of:

1. Specific measures for relief of the causative disorder.

2. Administration of corticosteroids, which may be of value in some cases when bleeding is troublesome. In general, steroids do not produce a remission as in idiopathic thrombocytopenia, and there is considerable difference of opinion as to a possible non-specific effect on capillary fragility resulting in a lessening or even temporary cessation of bleeding manifestations.

3. Platelet transfusion in selected cases (p. 393), particularly when the condition is acute and likely to be limited in duration.

4. *Splenectomy.* In most cases, splenectomy is not indicated. However, it may be indicated in those disorders in which treatment of the underlying disorder is unsuccessful in controlling the bleeding, provided that the immediate prognosis of the underlying disorder is reasonable. Thus, it may be indicated in hypersplenism with thrombocytopenic bleeding, in very occasional cases of myelofibrosis, in chronic lymphocytic leukaemia, in malignant lymphoma, and in aplastic anaemia with refractory thrombocytopenia causing troublesome bleeding.

Thrombocytopenia due to drugs and chemicals

Thrombocytopenia due to the toxic action of drugs and chemicals on the blood and marrow is not uncommon; most cases occur as a complication of drug therapy, but occasional cases are due to the toxic action of chemicals used in industry or in the home. Drugs that cause thrombocytopenia fall into two groups: (i) those that cause aplastic anaemia; and (ii) drugs that cause selective thrombocytopenia, i.e. thrombocytopenia without anaemia and neutropenia.

Table 14.4. *Drugs and thrombocytopenia*

Drugs that cause aplastic anaemia
Cytotoxic drugs
Chloramphenicol
Chlorothiazide
Tolbutamide, chlorpropamide
Organic arsenicals
Drugs that cause selective (immune) thrombocytopenia
Quinidine, quinine, α-methyldopa, digitoxin
Chlorothiazide, frusemide
Tolbutamide, chlorpropamide
Heparin
Meprobamate, diphenylhydantoin, carbamazepine, valproate
Sulphonamides, penicillins, cephalosporins, trimethoprim
Phenylbutazone, salicylates, chloroquine, gold, penicillamine
Antazoline
Phenobarbitone, phenothiazines
Para-aminosalicylic acid, rifampicin

Drugs that cause aplastic anaemia (Table 14.4) These drugs may cause either selective thrombocytopenia or thrombocytopenia as part of an aplastic anaemia. Thrombocytopenia is sometimes the first and only indication of marrow depression. If the drug is stopped as soon as it appears, anaemia and neutropenia may not develop; this is especially so with chlorothiazide, organic arsenicals, gold, and sulphonamides. The prognosis is much better when thrombocytopenia is the sole evidence of marrow depression than when pancytopenia develops.

Drugs that cause selective thrombocytopenia (Table 14.4) These are all low-risk drugs, purpura occurring only occasionally or rarely. More comprehensive lists of offending drugs are found in the monograph of Swanson & Cook (1977) and the review of Hackett *et al.* (1982).

Mechanism. The mechanisms responsible for severe drug-induced thrombocytopenia fall broadly into two groups: (i) those having a direct toxic effect on the bone marrow; and (ii) a hypersensitivity reaction in which the platelets are rapidly destroyed in the peripheral blood, possibly with associated impairment of platelet formation by megakaryocytes.

Direct toxic action on the marrow is probably responsible for the thrombocytopenia resulting from most of the drugs listed in Table 6.3, p. 123. Severe thrombocytopenia occurs only in a small percentage of patients under treatment, and its occurrence is determined by the *idiosyncrasy* of the patient to the particular drug. However, thrombocytopenia due to *ristocetin* appears to be due to a direct dose-related non-immune action of the drug on platelets.

The *hypersensitivity* reaction with actual destruction of platelets in the peripheral blood is classically seen in quinidine and quinine sensitivity. It was originally extensively studied by Ackroyd (1953) in relation to sedormid sensitivity. A single dose of these drugs administered to a person sensitive to them produces a profound fall in platelets, usually in a matter of hours, due to the action of a plasma factor.

Ackroyd proposed that the drug acts as a hapten, combines with the platelet, renders it antigenic, and results in the formation of antibody against the drug–platelet complex. On further drug administration, this antibody causes platelet agglutination, and in the presence of complement, lysis. A modification of this theory has been proposed, which suggests that the drug combines with a plasma protein rather than the platelet to form the antigen, which results in antibody formation. When the drug is re-administered, the antibody combines with the antigen (drug plus plasma protein) to form an immune complex which is adsorbed onto the surface of the platelet, resulting in its removal by the reticulo-endothelial system. According to this theory, the platelet is involved in the immune reaction as an innocent bystander' on which an extrinsic immune complex reacts. More recent studies suggest that both platelet membrane (glycoprotein Ib and glycoprotein IX) and plasma protein is required for antibody formation and for subsequent platelet damage, and it appears that von Willebrand factor is involved in this complex system.

Clinical features. There is usually a history of administration of the drug for days, weeks, or even months, followed by bleeding in a matter of hours up to several days following the last dose. In cases due to marrow depressing agents, e.g. gold, there is sometimes an interval of weeks or more between the last dose and the onset of bleeding. The bleeding is sometimes mild and limited to the skin, but frequently it is severe with extensive mucous membrane haemorrhage and *'blood blisters' in the mouth*, as well as skin petechiae and ecchymoses. Severe haemorrhage of sudden onset is especially characteristic of those drugs in which hypersensitivity can be demonstrated, especially quinidine, quinine, and digitoxin. With acute severe bleeding, constitutional symptoms are common—chills, headaches, generalized aches, fever, abdominal pain, nausea, vomiting, and itching of the skin. Withdrawal of the drug is followed by cessation of bleeding within a few hours or days. Quinidine purpura is more common in females than males.

Thrombocytopenia due to quinine is not as common as that due to quinidine, but it is of special importance because quinine is present in a number of commonly consumed drinks such as 'tonic' waters and other bitter drinks, and in certain proprietary medicines which may be self-administered. The term 'cocktail purpura' has been used to describe purpura occuring after ingestion of drinks (Belkin 1967).

A unique drug-induced thrombocytopenic syndrome is associated with heparin administration in 3–5 per cent of patients receiving the drug for more than 5–7 days. In a small proportion of individuals so affected, thrombocytopenia is accompanied by thrombosis, either venous or arterial, often widespread and resulting in severe morbidity and significant mortality. Usually, the patient's plasma contains an antibody which aggregates normal platelets in the presence of 0.5–1.0 U heparin/ml *in vitro*. A more sensitive laboratory test may be release of ^{14}C-labelled serotonin from platelets in a similar *in vitro* system (Sheridan *et al.* 1986). An early diagnosis is essential, and routine platelet counts should be carried out on patients receiving heparin for more than five days. Treatment consists of suspending heparin and administering dextran intravenously, and usually warfarin. There is hope that recently developed low molecular weight heparin analogues might not cross-react with the patient's antibodies, and will thus represent alternative and more effective therapy for this grave illness. The condition is reviewed by Chong (1987).

The *typical blood picture* is that of thrombocytopenia without anaemia or neutropenia. There may be a moderate leucocytosis during the bleeding. The bone marrow shows a normal or increased number of megakaryocytes, many of which show absent or reduced granularity.

The *diagnosis* is suggested by the history of drug ingestion, the severity of the bleeding manifestations, the presence of constitutional symptoms, and spontaneous remission on cessation of the drug. Typical response to a test dose establishes the diagnosis with certainty, but as test doses may produce dangerous bleeding they are unsafe and should be avoided.

Because of the importance of avoiding the offending drug in the future, special tests designed to support the diagnosis of causal relationship between the thrombocytopenia and the suspected drug should be carried out. These tests are commonly positive when the thrombocytopenia is due to quinidine, quinine, digitoxin, and heparin in which antibody-mediated hypersensitivity has been demonstrated to be the mechanism of the thrombocytopenia, but may be positive with other drugs, although less commonly so. The tests are discussed by Hackett *et al.* (1982). The demonstration of immunoglobulin binding to platelets in the presence of the offending drug will probably prove to be the most sensitive laboratory test. Other tests, in probable order of sensitivity, are the complement fixation test, platelet serotonin and platelet factor 3 release test, the clot retraction inhibition test, and platelet agglutination and lysis test. The platelet agglutination and lysis tests are relatively insensitive, and often give negative results when other tests are positive.

There is evidence that the timing of the investigation may be important in diagnosis; if tests are negative during the early thrombocytopenic stage they should be repeated after the platelet count has returned to normal. It is important to realize that a causal relationship between thrombocytopenia and a drug may not be demonstrated by *in vitro* tests in suspected cases, even if currently available tests are performed during both the thrombocytopenic and recovery phases. Thus, a negative result for a specific drug does not exclude it as a cause of the thrombocytopenia.

Occasionally, thrombocytopenic purpura first develops in the post-operative period; in such cases it may be due to sedatives, analgesics, or antibiotics, and infection should be excluded.

Prognosis. In selective thrombocytopenia, the platelet count returns to normal and the bleeding ceases within a few hours to a few days after stopping the drug; recovery is nearly always complete within 7–14 days. Occasionally, death occurs, usually from cerebral haemorrhage. Heparin-induced thrombocytopenia with thrombosis carries a worse prognosis. When thrombocytopenia occurs as part of an aplastic anaemia, the prognosis is that of aplastic anaemia (p. 126).

Treatment consists of: (a) immediate cessation of the offending drug. Once a patient has developed thrombocytopenia due to a particular drug they should never be given that drug or chemically related drugs again, and should carry a warning card to show to future medical attendants (Fig. 14.12); (b) the administration of corticosteroids in patients with severe bleeding, as for acute idiopathic thrombocytopenic purpura; and (c) blood transfusion to replace blood loss. It is probable that

---

Mr A.B. developed an acute thrombocytopenic purpura following the ingestion of quinine, due to his sensitivity (allergy) to this drug. Under no circumstances should he receive this drug again.

He has also been warned not to drink tonic waters or other drinks containing quinine and to inquire whether proprietary medicines he purchases contain quinine.

Fig. 14.12. *Warning card for a patient with thrombocytopenia due to quinine sensitivity.*

in cases caused by antibodies, transfused platelets are rapidly destroyed. Nevertheless, if bleeding appears to be life-threatening, platelet transfusion should be given (p. 393). Splenectomy is without beneficial effect and is contra-indicated.

Thrombotic thrombocytopenic purpura

Thrombotic micro-angiopathic haemolytic anaemia and thrombohaemolytic thrombocytopenic purpura, are synonyms for thrombotic thrombocytopenic purpura, a rare disorder characterized by the occurrence of fever, thrombocytopenic purpura, haemolytic anaemia, fluctuating neurological disturbances of variable nature, and renal disease. Any one of these features may be absent, and often all five are present only in the terminal stages. Abdominal pain and jaundice are not uncommon.

The disorder is of rapid onset, purpura or rapidly developing anaemia usually being the first manifestations. It may occur at any age, but is most common in young adults. The spleen may be palpable. Blood examination shows a severe haemolytic anaemia, thrombocytopenia, and leucocytosis, sometimes with a leukaemoid reaction; the morphological features of micro-angiopathic haemolytic anaemia are typically present (p. 207). The direct Coombs' test is usually negative. Bone marrow examination reveals erythroid and often myeloid hyperplasia, and a normal or slightly increased number of megakaryocytes; sections of aspirated marrow show diagnostic hyaline thrombi in a significant proportion. A polyclonal increase in immunoglobulins may be found. Laboratory evidence for disseminated intravascular coagulation is usually minimal or absent.

The aetiology is unknown; it appears to be related to the collagen diseases, and it is possible that hypersensitivity plays an aetiological role. Associations are recent infections, pregnancy, oral contraceptives, and a genetic susceptibility. At post mortem, multiple haemorrhages, usually petechial, are found macroscopically, while microscopically the characteristic feature is the presence in many organs of hyaline thrombi in the capillaries and terminal arterioles. The clinical manifestations are due to widespread intravascular platelet thrombi. The pathogenesis is not known, but evidence points to a vascular endothelial cell abnormality. Defective prostacyclin release, impaired fibrinolysis, and abnormal von Willebrand factor multimers in plasma, all related to endothelial functions, have been reported in this disease. A platelet agglutinating factor has also been described. The administration of plasma or cryoprecipitate can reverse some of the abnormalities.

Diagnosis can sometimes be established by demonstration of the typical thrombi in a biopsy specimen, for example from the gingiva. There is no definitive treatment. A number of empirical measures, including corticosteroids, splenectomy, and anticoagulants, appear ineffective in most instances. Recent experience confirms that plasmapheresis (and in some cases repeated plasma infusions) is of unequivocal benefit in most cases. Because of variable responses a combination of daily plasmapheresis, antiplatelet drugs, and corticosteroid in high dosage should be instituted on diagnosis. In earlier reports, the disease was almost uniformly fatal, usually within a matter of weeks. A growing number of cases (up to 75 per cent) surviving long periods have been recorded more recently, and clearly survival has been influenced by treatment. The disease is well reviewed by Amorosi & Ultmann (1966), Byrnes & Moake (1986), and Remuzzi (1987).

Neonatal and inherited thrombocytopenias

The platelet count of full-term newborns is only slightly lower than that of older children and adults. Premature infants, however, have lower platelet counts, and this should be borne in mind during the investigation of bleeding in a premature infant. Neonatal thrombocytopenia may be acquired or inherited, and presents at birth or within a few hours of birth. However, inherited disorders may not present clinically for several months or longer after birth; they may remain a problem throughout life (Table 14.5).

It should be remembered that petechiae not due to thrombocytopenia are quite commonly seen in

Table 14.5. *Neonatal and congenital thrombocytopenia*

Immune
Auto-immune: mothers with chronic idiopathic thrombocytopenia purpura
Iso-immune (allo-immune): platelet group incompatibility
Infections
Congenital or neonatal
Drug administration to mother
Congenital megakaryocytic hypoplasia
Isolated
Associated with congenital abnormalities or pancytopenia
Hereditary
Sex-linked: pure form, Aldrich's syndrome
Autosomal: dominant or recessive
Congenital leukaemia
Giant haemangioma

normal newborn infants; they are usually confined to the head and upper chest, and disappear in a short time; they are considered to be due to a temporary increase of venous pressure during delivery.

Immune thrombocytopenia

This may arise in cases in which the mother has suffered from idiopathic thrombocytopenic purpura, and is due to the transplacental passage of the antiplatelet auto-antibody from the mother to the fetus. It occurs in approximately 50 per cent of infants born to mothers who are thrombocytopenic at the time of delivery, but is less common when the mother's platelet count is normal. It may occur in infants of both splenectomized and non-splenectomized mothers (p. 385). The purpura appears within 24 hours of birth, is usually mild, and spontaneously disappears within several weeks; however, it is sometimes severe and may occasionally result in death.

Immune thrombocytopenia may also occur in infants from mothers who do not have idiopathic thrombocytopenic purpura. The infant possesses a platelet antigen lacking in the mother, usually PL^{A1}. Maternal antibodies directed against PL^{A1} (see p. 375) cross the placenta to the fetal circulation, and produce a condition known as iso-immune (allo-immune) neonatal thrombocytopenic purpura; this condition has been reported as the cause of about 20 per cent of cases of immune neonatal thrombocytopenia. In general, bleeding manifestations are more severe in the iso-immune than auto-immune thrombocytopenic purpuras. Thrombocytopenia may also occur in erythroblastosis fetalis; its mechanism is uncertain, but it is probably related to either the haemolysis or to exchange transfusion.

Drug ingestion by the mother

Two varieties of this form of neonatal thrombocytopenia exist. In one, neonatal thrombocytopenia is associated with immune drug-induced thrombocytopenia (p. 388) in the mother, with passage of the antibody across the placenta to act on the infant's platelets. In the second, the mother is not thrombocytopenic; this variety has been described particularly with thiazide drugs, especially when given for prolonged periods, e.g. up to three months, during pregnancy. It appears that the marrow of the affected infants is unduly susceptible to the drug.

Infection

Thrombocytopenia occurring at birth or in the first two days of life may result from almost any form of infection, but is particularly common in infections such as cytomegalic inclusion disease, disseminated herpes simplex infection, congenital toxoplasmosis, and congenital syphilis.

Megakaryocytic hypoplasia

Megakaryocytic hypoplasia occurs as an isolated phenomenon in an otherwise healthy child, or in association with a syndrome of congenital abnormalities. The congenital abnormalities most commonly associated with megakaryotyic hypoplasia include bilateral absence of the radii, the rubella syndrome, and pancytopenia with multiple congenital abnormalities (Fanconi's syndrome).

Inherited thrombocytopenias

A number of genetically distinct forms of inherited thrombocytopenia have been described. These include sex-linked thrombocytopenia, autosomal dominant, and autosomal recessive thrombocytopenia. These conditions produce life-long bleeding disorders of variable severity, and bleeding in the newborn is infrequent. Inherited thrombocytopenia occurring in the pure form may be associated with functionally abnormal platelets.

In three of the inherited disorders, distinctive features are present. *Aldrich's syndrome* is characterized by eczema, recurrent infections, and thrombocytopenia; most infants eventually die, by the age of three years. The *May–Hegglin* anomaly is familial, and characterized by thrombocytopenia (often mild and usually asymptomatic), with giant platelets and Döhle bodies in the cytoplasm of the granulocytes. The *Bernard–Soulier* syndrome, with giant platelets and functional defects, is also characterized by a degree of thrombocytopenia in most patients. The functional defects in these disorders are described in more detail on p. 395.

Platelet transfusion

Types of platelet preparation

The transfusion of viable, physiologically active platelets can be achieved:

1 with fresh whole blood;

2 with platelet-rich plasma (PRP) or platelet concentrates (PC) obtained from fresh whole blood;

3 with platelet concentrates prepared by plateletpheresis using a continuous or intermittent flow cell separator. Plateletpheresis has the decided advantage that a clinically useful transfusion can be achieved using platelets harvested from a single donor. A comparable infusion of platelets prepared from donor units of 500 ml whole blood necessitates pooling from about six donors (total 5–6 $\times$ 10^{11} platelets);

4 with autologous (own) platelets collected by plateletpheresis and stored frozen until required.

In the majority of cases, whatever the underlying disease, platelet concentrates are used. Associated anaemia may be treated by the transfusion of packed red cells. Fresh whole blood is more difficult to obtain and, in practice, is effectively replaced by the combination of packed red cells and platelet concentrates.

The methods of preparation of platelets are undergoing constant revision, but most currently employ an acidified anticoagulant solution and a closed system of plastic packs. Meticulous technique in the collection of the blood is of paramount importance in obtaining a satisfactory yield of platelets; in particular, any clotting must be avoided as the presence of even small amounts of thrombin can seriously damage platelets. Preparation is usually carried out at ambient room temperature (22°C) which results in a reasonable lifespan when re-infused into the patient, and allows longer storage before administration. With the introduction of newer plastics, the container bags allow rapid gas exchange, ensuring maintenance of pH greater than 6.0. The storage period is consequently longer, and platelets may remain viable for transfusion for up to seven days.

Clinical effect

The clinical effect is related to the number and viability of the platelets given, the mechanism of the thrombocytopenia (p. 377), and the presence or otherwise of significant splenomegaly. A poor response may also be due to associated infection, fever, consumption coagulopathy, or the presence of antibodies, either iso- (see below) or auto- (p. 375).

Platelet viability is determined by the time interval between collection and use, and by the care in preparation (see above). In general, the shorter the time between the commencement of withdrawal of the blood from the donor and the completion of transfusion in the recipient, the more effective is the transfusion. Thus, the time should be as short as possible.

The effect is determined by clinical assessment of the bleeding tendency, combined with estimation of the platelet count. A transfusion is regarded as successful when the bleeding manifestation for which it was given is controlled for a period of at least 48 hours. Control of the bleeding tendency commonly outlasts the rise in the platelet count when this occurs (it should be 10–20 $\times$ $10^9/l/m^2$

one hour post-transfusion for each unit of platelets infused). In some cases there is no significant rise despite clinical improvement in the bleeding.

Iso-(allo-)immunization and reactions

Platelets contain iso-antigens; to date, about a dozen have been identified. There are no naturally occurring iso-antibodies, and antibodies, when present, are the result of immunization by previous transfusion. Antibodies are most readily detected by complement fixation and platelet release techniques. The latter have been shown to be sensitive to iso-antibodies (Hirschman *et al.* 1973) and these have HLA (p. 478) or membrane glycoprotein specificities. Tests may be used to select compatible donors for platelet transfusion, but these are specialized and not widely applied at present. Direct cross-matching procedures are also described (Yam *et al.* 1984), but not widely practised.

Although immunization from previous platelet administration is clinically less of a problem than first anticipated, platelet iso-antibodies are readily formed, and may impair the effectiveness of repeated transfusions.

Where sensitive techniques are used, iso-immunization can be shown to occur after very few transfusions. For this reason, care should be taken in selecting donors for patients who may required prolonged support as, for example, in aplastic anaemia. This is especially the case if bone marrow transplantation is contemplated, when care must be taken to avoid immunization against HLA antigens. It is the basis for the increased use of single-donor platelet preparations from plateletpheresis of close relatives or HLA-identical individuals in such donors. Patients with acute leukaemia, on the other hand, who are undergoing treatment that is immunosuppressive seem less liable to develop antibodies, and may be sustained for long periods using platelets from ABO and Rh compatible donors.

Mild reactions with fever and chill are not uncommon, but serious transfusion reactions do not appear to occur; in patients with mild reactions complement-fixing platelet antibodies may be demonstrated *in vitro*, and there is failure of the transfusion to increase the platelet count. Marked reactions, when they occur, are probably due to the presence of associated leucocyte antibodies acting against transfused leucocytes.

Another serious hazard of platelet transfusion is transmission of virus, including human immunodeficiency virus (HIV) and hepatitis, but the risks are minimized by donor testing for hepatitis B antigen and HIV antibody.

Indications

Platelet transfusion should be limited to patients with severe thrombocytopenia with specific indications.

An important factor in determining the effectiveness and thus the indications for platelet transfusion is the mechanism of thrombocytopenia. In cases due to decreased marrow production, the platelets generally survive long enough to be effective, provided they are properly prepared and given in adequate numbers. However, in cases due to excess platelet destruction, they seldom survive sufficiently long to cause clinical improvement. Significant splenomegaly with sequestration and possibly destruction of platelets may also lessen effectivenss.

The indications are both surgical and medical; the surgical indication is often prophylactic.

Medical. In potentially self-limiting thrombocytopenias of short duration, e.g. due to drug reaction (especially when due to marrow depression), chemotherapy, radiation, and massive transfusion, platelet transfusion is indicated when there is serious bleeding.

In thrombocytopenia of longer duration, as in aplastic anaemia or bone marrow infiltration, platelet transfusion may be used temporarily to tide the patient over an exacerbation of bleeding. This is especially so when there is an acute additional factor which is depressing the platelet count and increasing clinical bleeding, e.g. infection in aplastic anaemia, chemotherapy in acute leukaemia, chemotherapy or radiation in lymphomas and chronic leukaemias. There is reasonable evidence that regular prophylactic platelet transfusions to individuals with platelet counts persistently lower than $20 \times 10^9/l$ will reduce the incidence of spontaneous haemorrhage and probably mortality (Higby *et al.* 1974).

Platelet transfusion is particularly indicated with suspected or proven internal bleeding, e.g. intracranial, thoracic, or peritoneal bleeding.

Surgical. Prophylactic transfusion may be indicated when significant bleeding is expected, as in patients with thrombocytopenia due to marrow insufficiency or depression, e.g. in aplastic anaemia, and lymphoma or leukaemia. In general, it is not indicated in splenectomy for idiopathic thrombocytopenic purpura, although it may be used in occasional cases (p. 385). Platelet transfusion is indicated for surgical procedures in patients with significant platelet dysfunction.

Qualitative platelet disorders

A bleeding disorder can result not only from a decrease in platelet number (quantitative defect), but also from an abnormality of function (qualitative defect). Qualitative defects may result in excessive bleeding, even though the platelet count is normal, which is the case in the majority of instances of disordered platelet function.

Special tests

Skin bleeding time (p. 377). The bleeding time is the most useful clinical test to confirm the presence of a suspected defect in platelet function. If the bleeding time is normal, a platelet abnormality is of limited clinical significance. In the presence of thrombocytopenia, prolongation of the bleeding time beyond that expected for the platelet count is suggestive of co-existing platelet dysfunction (see Fig. 14.9).

Morphology of platelets is of value in the diagnosis of a number of functional disorders, both congenital and acquired. Morphological features include size and shape, and the appearance of granules and other cytoplasmic features. The morphology may be assessed on routine blood smear, by fluorescent microscopy using specific stains or fluorescent antibodies, and by transmission electron microscopy to identify dense bodies, alpha granules, the microtubules, the surface-connected cannalicular system, and other ultrastructural details.

Platelet aggregation tests, based on the technique originally reported by Born in 1962, remain the cornerstone for defining functional defects in the clinical laboratory. Aggregation is carried out in transparent cuvettes at 37°C using stirred platelet-rich plasma. Agonists are added to individual fresh samples, the reagents being chosen to test different pathways of platelet activation. Aggregation causes a decrease in the turbidity of the platelet suspension. This decrease in turbidity (or increase in light transmission) is detected by a photo-electric cell and recorded on moving paper (Fig. 14.13). Numerous modifications have been made, including the automated, simultaneous measurement of adenosine diphosphate and triphosphate release by chemiluminescence, or the recording of aggregation of platelets in whole blood by measuring the changes in electrical impedance. The agonists commonly used are collagen, ADP, arachidonic acid, adrenaline, thrombin, and ristocetin.

Platelet factor 3 availability assay (PF3 availability). This assay measures the platelet contribution to clotting of blood, which can be substituted by a number of phospholipids. It is based on the shortening of the Russell's viper venom (or kaolin) clotting time due to the presence of platelets. Occasionally, patients have been described who have an isolated defect in PF3 availability but, for the most part, more specific tests of platelet function, in particular platelet aggregation, provide greater specificity, and the assay is not widely performed in routine laboratories.

Platelet adhesion, measured by retention of platelets in glass bead columns, has been superseded by more specific tests, especially in the diagnosis of von Willebrand's disease. This technique reflects a combination of adhesion and aggregation of platelets and, perhaps for this reason, is prone to artefact. Adhesion in glass bead columns is dependent on many factors, such as the anticoagulant used, the rate of perfusion of blood through the column, the type of tubing, and characteristics of the glass beads. Abnormal adhesion is common in thrombasthenia, Bernard–Soulier syndrome, von Willebrand's disease, myeloproliferative disorders,

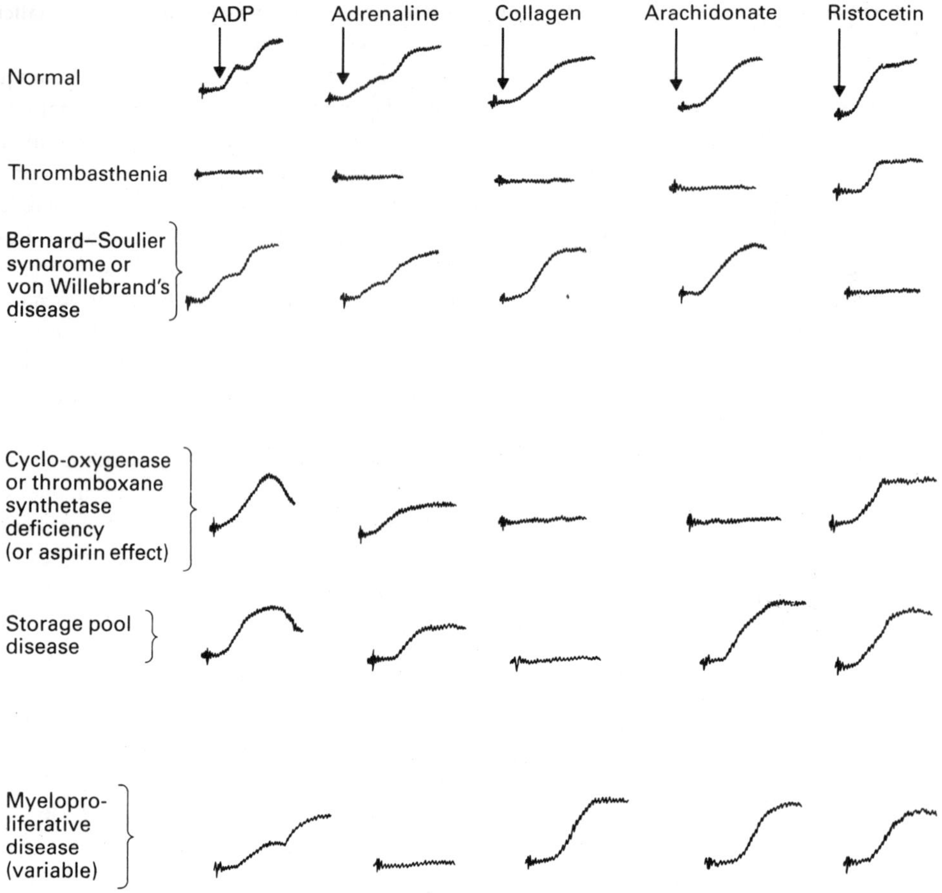

Fig. 14.13. *Tracings on moving paper illustrating the extent of platelet aggregation (vertical axis) with the passage of time (horizontal axis) following addition of agonists to an aggregometer containing platelets from normal subjects, and subjects with various qualitative platelet disorders. Traces indicate optical density changes in aggregometer caused by platelet aggregation following addition of agonist (↓).*

uraemia, and congenital aggregation disorders described below.

The *prothrombin consumption* test measures the residual prothrombin remaining in serum after the clotting of whole blood. The test depends on both the coagulation cascade and the presence of normal numbers of functional platelets. While useful as a screening test, more specific tests, particularly platelet aggregation, are more likely to define functional abnormalities, and for this reason many routine laboratories would not include it in their normal test profile. The technique is considered in more detail by Dacie & Lewis (1984).

Specialized techniques and research tools. There are now many sophisticated techniques for defining the physiology and biochemistry of platelet function in research laboratories. These include: (a) the identification and analysis of membrane receptors by electrophoresis and antibody probes; (b) measurement of secreted proteins, e.g. β thromboglobulin and platelet factor 4, using specific immuno-assays; (c) analysis of fatty acid metabolites, particularly those of arachidonic acid by radio-immunoassay or chromatograhic techniques; and (d) the measurement of intracellular calcium concentration changes by fluorescent markers. The application of these and other techniques has led to the better definition of functional defects over the past two decades.

Classification of platelet dysfunction

Both congenital and acquired disorders exist in which platelet functional defects are clearly defined. They may be classified according to aetiology (Table 14.6).

Table 14.6. *Classification of disorders of platelet function*

Congenital

Membrane receptor defects
Glycoprotein IIb/IIIa deficiency—Glanzmann's thrombasthenia
Glycoprotein Ib deficiency—Bernard-Soulier syndrome
Pseudo-von Willebrand disease

Enzyme defects
Phospholipase deficiency—aspirin-like defect
Cyclo-oxygenase deficiency—aspirin-like defect
Thromboxane synthetase deficiency

Granule defects
Storage pool deficiency
Alpha granule deficiency—Gray platelet syndrome

Platelet procoagulant activity defects

Acquired
Stem cell disorders—leukaemia, myelodysplasia, myeloproliferative
Drugs (p. 400, Table 14.7)
Dysproteinaemias—myeloma, macroglobulinaemia (p. 367)
Uraemia (p. 366)
Miscellaneous—auto-antibodies, disseminated intravascular coagulation (DIC), post-transfusion, etc.

Congenital qualitative platelet defects

THROMBASTHENIA (GLANZMANN'S DISEASE)

In 1918, Glanzmann described a bleeding disorder associated with a normal platelet count and defective clot retraction. It is a familial disorder, occurring in both sexes and transmitted as an autosomal recessive gene. The bleeding time is long in spite of a normal platelet count and normal platelet morphology. The platelets fail to aggregate in response to ADP, collagen, and thrombin, but do respond to ristocetin (Fig. 14.13). There is decreased or absent glass bead retention and platelet factor 3 availability with a defective release reaction. The defect is located in the membrane with a lack of glycoprotein IIb–IIIa complex, which is the point of attachment with fibrinogen, which in turn is required for platelet–platelet binding in the aggregation process. Clinically, the disorder is characterized by a tendency to bruise after even minor trauma, excessive and prolonged bleeding after cuts and abrasions, epistaxes, and menorrhagia which can be a very troublesome problem. Deep haematoma and haemarthroses are rare. The heterozygote is usually unaffected, although occasionally a mild bleeding tendency with easy bruising has been described.

BERNARD-SOULIER SYNDROME

This is a very rare, autosomal recessive disorder characterized by a severe bleeding tendency. The pattern of bleeding is similar to that of Glanzmann's thrombasthenia, and heterozygotes have normal haemostasis. The syndrome is characterized by a combination of moderate to severe thrombocytopenia, large platelets on peripheral blood smear, and a very prolonged skin bleeding time. The platelets aggregate with physiological agonists (although slowly with thrombin) but fail to 'agglutinate' with ristocetin, a similar pattern to that seen with classical von Willebrand's disease. The defect, however, lies in the deficiency of membrane glycoprotein Ib and associated glycoprotein IX. There may also be an abnormality of the glycoprotein V. The only available treatment of these patients, and indeed all of the congenital functional disorders, is the judicious use of platelet transfusion in the face of a bleeding episode or as prophylaxis for surgery. The major problem is then the development of antiplatelet iso-(allo-)antibodies, rendering further transfusions ineffective.

DEFECTS OF PLATELET ENZYMES

Familial deficiency of the enzymes, cyclo-oxygenase and thromboxane synthetase, involved in the metabolism of arachidonic acid and production of thromboxane A_2 have been reported. These are rare, and their genetic transmission uncertain. The bleeding defect is mild, and it is of clinical significance only in the case of serious trauma or surgery. The bleeding time is prolonged to a mild or moderate degree, and platelet aggregation to ADP, collagen, and arachidonic acid is abnormal. Differentiation from storage pool disease (see below) is achieved by studying the effects of arachidonic acid and endoperoxide analogues in aggregation, and identifying normal dense bodies and their contents. Platelet transfusion to cover trauma or surgery is usually the only therapy required.

GRANULE DEFECTS

Deficiencies of specific granules may occur independently—dense body deficiency (δ storage pool disease), Gray platelet syndrome (α granule deficiency)—together ($\alpha\delta$ storage pool disease), or as a component of a group of inherited diseases with multiple abnormalities.

The group of inherited disorders in which δ storage pool deficiency is one of a number of defects consists of Hermansky–Pudlack syndrome (oculocutaneous albinism, bleeding tendency, and pigmented macrophages in the bone marrow), Wiskott–Aldrich syndrome (thrombocytopenia, eczema, and immunodeficiency) and Chediak–Higashi syndrome (susceptibility to infection, thrombocytopenia, and defective pigmentation of skin and retina). Thrombocytopenia with absent radii is said to be associated with storage pool disease in some cases.

Storage pool disease (δ-SPD) causes a mild to moderate bleeding tendency similar to that induced by aspirin. Inheritance is autosomal dominant. Platelet aggregation with ADP and collagen is defective, but to arachidonic acid is normal. Absence of the dense bodies can be documented using electron microscopy, fluorescence with mepacrine-treated platelets, or by the grossly subnormal secretion of adenine nucleotides.

Gray platelet syndrome (α-SPD) is an extremely rare autosomal dominant disorder with a mild bleeding diathesis, epistaxis, easy bruising, and ecchymoses. The characteristics are prolongation of skin bleeding time, mild to moderate thrombocytopenia, and enlarged platelets with an unusual gray colour on routine peripheral blood film. The platelet lack the α granules, and are deficient in the constituents of these granules (p. 363). The defect is almost certainly one of granule 'packaging', as the plasma concentration of α granule proteins which are unique to megakaryocytes and platelets (e.g. β TG) is increased, suggesting synthesis in the marrow but subsequent leakage in the megakaryocyte or platelet. Marrow fibrosis is seen in this condition, and is presumably a consequence of elevated local concentrations of the platelet-derived growth factor and of other components that normally concentrate in the granule, destined for release at sites of tissue injury far from the site of synthesis.

Combined defects ($\alpha\delta$-SPD), with deficiencies in both major platelet granules, are described. Additional abnormalities in the metabolism of the platelet have been reported with these syndromes. Platelet functional defects are reviewed by Weiss (1980), George *et al.* (1984), and Hardisty & Caen (1987).

PLATELET PROCOAGULANT ACTIVITY DEFECTS

One patient has been described with a bleeding disorder characteristic of a plasma coagulation defect, prolonged bleeding following tooth extraction and tonsillectomy, and the development of spontaneous retroperitoneal haematoma. Her platelets were deficient in factor Va binding sites (Miletich *et al.* 1979). Isolated defects in PF3 availability have also been reported. These rare cases substantiate the role of platelets in plasma coagulation (pp. 363, 409) as opposed to their clearly defined primary haemostatic function.

Acquired platelet dysfunction

Secondary qualitative defects are seen in a heterogeneous group of disorders. Partial or complete defects in either aggregation, adhesion, or the release reaction may occur separately or together in the same patient.

In stem cell defects, platelet dysfunction is

common, frequently associated with thrombocytopenia. The *myeloproliferative disorders* (p. 318) have been most thoroughly studied, perhaps because of the paradox of both bleeding and thrombotic disease occurring in these diseases, not infrequently co-existing in the same patient. Each of the specific diseases, *polycythaemia rubra vera, thrombocythaemia*, and *myelofibrosis*, may be complicated by platelet dysfunction. The bleeding may be severe with ecchymoses, epistaxis, gastrointestinal bleeding, and excessive surgical bleeding. Frequently, the platelet count is abnormally high, and the complications of bleeding and thrombosis appear to be more common in patients with excessive platelet numbers. Nevertheless, in polycythaemia rubra vera the elevated haematocrit (by virtue of the increased viscosity) is a more important arbiter of thrombosis than the platelet count (p. 329).

The peripheral blood film often shows platelets with great variation in size; extremely large platelets and megakaryocyte fragments are particularly characteristic. Ultrastructural abnormalities are present, and vary widely. Megakaryocytes are usually markedly increased in number in the bone marrow, and again often show morphological abnormalities, with small immature forms.

Associated functional abnormalities are prolongation of the skin bleeding time and disordered platelet aggregation pattern. 'Spontaneous' aggregation is not uncommon. Absent aggregation with adrenaline is the most frequent defect, seen in two-thirds of cases. Both increased and decreased sensitivity to other platelet agonists, abnormal glycoprotein patterns, disorders of arachidonic acid metabolism, and granule abnormalities have all been well documented. Frustratingly, the *in vitro* abnormalities have rarely been shown to correlate with clinical behaviour. Further, the administration of aspirin to patients with polycythaemia rubra vera does not appear to prevent thrombotic complications, and probably increases the risk of haemorrhage. Reduction of the platelet count to normal by chemotherapy or [^{32}P] phosphorus is probably beneficial, and the risk of thrombosis is decreased by measures that keep the haematocrit below 45 per cent in cases of polycythaemia rubra vera.

Platelet function in *acute leukaemia* and *myelodysplastic syndromes* has been less extensively studied; significant thrombocytopenia is usually the overriding problem. However, similar functional defects to those described with the myeloproliferative disease are well recognized, and at times cause a haemostatic defect in the patient with normal or near normal platelet numbers.

A wide variety of *therapeutic drugs* and *dietary components* causes platelet dysfunction, for the most part resulting in a mild haemostatic defect with easy bruising and a mild to moderate prolongation of the skin bleeding time. These drugs should be avoided where possible in patients undergoing surgery, in patients receiving anticoagulants, and in the presence of thrombocytopenia. The major mechanisms of drug interference with platelet function, and examples of such agents, are shown in Table 14.7. The fortuitous activity of drugs in reducing platelet function has been harnessed in the therapy of occlusive vascular disease, and this aspect is considered in detail on p. 465.

The role of platelet dysfunction in *uraemia* has been described on p. 366. In *dysproteinaemias* (p. 367), coating of the platelet membrane and thrombogenic connective tissue by the paraprotein interferes with platelet adhesion and aggregation. The defect, reflected by a prolonged skin bleeding time, is correctable by plasmapheresis.

As indicated above (p. 381), *platelet auto-antibodies* may be associated with platelet dysfunction in the absence of thrombocytopenia. Platelet activation causing degranulation, but not excessive shortening of platelet survival time, may result in an acquired 'storage pool' deficiency and may be the common mechanism for dysfunction accompanying a number of situations, which include *disseminated intravascular coagulation (DIC), massive transfusion, thrombotic thrombocytopenic purpura, haemolytic uraemic syndrome, cardiopulmonary bypass*, and even *myeloproliferative* and *leukaemic diseases*.

Thrombocytosis and thrombocythaemia

Thrombocytosis is defined as an increase above normal values, i.e. greater than 400×10^9/l, in the

Table 14.7. *Drugs affecting platelet function*

Mechanism of effect	Examples	Clinically significant defect at therapeutic doses
Interference with arachidonate metabolism		
Phospholipase A inhibition	Mepacrine	No
Alteration of membrane phospholipid	Dietary eicosapentanoic acid (fish oil)	Yes
Cyclo-oxygenase inhibition	Acetylsalicylic acid	Yes
	Indomethacin	Yes
	Other NSAIDs	Variable
Thromboxane synthetase inhibition	Imidazole analogues	Yes
Thromboxane receptor antagonist		
Drugs that increase cyclic AMP levels directly		
Prostanoids	Prostacyclin and prostaglandin E_1	Yes
Phosphodiesterase inhibition (probably other mechanisms)	Dipyridamole, theophylline	No
Other mechanisms		
React at platelet membrane and other levels of platelet metabolism	Sulphinpyrazone	No
	Ticlopidine	Yes
	Antibiotics such as penicillin, carbenicillin (high dose)	Yes
	Dextran infusion	Yes
	Calcium channel blockers,	Probably not
	β adrenergic blockers,	Probably not
	hydroxychloroquine, alcohol, etc.	Probably not

number of platelets in the peripheral blood. The causes are listed in Table 14.8.

The association of a raised platelet count with a bleeding tendency may occur with the myeloproliferative disorders, polycythaemia vera and myelofibrosis, while in other cases it is the only abnormality, and is termed idiopathic thrombocythaemia (p. 334). Some of these cases subsequently develop the typical features of polycythaemia vera, or myelofibrosis (p. 334).

Reactive thrombocytosis rarely requires therapeutic intervention, except for treatment of the underlying condition. Thrombocythaemia, on the other hand, is a diagnosis with major implications. The distinction between the two categories is important in that patients with 'reactive' thrombocytosis should not be exposed to ^{32}P phosphorus or alkylating agents, whilst those with thrombocythaemia are at risk from both bleeding and thrombosis (Buss *et al.* 1985).

Idiopathic (haemorrhagic) thrombocythaemia

Essential or primary thrombocythaemia are synonyms for idiopathic (haemorrhagic) thrombocythaemia, a clinical syndrome characterized by repeated excessive bleeding, especially from the mucous membranes, and thrombotic changes, particularly in small vessels. Extremely high platelet counts may be seen. It is classified as one of the myeloproliferative disorders, and its pathological features often resemble those of myelofibrosis or polycythaemia vera.

Clinical features. The disorder occurs most often in middle and older age groups. The outstanding

Table 14.8. *Causes of thrombocytosis*

'Reactive' thrombocytosis
Haemorrhage—moderate increase in the platelet count may follow acute haemorrhage
Surgery and trauma, particularly fractures of bones
Iron deficiency anaemia (p. 42)
Splenectomy (p. 358)
Infection—occasionally
Non-infective inflammatory disorders including collagen diseases
Malignancy especially in Hodgkin's disease, carcinoma
Thrombocythaemia
Polycythaemia vera and myelofibrosis (p. 318)
Idiopathic thrombocythaemia (p. 400)
Chronic granulocytic leukaemia (p. 259)
Myelodysplastic syndromes (p. 258)

symptom is bleeding of varying severity, and small blood vessel occlusion. Gastrointestinal bleeding is most common, but haematuria, haemoptysis, menorrhagia, and bleeding after minor trauma and surgery are also common. Spontaneous bruising occurs, and large haematomas form after only mild trauma. Petechiae are rare. Thrombosis is a common complication and particularly affects toes, feet, fingers, and the cerebral circulation, but may occur at any site (Schafer 1984). Splenectomy is common, and the liver may be enlarged. Occasionally, splenomegaly is absent; if Howell–Jolly bodies are present in the peripheral blood, then infarction/atrophy of the spleen is probable. There is an increased incidence of peptic ulceration and of gout.

The bone marrow is hyperplastic with a gross increase in megakaryocytes; hyperplasia of the myeloid and erythroid series is common. Most megakaryocytes appear normal, but often immature and abnormal forms are present. Sometimes, marrow trephine shows areas of fibrosis.

Blood picture. The outstanding feature is an increase in the platelet count, which is usually over $1000 \times 10^9/l$, and often much higher. Abnormalities of morphology are usual with irregular and giant forms. Defects of platelet function are present in most cases (p. 399). A moderate leucocytosis, may be seen. There may be a moderate shift to the left, with 1–3 per cent myelocytes. The neutrophil alkaline phosphatase is usually increased. The red cell picture is variable with normal values, anaemia, or mild polycythaemia; anisocytosis and poikilocytosis may be present.

Treatment. The incidence and severity of bleeding is broadly related to the increase in platelet count; a defect of platelet function also contributes. Treatment, therefore, is aimed at reducing the platelet count to normal or near normal. This may be achieved by the administration of ^{32}P (a dose of 3–4 millicuries, 111–148 Mbq, is usually sufficient to reduce the platelets in several weeks) or by the use of busulphan. As these agents are leukaemogenic they should be reserved for use in older patients. Hydroxyurea and pipobroman have all been used with success, as in the treatment of polycythaemia vera and may be preferable (p. 329). A good discussion of therapeutic options is provided by Schafer (1984). Plateletpheresis and aspirin are of some value in special situations. Splenectomy is contra-indicated as it causes a further rise in platelet count and may aggravate the bleeding tendency.

Course and prognosis. The disorder usually remains quiescent for long periods after treatment, or may run a chronic course over a number of years. The patient may die from haemorrhage or thrombosis, or from the more usual complications of the myeloproliferative disorders, acute leukaemia or marrow failure.

References and further reading

Books and monographs

Bloom, A.L. & Thomas, D.P. (Eds) (1987) *Haemostasis and Thrombosis*, 2nd Ed., Churchill Livingstone, Edinburgh.

Colman, R.W., Hirsh, J. & Marder, V. (Eds) (1987) *Hemostasis and Thrombosis*, 2nd Ed., Lippincott, Philadelphia.

Dacie, J.V. & Lewis, S.M. (1984) *Practical Haematology*, 6th Ed., Churchill Livingstone, London.

De Gruchy, G.C. (1975) *Drug-induced Blood Disorders*, Blackwell Scientific Publication, Oxford.

Gordon, J.L. (Ed.) (1981) *Platelets in Biology and Pathology*, 2nd Ed., North Holland, Amsterdam.

Harker, L. & Zimmerman, T.S. (Eds) (1983) *Measurements of Platelet Function*, Churchill Livingstone, Edinburgh.

McMillan, R. (Ed.) (1983) *Immune Cytopenias*, Churchill Livingstone, Edinburgh.

Spaet, T.H. (Ed.) (1972, 1974, 1976, 1978, 1980, 1982, 1984) *Progress in Hemostasis and Thrombosis*, Vols. 1–7, Grune & Stratton, New York.

Verstraete, M., Vermylen, J., Lijnen, R. *et al.* (1987) *Thrombosis and Haemostasis 1987*, Leuven University Press, Belgium.

Haemostasis, platelets, and vessel wall

Burch, J.W. & Majerus, P.W. (1979) The role of prostaglandins in platelet function. *Semin. Hematol.* **16**, 196.

Chesterman, C.N. & Berndt, M.C. (1986) Platelet and vessel wall interaction and the genesis of atherosclerosis. *Clin. Haemat.* **15**, 323.

Haslam, R.J. (1987) Signal transduction in platelet actiation. In: Verstraete, M., Vermylen, J., Lijnen, R. & Arnout J. (Eds) *Thrombosis and Haemostasis 1987*, p.147, Leuven University Press, Belgium.

Kitchens, C.S. & Pendergast, J.F. (1986) Human thrombocytopenia is associated with structural abnormalities of the endothelium that are ameliorated by glucocorticosteroid administration. *Blood*, **67**, 203.

Kitchens, C.L. & Weiss, L. (1975) Ultrastructural changes of endothelium associated with thrombocytopenia. *Blood*, **46**, 567.

Macfarlane, R.G. (1941) Critical review: the mechanism of haemostasis. *Quart. J. Med.* **33**, 1.

Miyazono, K., Okabe, T., Urabe, A. *et al.* (1987) Purification and properties of an endothelial cell growth factor from human platelets. *J. Biol. Chem.* (in press)

Sixma, J.J. (1987) Platelet adhesion in health and disease. In: Verstraete, M., Vermylen, J., Lijnen, R. & Arnout, J. (Eds) *Thrombosis and Haemostasis 1987*, p.127, Leuven University Press, Belgium.

Vascular disorders and non-thrombocytopenic purpura; the symptomatic vascular purpuras; miscellaneous purpuras

Ackroyd, J.F. (1953) Allergic purpura, including purpura due to foods, drugs and infections. *Am. J. Med.* **14**, 605.

Allen, D.M., Diamond, L.K. & Howell, A. (1960) Anaphylactoid purpura in children (Schonlein-Henoch syndrome). Review with a follow-up of the renal complications. *Am. J. Dis. Child.* **99**, 833.

Bick, R.L. (1979) Vascular disorders associated with thrombohaemorrhagic phenomena. *Semin. Thromb. Hemostas.* **5**, 167.

Chandler, D. & Nalbandian, R.M. (1966) DNA autosensitivity. *Am. J. Med. Sci.* **251**, 145.

Cream, J.J., Gumpel, J.M. & Peachey, R.D.G. (1970) Schonlein–Henoch purpura in the adult. *Quart. J. Med.* **39**, 461.

Cupps, T.R. & Fauci, A.S. (1981) *The Vasculitides*, Saunders, Philadelphia.

Defreyn, G., Vergara Douden, M., Machin, S.J. *et al.* (1980) A plasma factor in uraemia which stimulates prostacyclin release from cultured endothelial cells. *Thromb. Res.* **19**, 695.

Fernandez, F., Goudable, C., Sie, P. *et al.* (1985) Low haematocrit and prolonged bleeding time in uraemic patients: effect of red cell transfusions. *Brit. J. Haemat.* **59**, 139.

Gardner, F.H. & Diamond, L.K. (1955) Autoerythrocyte sensitization. A form of purpura producing painful bruising following auto-sensitization of red blood cells in certain women. *Blood*, **10**, 675.

Goodman, R.M., Levitsky, J.M. & Friedman, I.A. (1962) The Ehlers–Danlos syndrome and multiple neurofibromatosis in a kindred of mixed derivation, with special emphasis on haemostasis in the Ehlers–Danlos syndrome. *Am. J. Med.* **32**, 976.

Harrison, D.F.N. (1964) Familial haemorrhagic telangiectasia. *Quart. J. Med.* **33**, 25.

Hjort, P.F., Rapaport, S.I. & Jorgensen, L. (1964) Purpura fulminans. Report of a case successfully treated with heparin and hydrocortisone. Review of 50 cases from the literature. *Scand. J. Haemat.* **1**, 169.

Horowitz, H.I., Stein, I.M., Cohen, B.D. *et al.* (1970) Further studies on the platelet-inhibiting effect of guanidinosuccinic acid and its role in uremic bleeding. *Am. J. Med.* **49**, 336.

Janson, P.A., Jubelirer, S.J., Weinstein, M.J. *et al.* (1980) Treatment of the bleeding tendency in uremia with cryoprecipitate. *New Engl. J. Med.* **303**, 1318.

Lackner, H. & Karpatkin, S. (1975) On the 'easy bruising' syndrome with normal platelet count. A study of 75 patients. *Ann. Int. Med.* **89**, 190.

Lee, S.L. & Miotti, A.B. (1975) Disorders of hemostatic function in patients with systemic lupus erythematosus. *Semin. Arth. Rheumat.* **4**, 241.

Liu, Y.K. Kosfeld, R.E. & Marcum, S.G. (1984) Treatment of uraemic bleeding with conjugated oestrogen. *Lancet*, **ii**, 887.

Livio, M., Marchesi, D., Remuzzi, C. *et al.* (1982) Uraemic bleeding: role of anaemia and the beneficial effect of red cell transfusions. *Lancet*, **ii**, 1013.

Mannucci, P.M. Remuzzi, G., Pusineri, F. *et al.* (1983) Deamino-8-D-arginine vasopressin shortens the bleeding time in uremia. *New Engl. J. Med.* **308**, 8.

McConkey, B., Fraser, G.M. & Bligh, A.S. (1962) Osteoporosis with purpura in rheumatoid disease: prevalence and relation to treatment with corticosteroids. *Quart. J. Med.* **31**, 419.

McPherson, R.A., Onstad, J.W., Ugaretz, R.J. *et al.* (1977) Coagulopathy in amyloidosis: combined deficiency of factors IX and X. *Am. J. Hemat.* **3**, 225.

Nicolaides, S.H. (1967) Spontaneous bruising. *Lancet*, **ii**, 370.

Rabiner, S.F. & Molinas, F. (1970) The role of phenol and phenolic acids on the thrombocytopathy and defective platelet aggregation of patients with renal failure. *Am. J. Med.* **49**, 346.

Ratnoff, O.D. & Agle, D.P. (1968) Psychogenic purpura: a re-evaluation of the syndrome of autoerythrocyte sensitization. *Medicine*, **47**, 475.

Remuzzi, G., Marchesi, D., Livio, M. *et al.* (1978). Altered platelet and vascular prostaglandin generation in patients with renal failure and prolonged bleeding times. *Thromb. Res.* **13**, 1007.

Saunders (1960) p. 14–31.

Scarborough, H. & Shuster, A. (1960) Corticosteroid purpura. (Preliminary communication). *Lancet*, **i**, 93.

Schuster, S. & Scarborough, H. (1961) Senile purpura. *Quart. J. Med.* **30**, 33.

Stewart, J.H. & Castaldi, P.A. (1967) Uraemic bleeding: reversible platelet defect corrected by dialysis. *Quart. J. Med.* **36**, 409.

Tattersall, R.N. & Seville, R. (1950) Senile purpura. *Quart. J. Med.* **19**, 151.

Waldenström, J. (1952) Three new cases of purpura hyperglobulinaemia: a study in long standing benign increase in serum globulin. *Acta Med. Scand.* Suppl. 226, **142**, 931.

Platelets, thrombocytopenia, and platelet functional defects

Ackroyd, J.F. (1953) Allergic purpura, including purpura due to foods, drugs and infections. *Am. J. Med.* **14**, 605.

Ahn, Y.S., Harrington, W.J., Seelman, R.C. *et al.* (1974) Vincristine therapy of idiopathic and secondary thrombocytopenias. *New Engl. J. Med.* **291**, 376.

Ahn, Y.S., Harrington, W.J., Mylvaganam, R. *et al.* (1984) Slow infusion of vinca alkaloids in the treatment of idiopathic thrombocytopenic purpura. *Ann. Int. Med.* **100**, 192.

Ahn, Y.S., Harrington, W.J., Simon, S.R. *et al.* (1983) Danazol for the treatment of idiopathic thrombocytopenic purpura. *New Engl. J. Med.* **308**, 1396.

Amorosi, E.L. & Ultmann, J.E. (1966) Thrombotic thrombocytopenic purpura. Report of 16 cases and review of the literature. *Medicine*, **45**, 139.

Aster, R.H. & Keene, W.R. (1969) Sites of platelet destruction in idiopathic thrombocytopenic purpura. *Brit. J. Haemat.* **16**, 61.

Bayer, W.L., Sherman, F.E., Michaels, R.H. *et al.* (1965) Purpura in congenital and acquired rubella. *New Engl. J. Med.* **273**, 1362.

Becker, G.A. & Aster, R.H. (1972) Short term platelet preservation of 22°C and 4°C. *Blood*, **40**, 593.

Belkin, G.A. (1967) Cocktail purpura; an unusual case of quinine sensitivity. *Ann. Int. Med.* **66**, 583.

Berney, S.I., Metcalfe, P., Wathen, M.C. *et al.* (1985) Posttransfusion purpura responding to high dose intravenous IgG: further observations on pathogenesis. *Brit. J. Haemat.* **61**, 627.

Born, G.V.R. (1962) Aggregation of blood platelets by adenosine diphosphate and its reversal. *Nature*, **194**, 927.

Bouroncle, B.A. & Doan, C.A. (1966) Refractory idiopathic thrombocytopenic purpura treated with imuran. *New Engl. J. Med.* **275**, 630.

Brearley, R.L. & Rowbotham, B. (1984) High dose gammaglobulin for idiopathic thrombocytopenic purpura. *Austr. N.Z. J. Med.* **14**, 67.

Brecher, G. & Cronkite, E.P. (1950) Morphology and enumeration of human blood platelets. *J. Appl. Physiol.* **3**, 365.

Brizel, H.E. & Raccuglia, G. (1965) Giant haemangioma with thrombocytopenia. *Blood*, **26**, 751.

Bull, B.S., Schneiderman, M.A. & Brecher, G. (1965) Platelet counts with the Coulter counter. *Am. J. Clin. Path.* **44**, 678.

Burgess, M.A., Hirsh, J. & De Gruchy, G.C. (1969) Acute thrombocytopenic purpura due to quinine sensitivity. *Med. J. Aust.* **1**, 453.

Bussel, J.B. & Hilgartner, M.W. (1984) The use and mechanism of action of intravenous immunoglobulin in the treatment of immune haematologic disease. *Brit. J. Haemat.* **56**, 1.

Byrnes, J.J. & Moake, J.L. (1986) Thrombotic thrombocytopenic purpura and the haemolytic uraemic syndrome: evolving concepts of pathogenesis and treatment. *Clin. Haemat.* **15**, 413.

Chong, B.H. (1987) Heparin-induced thrombocytopenia. *Haemat. Rev.* (in press).

Cines, D.B. & Schreiber, A.D. (1979) Immune thrombocytopenia. Use of a Coombs' antiglobulin test to detect IgG and C_3 on platelets. *New Engl. J. Med.* **300**, 106.

Clancy, R., Jenkins, E. & Firkin, B.G. (1972) Qualitative platelet abnormalities in idiopathic thrombocytopenic purpura. *New Engl. J. Med.* **286**, 622.

Colvin, B.T. (1985) Thrombocytopenia. *Clin. Haemat.* **14**, 661.

Court, W.S., Bozeman, J.M., Soong, S-J. *et al.* (1987) Platelet surface-bound IgG in patients with immune and nonimmune thrombocytopenia. *Blood*, **69**, 278.

Evans, R.S., Takahashi, K., Duane, R.T. *et al.* (1951) Primary thrombocytopenic purpura and acquired haemolytic anaemia. Evidence for a common etiology. *Arch. Int. Med.* **87**, 48.

Fehr, J., Hofmann, V. & Kappeler, C.M. (1982) Transient reversal of thrombocytopenia in idiopathic thrombocytopenic purpura by high-dose intravenous gamma globulin. *New Engl. J. Med.* **306**, 1254.

Filip, D.J. & Aster, R.H. (1978) Relative hemostatic effectiveness of human platelets stored at 4°C and 22°C. *J. Lab. Clin. Med.* **91**, 618.

Firkin, B.G., Wright, R., Miller, S. *et al.* (1969) Splenic macrophages in thrombocytopenia. *Blood*, **33**, 240.

Fountain, J.R. & Losowsky, M.S. (1962) Haemorrhagic thrombocythaemia and its treatment with radio-active phosphorus. *Quart. J. Med.* **31**, 207.

George, J.N., Nurden, A.T. & Philips, D.R. (1984) Molecular defects in interactions of platelets with the vessel wall. *New Engl. J. Med.* **311**, 1084.

Hackett, T., Kelton, J.C. & Roberts, P. (1982) Drug induced platelet destruction. *Semin. Thromb. Hemostas.* **8**, 116.

Hanson, P.M. & Ginsberg, M.H. (1981) Immunological reactions of platelets. In: Gordon, J.L. (Ed.) *Platelets in Biology and Pathology*, 2, p.265, Elsevier/North-Holland.

Hardisty, R.M. & Caen, J.P. (1987) Disorders of platelet function. In: Bloom, A.L. & Thomas, D.P. (Eds) *Haemostasis and Thrombosis*, 2nd Ed., p.365, Churchill Livingstone, Edinburgh.

Harker, L. (1978) Platelet survival time: its measurement and use. In: Spaet, T.H. (Ed.) *Progress in Hemostasis and Thrombosis*, Vol. 4, p.321, Grune & Stratton, Florida.

Harker, L.A. & Slichter, S.J. (1972) The bleeding time of a screening test for evaluation of platelet function. *New Engl. J. Med.* **287**, 155.

Harrington, W.J. & Arimura, G. (1961) Immunological aspects of platelets. In: *Blood Platelets*, Henry Ford Hospital International Symposium, Little, Brown & Company, Boston.

Harris, E.N., Gharavi, A.E., Hegde, U. *et al.* (1985) Anticardiolipin antibodies in autoimmune thrombocytopenic purpura. *Brit. J. Haemat.* **59**, 231.

Hegde, U.M., Gordon Smith, E.C. & Worlledge, S. (1977) Platelet antibodies in thrombocytopenic patients. *Brit. J. Haemat.* **35**, 113.

Higby, D.J., Cohen, E., Holland, J.F. *et al.* (1974) The prophylactic treatment of thrombocytopenic leukemia patients with platelets: a double blind study. *Transfusion*, **14**, 440.

Hirschmann, R.J., Yankee, R.A., Coller, B.S. *et al.* (1973) Sensitive methods for the detection and characterization of platelet iso-antibodies. *Thromb. Diath. Haemorrh.* **29**, 408.

I.C.S.H. Panel on diagnostic application of radio-isotopes in hematology (1977) Recommended methods for radioisotope platelet survival studies. *Blood*, **50**, 1137.

Karpatkin, S., Strick, N., Karpatkin, M.B. *et al.* (1972) Cumulative experiences in the detection of anti-platelet antibody in 234 patients with idiopathic thrombocytopenic purpura, systemic lupus erythematosus and other clinical disorders. *Am. J. Med.* **52**, 776.

Kelton, J.G. (1983) Management of the pregnant patient with idiopathic thrombocytopenic purpura. *Ann. Int. Med.* **99**, 796.

Kunicki, T.J. & Newman, P.J. (1986) The biochemistry of platelet-specific alloantigens. *Curr. Stud. Haematol. Blood Transf.* **52**, 18.

Laros, R.K. & Kagan, R. (1983) Route of delivery for patients with immune thrombocytopenic purpura. *Am. J. Obstet. Gynec.* **148**, 901.

Lindenbaum, J. & Hargrove, R.L. (1968) Thrombocytopenia in alcoholics. *Ann. Int. Med.* **68**, 526.

Lusher, J.M. & Iyer R. (1977) Idiopathic thrombocytopenic purpura in children. *Semin. Thromb. Hemostas.* **3**, 175.

Malmsten, C., Hamberg, M., Svensson, J. *et al.* (1975) Physiological role of an endoperoxide in human platelets: hemostatic defect due to platelet cyclooxygenase deficiency. *Proc. Natl. Acad. Sci. U.S.A.* **72**, 1446.

McMillan, R. (1981) Chronic idopathic thrombocytopenic purpura. *New Engl. J. Med.* **304**, 1135.

McVerry, B.A. (1985) Management of idiopathic thrombocytopenic purpura in adults (Annotation). *Brit. J. Haemat.* **59**, 203.

Mielke, C.H., Kaneshiro, I.A., Mather, J.M. *et al.* (1969) The standardized Ivy bleeding time and its prolongation by aspirin. *Blood*, **34**, 204.

Miletich, J.P., Kane, W.H., Hofmann, S.L. *et al.* (1979) Deficiency of factor Xa–factor Va binding sites on the platelets of a patient with a bleeding disorder. *Blood*, **54**, 1015.

Moncada, S. & Vane, J.R. (1979) Arachidonic acid metabolites and the interactions between platelets and blood-vessel walls. *New Engl. J. Med.* **300**, 1142.

Morley, A. (1969) A platelet cycle in normal individuals. *Austr. Ann. Med.* **18**, 127.

Murphy, M.F., Metcalfe, P., Waters, A.H. *et al.*. (1987) Incidence and mechanism of neutropenia and thrombocytopenia in patients with human immunodeficiency virus infection. *Brit. J. Haemat.* **66**, 337.

Newland, A.C., Treleaven, J.G., Minchinton, R.M. *et al.* (1983) High-dose intravenous IgG in adults with autoimmune thrombocytopenia. *Lancet*, **i**, 84.

Nurden, A.T. & Caen, J.P. (1974) An abnormal platelet glycoprotein pattern in three cases of Glanzmann's thrombasthenia. *Brit. J. Haemat.* **28**, 253.

Nurden, A.T. & Caen, J.P. (1979) The different glycoprotein abnormalities in thrombasthenic and Bernard–Soulier platelets. *Semin. Hematol.* **16**, 234.

Oksenhendler, E., Bierling, P., Farcet, J.P. *et al.* (1987) Response to therapy in 37 patients with HIV-related thrombocytopenic purpura. *Brit. J. Haemat.* **66**, 491.

Pizzuto, J. & Ambriz, R. (1984) Therapeutic experience on 934 adults with idiopathic thrombocytopenic purpura: multicentric trial of the cooperative Latin American Group on Hemostasis and Thrombosis. *Blood*, **64**, 1179.

Polycythaemia Study Group (1986) p. 14–93.

Remuzzi, G. (1987) Thrombotic thrombocytopenic purpura. In: Verstraete, M., Vermylen, J., Lijnan, H.R. & Arnout, J. (Eds) *Thrombosis and Haemostasis 1987*, p.673, Leuven University Press, Belgium.

Rowan, R.M., Allan, W. & Prescott, R.J. (1972) Evaluation of an automatic platelet counting system utilizing whole blood. *J. Clin. Path.* **25**, 218.

Schiffer, C.A., Aisner, J. & Wiernk, P.H. (1978) Frozen autologous platelet transfusion for patients with leukemia. *New Engl. J. Med.* **299**, 7.

Sheridan, D., Carter, C. & Kelton, J.G. (1986) A diagnostic

test for heparin-induced thrombocytopenia. *Blood*, **67**, 27.

Slichter, S.J. & Harker, L.A. (1976) Preparation and storage of platelet concentrates. II. Storage variables influencing platelet viability and function. *Brit. J. Haemat.* **34**, 403.

Sultan, Y., Delobel, J., Jeanneau, C. *et al.* (1971) Effect of periwinkle alkaloids in idiopathic thrombocytopenic purpura. *Lancet*, **i**, 496.

Sullivan, L.W., Adams, W.H. & Yong, K.L. (1977) Induction of thrombocytopenia by thrombophoresis in man: patterns of recovery in normal subjects during ethanol ingestion and abstinence. *Blood*, **49**, 197.

Sussman, L.N. (1967) Azathioprine in refractory idiopathic thrombocytopenic purpura. *J. Am. Med. Ass.* **202**, 259.

Swanson, M. & Cook, R. (1977) *Drugs, Chemicals and Blood Dyscrasias*, Drug Intelligence Publications, Illinois.

Thatcher, G.L. & Clatanoff, D.V. (1968) Splenic haemangioma with thrombocytopenia and afibrinogenaemia. *J. Pediat.* **73**, 345.

Territo, M., Finkelstein, J., Oh, W. *et al.* (1973) Management of autoimmune thrombocytopenia in pregnancy and in the neonate. *Obstet. Gynec.* **41**, 579.

Von Behrens, W.E. (1975) Mediterranean macrothrombocytopenia. *Blood*, **46**, 199.

Weiss, H.J. (1980) Congenital disorders of platelet function. *Semin. Hematol.* **17**, 228.

Weiss, H.J., Witte, L.D., Kaplan, K.L. *et al.* (1979) Heterogeneity in storage pool deficiency: studies on granule-bound substance in 18 patients including variants deficient in α-granules, platelet factor 4, β-thromboglobulin and platelet-derived growth factor. *Blood*, **54**, 1296.

Yam, P., Petz, L.D., Scott, E.P. *et al.* (1984) Platelet crossmatch tests using radiolabelled staphylococcal protein A, or peroxidase antiperoxidase in alloimmunized patients. *Brit. J. Haemat.* **57**, 337.

Young, R.C., Nachman, R.L. & Horowitz, H.I. (1966) Thrombocytopenia due to digitoxin. *Am. J. Med.* **41**, 605.

Thrombocytosis and thrombocythaemia

Boxer, M.A., Braun, J. & Ellman, L. (1978) Thromboembolic risk of postsplenectomy thrombocytosis. *Arch. Surg.* **113**, 808.

Brusamolino, E., Canevari, A., Salvaneschi, L. *et al.* (1984) Efficacy trial of pipobroman in essential thrombocythemia: A study of 24 patients. *Cancer Treat. Rep.* **68**, 1339.

Buss, D.H., Stuart, J.J. & Lipscomb, G.E. (1985) The incidence of thrombotic and hemorrhagic disorders in association with extreme thrombocytosis: an analysis of 129 cases. *Am. J. Hemat.* **20**, 365.

Case, D.C., Jr. (1984) Therapy of essential thrombocythemia with thiotepa and chlorambucil. *Blood*, **63**, 51.

Colman, R.W., Sievers, C.A. & Pugh, R.P. (1966) Thrombocytophoresis: a rapid and effective approach to symptomatic thrombocytosis. *J. Lab. Clin. Med.* **68**, 389.

Cronberg, S., Nilsson, I.M. & Gydell, K. (1965) Haemorrhagic thrombocythaemia due to defective platelet adhesiveness. *Scand. J. Haemat.* **2**, 208.

Davis, W.M. & Mendez Ross, A.O. (1973) Thrombocytosis and thrombocythemia: The laboratory and clinical significance of an elevated platelet count. *Am. J. Clin. Path.* **59**, 243.

Fountain, J.R. & Losowsky, M.S. (1962) Haemorrhagic thrombocythaemia and its treatment with radio-active phosphorous. *Quart. J. Med.* **31**, 207.

Gunz, F.W. (1960) Haemorrhagic thrombocythaemia. *Blood*, **15**, 706.

Jabaily, J., Iland, H.J., Laszlo, J. *et al.* (1983) Neurologic manifestations of essential thrombocythemia. *Ann. Int. Med.* **99**, 513.

Kessler, C.M., Klein, H.G. & Havlik, R.J. (1982) Uncontrolled thrombocytosis in chronic myeloproliferative disorders. *Brit. J. Haemat.* **50**, 157.

Kan-Yu, K. (1978) Platelet hyperaggregability and thrombosis in patients with thrombocythemia. *Ann. Int. Med.* **88**, 7.

Orlin, J.B. & Berkman, E.B. (1980) Improvement of platelet function following plateletpheresis in patients with myeloproliferative diseases. *Transfusion*, **20**, 540.

Schafer, A.I. (1984) Bleeding and thrombosis in the myeloproliferative disorders. *Blood*, **64**, 1.

Talpaz, M., Mavligit, G. & Keating, M. *et al.* (1983) Human leukocyte interferon to control thrombocytosis in chronic myelogenous leukemia. *Ann. Int. Med.* **99**, 789.

Chapter 15
Coagulation Disorders

The coagulation mechanism is one of the components of the haemostatic mechanism (p. 360). It comprises three separate, though related, systems: the coagulation system, the coagulation-inhibitory system, and the fibrinolytic system. Pathological disturbances may occur in any one or more of these systems and lead to a bleeding tendency or intravascular coagulation, or to a combination of the two, depending on a wide variety of factors. A bleeding tendency occurs when there is a deficiency of clotting factors, inhibition of the coagulation process, or excessive activity of the fibrinolytic system.

Although haemorrhagic disorders due to abnormalities of coagulation are relatively uncommon, their early recognition and accurate diagnosis is important as there are specific forms of treatment for many of them. The congenital coagulation disorders are listed in Table 15.5 (p. 420) and the acquired disorders in Table 15.9 (p. 435); the latter are more common.

The chapter opens with an account of the physiology of blood coagulation. This is followed by a discussion of the pathogenesis of the coagulation disorders and of the principles of the laboratory tests used in the investigation of a patient with a suspected coagulation disorder. The individual coagulation disorders are then discussed. Finally, a scheme for the investigation of a patient with a haemorrhagic disorder is summarized.

The physiology of blood coagulation

The essential role of the coagulation mechanism is carried out by the coagulation factors. The coagulation-inhibitory and the fibrinolytic systems have the important functions of preventing accidental intravascular clotting and of maintaining the patency of the vascular lumen after intravascular clotting has occured. The inter-relationship of these three mechanisms may be represented diagrammatically, as in Fig. 15.1.

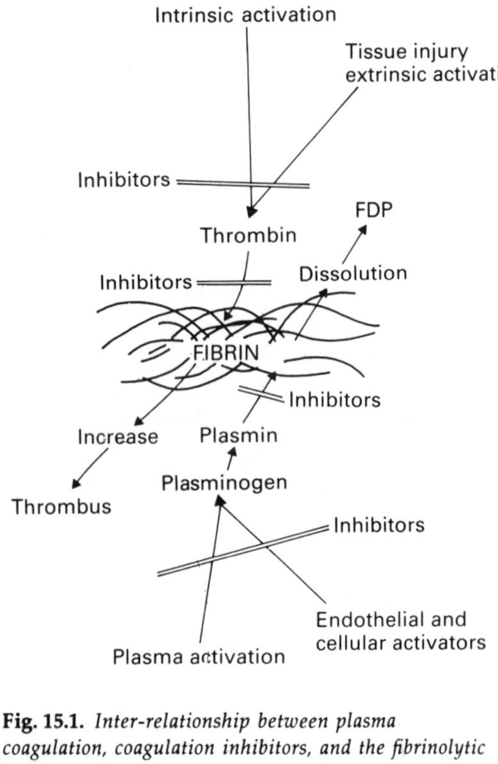

Fig. 15.1. *Inter-relationship between plasma coagulation, coagulation inhibitors, and the fibrinolytic system.*

The coagulation system

The main *function* of the coagulation system is, in the event of injury, to produce thrombin, which firstly aids the activation of platelets in haemostasis, secondly forms a stable fibrin network from circulating fibrinogen, and thirdly stimulates coagulation inactivating mechanisms, thus limiting the process to the vicinity of the injury. The *components* of the system are: (a) the plasma protein coagulation factors, calcium, and platelets, all of which are present in the circulating blood; (b) certain surfaces not normally in contact with the circulating blood; and (c) lipoprotein derived from injured tissue cells and termed 'tissue factor'.

PLASMA PROTEIN COAGULATION FACTORS

The factors and their most important features are listed in Table 15.1. They are present in the plasma in trace to small amounts and, although difficult to isolate in pure form, they can be identified and quantitated by characteristic behaviour in *in vitro* tests.

Factors II, VII, IX, X, XI, XII, and pre-kallikrein are inactive precursors of serine proteases, all retaining considerable homology with trypsin, which is one of the earliest evolutionary prototypes (de Haen *et al.* 1975). The carboxy-terminal region is similar in all the serine proteases, consists of about 250 amino-acid residues, and contains the active site region. The vitamin K-dependent factors (II, VII, IX, and X) show considerable identity of the amino-terminal region, containing 10–12 carboxy glutamic acid residues essential for Ca^{++}-mediated phospholipid binding. The inactive zymogens are activated by limited proteolysis, often accompanied by the release of an activation peptide. Each of the active coagulation factors has a considerable degree of specificity for its substrate, this specificity being conferred by the 'binding pocket' and the conformation of the protein as a whole, which probably limits its substrate recognition (reviewed by Lammle & Griffin 1985; Zur & Nemerson 1987; Berrettini *et al.* 1987).

Factors V and VIII are larger glycoproteins; factor V has a molecular weight of approximately 330 000, and factor VIII 360 000. Activation of these factors is

Table 15.1. *Plasma protein coagulation factors*

Factors		Plasma concentration (mg/ml)	Bleeding disorder: Congenital	Bleeding disorder: Acquired	Laboratory diagnosis: APTT	PT	TCT
Contact*	XII	3×10^{-2}	—	—	+	–	–
	XI	$4–6 \times 10^{-3}$	Rare, mild		+	–	–
Vitamin K dependent†	X	1×10^{-2}	Rare, mild	Neonates	+	+	–
	IX	5×10^{-3}	Uncommon, variable	Liver disease and	+	–	–
	VII	$5–10 \times 10^{-4}$	Rare, variable	vitamin K deficiency	–	+	–
	II	1×10^{-1}	Rare, mild		+	+	–
Antihaemophilic A	VIII	$1–2 \times 10^{-4}$	Uncommon, variable	DIC	+	–	–
Von Willebrand factor		$5–20 \times 10^{-3}$	Uncommon, variable	—	+	–	–
	V	1×10^{-2}	Rare, variable	DIC	+	+	–
Fibrinogen	I	2–5	Rare	DIC, fibrinolysis	+	+	+
Fibrin stabilizing	XIII	8×10^{-3}	Defective wound healing	—	–	–	–

*Pre-kallikrein and high molecular weight kininogen are also involved (see text).
†Neonatal deficiency may involve all four of these factors.
APTT = activated partial thromboplastin time.
PT = prothrombin time.
TCT = thrombin clotting time.
DIC = disseminated intravascular coagulation.

also achieved by limited proteolytic cleavage, resulting in the formation of two non-covalently associated peptides derived from the amino-terminal and carboxy-terminal portions of the inactive molecule, in the case of factor Va being of molecular weight of 94 000 and 74 000 respectively. There is substantial homology between the heavy and light chains of factor Va and factor VIIIa (Zimmerman & Fulcher 1985; Mann *et al.* 1987).

Von Willebrand factor forms a non-covalent complex with factor VIII, thus preventing more rapid removal of the coagulation protein from the plasma. The other contributions of von Willebrand factor to haemostasis also relate to its adhesive properties, mediating adhesion of platelets to the subendothelial tissues (p. 361) and involvement in platelet aggregation (p. 362). Von Willebrand factor circulates as heterogeneous collections of oligomers ranging from the dimer of 500 000 to species of greater than 10 000 000 (Zimmerman & Meyer 1987, Sadler 1987).

Factor I or fibrinogen, is an asymmetrical protein consisting of three pairs of dissimilar polypeptide chains, $A\alpha_2$, $B\beta_2$, and γ_2, linked by disulphide bonds. The molecular weight of fibrinogen is 340 000. The amino-terminal segments of all six chains are probably clustered in a central domain with fibrinopeptides A and B protruding. The proteolytic cleavage of fibrinogen by thrombin, with the release of the fibrinopeptides, is responsible for the spontaneous polymerization of fibrin molecules to form an insoluble network. For a more detailed discussion see Doolittle (1987).

Factor XIII is an inactive pro-enzyme composed of two pairs of polypeptide chains (a_2b_2). A platelet factor XIII consists of only two 'a' chain subunits. Factor XIII is activated to a calcium-dependent transglutaminase by thrombin cleavage of a small peptide from the amino-terminal end of the 'a' subunits. The transglutaminase activity of factor XIIIa is primarily directed to forming isopeptide bonds between lysine and glutamine residues of the fibrin γ chains to form γ–γ dimers, and the α chains to form polymers. These reactions, termed cross-linking or stabilization, make fibrin resistant to plasmin attack and confer structural stability.

The liver hepatocyte is the site of synthesis of most of the coagulation proteins. Vitamin K is required to convert the inactive forms of factors II, VII, IX, and X in the liver to their active forms by carboxylation of amino-terminal clusters of glutamic acid residues to γ-carboxy glutamic acid. Factor VIII is probably synthesized in hepatic sinusoidal endothelial cells. Von Willebrand factor is synthesized in vascular endothelium and bone marrow megakaryocytes. Plasma factor V is derived from hepatic synthesis, while platelet factor V is probably synthesized in megakaryocytes. Factor XIII is similarly disposed.

Synthesis of these proteins is controlled by autosomal genes, with the exception of factor VIII and factor IX where sex-linked genes operate. Inherited deficiency states usually result from the production of a defective molecule, although complete or partial failure of synthesis may occur in some cases. Autosomal recessive inheritance probably explains the extreme rarity of most disorders; the disorders in which factor VIII or factor IX are inherited in the sex-linked manner (haemophilia A and haemophilia B) are relatively much more common.

Fibrinogen concentration may be measured directly as clottable protein, but the other coagulation proteins are usually expressed in units of activity compared to that of a pool of normal plasma. Immunoreactive protein levels can also be measured. It is a general rule that the haemostatic efficiency of the coagulation system is not impaired until the activity of one or more clotting factors is less than 30 per cent of normal (0.3 U/ml).

CALCIUM

Calcium ions are essential in low concentrations for normal blood coagulation, both in the binding of coagulation factor complexes to phospholipid and in the dependency of some coagulation enzymes. When blood is collected for coagulation tests it must be prevented from clotting by the addition of a suitable concentration of a calcium-binding chemical, e.g. sodium citrate. When coagulation tests are performed on the separated plasma an appropriate amount of calcium chloride must be added to permit clotting to proceed.

There is no evidence that coagulation disorders result from pathological reduction in ionized calcium. Nevertheless, transient prolongation of the whole blood clotting time has been observed with very rapid blood transfusion of citrated blood (p. 446).

PLATELET LIPID (PLATELET FACTOR 3) AND MEMBRANE BINDING SITES FOR COAGULATION FACTORS

During haemostasis, activated platelets provide negatively charged phospholipid on the membrane surface, a site for binding Ca^{++} which in turn binds prothrombin and the other vitamin K-dependent coagulation factors. Other specific binding sites appear on the platelet surface during the process of aggregation. Factor Va is bound to the platelet surface, providing binding sites for factor Xa. This congregation of components facilitates the *local*, rapid activation of prothrombin to thrombin. In coagulation tests, a substitute for platelet factor 3 is necessary, and lipids of animal or vegetable origin are commonly used.

FOREIGN SURFACES

The fact that the blood remains fluid in the blood vessels is partly due to the fact that normal vascular endothelium does not promote blood coagulation. Foreign surfaces, both endogenous and exogenous, promote clotting in varying degree; this appears to depend upon the surface electrical charge and the property of wettability. The inactive coagulation factor XII (Hageman factor) is activated by contact with foreign surfaces, and thus the coagulation process is initiated. Coagulation may be initiated in the intravascular space by such foreign surfaces as tumour cells, disrupted villi as in accidental antepartum haemorrhage, and endothelial cells damaged by trauma and infarction. Potent activators include sulphated glycospholipids and sulphatides. Some silicone surfaces and a number of plastics have a negligible or very weak effect in promoting blood clotting; this property is particularly desirable for intravenous prostheses, catheters, and extracorporeal equipment, e.g. heart–lung machines.

In the past, a number of blood clotting tests were insensitive or unreliable due to the inconstant activation of the clotting process by the glass tubes; however, the addition of one of a number of surface active agents, e.g. kaolin, celite, or ellagic acid to plasma, shortly before testing, results in constant activation of the process and thus great improvement in sensitivity of the tests, e.g. activated partial thromboplastin time test (p. 415).

TISSUE FACTOR (TISSUE THROMBOPLASTIN)

Damaged tissue cells expose a lipoprotein called tissue factor, which promotes blood coagulation. Induction of tissue factor expression on the surface of monocytes and vascular endothelium by a number of stimuli, including lipopolysaccharide (endotoxin), interleukin-I, and tumour necrosis factor, has also recently been shown. This would provide a mechanism for fibrin formation in inflammatory lesions and tumours as well as after trauma.

Tissue factor consists of a single protein species, apoprotein III, in a complex with a mixture of phospholipids. The protein is oriented across the cell membrane, with a short intracytoplasmic domain. Only in combination with phospholipids, phosphatidylcholine, phosphatidylethanolamine, and phosphatidylserine does apoprotein III maintain its procoagulant activity. Tissue factor probably represents the cell surface receptor for factor VII. Factor VII itself is unlike the other coagulation factors in that it appears to circulate in a partially activated form. For the full expression of its activity and the initiation of coagulation, however, it requires binding to tissue factor, which of course is not normally exposed to the circulating blood. For further detail, refer to Berrettini *et al.* (1987).

The theory of blood coagulation

Coagulation was originally conceived as a process initiated by the release of an activating substance (thromboplastin) from platelets and tissue cells (Morawitz 1905) with a simple scheme which can be illustrated in the following way:

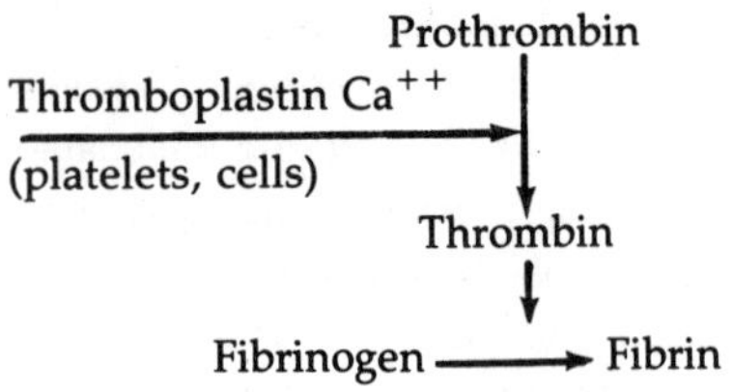

With the development of knowledge about individual clotting factors, the classical theory has undergone considerable modification. It is now known that inactive prothrombin is converted to thrombin by the products formed during earlier stages of coagulation, and which can be brought about by two well-defined sets of reactions known as the extrinsic and intrinsic pathways.

REACTION SEQUENCE

A scheme of coagulation sequences is shown in Fig. 15.2. A number of explanatory notes may help an appreciation of this complex system.

The mechanism of *contact activation* is poorly understood. Surface-bound factor XII becomes susceptible to limited cleavage by kallikrein and also ultimately to auto-activation by factor XIIa itself. The same activating surfaces result in high molecular weight kininogen acting as a non-enzymatic

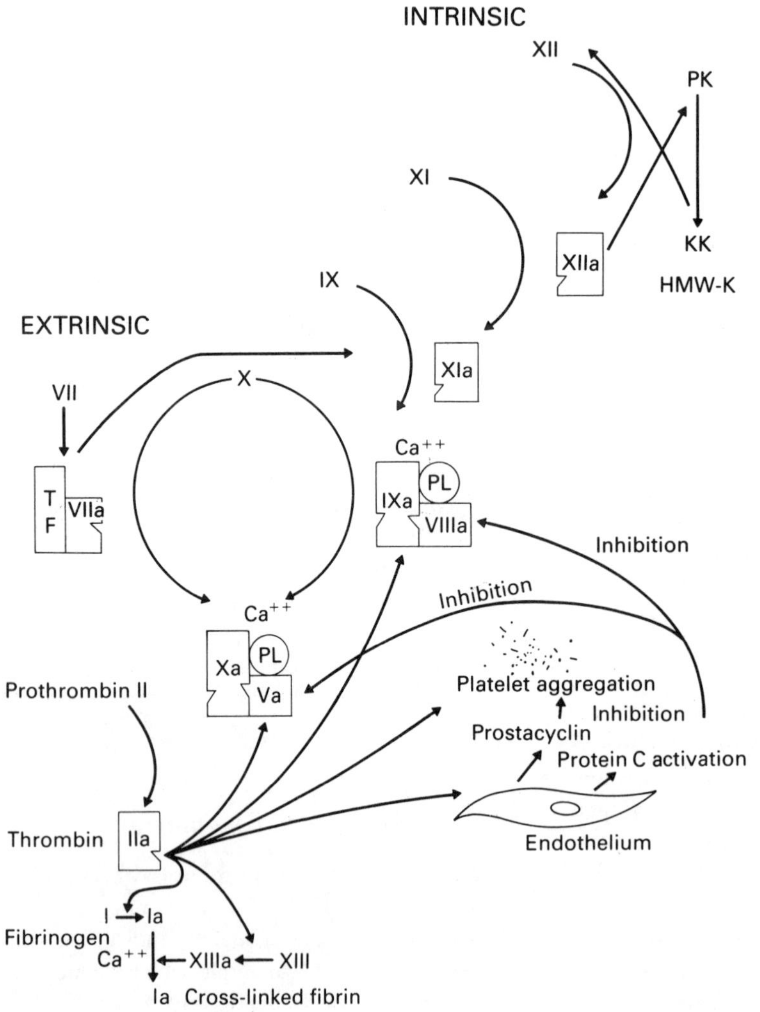

Fig. 15.2. *Proposed reaction sequence in coagulation. It is of interest that components of both the kallikrein and the kinin system are required for the effective operation of factor XII and for activation of factor XI in the test tube, and yet deficiencies in these systems do not result in a clinical bleeding tendency. PK = pre-kallikrein, KK = kallikrein, HMW-K = high molecular weight kininogen, TF = tissue factor, PL = phospholipid.*

co-factor, which interacts with both factor XII and plasma pre-kallikrein with the ultimate reciprocal activation of both. High molecular weight kininogen is also a co-factor for the activation of factor XI by factor XIIa. The contact system may activate a number of other enzyme systems, including the fibrinolytic and the kinin. Paradoxically, deficiency of factor XII, high molecular weight kininogen, and pre-kallikrein (Fletcher factor), while prolonging the coagulation times dependent on contact activation in the test tube, *do not* result in a clinical bleeding disorder (reviewed by Ratnoff & Saito 1979).

Factor IXa is formed by the proteolytic activation of factor IX by factor XIa in the classical *'intrinsic'* system. It is clear, however, that factor IX may also be activated by the VIIa–tissue factor complex of the *'extrinsic'* system; thus the distinction between the two enzyme cascades becomes artificial. Despite the blurring of this distinction between intrinsic and extrinsic pathways, proper functioning of both is required for normal haemostasis.

Factor IXa forms a complex with factor VIIIa, Ca^{++}, and phospholipid to complete the factor X activator, termed 'tenase'. A similar complex is assembled by factor Xa, factor Va, Ca^{++}, and phospholipid to form the prothrombin activator 'prothrombinase'. The reactions are massively accelerated on the surface of activated platelets, and probably other activated cells including the vascular endothelium.

Thrombin has multiple functions which are not all shown in Fig. 15.2. Note, however, the positive amplification of coagulation by thrombin activation of factor V and VIII. At the same time, thrombin activation of protein C (p. 412) and of vascular prostacyclin release has an opposing function to limit the coagulation process.

INHIBITORS OF COAGULATION

The *natural inhibitors* of coagulation provide a mechanism to limit clotting to the vicinity of tissue injury. A number of these inhibitors bear homology to the inhibitors of fibrinolysis and constitute a superfamily of proteins known as *'serpins'*. This group of inhibitors functions by offering their active protease an alternative high-affinity substrate that resists complete cleavage (Carrell *et al.* 1987). They form a stoichiometric complex with the target protease, the complex being subsequently catabolized and cleared from the circulation. Thus the inhibitors are consumed in the process of coagulation, as are coagulation factors, and this is important when considering massive thrombosis or disseminated intravascular coagulation.

Table 15.2 lists the major inhibitors of coagulation and some of their features. *Antithrombin III* is the major antithrombin activity, contributing about 70 per cent of the capacity of plasma, but it also inhibits factor XIIa, XIa, IXa, and in particular Xa. Inhibition of coagulation factors by antithrombin III is greatly enhanced by the presence of heparin, primarily due to acceleration of both the cleavage and the complexing of the protease to the inhibitor. Antithrombin III is synthesized by hepatocytes and the vascular endothelium.

Heparin co-factor II selectively inhibits thrombin,

Table 15.2. *Inhibitors of blood coagulation*

Inhibitor	Plasma concentration (mg/ml)	Deficiency associated with thrombosis	Target coagulation factor
Serine protease inhibitors			
Antithrombin III	$1–1.5 \times 10^{-1}$	Yes	Xa, thrombin
Heparin co-factor II	—	?	Thrombin
α_2 macroglobulin	2.5	?	Thrombin, kallikrein
Protein C system			
Protein C	4×10^{-3}	Yes	Factors Va, VIIIa
Protein S	$3–4 \times 10^{-2}$	Yes	Co-factor for activated protein C

and its activity is enhanced by heparin and by other proteoglycans, particularly dermatin sulphate, a major component of the vascular wall. *Alpha$_2$ macroglobulin* may contribute to overall anticoagulant activity, but the physiological significance is not known.

Protein C, a vitamin K-dependent protein, is a potent inactivator of factor Va and factor VIIIa when it is itself activated by thrombin with a co-factor expressed on the plasma membrane of vascular endothelium (Esmon & Owen 1981) termed *thrombomodulin*. Factor Va–light chain also enhances the activation of protein C. A further vitamin K-dependent glycoprotein, protein S promotes binding of activated protein C to lipid and platelet surfaces, thus enhancing anticoagulant activity.

The protein C–thrombomodulin system is thus localized to the endothelium, an appropriate site to limit coagulation and thrombosis. Antithrombin III and heparin co-factor II have also the potential for local enhancement due to the glycosaminoglycan concentration in the vessel wall.

Other naturally occurring inhibitors are fibrin itself, which binds thrombin, and the breakdown products of fibrinogen and fibrin produced by the action of the fibrinolytic enzyme, plasmin. These are known as fibrin(ogen) degradation products, and have a potent antithrombin action when present in high concentrations. The natural anticoagulants are reviewed by Salem (1986).

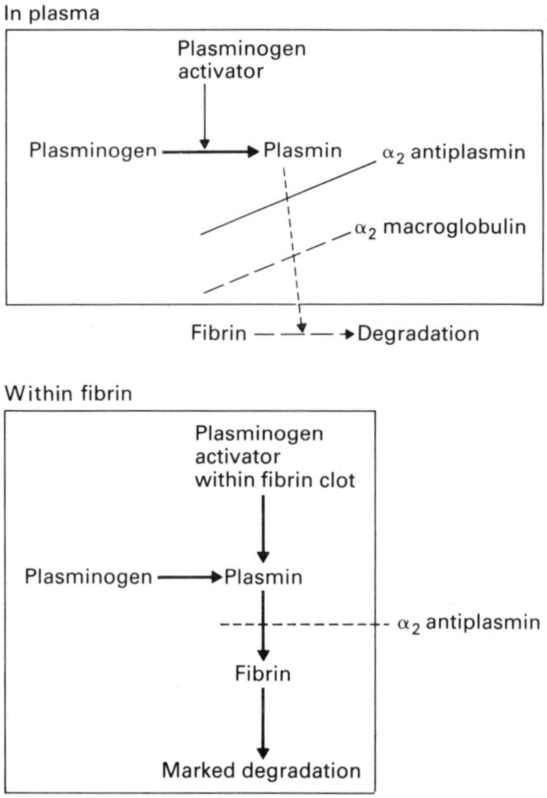

Fig. 15.3 *Diagrammatic representation of the fibrinolytic system. The kinetics of the interactions are in favour of fibrin breakdown by plasmin when both activator and plasminogen are absorbed on to fibrin. The kinetics are in favour of plasmin inhibition by α_2 antiplasmin if plasminogen is activated in plasma.*

The plasma fibrinolytic system

The physiological function of the fibrinolytic enzyme system is to digest intravascular deposits of fibrin (thrombi) in both large and small vessels and extravascular fibrin present in haemostatic plugs and in inflammatory exudates.

A simplified scheme of the fibrinolytic system is shown in Fig. 15.3.

PLASMINOGEN–PLASMIN SYSTEM

Plasminogen is a glycoprotein of molecular weight 90 000 which is synthesized in the liver. It is converted enzymatically by plasminogen activators to the fibrinolytic enzyme, plasmin. This enzyme not only digests fibrin (the desired physiological effect) but also digests fibrinogen and the clotting factors V and VIII.

Activators

Plasminogen activator is present in the tissue (tissue plasminogen activator), in plasma, and in urine (urokinase). Tissue plasminogen activator is localized in the vascular endothelium of veins, capillaries, and pulmonary arteries, and in the microsomal fraction of cells. Tissue plasminogen activator is released into the bloodstream in response to a number of stimuli, including ischaemia, vaso-active drugs, and exercise. Released activator is inactivated rapidly in the bloodstream by complexing to tissue plasminogen activator inhibitors, and has a half-life of about five minutes.

The major tissue plasminogen activator inhibitors are synthesized in the liver and in vascular endothelium, but about 30 per cent of the total is probably megakaryocyte-derived and is stored in platelet α granules. The activator in the urine, urokinase, differs structurally from tissue plasminogen activator, and is produced primarily in the kidneys and excreted in the urine where it may help to maintain urinary tract patency. Endothelial urokinase probably contributes a small proportion of plasma activator activity. Factor XIIa not only initiates coagulation, but also accelerates the conversion of plasminogen to plasmin via a pro-activator, almost certainly kallikrein. This enzyme, together with factor XII fragments, may also react in the plasma kinin system, influencing vessel tone and permeability.

Fibrinolysis

When clotting occurs, a small amount of plasminogen is trapped in the fibrin strands. Plasminogen activator, released locally from the vascular endothelium or traumatized tissues, binds to the fibrin of the thrombus and converts plasminogen to plasmin, itself bound to its substrate fibrin, and in this conformation protected from its otherwise highly effective inhibitor α_2 antiplasmin. Fibrin is thus digested. There is little or no plasma fibrinolytic activity because plasmin that is formed in the bloodstream from activation of plasma plasminogen is rapidly inactivated by circulating α_2 antiplasmin unless there is a gross excess (see below). Alpha$_2$ macroglobulin also acts as a secondary plasmin inhibitor in the presence of excess plasmin. The physiology of fibrinolysis is reviewed by Collen (1980).

The pathogenesis of coagulation abnormalities

From a consideration of the physiology of coagulation it is evident that impairment of coagulation, and thus a haemorrhagic tendency, may result from one or more of the following mechanisms.

Deficiency of one or more blood coagulation factors

Deficiency may be due either to defective synthesis or excessive utilization with normal synthesis. *Defective synthesis* of the plasma protein coagulation factors results from many causes: (a) genetic causes which usually lead to the deficiency or reduced activity of a single coagulation factor; (b) deficiency of vitamin K or its antagonism by the oral anticoagulants; (c) severe disease of liver; and (d) rarely in association with other diseases. Excessive utilization of some coagulation factors occurs with intravascular coagulation (p. 442) and in some cases of pathological fibrinolysis.

Inhibition of coagulation by acquired inhibitors

Changes in the naturally occurring inhibitors do not cause pathological inhibition of coagulation. However, in certain circumstances, abnormal inhibitors appear and interfere with blood coagulation.

Acquired inhibitors of coagulation, although rare, are well recognized and are usually auto-antibodies with specificity for a particular coagulation factor. This is in contrast to the naturally occurring inhibitors whose action is against the active intermediate products of coagulation. Monoclonal immunoglobins produced in multiple myeloma and Waldenström's macroglobulinaemia may interfere with coagulation reactions, particularly fibrin polymerization, in a non-specific fashion. The syndromes associated with acquired inhibitors are described on p. 447.

It should be noted also that the fibrinogen and fibrin breakdown products which occur in acute pathological fibrinolysis are potent, though transient, inhibitors of fibrin polymerization and thus blood clotting.

Fibrinolysis

In certain uncommon conditions, large amounts of tissue activator may be released into the bloodstream, producing a transient but marked hyperplasminaemic state. Abnormal bleeding may then occur because: (a) fibrin which is present in wounds

Table 15.3. *Laboratory screening tests in disorders of coagulation*

	Deficiency of coagulation factors												Presence of inhibitors			
	Prothrombin	Factor VII	Stuart–Prower	Christmas factor	Hageman	PTA	Pro-accelerin	Fibrinogen	Anti-haemophilic	Fibrin stabilizing	Platelet number	Platelet lipid	Intrinsic prothrombin activator system	Extrinsic prothrombin activator system	Thrombin–fibrinogen system	DIC and fibrinolysis
Coagulation tests	II	VII	X	IX	XII	XI	V	I	VIII	XIII						
Activated partial thromboplastin time	+	−	+	+	+	+	+	+	+	−	−	−	+	+	+	+
One-stage prothrombin time	+	+	+	−	−	−	+	+	−	−	−	−	−	+	+	+
Thrombin clotting time	−	−	−	−	−	−	−	+	−	−	−	−	−	−	+	+
Clot solubility test	−	−	−	−	−	−	−	−	−	+	−	−	−	−	−	−
Fibrinogen/fibrin degradation products	−	−	−	−	−	−	−	−	−	−	−	−	−	−	±	+

+ = abnormal result; − = abnormality not detected by this test. Other tests such as prothrombin consumption, fibrinogen assay and thromboplastin generation may be used in some laboratories. DIC = disseminated intravascular coagulation.

or haemostatic plugs is rapidly digested; (b) the products of fibrinogen and fibrin digestion (breakdown products) act as anticoagulants which interfere with fibrin clot formation and platelet function; and (c) the plasmin digests fibrinogen and factors V and VIII.

Miscellaneous

Congenital and acquired disorders of platelets (p. 395) sometimes result in the diminished availability of platelet factor 3 *in vitro* or other platelet procoagulant activity.

In patients with primary and secondary polycythaemia, abnormal bleeding not uncommonly complicates surgery. The bleeding probably results from an abnormally high concentration of red cells in the haemostatic plug, disordered platelet function, the effect of sludging in small vessels, and, occasionally, disseminated intrasvascular coagulation.

The diagnosis of coagulation disorders

A scheme for the investigation of patients with bleeding disorders, including coagulation disorders, is given on p. 449 (Table 15.12). The diagnosis of a coagulation abnormality may be strongly suspected from the clinical assessment, but requires confirmation by laboratory investigations.

Clinical assessment

The importance of careful history taking and physical examination cannot be overemphasized. In a number of acquired coagulation disorders, and in some congenital ones, a presumptive diagnosis can be made from clinical features; occasionally, it is necessary to act on this diagnosis when life-threatening bleeding demands appropriate emergency treatment before the results of laboratory tests are available. Accurate clinical information is of the greatest value to the laboratory, for both the selection of tests and their interpretation.

Laboratory tests (Table 15.3, Fig. 15.4)

The laboratory tests used in the investigation of suspected coagulation disorders belong to two groups: *screening* tests, and *special* tests, including factor assays. The most commonly used tests are described below, and brief comments are given on their significance; more detailed information may be obtained by consulting Austen & Rhymes (1975), Dacie & Lewis (1984), Bloom & Thomas (1987), and Colman *et al.* (1987).

SCREENING TESTS

As no single test is sufficiently specific to detect all types of coagulation abnormality, it is usually necessary to perform a number of tests; most

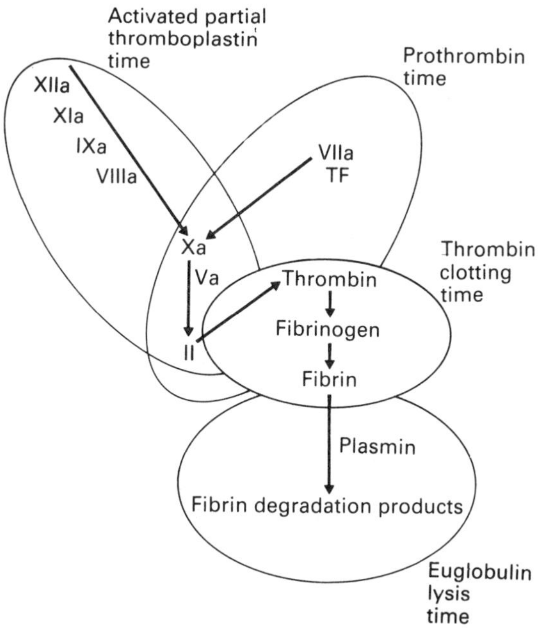

Fig. 15.4. *Scheme of blood coagulation showing parts of the mechanism examined by common tests.*

laboratories are now capable of performing a range of tests which are sufficiently sensitive to detect clinically significant abnormalities.

The one-stage prothrombin time (Quick's method)

This test determines the time plasma takes to clot after tissue factor (usually an extract of brain) and calcium are added. The normal range varies with the particular tissue factor used; for this reason, plasma from a normal subject must be tested at the same time. The patient's results are not regarded as abnormal unless the clotting time is more than two seconds longer than the control time. The preferred method of expression of the result is the ratio of patient to control clotting time. The upper limit of normal is 1.2.

In addition to sensitivity to prothrombin levels, the test detects deficiency of factors V, VII, X, fibrinogen, and the presence of some inhibitors. The areas of sensitivity of the major screening tests are shown in Fig. 15.4. When it is necessary to distinguish between factor deficiencies and the presence of inhibitors, the test is repeated on the patient's plasma after adding a small volume (20 per cent) of normal plasma; the clotting time is almost completely corrected when the abnormality is due to deficiency, but is poorly corrected when inhibitors are present.

The is a most useful test for investigating coagulation abnormalities, as it is sensitive and, in general, reliable. A normal result excludes abnormality in that portion of the coagulation mechanism which the test examines; however, it is not a sensitive index of fibrinogen deficiency. Falsely abnormal results most commonly occur in patients with polycythaemia; this results from the fact that the sample of the patient's plasma tested contains an excess of chemical anticoagulant, unless allowance has been made for the high haematocrit when the blood sample is first taken. Concurrent oral anticoagulant or heparin therapy may also cause an abnormal result.

The activated partial thromboplastin time

This test determines the time which plasma, previously incubated with kaolin or other surface active agents (which activate the surface contact clotting factors, factors XII, and XI), takes to clot in the presence of an optimum amount of platelet lipid substitute and calcium. The portion of the coagulation mechanism that is examined by this test is shown in Fig. 15.4. Normal plasma must be tested at the same time, and usually takes 35–45 seconds to clot. An abnormal result is indicated when the patient's clotting time is ten or more seconds longer than the control time.

Interpretation of the result is made in conjunction with the results obtained in the one-stage prothrombin time test. When the latter test is normal, an abnormal result in this test usually indicates deficiency of either factor VIII or factor IX, but rare deficiencies of factors XII, XI, pre-kallikrein, or high molecular weight kininogen, and also the presence of inhibitors, must be considered.

This test is very sensitive and, in general, a normal result may be taken as indicating that there is no clinically significiant deficiency of the above clotting factors. Normal results may be falsely obtained when blood samples are contaminated with tissue juices due to difficult venepuncture.

It should be noted that this test does not measure platelet factor 3 activity, as a platelet substitute is used in the test. A simple modification, in which kaolin is added to platelet-rich plasma without any extraneous lipid, is available for this purpose.

Thrombin clotting time

This test determines the time plasma takes to clot after the addition of a solution of thrombin. The concentration of thrombin solution is adjusted to clot normal plasma in 15 seconds. When the patient's plasma takes more than 18 seconds to clot, the result is regarded as abnormal. In addition to determining the clotting time, the quality of the clot must be observed and compared with the normal clot.

Prolongation of the clotting time may result either from hypofibrinogenaemia or from the presence of inhibitors, including heparin and fibrin breakdown products. Inhibitors may be suspected when the addition of the patient's plasma to normal plasma causes prolongation of the clotting time. Failure to obtain a clot may result from complete deficiency of fibrinogen or the presence of very potent inhibitors of the thrombin–fibrinogen reaction. Distinction between these may be made by using a more potent thrombin solution.

Screening tests for detecting increased fibrinolysis

These include the whole blood clotting time and observation for clot lysis, and more specialized procedures as in Table 15.3 (p. 414). A simple test for fibrin degradation products, using latex particles coated with antibody to fibrinogen degradation products, has gained wide acceptance in the investigation of mild degrees of fibrinolytic activity. Recent developments include immuno-assays specific for the plasmin degradation products of cross-linked fibrin. Thus, products detected by these assays must be derived from clot or thrombus, fibrinogen and its degradation products not being recognized by the antibodies employed in the system (Rylatt *et al.* 1983).

SPECIAL TESTS

Special tests are required: (a) to identify the deficient coagulation factor; (b) to determine the concentration or activity and so degree of deficiency; and (c) to detect and quantitate immune inhibitors of coagulation. These tests are now widely available and can be performed in most large hospital haematology departments. They include other procedures such as the prothrombin consumption test, coagulation factor assays, and platelet function tests. Although of considerable historical interest, the thromboplastin generation test is confined to more specialized centres as specific assays are available for most coagulation factors. Some coagulation laboratories perform highly specialized procedures to clarify the nature of some inherited disorders, to detect carriers amongst the female relatives, and to assist in the management of severe bleeding in haemophilia and the inhibitor state.

General principles in the treatment of coagulation disorders

Four main points should be considered in the management of patients with coagulation disorders; they are: (a) the treatment of the underlying cause; (b) correction of the abnormality with drugs and replacement transfusions; (c) treatment at the bleeding site; and (d) general supportive measures. An accurate diagnosis is most important, as treatment of the individual disorders differs considerably. The remaining part of this section summarizes the various measures that are used; further details are given in discussion of the individual disorders.

Treatment of the underlying causative disorder

Most of the acquired coagulation disorders are secondary to an underlying disorder, and recognition and treatment of the underlying condition often results in relief or cure of the coagulation abnormality. The disorders include: (a) biliary tract obstruction and intestinal diseases which cause malabsorption of vitamin K (p. 436); (b) liver disease in which there is impaired synthesis of coagulation factors (p. 437); (c) the ingestion of oral anticoagulant drugs or administration of heparin therapy (p. 439); and (d) many disorders which cause the defibrination syndrome and pathological fibrinolysis (Table 15.11, p. 442).

Correction of the coagulation abnormality with drugs and transfusion replacement therapy

Drugs that are useful in the correction of coagulation abnormalities are usually specific and of value only in a limited number of disorders. They include vitamin K (p. 442), protamine sulphate (p. 442), calcium gluconate, antifibrinolytic agents, e.g. ε amino-caproic acid (p. 445), and the kallikrein inhibitor trasylol (p. 445), heparin (p. 446), desamino-8-D-arginine vasopressin (p. 431), androgens (p. 431), and topical haemostatics such as thrombin.

Replacement Therapy has the object of achieving rapid correction of the deficiency of one or more coagulation factors. Factors may be given in the form of whole blood, fresh frozen plasma, or one of the various concentrates of factor VIII or factors II, VII, IX, and X. Table 15.4 lists the types of blood products that are used and their special indications.

The *broad indications* for replacement therapy are: (a) early treatment of spontaneous bleeding episodes; (b) established severe or prolonged wound and tissue bleeding; and (c) control of bleeding during and after surgery and trauma. Long-term prophylactic replacement therapy in the inherited disorders, especially severe haemophilia A and Christmas disease, may be beneficial, but is generally not practised in view of the storage of materials and the possible increased risk of development of inhibitors due to antibody formation.

The *type of blood* product indicated depends on a number of considerations, including the diagnosis of the bleeding disorder, the type and site of bleeding, the availability of the different blood products, and response to therapy as judged clinically and by laboratory tests.

Irrespective of the type of coagulation abnormality, acute blood loss must always be replaced with adequate amounts of blood, either as whole blood or appropriate fractions. When there is no indication for whole blood, and it is necessary to institute or maintain corrections of the clotting factor deficiency, this can usually be achieved by the transfusion of fresh frozen plasma or an appropriate concentrate. Platelet concentrates may also be required if there is associated thrombocytopenia.

Concentrates of fibrinogen, factor VIII, and a mixture of factors II, VII, XI, and X (PPSB), or II, XI, and X (prothrombinex), are indicated in many bleeding episodes in patients with known deficiencies of these factors. If insufficient amounts are available, fresh frozen plasma must be used. There is also a growing tendency to encourage home therapy with concentrates, after appropriate instruction of the family (Levine & Britten 1973). This requires careful supervision under the direction of established haemophilia treatment centres.

The *amount of material* which should be given at a

Table 15.4. *Haemostatic blood products*

Blood product	Special properties	Clinical indications
Fresh whole blood	Platelets, all coagulation factors, red blood cells	When whole blood is required in liver disease, disseminated intravascular coagulation, acute pathological fibrinolysis, massive blood replacement, haemophilia A, and when the diagnosis is uncertain in congenital bleeders
Platelet concentrates	Platelets	Thrombocytopenic bleeding
Fresh frozen plasma (FFP)	All coagulation factors	Congenital and acquired coagulation disorders
Factor VIII concentrates (a) low or intermediate potency, cryoprecipitate	Factor VIII and fibrinogen	Indications p. 429. Only in haemophilia A (never use in haemophilia B)
(b) high potency human factor VIII, animal factor VIII	Factor VIII	Specially valuable in major surgery and when antifactor VIII inhibitors are present
PPSB (factors II, VII, IX, X)* Prothrombinex (factors II, IX, X)*		Severe bleeding in liver disease, haemophilia B, and other congenital factor deficiencies. Sometimes in the treatment of patients with factor VIII inhibitor
Fibrinogen	Factor I	Acute disseminated intravascular coagulation and acute pathological fibrinolysis in addition to other replacement therapy (p. 445)

*Some preparations have been thrombogenic, and care is required in their use.

single transfusion depends on the severity of the coagulation defect, the amount of tissue damaged, and the site of bleeding. In general, the most important factor for determining the amount to be given is the extent of tissue damage. When it is not great, as in spontaneous episodes of bleeding and following mild trauma, a single transfusion of plasma amounting to 7–10 ml/kg bodyweight usually arrests bleeding. When tissue damage is greater or bleeding is present in a dangerous site, e.g. the tongue, it is usual to give twice this amount. In major trauma, including surgery, greater correction of the coagulation abnormality is usually required, and it is then necessary to use concentrates of clotting factors to avoid fluid overload. Treatment with concentrates should be controlled with factor assays, and the amount required adjusted accordingly. Detailed dosage schedules are available (Biggs 1978, Bloom & Thomas 1987, and see p. 431).

The *duration* of replacement therapy depends on the cause of the bleeding disorder, the severity of tissue damage, and the response to treatment. Frequently, a single transfusion arrests bleeding due to minimal tissue damage in patients with very severe coagulation abnormalities. When tissue damage is greater, and other treatment is ineffective in correcting the underlying cause, it is usually advisable to repeat the transfusion at intervals of 24 hours or less for several days.

Following major surgery, it is essential to continue correction of the coagulation abnormality until healing occurs; it is usually essential to monitor replacement therapy and adjust the dose and its frequency according to the results of laboratory tests.

The *rate of administration* should be rapid in order to obtain high peak blood concentrations of the deficient clotting factor and thus optimum haemostatic effect.

Mild *complications* of plasma component infusions include pyrogenic and allergic reactions, usually transient and requiring no specific treatment. Occasionally, antihistamine or even hydrocortisone and adrenaline may be required. Potentially more sinister is the very high incidence of laboratory evidence of *hepatitis* in patients receiving regular component therapy (Spero *et al.* 1978). The majority of severely haemophilic patients have antibody to hepatitis B surface antigen and a smaller proportion (about 10 per cent) are hepatitis B antigen positive. Most have persistently elevated liver enzyme concentrations, and biopsy evidence of liver disease is frequently present in the comparatively small numbers of patients studied. The long-term significance of these abnormalities is not known, but clearly administration of concentrates prepared from massive donor pools should be avoided where possible in the mildly affected patient, and vaccination of unexposed patients with hepatitis B vaccine should be undertaken. This clearly leaves patients exposed to non-A, non-B hepatitis.

Finally, cases of *acquired immunodeficiency syndrome* have occured in haemophilic patients who have been infected with the causative virus (HIV) in contaminated plasma fractions. Most haemophilic patients receiving replacement therapy have laboratory abnormalities associated with immunodeficiency, and circulating antibodies to HIV. With donor screening for HIV and heat treatment of factor concentrates, the risks of seroconversion are *now* very small.

Because of the risks of infection and the expense of preparing coagulation factor concentrates, the recent successful cloning of the gene for factor VIII is an exciting advance. Its expression in mammalian cells indicates the possibility of recombinant DNA-factor VIII becoming available for therapeutic use in the near future. The product is presently undergoing tests in humans, and this and other issues are recently reviewed by Roberts & Macik (1987).

Local treatment at the bleeding site

WOUNDS AND MUCOUS MEMBRANE BLEEDING

Treatment at the bleeding site is particularly important in the case of minor wounds, as appropriate treatment usually prevents prolonged bleeding and the need for replacement therapy. The measures are pressure, topical haemostatics, and immobilization.

Local pressure assists in the arrest of bleeding by raising tissue tension, and may be applied digitally, with pressure dressings and with sutures. However, haemostasis is much more certainly achieved when topical haemostatics are used in conjunction with pressure.

The most useful type of *topical haemostatics* are vasoconstrictor drugs, which may be used either alone or in combination with the clotting agent, thrombin. The topical application of solutions of adrenaline in high concentration (0.5–1 per cent) has been found to be both safe and effective. Initially, a temporary adrenaline-moistened dressing is applied with pressure to the wound for about five minutes and repeated at intervals until bleeding has stopped or is greatly reduced; a permanent dressing is then applied. If bleeding tends to recur, thrombin is applied to the wound which should have been rendered relatively blood-free with vasoconstrictor drugs as the natural antithrombins in the spilled blood rapidly destroy the applied thrombin. Thrombin is usually in aqueous solution (1000 units of thrombin per ml); it may also be dissolved in the solution of adrenaline.

The usual indications for suturing wounds apply, but bleeding should be controlled with topical haemostatics; replacement therapy should be given if repeated attempts at local haemostasis fail, or in the case of a very large and deep wound.

The *immobilization* of wounds by bandaging, and if necessary with splinting, helps to prevent recurrence of bleeding. Unless contra-indicated, wounds should remain undisturbed until healing is judged to have occurred; sutures should generally be allowed to remain in position much longer than usual.

When small wounds of mucous membrane cannot be immobilized, e.g. lacerations of the tongue, repeated application of local haemostatics usually prevents recurrence; initially, applications should be made at short intervals, and then several times a day until healing is evident.

HAEMATOMAS AND HAEMARTHROSIS

In an attempt to prevent or limit bleeding, local pressure should be applied early to the site after accidental contusion or puncture; however, if bleeding progresses, pressure should not be excessively increased as it is usually ineffective and aggravates pain. Usually, bleeding into the tissues is self-limited, but continued bleeding may lead to symptoms that demand its arrest by replacement therapy.

The most useful local measures in this type of bleeding are elevation and immobilization of the part. Aspiration of haematomas is generally contra-indicated unless it is certain that loculation has occurred, and then should be done only after correction of the abnormality in coagulation. Aspiration of joints (Biggs 1978) is sometimes performed, although it is not universally recommended, and is largely confined to the knees. More rapid resolution of haemarthroses with earlier ambulation may be achieved, but aspiration must always be preceded by coagulation factor replacement.

General supportive measures and care

During the acute and convalescent stages of a bleeding episode, it is necessary to institute measures that aid in the arrest of bleeding, promote healing, and return the patient to normal activity. Relief of pain, anxiety, and hypovolemia aid in the arrest of bleeding. Return to normal activity is helped by the correction of iron deficiency resulting from blood loss, and by physiotherapy when indicated.

Congenital and long-standing acquired coagulation disorders require the adoption of special measures to prevent unwarranted psychological and social complications, for appropriate emergency care of acute episodes of bleeding, and for hereditary counselling in the congenital disorders. The adoption of such measures has avoided much of the invalidism once associated with severe bleeding disorders. Further details are given on p. 427.

Clinical disorders due to coagulation abnormalities

The clinical disorders due to coagulation abnormalities are described in this section under two headings: *congenital* coagulation disorders, and *acquired* coagulation disorders. As the clinical manifestations of defective coagulation are, in general, similar in the different types of coagulation disorder, a detailed description of the haemorrhagic symptoms is given in the discussion of haemophilia which follows.

Congenital coagulation disorders

Congenital coagulation disorders (Table 15.5) are rare; the most common is haemophilia A (congenital factor VIII deficiency) which has an estimated birth incidence in different countries ranging from 1 in 10 000 to less than 1 in 100 000.

These disorders are almost invariably due to deficient activity of a single coagulation factor, which results from a genetically determined abnormality in synthesis. In congenital hypoprothrom-

Table 15.5. *Congenital coagulation disorders*

The haemophilias
Haemophilia A (classical haemophilia)
Haemophilia B (Christmas disease)
Von Willebrand's disease
Other congenital deficiency disorders
Fibrinogen (factor I) absence or deficiency
Prothrombin (factor II) deficiency
Factor V deficiency
Factor VII deficiency
Factor X (Stuart factor) deficiency
Factor XI (plasma thromboplastin antecedent) deficiency
Factor XII (Hageman factor) deficiency
Factor XIII (fibrin-stabilizing factor) deficiency
Fletcher factor (pre-kallikrein) deficiency
Fitzgerald factor (high molecular weight kininogen) deficiency

binaemia, variant forms have been described in different families on the basis of electrophoretic mobility. Von Willebrand's disease involves factor VIII deficiency similar to that occurring in haemophilia A in terms of coagulant activity, but other functions associated with von Willebrand factor and influencing platelet activity are also lacking, giving a condition with multiple haemostatic defects. There are rare instances of congenital deficiency of more than one factor, such as factors V and VIII.

Haemophilia A and haemophilia B

Haemophilia was the first haemorrhagic disorder to be accurately described when it was recognized as an hereditary bleeding disorder of males which is transmitted by healthy women. Until 1952, it was thought that the coagulation abnormality in haemophilia was always caused by the deficiency of the blood clotting factor antihaemophilic factor (AHF or factor VIII), but it was then found that the blood of some patients was deficient in a previously unrecognized clotting factor which was called plasma thromboplastin component or Christmas factor (PTC or factor IX). The term *haemophilia A* is now used to describe the disorder when factor VIII is deficient, and *haemophilia B* to describe the disorder when factor IX is deficient. Haemophilia A is seven times more common than haemophilia B.

Synonyms for haemophilia A are true haemophilia and classical haemophilia; those for haemophilia B are Christmas disease and plasma thromboplastin component (PTC) deficiency.

Inheritance. Haemophilia A and haemophilia B are genetically unrelated, but both are inherited as sex-linked recessive characters because the genes for the disorders are carried by the X chromosome. Thus females carrying a gene for haemophilia on one of their two X chromosomes transmit the gene to half of their female offspring and to half of their male offspring according to the laws of chance. On the other hand haemophiliacs, having only one X chromosome, transmit the gene to all their female offspring, but to none of their male children.

Males who inherit a gene for haemophilia invariably have deficiency of the corresponding coagulation factor. The concentration of the clotting factor in their plasma ranges from complete deficiency to as high as 30 per cent of normal. Related males with haemophilia have a similar, and usually identical, concentration of the deficient clotting factor in their blood; it does not vary with age. It can therefore be concluded that in addition to the two types of haemophilia being genetically distinct, the plasma concentration of the clotting factor concerned is also genetically controlled, and that there are different grades of haemophilia.

In about 30 per cent of cases, usually with severe haemophilia, evidence of inheritance is lacking. This is presumably due to recent gene mutation which causes the mother to become a carrier, or alternatively after several generations of carrier daughters.

Females carrying a gene for haemophilia are called *carriers.* A small proportion of carriers, especially of haemophilia B, have a very mild tendency to bleed and a subnormal concentration of the relevant clotting factor in their blood. Rarely, the deficiency of the clotting factor is sufficiently severe to cause a moderate bleeding tendency. Women in families with haemophilia often wish to know if they are *carriers.* When tests show a discrepancy between factor VIII activity and von Willebrand factor levels (normally quantitatively related), a woman can be a suspect as a carrier of haemophilia A. The same cannot be said for haemophilia B, and in neither condition does a normal result exclude the possibility of the carrier state (Bennett & Ratnoff 1973).

Genetic analysis using a DNA probe that detects a very polymorphic region of the X chromosome, closely linked to haemophilia A, is reported to be informative in more than 90 per cent of families with the disease (Oberle *et al.* 1985). This technique can be used in both carrier detection and in prenatal diagnosis using chorionic biopsy or fetal blood collection. Similar probes are available for investigation of carrier status in haemophilia B (Gianelli *et al.* 1984) and in von Willebrand's disease (Sadler 1987).

Incidence. The frequency of haemophilia varies in different races; the highest incidence is reported in populations of British and northern European ancestry. In Australia, the incidence is 1 per 5000 male births; the reported incidence in other countries is usually lower.

Clinical features

The bleeding tendency usually appears in infancy, sometimes during the first weeks of life, but in mild cases it may not become apparent until adolescence or even adult life.

SEVERITY OF THE BLEEDING TENDENCY

The clinical manifestations vary in severity from patient to patient, but they tend to be the same in related haemophiliacs. The clinical severity is closely, but not absolutely, related to the concentration of the deficient factor. When the concentration of the clotting factor is less than one per cent of normal, symptoms are usually severe; when it is between one and three per cent, the symptoms are usually moderately severe. They are usually mild when the concentration is more than three per cent of normal, except after surgery and severe trauma. The severity of the symptoms in haemophilia A and haemophilia B are similar for corresponding concentrations of the deficient clotting factor.

VARIABILITY OF THE BLEEDING TENDENCY

Although the concentration of the deficient factor remains the same in an individual, the clinical course of most haemophiliacs with severe deficiency, and some with moderate deficiency, is characterized by fluctuations in the severity of the bleeding tendency. During a peroid of an increased tendency to bleed, patients exerience bleeding into the tissues after the slightest injury, and may even bleed spontaneously. During a phase of reduced tendency to bleed, they can withstand quite severe contusions without ill effect. These phases vary in degree and duration; and increased tendency to bleed commonly lasts for weeks or months, and on occasions may persist for years. In contrast to tissue bleeding, wound bleeding does not appear to be less severe during a quiescent phase. The cause of the fluctuations in the bleeding tendency is unknown but is also observed in other hereditary haemorrhagic disorders. The active phases tend to be less prominent when emotional disturbances have been resolved, and also after puberty.

TYPE AND SITE OF BLEEDING

Wound bleeding is the characteristic symptom of all haemophiliacs. It is usually slow and persists for days to weeks in spite of the presence of large clots. The onset of bleeding may be immediate, but is commonly delayed for hours or even days, particularly in mild haemophilia. Recurrence of bleeding after haemostasis has apparently occurred is particularly common.

Tissue bleeding. Spontaneous bleeding may occur into almost every tissue of the body, but is more common in some sites than others; it occurs frequently in patients with severe dificiency, infrequently in moderate deficiency, and rarely in mild deficiency. Injuries causing contusion, ligamentous strains, or rupture of muscle fibres result in excessive bleeding at the site of injury in all but very mild haemophiliacs.

The extent of bleeding depends on the amount of tissue damaged, the concentration of the clotting factor, and the presence or absence of an active phase of bleeding. Bleeding into the tissues causes the formation of haematomas which vary in blood content from a few millilitres to several litres. The size of haematomas and the complications which arise from them are greatly reduced by early replacement therapy.

In addition to pain and swelling, there may develop fever, anorexia, leucocytosis, and anaemia of moderate to severe degree. Retroperitoneal (Fig. 15.5) and mesenteric bleeding is relatively common; in severe deficiency, intra-abdominal bleeding is a much more frequent cause of abdominal pain than is acute appendicitis.

Skin. A tendency to bruise excessively after slight injury is noted by most haemophiliacs, but spontaneous bleeding into the skin and subcutaneous tissues is common only in severe deficiency. Superficial abrasions rarely cause excessive bleeding, but lacerations and contused wounds are frequently followed by prolonged and troublesome bleeding lasting many weeks. Petechial bleeding is rare.

Mouth and nose. Bleeding from lacerations of the tongue and the frenum of the upper lip is common in children. Bleeding from the gums is uncommon during primary dentition, but is sometimes trouble-

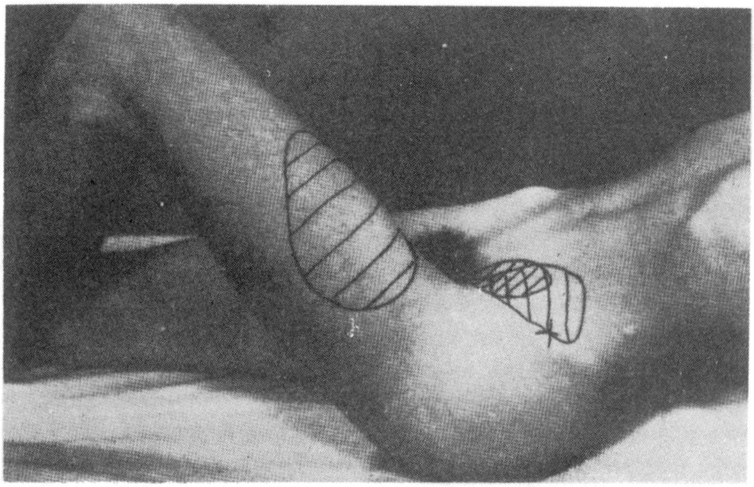

Fig. 15.5. *Retroperitoneal haemorrhage in severe haemophilia A. The boy, aged 15 years, developed pain in the left lower abdomen and difficulty with walking three days before the photograph was taken. Twelve hours after onset of pain there was abdominal tenderness, flexion of the left hip, and a small area of anaesthesia on the front of the thigh. The photograph shows the fully developed signs characteristic of a haemorrhage involving the left psoas muscle and lumbar plexus; there was an area of hyperasthesia in the inguinal region (small oval area of diagonal hatching), diminished left patellar reflex, and quadriceps weakness. The area of anaesthesia on the front of the thigh had increased in size, and a mass had appeared in the left iliac fossa (horizontal hatched area over abdomen). Complete recovery with disappearance of all physical signs occurred in three weeks.*

some during the shedding of these teeth. Bleeding from the sockets after tooth extraction is almost invariable, and in mild haemophiliacs is often the first and sometimes the only manifestation of the disease. In severe haemophilia, spontaneous epistaxis and bleeding into the muscular tissues of the tongue are not uncommon.

Synovial joints. Prior to effective replacement therapy, patients with severe haemophilia suffered recurring haemorrhage into joint spaces (Fig. 15.6). It is less likely in moderate haemophilia, and may never occur in mild haemophilia. Haemarthroses may occur spontaneously, but usually result from a minor joint strain or from a direct injury; they

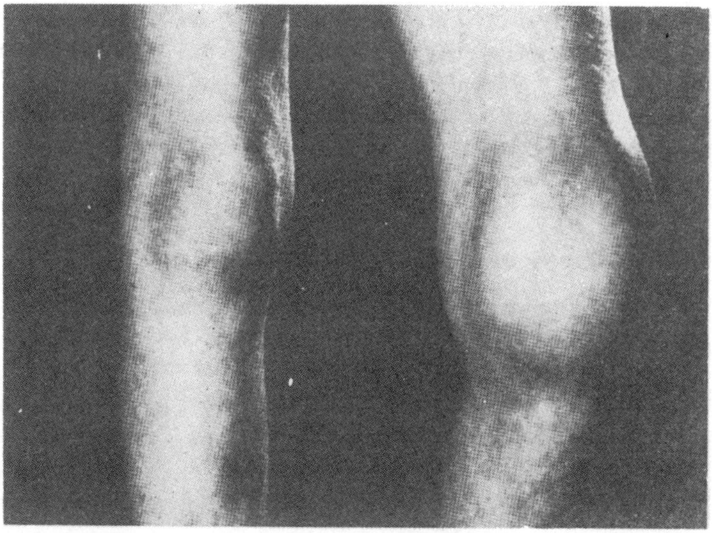

Fig. 15.6. *Haemarthrosis of the knee joint in haemophilia. The boy, aged nine years, with severe haemophilia B developed haemarthrosis without known injury.*

happen most frequently during an active phase of bleeding. The pain and disability of a haemarthrosis depend on the rapidity and duration of bleeding, and vary from mild to very severe; commonly, the acute symptoms persist for 3–4 days, but recovery may take weeks. In infants, the ankle joints are most commonly affected, but in older children and adults the knees are most frequently affected. The elbows are next most commonly involved, while the shoulder, wrist, hip, and finger joints are affected less frequently. The synovial joints of the spinal column are affected only rarely. Unless haemophilia has been diagnosed previously, rheumatic fever, septic arthritis, and acute osteomyelitis may be diagnosed in error. Chronic arthritis commonly develops in joints that have been the site of recurring haemorrhages.

Central nervous system. Intracranial haemorrhage, either extra- or intracerebral, is not uncommon, particularly in severe haemophilia. In children, it occurs most commonly after head injury, but in adults it is usually spontaneous. Bleeding into the spinal cord or canal is rare.

Urogenital and gastrointestinal tracts. Haematuria is a not uncommon symptom of some patients with severe haemophilia, in whom it usually occurs without apparent cause. Bleeding usually lasts for 7–14 days, and is sometimes accompanied by ureteric colic due to the passage of clots. It is very rare in mild haemophilia, except after trauma. Haematemesis and bleeding *per rectum* are not uncommon, but rarely occur in the absence of other symptoms. Gastrointestinal bleeding is commonly the result of ingestion of aspirin or alcohol; occasionally it occurs as a complication of a peptic ulcer or erosion of the mucosa due to an intramural haematoma.

COMPLICATIONS OF HAEMORRHAGE

The incidence and severity of complications is greatly lessened by early and adequate treatment.

Pain is the most common and disturbing symptom of haemophiliacs, particularly those with severe disease. Local pain is due to the increasing pressure in a haematoma caused by persistent bleeding; commonly there is little difficulty in diagnosing the cause of the pain, as local swelling is usually evident. Referred pain results from the pressure effects of haematomas on peripheral nerves, and nerve roots or trunks; this may be suspected when pain is severe and local swelling is absent. Visceral-type pain most commonly results from intramural haematomas of the intestinal wall; occasionally it is due to mediastinal haemorrhage. Early replacement therapy usually produces rapid relief of referred and visceral pain—a point of importance in diagnosis.

Anaemia frequently develops in patients with severe and moderate haemophilia, and is due to blood loss. When blood loss is acute, the anaemia is normocytic in type or is slightly macrocytic due to the increased reticulocyte count; with chronic loss, hypochromic anaemia due to iron deficiency may develop. In young children, multiple haematomas may cause temporary deviation of iron into the tissues, and can lead to the occurrence of a hypochromic anaemia in the absence of blood loss. During episodes of bleeding, the haemoglobin usually falls to 7–9 g/dl but sometimes, especially with insidious bleeding, values may fall rapidly to 5 g/dl or less; this occurs particularly in small children. Haemoglobin estimations should therefore be performed daily during acute bleeding episodes, as it is not always easy to assess clinically the amount of blood lost. A moderate leucocytosis accompanies active bleeding, especially into the tissues. When large haematomas are present, the serum bilirubin may be increased.

Constitutional disturbances. Bleeding into the tissues and joint spaces frequently causes marked elevation of the temperature within 24 hours, which may persist for a week or more. It is usually accompanied by severe anorexia and malaise, which can persist until the haematoma resolves. These constitutional disturbances, when accompanied by a leucocytosis, may be misinterpreted as being due to a septic condition; the differentiation is sometimes difficult.

Chronic haemophilic arthritis. Permanent joint damage usually results from repeated haemorrhages into a joint, but may follow a single haemorrhage. The limitation of movement is usually due to fibrous adhesions within the joint, but may be due to osteophytic outgrowths. In the early stages the radiological changes are slight, but in the later stages the joint space becomes narrow and the adjacent bone ends are enlarged by osteophytic outgrowths; cyst-like rarefactions sometimes occur in the adjacent bone. In the knee joint, the intercondylar notch is enlarged; in the hips, the changes at the upper end of the femur may resemble those seen in Perthes' disease. In severe haemophilia, it is usual for several joints to become affected, but in rare cases no arthritis is clinically detectable. In the less severe grades of haemophilia, chronic arthritis is uncommon.

Pressure effects and sequelae of haematomas. The most serious complications of haemophila result from the pressure of haematomas on sensitive or vital structures. Compression of peripheral nerves is common, and results in transient or prolonged paresis, anaesthesia, or hyperaesthesia. The femoral nerve and other branches of the lumbar plexus are most often affected (see Fig. 15.5). A condition resembling Volkmann's ischaemic contracture is not an uncommon complication of a haematoma in the muscles of the forearm (Fig. 15.7). Less commonly, compression of blood vessels results in gangrene of the distal part of a limb. Respiratory embarrassment is a relatively uncommon but serious complication; it may result from an obstruction of the nasopharynx by a haematoma of the tongue or from a haematoma of the larynx, due either to blood spreading down fascial planes after tooth extraction or to local trauma. Complete intestinal obstruction due to an intramural haemorrhage is a severe but uncommon complication. Mediastinal and intrapleural haemorrhage are rare complications which may cause cardiac tamponade or respiratory failure. Recurring subcortical or medullary haemorrhage in bones leads to the formation of pseudotumours (Fig. 15.8) which slowly increase in size over years. Necrosis of the skin sometimes results from the pressure of an underlying haematoma; it also results from thermal and other injuries, when there is anaesthesia following nerve compression (see Fig. 15.5).

Diagnosis

The diagnosis can usually be suspected from the clinical and hereditary features, but is established with certainty only with the aid of laboratory tests.

Clinical and hereditary features. The clinical features of most importance are the sex, the age of onset, and the type of bleeding; the hereditary feature of importance is evidence of sex-linked

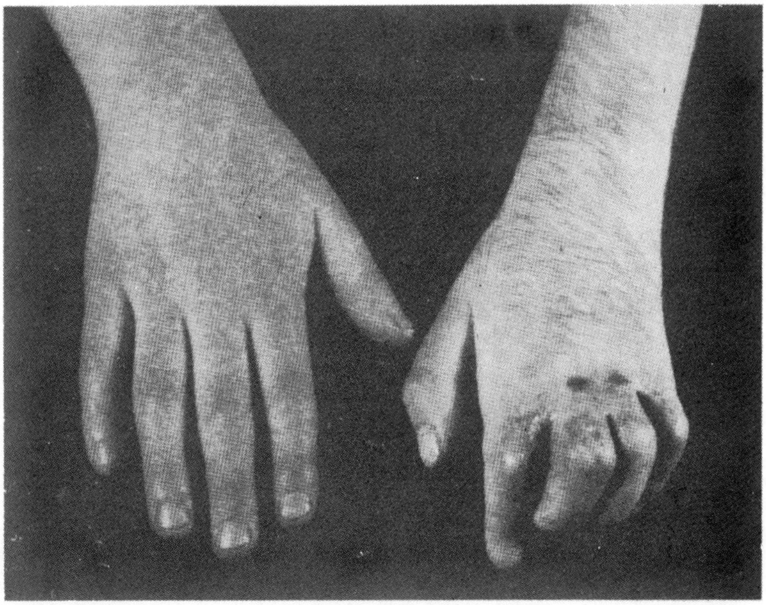

Fig. 15.7. *Volkmann's ischaemic contracture in haemophilia. This photograph shows a claw-hand deformity resulting from a haematoma of the left forearm. There was also anaesthesia of the hand due to nerve involvement by the haematoma; this led to a severe burn which required skin grafting. From a boy aged eight years with haemophilia B.*

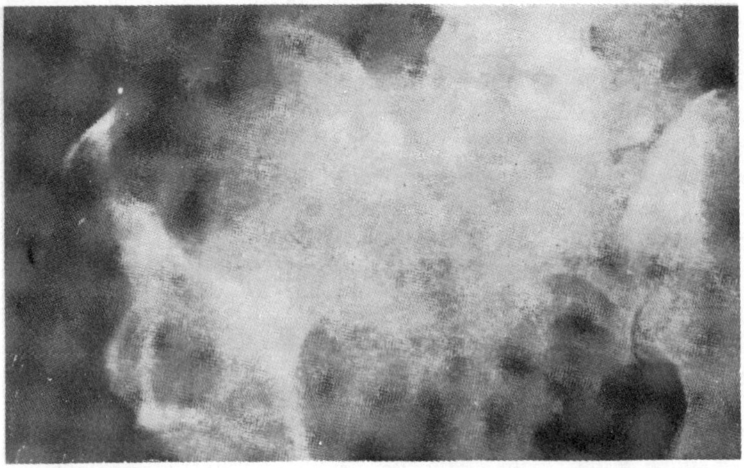

Fig. 15.8 *Haemophilic pseudotumour of bone. This X-ray from a man with haemophilia A shows a large pseudotumour of the right ileum resulting from haemorrhage into the bone; areas of destruction and calcification are well seen. There is loss of definition of the right sacroiliac joint due to extension of the haemorrhage into the soft tissues.*

recessive inheritance. The diagnosis is therefore strongly suggested by the onset in a male child of an abnormal bleeding tendency with the characteristics of a coagulation disorder (p. 422) and a history of bleeding in male relatives on the maternal side of the family. In severe haemophilia, the onset of ecchymoses, prolonged bleeding from lacerations and other wounds, and bleeding into the deep tissues and joints usually commences before the age of two years; on the other hand, in mild haemophilia symptoms may not appear until adolescence or adult life when abnormal bleeding follows tooth extraction or surgery.

As the hereditary aspects are so important, a detailed family history must be taken and a family tree drawn for accurate reference. It should be recalled that severe haemophilia frequently occurs in the absence of a previous family history of bleeding. In mild haemophilia, careful inquiry usually reveals episodes of abnormal bleeding in male relatives who do not necessarily regard themselves as being bleeders; abnormal bleeding after tooth extraction is the most common symptom.

Laboratory findings. The diagnosis of haemophilia A or haemophilia B requires the demonstration of deficiency of factor VIII or factor IX, respectively, in the patient's plasma. However, all the clinical and laboratory findings must be considered before the diagnosis is accepted because deficiency of factor VIII occurs also in von Willebrand's disease, and deficiency of factor IX occurs in newborn infants, liver disease, and vitamin K deficiency.

The tourniquet test is usually normal but, because of the possibility of causing a haematoma in the forearm, it is unwise to perform this test when severe haemophilia or other severe coagulation abnormalities are suspected. The skin bleeding time is usually normal; the platelet count is normal, and the platelets are morphologically normal.

Screening tests for the detection of coagulation abnormalities give the following results. The activated partial thromboplastin time is typically prolonged in all grades of haemophilia, except the mildest or when the patient has recently received transfusion with fresh blood, or with poorly collected blood samples. In severe haemophilia, the clotting time is usually in excess of 100 seconds, and in mild haemophilia is usually 10–20 seconds longer than the control time. The one-stage prothrombin and thrombin clotting times are normal.

Special laboratory tests should be performed in all cases to establish accurately the nature of the coagulation abnormality, as may be done with specific factor assays. In the unusual situation where these are not available, a thromboplastin generation test could be used to distinguish between factor VIII and factor IX deficiency. It is also important to exclude the presence of a coagulation inhibitor.

In families with haemophilia, an early diagnosis in the neonate is often desired by mothers who are potential carriers of haemophilia. When it is known that the bleeding disorder is haemophilia A, the diagnosis can be established by using assay techniques on blood obtained from the umbilical cord at birth, or within a few days from blood obtained by heel puncture; this is possible as factor VIII is not placenta-permeable, and blood concentrations of the factor present at birth are relevant. Pre-natal diagnosis is also available, using fetoscopic blood sampling and either immunoradiometric assay for factor VIII (coagulant portion) or microtechniques for factor VIII coagulant activity. Gene probes for random fragment length polymorphism using trophoblast tissue or fetal blood may shortly prove more acceptable (p. 421). In the case of haemophilia B, tests should be deferred for 4–6 weeks as factor IX and other vitamin K-dependent factors (p. 436) may be low at birth and slow in rising to normal levels.

Troublesome bleeding rarely results when superficial veins are punctured to obtain blood specimens provided that moderate pressure is applied to the puncture site for five minutes; puncture of deep veins, e.g. femoral vein, and the ear-lobe should be avoided in patients with bleeding disorders, as prolonged bleeding may result from difficulty in maintaining pressure at these sites.

Course and prognosis

Prior to the advent of blood transfusion and replacement therapy, about 90 per cent of patients with severe haemophilia died before reaching adult life, either from exsanguination or from the pressure of a haematoma on a vital structure. Patients with moderate and mild haemophilia often died from an unrelated disease, but when death did result from bleeding, it was usually caused by severe accidental trauma or by surgery.

In *severe* haemophilia, several to 50 or more attacks of bleeding may occur in the course of a year; however, the severity of the attacks and their complications has been remarkably diminished with replacement therapy. Thus, the great majority of patients with severe haemophilia, and practically all with moderate haemophilia, may now expect to live well into adult life, to earn their own living, and to raise a family. The frequency of attacks of bleeding is less in those who develop appropriate attitudes.

The most serious hazards for a haemophiliac are *intracerebral bleeding* and the development of *resistance to replacement therapy*. The occurrence of severe headache, particularly in adult haemophiliacs, is commonly due to intracerebral bleeding; mortality is high, but is reduced when replacement therapy is commenced early. Although there is no increase in the tendency to bleed or in the frequency of attacks when immune inhibitors of coagulation develop, resistance, either partial or complete, occurs; when inhibitors are weak, it is found that increased dosage of replacement therapy is effective. However, when they are potent, replacement therapy is usually ineffective and surgery is very hazardous.

Management

The management of haemophilia is considered under the following headings: general aspects; treatment of bleeding; surgery; and special therapeutic measures.

GENERAL ASPECTS

Below are described the many factors that must be considered when giving a prognosis and when advising on the upbringing of a haemophilic child.

Psychologial factors and personality development. During the past 20 years, there has been increasing realization that the bleeding tendency is aggravated by acute emotional disturbances; it is also believed by many that the course of the disorder is less severe in haemophiliacs who have developed a healthy personality and who do not identify themselves as being significantly handicapped or abnormal. A number of observations indicate that such development is influenced in childhood by parental attitudes (Mattisson & Gross 1966). Mothers, in particular, experience guilt over having borne a diseased child, and may either reject or over-protect him; this commonly leads to social maladjustment, and thus failure to cope with environmental stresses. Guilt may be prevented or overcome by giving a good, not unwarranted, prognosis and by planning for her child's immediate and long-term medical care, schooling, leisure activities, and vocational training. In particular, it is important that parents avoid discouraging restrictions. When patients attend frequently with unaccountable attacks of bleeding, it is commonly found that there is an underlying emotional disturbance, the cause of which should be sought and relieved. The doctor and others who are responsible for various aspects in the upbringing of the child should take particular care to avoid measures that could directly or indirectly lead to loss of the self-confidence which has been gained by earlier good management.

Schooling. Most severe haemophiliacs are able to attend kindergarten and ordinary schools; although most teachers are at first fearful, they too become confident with parent's assistance and the knowledge that bleeding attacks rarely result from injuries received while at school. It should be accepted by both the school authorities and the parents that any harm which might befall a child while at school is a very small price to pay for the advantages which might otherwise be denied him. Physical activities should not be restricted, except to avoid severe injury; older children take pride in protecting, but not restricting, haemophilic children. 'Body-contact' sports, e.g. football and basketball, and games played with hard balls, e.g. cricket and baseball, should be avoided. On the other hand, even severe haemophiliacs should be encouraged to participate in active but not violent exercise, e.g. swimming, cycling, tennis, and walking; good physical condition seems to reduce incidents of bleeding from sudden accidental strains.

Vocational guidance. As children with severe haemophilia are likely to develop some physical disabilities, education should be planned to enable them to choose a sedentary occupation, should this become necessary. However, vocational guidance to 'safe' work, rather than work in accordance with interests and abilities, leads to job dissatisfaction and sometimes aggravation of the bleeding tendency.

Emergency medical care. Parents should be taught that bleeding in haemophilia is not suddenly life-threatening, and how to apply local therapy until medical care is available. Appropriate medical care should be available within a few hours because, when indicated, replacement therapy is of particular value when given early. Self-administration of factor VIII concentrate, or administration by parents in the case of younger children, has dramatically reduced hospitalization, outpatient visits, and associated costs. Thus, where possible, severe haemophiliacs should be taught all aspects of self-administration to cover minor haemorrhages. Haemophiliacs should be provided with a card containing details of their diagnosis for use in an event of accident; such a card is particularly important for mild haemophiliacs, as verbal statements concerning the diagnosis occasionally are not heeded by dentists and surgeons.

Special institutions. In some countries, residential schools with facilities for giving replacement therapy have been developed, or are advocated. While certain advantages are evident, they have the disadvantage of unduly emphasizing disability. Special facilities exist in many hospitals for the general care of haemophiliacs, for replacement therapy, and for other specialized care. In such hospitals, the availability of emergency care at all times is a major factor in minimizing the complications of bleeding and thus incapacity for work.

Lay haemophilia organizations exist in most countries, and are useful sources of general information; some can provide financial and other assistance for haemophilic members.

Other measures. Careful dental hygiene and regular dental examination are important. Prophylactic immunization, including hepatitis B, should be given early. A very fine gauge needle should be used, and pressure applied to the injection site for at least five minutes. When possible, medication should be given orally; intramuscular injections should be avoided unless the coagulation abnormality has been corrected by replacement therapy.

Older haemophiliacs should be warned against neglecting medical care through over-confidence or on account of social and business pressures.

TREATMENT OF BLEEDING

The general principles in the treatment of bleeding are outlined on p. 417; the particular aspects that apply to management in haemophiliacs are discussed in more detail below.

General supportive measures

Although most attacks of bleeding can be treated without admission to hospital, care in hospital is usually desirable in cases of infants and small children; this permits closer observation, relieves anxious parents of undue responsibility, and permits them to gain confidence and to be instructed in general management. While many types of bleeding, including haemarthrosis of weight-bearing joints, require treatment in hospital, the period of hospitalization should be kept as short as possible with the object of maintaining confidence and of encouraging early return for treatment in future attacks of bleeding. Analgesics may be used to relieve pain, but not as a substitute for replacement therapy; aspirin and other drugs affecting platelet function should avoided because of the increased risk of bleeding, particularly from the gastrointestinal tract.

Local haemostatic measures

Bleeding from small wounds and other accessible sites can usually be arrested with local treatment; the measures used are discussed in detail on p. 419. In haemophilia, epistaxis can usually be controlled by external digital pressure applied just below the nasal bones for 5–15 minutes. If bleeding persists, adrenaline is carried to the bleeding area on a light cotton-wool pack and digital pressure is re-applied. Rarely, packing with ribbon gauze soaked in a thrombin–adrenaline mixture is required to arrest intractable bleeding; after its removal, vasoconstrictor drops or spray are used for several days.

Replacement therapy

Replacement therapy has been discussed on p. 417. In the past, its use was restricted to life-threatening or long-standing attacks of bleeding because of the fear of patients developing resistance to replacement therapy as the result of stimulating specific inhibitors against the deficient clotting factor, and because of the development of allergic reactions to donors' plasma proteins. It is now recognized that although about 5–10 per cent of patients develop immune inhibitors, the advantages of replacement therapy are so great in the majority of patients that restrictions are not warranted when the therapeutic indications exist.

The usual complications of frequently transfused patients (p. 480) are commonly observed. It is especially important to observe the usual precautions in the cross-matching and administration of blood in a patient receiving repeated blood transfusions (p. 476). Conservation of the veins is of the utmost importance.

Indications. The general indications for replacement therapy have been discussed on p. 417. The particular indications in haemophilia for the treatment of established bleeding are as follows: (a) to prevent the extension of haematomas in sites which endanger life, e.g. the throat, chest, abdomen, and central nervous system; (b) to prevent or limit peripheral nerve and muscle damage by haematomas, e.g. in the muscles of the forearm (see Fig. 15.7) and in the psoas muscle (see Fig. 15.5); (c) to arrest prolonged bleeding from mucous membranes and wounds which cannot be otherwise controlled; and (d) to arrest bleeding into tissues and other spaces which progresses to the stage of causing severe pain. Replacement therapy should be given in preference to analgesics when pain is obviously due to bleeding into tissues and joints, and for diagnostic purposes when the cause of the pain is uncertain. When replacement therapy is given early in an episode of bleeding, pain is usually relieved in an hour or two; this most certainly indicates the arrest of bleeding, as reduction in local signs usually follows. On the other hand, when replacement therapy is delayed, relief of pain and swelling is slow and may take many days. The incidence of complications is also greatly increased when treatment is delayed.

Prophylactic replacement therapy is also indicated after severe injury, particularly head injury, and also for surgery and tooth extraction.

Type of blood product indicated. The different types of blood product that may be used for treatment in haemophilia A and haemophilia B are listed in Table 15.4, p. 418. The products include whole blood, plasma, and concentrates containing factor VIII or factor IX. It is essential that the blood product used contains the required clotting factor and that it is present in the appropriate amount.

The choice of material to be used in treating or preventing bleeding episodes depends in part on the availability of concentrates, cryoprecipitate, or fresh frozen plasma, and on the severity of the particular bleed. There is a growing tendency to increase the amount of concentrates produced as blood components are more effectively utilized. Cryoprecipitate provides a useful alternative to plasma if high yields of factor VIII activity can be attained. More highly purified concentrates prepared by plasma fractionation are more expensive to produce and carry a greater risk of viral contamination, but have an important place in haemophilia treatment.

The accent in management must be on the earliest possible administration of plasma or concentrate after the onset of a bleeding episode. Home therapy with factor VIII concentrate provides the most efficient method of ensuring early treatment. The alternative to self- or family-administered home treatment is easy access to a treatment centre where prompt attention is available.

If concentrates or cryoprecipitate are not available, fresh frozen plasma is effective and safe in most instances of spontaneous bleeding of relatively minor degree. The disadvantages of plasma are the large volumes required and the frequent occurrence of allergic reactions. Nevertheless, in acute haemarthrosis and haematomas, a dose of plasma between 7 and 15 ml/kg given over a period of 30–60 minutes often effectively arrests bleeding and relieves pain. This dose normally needs to be repeated at intervals of 12–24 hours until it is clear that the episode is controlled. Because of the risk of allergic reactions, it is advisable to give an antihistamine intravenously at the beginning of infusion, and corticosteroids should be available if required.

The indications for concentrates include: (a) home therapy; (b) severe bleeding episodes or extensive tissue damage, and especially central nervous system bleeding; (c) failure of the expected response to plasma or severe allergic reactions; and (d) prophylaxis for surgery.

Failure to obtain the expected improvement after several administrations of plasma or concentrates should raise suspicion that resistance to therapy may be due to the development of an acquired inhibitor; coagulation tests should therefore be performed soon after a dose of therapy. Such inhibitors may pose a very great problem. A number of approaches have been devised including: (a) increasingly frequent infusions of high dose factor VIII concentrates; (b) repeated plasmapheresis to reduce the inhibitor (antibody) concentration; (c) infusion of factor IX concentrates, which in some cases appear to bypass the factor VIII lack and reduce the bleeding tendency; (d) the use of animal factor VIII concentrates, if available, for short-term administration (see p. 447 for further details).

The dosage of a concentrate to be used is determined by the potency of the material and the severity of the episode being treated. Cryoprecipitate, as generally prepared, has an activity approximating 100 units per bag; 400–600 units is the minimal dose required for a minor episode, and as much as 1000 units repeated 12-hourly may be required for more severe episodes or during surgery. Other concentrates containing factor VIII, factor IX, and related clotting factors have the concentrations shown on the container in either units of factor activity or as a plasma volume equivalent. This allows easy assessment of the dose required. As a general rule, an infusion of 1 unit factor VIII per kilogram bodyweight raises the plasma level by 0.02 U/ml. For factor IX, 1 unit concentrate per kilogram bodyweight results in a rise of 0.01 U/ml plasma.

The use of replacement therapy, including concentrates, is well summarized by Biggs (1978), Kaspar & Dietrich (1985), and Rizza & Jones (1987).

SURGERY

The availability of concentrates of clotting factors has rendered surgery in haemophiliacs almost as safe as for normal subjects. *General surgery* should be avoided whenever possible, but when necessary, it should be carried out in a centre that has the laboratory facilities for monitoring the response to replacement therapy. Before surgery, it is essential to perform *in vitro* and *in vivo* tests to ensure that the patient has not developed a specific inhibitor of clotting. Doses of the concentrate are usually given at 12-hourly intervals in haemophilia A, and at 24-hour intervals in haemophilia B; the dose must be adequate to increase factor levels to the normal range (0.5–1.0 U/ml) during surgery and to maintain levels of 0.4 U/ml or more until wound healing is established. Very rarely, immune inhibitors appear during convalescence; in such cases, massive doses of concentrates may be required to prevent bleeding.

Minor procedures, including tooth extraction, should also be carried out in hospitals that provide special care for haemophiliacs. Usually, replacement therapy is required on a lesser scale than for general surgery, particularly when blood can harmlessly escape to the surface in the event of excessive bleeding, and when topical haemostatic measures can be applied concurrently. Occasionally, intensive replacement therapy is indicated, e.g. for lumbar puncture, because of the risk of nervous system bleeding.

Dental extraction is commonly required in haemophiliacs; various regimens have been used to prevent bleeding, including massive replacement therapy as in general surgery. Experience suggests that the following regimen is a satisfactory compromise when extraction of up to four tricuspid teeth is necessary: care in hospital, re-assurance and sedation when necessary, pre-extraction replacement therapy with plasma (12 ml/kg) or cryoprecipitate 600–800 units, local anaesthesia, gentle extraction, insertion of catgut sutures, and local pressure. There should be acceptance by the doctor and the patient that moderate bleeding may occur, is without danger, and can be permanently arrested when replacement therapy is given on the seventh or eighth day after extraction.

The fibrinolytic inhibitors, ε amino-caproic acid (EACA) or tranexamic acid, are commonly administered concurrently to reduce factor VIII requirements. A satisfactory regimen consists of EACA taken orally in a dose of 5 g four times daily for one week, starting on the day of the extraction. With this management, some patients with severe haemophilia experience no bleeding, and sockets heal without further treatment; more commonly, such patients can be discharged on the tenth day when healing of the sockets is well advanced and recurrence of bleeding is unlikely.

Warning is necessary that no attempt should be made to arrest wound or tooth socket bleeding with very tight sutures or excessive external pressure as these procedures are usually ineffective and cause the lost blood to infiltrate tissues.

Desamino-8-D-arginine vasopressin (DDAVP). The plasma concentration of factor VIII increases in response to a number of physiological stimuli, including exercise, and to pharmacological agents including adrenaline and vasopressin (Mannucci *et al.* 1975). Plasminogen activator, and probably prostacyclin, are also liberated by vasopressin. The mechanism is unknown, but it does not appear to be due to vaso-activity nor to the release of a neuropeptide with secondary effect. The vasopressin analogue DDAVP has comparatively few side-effects—mild flushing and tachycardia. Administered intravenously in a dose of 0.3 μg/kg bodyweight, factor VIII activities (including von Willebrand factor) rise to 3–5 times baseline within 60–120 minutes, sufficient to treat minor bleeding or minor surgery in mild to moderate haemophiliacs and in patients with von Willebrand's disease. The dose may be repeated within a few hours, but tachyphylaxis develops. The concomitant fibrinolytic response can be aborted with an antifibrinolytic agent given simultaneously (*Lancet* Editorial 1983).

Androgen therapy. Androgen administration has been shown to be effective in elevating blood levels of proteins in other congenital deficiency states, namely hereditary angioedema and α_1 antitrypsin deficiency. A recent report indicates that the attenuated androgen danazol (600 mg/day) raises significantly the levels of factor VIII and factor IX in the small number of haemophilic and Christmas disease patients tested (Gralnick & Rick 1983). Kaspar & Boylen (1985) were unable to reproduce these results. The long-term clinical implications are awaited.

SPECIAL THERAPEUTIC MEASURES

Corticosteroid therapy. A condition resembling acute synovitis sometimes occurs after an attack of acute haemarthrosis. The administration of prednisone appears to be beneficial.

Physiotherapy. Although early replacement therapy has largely avoided the severe muscle wasting and joint deformities previously encountered, physiotherapy and splinting must be used when indicated.

Orthopaedic care. Long-standing deformities which have resulted from neglect can usually be improved or corrected with traction, splinting, and with increasing frequency, reconstructive surgery.

Von Willebrand's disease

Von Willebrand's disease is an inherited disorder of haemostasis which clinically resembles haemophilia. It is inherited as an autosomal dominant character (occasionally recessive) and affects both sexes. In the majority of cases, the bleeding tendency is of mild degree and is often limited to easy bruising, epistaxis—particularly with upper respiratory infections—and troublesome bleeding for up to 36 hours after minor lacerations and tooth extraction. This mild form was often difficult to diagnose with certainty in the past, and some patients were regarded as suffering from an ill-defined condition known as hereditary capillary fragility or vascular pseudohaemophilia. More severely affected patients have troublesome bleeding such as menorrhagia and spontaneous bleeding disorders, as are found in severe haemophilia. These patients are at serious risk from surgery and trauma. The most important clinical features of von Willebrand's disease and mild haemophilia are compared with the simple easy bruising syndrome in Table 15.6, and the most important laboratory features of these disorders are compared in Table 15.7.

Von Willebrand's disease is characterized by: (a) a defect of platelet function giving rise to a long bleeding time; and (b) a coagulation defect due to deficiency of factor VIII activity in the plasma. The diagnostic features are as follows:

prolonged bleeding time;

defective or absent platelet aggregation with ristocetin;

Table 15.6. *Comparison of the clinical features of mild haemophilia, von Willebrand's disease, and the simple, easy bruising syndrome*

Feature	Mild haemophilia	von Willebrand's disease	Simple, easy bruising
Relative incidence	Uncommon	Moderately uncommon	Common
Sex	Males	Males & females	Mostly females
Family history of bleeding	Usual	Usual	Unusual
Inheritance	Sex-linked recessive	Autosomal dominant (or recessive)	Nil
Symptom			
Ecchymoses	Rare	Small, frequent	Small, frequent
Epistaxis	Rare	Common	Infrequent
Traumatic or surgical bleeding			
Onset	Delayed	Immediate	Usually none
Duration	Days to week	1–2 days but may recur	—
Minor lacerations	Rare	Usual	Rare
Tooth extraction	Usual	Usual	Rare
Menstrual loss	—	Excessive	Normal to mildly increased
Haematomas and haemarthrosis	Uncommon	Uncommon	Do not occur

Table 15.7. *Comparison of laboratory tests in mild haemophilia A, von Willebrand's disease, and the easy bruising syndrome*

Test	Mild haemophilia	von Willebrand's disease	Easy bruising
Bleeding time	Normal	Prolonged or normal	Rarely prolonged
Tourniquet test	Negative	Sometimes positive	Sometimes positive
Platelet aggregation			
ADP	Normal	Normal	Normal
Adrenaline	Normal	Normal	Abnormal
Collagen	Normal	Normal	Sometimes abnormal
Ristocetin	Normal	Abnormal	Normal
Prothrombin time	Normal	Normal	Normal
Activated partial thromboplastin time	Abnormal	Abnormal	Normal
Factor VIII activity	Reduced	Normal or reduced	Normal
von Willebrand antigen	Normal	Normal, reduced or absent	Normal
Factor IX activity	Normal	Normal	Normal

reduced ristocetin co-factor activity in plasma;
normal or decreased von Willebrand/factor VIII antigen in plasma;
normal or decreased factor VIII activity in plasma.

The tourniquet test is often positive, and the platelet count is normal. Not all of the laboratory diagnostic features listed may be present. It may be necessary to extend the investigation to other family members to aid in diagnosis. The precision of laboratory investigations has been greatly improved with the introduction of ristocetin as an aggregating agent of platelets. Howard & Firkin (1971) showed that this substance requires a factor, lacking in the plasma of patients with von Willebrand's disease, to cause platelet aggregation. Further advances have been in the use of immunodiffusion or immunoelectrophoretic techniques to assay for von Willebrand antigen. In von Willebrand's disease, factor VIII activity and von Willebrand factor classically vary together, whereas in haemophilia, factor VIII activity may be low or absent when von Willebrand factor is present in normal or increased amounts. The relationship of the two proteins is depicted in Fig. 15.9

Variant forms of von Willebrand's disease (Table 15.8) have been described, for example with normal factor VIII activity (Holmberg & Nilsson 1973), the principal abnormality being in the von Willebrand factor function affecting platelet function. The major variant (type II) of von Willebrand's disease exhibits the clinical pattern of the classical (type I) disorder. There is, however, normal factor VIII coagulation activity and quantitatively normal von Willebrand factor antigen. The ristocetin co-factor activity of this protein is abnormal, and this is related to various physicochemical characteristics which include the ability to form multimers and differences in the carbohydrate side-chains. Some authors segregate 'severe' von Willebrand's disease as type III, in part because the transmission is

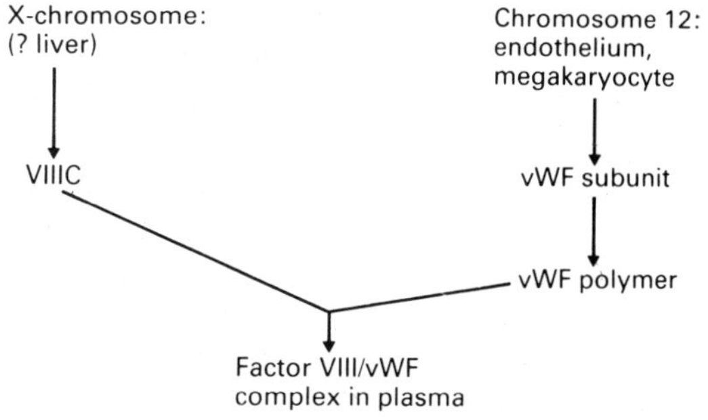

Fig. 15.9. *Relationship between factor VIII and von Willebrand factor.*

Table 15.8. *Varieties of von Willebrand's disease*

Type I (classical)	VIII : C low vWF : Ag low vWF : Rc low
Type II A	VIII:C normal or low vWF : Ag normal or low (abnormal electrophoresis) vWF : Rc very low (prolonged BT)
Type II B	as above vWF : Rc normal or low
Type III (severe)	as in type I but all activities very low or absent (recessive transmission)

VIII : C = Factor VIII activity (coagulant)
vWF : Ag = von Willebrand antigen.
vWF : Rc = Ristocetin co-factor.
BT = bleeding time.

typically recessive (Ruggeri 1987). The complexity of the disease is indicated by the identification of at least 22 different subtypes on the basis of phenotype of the von Willebrand protein (Ruggeri 1987).

Correction of the various abnormalities in von Willebrand's disease, after plasma transfusion, follows a complex pattern. The bleeding time, platelet glass bead retention, and aggregation with ristocetin are corrected for a short period of time, only about 6–12 hours. The factor VIII activity, however, often increases beyond the levels explicable on the basis of the amount infused. This endogenous factor VIII activity rises to a maximum over 24 hours, and falls gradually to the resting level. The same pattern follows transfusion of normal serum or plasma from severe haemophilia A patients, both lacking factor VIII activity (Larrieu *et al.* 1968). The precise explanation for these findings is unknown, but may represent a stimulation to synthesize factor VIII. The von Willebrand factor functions remain clinically important, and thus the bleeding time is a better clinical parameter to monitor treatment than measurement of factor VIII.

Treatment of bleeding requires local measures and the use of fresh frozen plasma or concentrates of factor VIII, such as cryoprecipitate. Local treatment may be sufficient for minor trauma, and the use of oestrogen/progestogen preparations to regulate the menstrual cycle often helps to control menorrhagia.

Other congenital disorders

Congenital fibrinogen (factor I) deficiency

In this rare disorder there is almost complete absence of fibrinogen in the plasma. It affects both sexes, and is inherited as an autosomal recessive character. The haemorrhagic tendency resembles that of moderate haemophilia. Bleeding most commonly follows trauma, especially severe trauma, but may occur spontaneously. Small lacerations frequently do not bleed excessively. In women, menstruation is usually normal. The characteristic laboratory finding is the failure of a clot to appear in the whole blood clotting time, the one-stage prothrombin time, and activated partial thromboplastin time and the thrombin time tests; the thromboplastin generation test is normal, and assay tests show that only fibrinogen is deficient. By biochemical methods, it appears that fibrinogen is completely absent, but immunological methods may reveal trace amounts of fibrinogen. Partial deficiency of fibrinogen, hypofibrinogenaemia, also occurs, probably representing the heterozygous state, and does not cause a haemostatic defect.

The general treatment is along the lines described on p. 417; accessible bleeding points usually respond to vasoconstrictor drugs, pressure, and, if necessary, suture. Blood transfusion may be required if blood loss has been great.

Inherited dysfibrinogenaemia. A steadily increasing number of families with functionally abnormal fibrinogen has been recorded; more than 80 are now described. Only a proportion bleed excessively, some show a tendency to wound breakdown, and a very few are reported to have a thrombotic tendency.

Congenital deficiency of factor II (prothrombin), factor V, factor VII, or factor X

Congenital deficiency of these factors is very rare. The bleeding tendency usually commences in infancy or childhood. The disorders affect both sexes, and appear to be inherited as autosomal recessive characters. The haemorrhagic symptoms are similar to those of moderate haemophilia. Several variants of prothrombin deficiency have been described, and all have been due to the presence of a defective coagulant protein. Combined deficiency of factors V and VIII have been reported (Seligsohn & Ramot 1969). This defect may result from an underlying lack of protein C inhibitor, allowing activated protein C to destroy circulating factors Va and VIIIa (Marlar & Griffin 1980), although this notion has not been confirmed. Other combined deficiency diseases are reviewed by Soff & Levin (1981).

Factor XI deficiency

This congenital disorder resembles moderate to mild haemophilia. It is transferred as an autosomal recessive character and affects both sexes; it is rare, and has been found most commonly in Jews. The laboratory findings include an abnormal activated partial thromboplastin time, and the deficiency is proven in a specific assay for factor XI. Without this step, the abnormality may be difficult to distinguish in the laboratory from factor XII deficiency. Bleeding is usually not severe, but may be controlled by transfusion of plasma or of the supernatant from cryoprecipitate.

Factor XII (Hageman factor) deficiency

Congenital deficiency of Hageman factor is characterized by the absence of a clinical haemorrhagic tendency despite prolongation of the whole blood coagulation time and the activated partial thromboplastin time. Most patients with this disorder have been discovered on routine laboratory testing. No treatment is required, and the patients may safely undergo surgical operations without special precautions. *Fletcher factor* (pre-kallikrein) and *Fitzgerald factor* (high molecular weight kininogen) deficiencies produce similar laboratory abnormalities without clinical significance, and are extremely rare.

Factor XIII (fibrin-stabilizing factor) deficiency

Congenital deficiency of fibrin-stabilizing factor causes haemorrhagic symptoms similar to mild and moderate grades of haemophilia. The congenital defect has been observed in a number of families, and bleeding from the umbilical stump after birth is a characteristic feature. The healing of wounds has been stated to be less satisfactory than in other coagulation defects. The bleeding time, platelet count, and the usual coagulation tests are normal. The diagnosis is established by demonstrating that the patient's blood clot dissolves in solutions of urea or monochloracetic acid. Bleeding is treated by local measures and the transfusion of fresh frozen plasma. Factor XIII has a long plasma half-life, and plasma transfusion corrects the bleeding tendency for several days.

Acquired coagulation disorders

Bleeding due to an acquired defect of coagulation (Table 15.9) is not uncommon in clinical practice. Because the bleeding is often associated with an underlying causative disorder, it frequently occurs as a complication of a condition already under treatment by a physician or surgeon. The most common causes are liver disease, anticoagulant therapy, and vitamin K deficiency. In these disorders, the bleeding is usually of mild to moderate severity, although it is occasionally severe. However, it is of particular clinical importance as it may aggravate or precipitate bleeding from a pre-existing local lesion, and may also cause bleeding to occur with minor therapeutic and diagnostic procedures, e.g. intramuscular injection and biopsy, as well as with surgical procedures. It is now well

Table 15.9. *Acquired coagulation disorders*

Vitamin K deficiency
Liver disease
Anticoagulant drugs
Disseminated intravascular coagulation (DIC)
Acute primary fibrinolysis
Massive transfusion of stored blood
Circulating inhibitors of coagulation

recognized that disseminated intravascular coagulation contributes to the bleeding in a wide variety of disorders (p. 442) and, especially when associated with surgery or childbirth, may cause catastrophic bleeding.

Vitamin K deficiency

Vitamin K is a fat-soluble vitamin which is essential for the synthesis by the liver of functional prothrombin (factor II), factor VII, factor IX, and factor X (see Table 15.1, p. 407). The vitamin K-dependent step is the formation of γ carboxyglutamic acid residues which are required for Ca^{++} binding associated with phospholipid binding. Vitamin K is obtained in part from food, especially green leaves, and in part from the bacterial flora in the bowel which synthesizes the vitamin; either source can compensate for a deficiency of the other. In practically all cases, deficiency of vitamin K in adults results from a clinically recognizable cause; it appears unlikely ever to be due to simple dietary deficiency. Following failure of absorption, vitamin K deficiency develops rapidly within 1–3 weeks, as the body stores are small. In practice, deficiency of vitamin K is confirmed by showing that the prolonged one-stage prothrombin time test is rapidly corrected in 6–24 hours after the parenteral administration of vitamin K.

Aetiology of vitamin K deficiency

Vitamin K deficiency occurs in three disorders:

DISORDERS THAT IMPAIR FAT ABSORPTION

Obstructive jaundice and biliary fistula. The main cause of vitamin K deficiency is biliary obstruction or fistula, which leads to impaired absorption due to the lack of bile salts; in long-standing obstruction, hepatic damage may develop, and thus the normal response is impaired following vitamin K administration.

Coeliac disease (gluten enteropathy), pancreatic disease, and related disorders. Intestinal disorders that cause malabsorption of fat and other food constituents sometimes lead to the impaired absorption of vitamin K, and thus to a coagulation disorder. In rare cases, abnormal bleeding may be the presenting symptom of these disorders.

STERILIZATION OF THE BOWEL BY ANTIBIOTIC DRUGS

Rarely, vitamin K deficiency has been observed in patients receiving prolonged treatment with oral antibiotics. In these cases, the deficiency has been attributed to the combined effects of a diet low in vitamin K and to loss of the normal bowel flora which synthesizes the vitamin.

HAEMORRHAGIC DISEASE OF THE NEWBORN

This disorder, which occurs during the first few days of life, is due to a defect in the synthesis of vitamin K-dependent clotting factors. This results from one or more of the following causes: reduced stores of vitamin K, functional immaturity of the liver, lack of bacterial synthesis of vitamin K, and as a consequence of the administration of certain drugs to the mother. Thus, it has been described after the administration to the mother of oral anticoagulants, and also anticonvulsant drugs and large doses of aspirin.

Treatment

Measures used in the treatment of vitamin K deficiency are:

- correction of the causative disorder;
- administration of vitamin K (see below);
- replacement therapy when bleeding is severe (p. 417).

VITAMIN K

A large number of vitamin K preparations is available; they fall into two broad groups: vitamin K_1, formerly available only as a naturally occurring fat-soluble compound, but now available as a water-soluble compound; and synthetic analogues of vitamin K.

Vitamin K_1 is available in 10 mg tablets for oral administration, e.g. *Konakion* tablets, and in ampoules for intravenous use, e.g. *Aquamephyton*

(1 ml ampoules of 10 mg, 5 ml of 50 mg) and *Konakion* (0.5 ml ampoules of 1 mg, 1 ml of 10 mg). An oral preparation of drops is also available.

The synthetic analogues include menaphthone (BP), which is well known as menadione (USP), and acetomenaphthone; they are available in 1, 5, and 10 mg tablets. The snythetic analogues for intramuscular and intravenous use include menadoxime (*Kapilin*), the disphosphoric acid esters (*Kappadione*), and menadione sodium bisulphite.

Vitamin K_1 is the most potent and rapidly acting vitamin K preparation. If there is no associated hepatic dysfunction, its administration is followed by an increase in the prothrombin value above the minimal level required for haemostasis within 3–4 hours, and usually a return to normal in about 24 hours. It is therefore the preparation of choice in patients with 'hypoprothrombinaemia' who are actively bleeding.

A disadvantage of vitamin K_1 is that it is relatively expensive, and thus the cheaper synthetic analogues have often been preferred when there is hypoprothrombinaemia without bleeding, e.g. in obstructive jaundice and for prolonged therapy in patients with malabsorption. However, there is some doubt about the efficacy of these agents, and vitamin K_1 is being increasingly used, irrespective of whether or not bleeding is present.

The dose of vitamin K_1 for the treatment of bleeding in adults is 10–20 mg, given either intramuscularly or intravenously. When the intravenous route is used (reserved for potentially fatal haemorrhage), the drug should be diluted with blood and given slowly at a rate not exceeding 5 mg per minute. When the intramuscular route is used, vitamin K should be given through a narrow-gauge needle, and pressure applied over the injection site for at least five minutes. The arm rather than the buttock should be used, as bleeding is readily observed. The usual dose of the synthetic analogues given to correct hypothrombinaemia is 5–10 mg three times a day, either orally or parenterally.

The response to therapy should be determined in all cases by repeating the prothrombin time test 24 hours after the commencement of treatment; failure to obtain correction or marked improvement in the prothrombin time suggests that there is hepatic disease or that absorption of the drug has not occurred if the drug has been given orally.

As prophylaxis against haemorrhagic disease of the newborn, it is not uncommon practice in many centres to administer vitamin K_1 shortly after birth to both premature and full-term infants. When there is active bleeding and the prothrombin time is prolonged, vitamin K_1 is given parenterally in a dose of 1–2 mg; this dose is repeated every six hours. If the bleeding is not rapidly controlled, the vitamin K_1 should be supplemented by transfusion with fresh whole blood or fresh frozen plasma. It should be noted that vitamin K_1 does not cause red cell haemolysis in infants with glucose-6-phosphate dehydrogenase deficiency (p. 186); on the other hand, the synthetic analogues of vitamin K may produce haemolysis with possible kernicterus, and are thus best avoided in infants.

Liver disease

In liver disease, there is not uncommonly some derangement of the coagulation mechanism as shown by laboratory tests. Bleeding, when it occurs, is usually mild or moderate in degree. Troublesome or severe bleeding is relatively uncommon except: (a) when minor procedures, e.g. intramuscular injections, liver biopsy, etc., are performed; (b) when there is a local lesion, either related to the liver disease, e.g. varices, or unrelated, e.g. peptic ulcer; (c) in patients with cirrhosis during and after abdominal surgery, especially shunting operations; (d) in acute fulminating hepatitis; and (e) in the terminal phases of chronic liver disease, especially cirrhosis. Occasionally, prolonged bleeding after trauma is the first sign of severe liver disease.

In a patient with liver disease who is bleeding, the contribution and severity of the coagulation defect is assessed by estimation of the one-stage prothrombin time. If it is the main factor (see below), the prothrombin time is prolonged and this is not reversed by the administration of vitamin K.

Pathogenic factors in bleeding

A number of factors may contribute to the haemostatic defect in liver disease. These include defective synthesis of clotting factors, thrombocytopenia, increased fibrinolytic activity, and, rarely, defibrination. The contribution of each of these factors differs, depending on the associated clinical circumstances. However, defective synthesis is usually the most important factor.

Defective synthesis of coagulation factors. The liver is the site of synthesis of clotting factors I, II, V, VII, IX, and X, and probably factors XI, XII, and XIII. The synthesis of coagulation factors is not equally depressed in liver disease. Thus, the activity of the vitamin K-dependent factors (II, VII, IX, and X), appear to be the first to be affected; depression of factor V activity usually occurs only in severe liver disease, and hypofibrinogenaemia only in very severe liver disease. Malabsorption of vitamin K due to impairment of bile salt secretion may occur in some cases of parenchymatous liver disease, and may be an additional contributing pathogenetic factor.

Thrombocytopenia. Thrombocytopenia in liver disease is usually associated with portal hypertension and congestive splenomegaly. It may, however, occur in patients with acute alcoholic liver disease in the absence of portal hypertension (p. 386), and in patients with fulminating hepatitis.

Increased fibrinolytic activity. The liver is the site of synthesis of plasminogen and of antiplasmins. In addition, it plays an important role in clearing plasminogen activators from the bloodstream. Increased fibrinolytic activity may occur in liver disease as a result of the combined effects of impaired clearance of the plasminogen activators and decreased synthesis of antiplasmin. In practice, fibrinolysis appears to contribute to bleeding in liver disease mainly in patients with cirrhosis when subjected to surgery.

Intravascular coagulation (p. 442). The liver is the site of clearance and inactivation of some clotting factors. Inhibitors of coagulation, in particular antithrombin III and the vitamin K-dependent protein C, are synthesized in the liver, and their circulating levels may be reduced in liver disease. There is evidence for abnormally rapid consumption of coagulation proteins in cirrhotic patients. Despite these factors, intravascular coagulation is only infrequently a major factor in the haemostatic defect in patients with severe liver disease. Patients are, however, at risk from treatment with prothrombin concentrates, which have been shown to induce intravascular coagulation in some cases.

Bleeding in hepatitis

Acute hepatitis. Patients with acute infective hepatitis do not usually bleed abnormally and have, at most, a mild coagulation defect. Patients in whom the disease is severe usually have a prolonged one-stage prothrombin time and a prolonged activated partial thromboplastin time; these may be associated with a significant bleeding tendency, and are not corrected by vitamin K_1 administration. Patients with *acute fulminating hepatitis* usually have a marked coagulation defect, often with a severe factor V deficiency, hypofibrinogenaemia, and sometimes with severe thrombocytopenia; in these patients, diffuse bleeding from skin and mucous membranes, and large haematomas, frequently occur.

Chronic hepatitis. A number of factors, including deficiencies of coagulation factors, thrombocytopenia, and defective platelet function, may contribute to the haemostatic defect in chronic hepatitis. This defect is usually only mild to moderate, but it may aggravate bleeding from a local lesion such as oesophageal varices or peptic ulcer, or it may predispose to serious surgical and post-surgical bleeding. Increased fibrinolytic activity may be an important contributing factor to bleeding when patients with chronic hepatitis undergo surgery, especially shunt operations. In addition, the haemostatic defect may be aggravated in patients who have severe gastrointestinal tract bleeding or surgical bleeding, by transfusion with large volumes of stored blood.

Treatment

GENERAL PRINCIPLES

Treatment of the liver disease should be instituted. The general principles of treatment of each of the possible contributing factors are as follows.

Coagulation defect. The majority of patients do not

respond to vitamin K_1 administration, but in some a slow response may be obtained after daily administration of 50 mg for 4–5 days. The coagulation defect can be improved by infusions of fresh plasma; however, this is limited because large volumes are required. Concentrates of factors II, VII, IX, and X are available, but must be used with caution in patients with liver disease. These concentrates may contain activated coagulation factors and are capable of inducing intravascular coagulation. The patients may have a deficiency of antithrombin and reduced ability to clear activated factors from the circulation. The use of concentrates must therefore be followed with careful laboratory control, and it is probably advisable in most cases to use fresh frozen plasma, despite its limitations.

Thrombocytopenia. Platelet concentrates prepared from 3 to 6 units of fresh blood may be used to treat patients with severe thrombocytopenia. Unfortunately, the effectiveness of transfused platelets is reduced, because the platelets are rapidly sequestered in the enlarged spleen.

Increased fibrinolytic activity. This is most commonly seen in patients with chronic hepatitis during or after surgery. It may be a manifestation of disseminated intravascular coagulation, and laboratory investigation is required to establish that fibrinolysis is the major process. If fibrinolysis is considered to be the chief cause of bleeding, one of the inhibitors—ε amino-caproic acid (EACA) or aprotinin (Trasylol)—should be administered (p. 445). Concurrent replacement of fibrinogen, coagulation factors, and plasma antithrombin with fresh frozen plasma, may also be advisable.

Prophylaxis. The severity of the haemostatic defect should be assessed in patients with liver disease when liver biopsy or surgery is contemplated. In the absence of bruising or bleeding, the bleeding time, platelet count, activated partial thromboplastin time, and prothrombin time serve as a useful guide to the likelihood of post-traumatic bleeding. If the partial thromboplastin time is significantly prolonged (> 50 when the control range is 30–45 seconds), the prothrombin ratio (patient : control) is greater than 1.5, the platelet count is less than 100×10^9/l, and the bleeding time is prolonged, an attempt should be made to correct the defects by transfusion of plasma and/or platelet concentrates before liver biopsy or surgery is performed.

ESTABLISHED BLEEDING

The nature and severity of the underlying haemostatic defect should be assessed and then treated according to the general principles outlined above. Approximately 50 per cent of patients with cirrhosis who bleed from oesophageal varices have a demonstrable coagulation abnormality. Although this abnormality is often mild, it may nevertheless contribute to the bleeding caused by the varices and thus should be treated. When large amounts of blood are required for replacement therapy, it is important to supplement the stored blood with fresh blood or fresh frozen plasma and platelet concentrates. As with any massive transfusion, it is good practice to give fresh frozen plasma and/or platelet concentrates when large volumes of stored blood are required.

Anticoagulant drugs

The anticoagulant drugs in clinical use are heparin and the vitamin K antagonists. Heparin inhibits the formation of thromboplastin and the action of thrombin (p. 411). It is not absorbed from the gastrointestinal tract and must therefore be given by injection. Heparin has an immediate anticoagulant effect which lasts from 1 to 6 hours after intravenous injection, depending on the dose given; when give subcutaneously, the effect lasts longer because of the time taken for absorption into the bloodstream. Heparin is converted in the liver to a less active form, which is then excreted in the urine.

The vitamin K antagonists include the coumarin and indanedione derivatives. These drugs suppress an essential step in the synthesis of active vitamin K-dependent clotting factors (factors II, XII, IX, and X) by the liver (p. 436). The anticoagulant effect is therefore delayed until the existing circulating clotting factors are cleared from the bloodstream. This delay is approximately 36–48 hours with warfarin (*Coumadin, Marevan*). The anticoagulant effect of warfarin and phenindione (*Dindevan*) given in therapeutic doses lasts for up to two days, and that of phenprocoumon (*Marcoumar*) for four days. However, in cases of overdose the anticoagulant effect may persist even longer. The coumarins are metabolized in the liver and excreted in the urine in an inactive form. Although patients with impaired liver function show increased sensitivity to the coumarins, the biological half-life of these drugs does not appear to be increased in patients with cirrhosis (Aggelar & O'Reilly 1966). The danger of hypersensitivity reactions is considerable with phenindione, which may cause skin rashes, agranulocytosis, jaundice, diarrhoea, and renal damage.

Control of anticoagulant therapy

Heparin therapy can be controlled by measuring the whole blood clotting time or the activated partial thromboplastin time. When heparin is given by continuous intravenous infusion, the whole blood clotting time should be maintained at 2–3 times the normal value. The corresponding prolongation of the activated partial thromboplastin time is 1.5–2.5 times the normal value (Pitney 1982). When heparin is given by intermittent injection, the clotting time should be approximately 1.5–2 times the normal value at the time the next injection is due.

Oral anticoagulant therapy is controlled either by the one-stage prothrombin time test or by the thrombotest. The therapeutic range for the one-stage prothrombin time is a ratio of patient to control of 2.0–4.0 (based on the international normalized ratio), and for the thrombotest is 6–15 per cent of normal. There are, however, local variations due to the lack of standardization of laboratory technique. The laboratory control of anticoagulant therapy is discussed in detail on pp. 467–8 and by Pitney (1982), Gallus & Hirsh (1976), the ICTH/ICSH report of the expert panel on oral anticoagulant control (1979) and Poller (1982). There is considerable individual variation in response to both heparin and the oral anticoagulants. In addition, the response to the drugs may be modified by a number of known endogenous and exogenous factors (Table 15.10).

Bleeding during anticoagulant therapy

Bleeding during anticoagulant therapy may be due to *overdosage*, either absolute or relative (see factors

Table 15.10. *Factors that interfere with control of oral anticoagulant therapy*

Drugs*		Other factors	
Potentiating	*Inhibiting*	*Potentiating*	*Inhibiting*
Salicylates	Barbiturates	Diarrhoea	Hereditary resistance
Sulindac	Carbamazepine		
Phenylbutazone	Chloral hydrate	Alcohol	
Indomethacin	Griseofulvin	Hepatitis	Malignancy
Sulphonamides	Spironolactone	Congestive cardiac failure	
Amiodarone			
Sulphinpyrazone	Glutethimide	Septicaemia	
Clofibrate	Ethchlorvynol	Prolonged hypotension	
Thyroxine	Cimetidine		
Oxymetholone		Acute renal failure	
Nortriptyline			
Allopurinol			
Cholestyramine			
Broad-spectrum antibiotics			

*This list of drugs is not exhaustive.

affecting response), or to a *local lesion*. In the best of hands, the incidence of major bleeding is very low, about 1 in 25 years of treatment (Poller 1982). Commonly, it results from minor trauma or therapeutic procedures, e.g. intramuscular injection. When a person on anticoagulant therapy develops bleeding manifestations, either local or general, the laboratory test being used for control must be performed. If bleeding is confined to one site, and the result of the test indicates the the anticoagulant effect is within the desired therapeutic range or is suboptimal, a local lesion predisposing to bleeding should be considered. Thus, when haematuria occurs without other bleeding manifestations, the possibility of a local renal lesion, such as renal calculus, should be considered, or if haematemesis and melaena occur, the possibility of a peptic ulcer or neoplasm. However, if the tests indicate that the anticoagulant effect is greater than desired (prothrombin ratio > 4.0, or thrombotest < 5 per cent), overdosage is more likely to be the cause of bleeding, especially if the bleeding occurs from more than one site.

Overdosage usually causes serious spontaneous bleeding, such as macroscopic haematuria, retroperitoneal haemorrhage, and cerebral haemorrhage, only when the coagulation tests are outside the therapeutic range for prolonged periods of time.

Increased susceptibility. Serious spontaneous bleeding most commonly occurs when an anticoagulant drug is given in the usual therapeutic dose to a patient with an increased susceptibility to the drug. Thus, it is important to be constantly aware of the factors that may alter the susceptibility to these drugs, especially in patients on long-term therapy.

Variation in susceptibility to oral anticoagulants may be caused by drugs and other factors, including a number of diseases (see Table 15.10). The drugs most commonly responsible for increased sensitivity are aspirin, the oral antibiotics, and phenylbutazone. Increased sensitivity to the oral anticoagulants also occurs in patients with impaired hepatic function, e.g. due to hepatitis, excessive alcohol intake, congestive cardiac failure, septicaemia, or prolonged hypotension, and in patients with diarrhoea, because this may be associated with impaired synthesis of vitamin K as well as impaired absorption.

Increased sensitivity to heparin may occur in patients with liver disease, severe renal disease, and oliguria, and in patients with peripheral circulatory failure.

There is an increased risk of cerebral haemorrhage in patients with severe hypertension, bacterial endocarditis, and with a recent thrombotic stroke, even though the clotting tests are within the therapeutic range. Patients over the age of 65 years show an increased tendency to bleed, both because they commonly have associated arterial disease and because their dosage requirements are often low.

Accidental overdose. Heparin is available in ampoules containing 1000, 5000, and 25 000 units per ml, and accidental overdosage may occur if these doses are confused. Accidental overdosage with oral anticoagulants most commonly occurs due to confusion over tablets in the early stages of treatment. This can be avoided by careful counselling about dosage and the use of a suitable anticoagulant book.

Deliberate overdosage. Occasionally, bleeding results from concealed self-medication, usually in members of the medical and para-medical professions, and from suicidal or criminal poisoning (O'Reilly & Aggeler 1966).

The cause of the abnormal bleeding in patients is sometimes elicited by inquiry about drug ingestion. When drug ingestion is not admitted, it may be strongly suspected by finding deficiency of all the four vitamin K-dependent clotting factors and confirmed by analysis of the patient's plasma. Overdose of phenindione may be suspected from the presence of an orange–pink pigment in the urine and sometimes in the plasma.

Surgery and anticoagulant therapy. In general, surgery should not be performed while patients are on full anticoagulant therapy. When a patient on an anticoagulant requires surgery, and the anticoagulant therapy is not mandatory, the drug should be ceased, and if the surgery is urgent the appropriate antidote given. If anticoagulation is essential it may be preferable to change to heparin (either full or low dosage) during the peri-operative period, as this affords the greatest control over the haemostatic defect. Many surgical procedures, however, have been carried out in patients on oral anticoagulant therapy without significant increase in haemorrhage, but great care with surgical haemostasis is obviously important. The problem is discussed in greater detail by Cade *et al.* (1979). Low-dose heparin, and other antithrombotic approaches used during surgery as prophylaxis against venous thrombo-embolism, are reviewed on p. 466.

Treatment

Bleeding during heparin therapy is treated by administration of protamine sulphate, a strongly basic agent which combines with and inactivates heparin. Protamine sulphate is available as an intravenous preparation in 5 ml ampoules containing 50 mg per ampoule. One milligram of protamine neutralizes approximately 1 mg (100 units) of heparin. When reversal of the effect of heparin is required within minutes of its intravenous injection, a full neutralizing dose of protamine (1 mg protamine to 100 units heparin) should be given. The effectiveness of the neutralization with protamine sulphate should be checked by estimating the clotting time or the activated partial thromboplastin time. The administration of protamine sulphate may have to be repeated because the drug is cleared from the bloodstream more rapidly than heparin. When heparin given subcutaneously has to be neutralized, protamine sulphate should be given in a neutralizing dose which is equivalent to 50 per cent of the last heparin dose, and this may have to be repeated. The exact dose of protamine required to produce neutralization can be worked out by performing a heparin neutralization test, but this test is not always available, and the approach outlined above is satisfactory in clinical practice.

Bleeding during oral anticoagulant therapy. If bleeding is severe, vitamin K_1 in a dose of 25 mg should be given intravenously. Precautions should be taken to give the drug slowly, at a rate not exceeding 5 mg per minute. Rapid administration may produce flushing, vertigo, tachycardia, hypotension, dyspnoea, and sweating. Reversal of the anticoagulant nevertheless takes some hours to achieve, and immediate replacement of the vitamin K-dependent factors with infusion of a concentrate or with fresh frozen plasma may be necessary (Taberner *et al.* 1976). When there is no bleeding, but the prothrombin time or thrombotest is below the generally accepted safe level and reversal is indicated, it can usually be achieved by the oral administration of 5 mg vitamin K_1 or intramuscular injection of 1–2 mg. Subsequent anticoagulation with oral agents becomes difficult if larger doses of vitamin K are used.

Disseminated intravascular coagulation

Defibrination syndrome and *consumption coagulopathy* are synonyms for disseminated intravascular coagulation, a haemorrhagic disorder in which diffuse intravascular clotting causes a haemostatic defect resulting from the utilization of coagulation factors and platelets in the clotting process. For this reason, it is often called consumption coagulopathy. Disseminated intravascular coagulation may complicate a variety of clinical conditions (Table 15.11). It may be acute, subacute, or chronic.

Table 15.11. *Causes of disseminated intravascular coagulation*

Acute
Obstetrical accidents
abruptio placentae
amniotic fluid embolism
abortion
Surgery, especially of the heart and lung
Haemolytic transfusion reaction
Septicaemia, especially Gram-negative and meningococcal
Pulmonary embolism
Snake bite
Hypersensitivity reactions
Heatstroke
Subacute or chronic
Disseminated or localized carcinoma
Septicaemia
Acute leukaemia (particularly promyelocytic)
Fetal death *in utero*
Purpura fulminans
Giant haemangioma

Pathogenesis

Disseminated intravascular coagulation may be caused by: (a) the release or entry of tissue factors that act as coagulants into the bloodstream; and (b) extensive endothelial damage. Coagulants are normally inactivated by naturally occurring circulating inhibitors, and are cleared by the reticulo-endothelial system. Thus, the occurrence of intravascular coagulation is augmented by stasis (which prevents the circulating inhibitors from reaching the coagulants) and by reticulo-endothelial blockade.

Experimental intravascular coagulation. The mechanism and consequences of defibrination can best be understood by considering the changes that occur during experimentally induced defibrination. Intravascular coagulation can be produced experimentally by infusing thrombin, tissue extracts, red cell lysates, or bacterial endotoxin into an animal. This initiates the clotting process (as shown at first by a shortening of the coagulation time), but as the process continues the blood becomes incoagulable because platelets, fibrinogen, and factors II, V, and VII are consumed by the clotting. Widespread intravascular fibrin deposition can usually be demonstrated in the animals soon after defibrination is induced, but these deposits are no longer evident days after induction, presumably because they are digested by the fibrinolytic system which is activated as a secondary phenomenon.

If the fibrinolytic inhibitor ε amino-caproic acid (EACA) is given to the animals early in the stage of intravascular coagulation, widespread thrombosis occurs with necrotic infarction of many organs, a process resembling the generalized Schwartzmann reaction. This observation suggests the activation of the fibrinolytic mechanism which occurs as a consequence of defibrination is an important protective mechanism. The secondary increase in fibrinolytic activity is localized to the site of the intravascular clotting and does not usually result in plasma fibrinolytic activity. The local breakdown of fibrin results in the formation of fibrin breakdown (split) products which then circulate in the bloodstream. Their presence may contribute to the coagulation defect and influence the clotting tests (p. 413).

The mechanism of the secondary fibrinolysis is uncertain; it may result from activation of the fibrinolytic system by active factor XII (Hageman factor), but more likely from release of tissue plasminogen activator due to endothelial damage which is produced by disseminated intravascular thrombosis or by the initial insult. Experimental aspects of disseminated intravascular coagulation are reviewed by Chesterman (1978) and Muller-Berghaus (1987).

Aetiology

Intravascular coagulation may occur as a complication of a number of disorders and clinical situations. (see Table 15.11). The process may be localized or diffuse, depending on the stimulus. Clearly a number of different 'triggers' exist, and these include tissue factors and cellular material (e.g. tumours, trauma, obstetric accidents), bacterial endotoxin, and antigen–antibody complexes (mismatched transfusion). The tissue localization may be influenced by factors such as vascular tone, organ perfusion, hydration, and local inflammation.

Clinical features

There are two main clinical features of disseminated intravascular coagulation: *bleeding,* which is the most common clinical manifestation, and *organ damage* due to the ischaemia caused by the effect of the widespread intravascular thrombosis, e.g. on the kidney and brain. Thus renal failure due to small-vessel occlusion with fibrin deposits may occur in post-partum or post-surgical patients, and as a complication of septicaemia. In addition, microangiopathic haemolytic anaemia may occur in association with subacute defibrination states which complicate disseminated carcinoma (p. 208). Occasionally, the thrombotic process affects large vessels, e.g. causes venous thrombosis and arterial thrombosis, and in these patients the thrombotic manifestations may occur with or without evidence of bleeding.

It should be realized, however, that minor degrees of intravascular coagulation not uncommonly occur with a number of the disorders listed in Table 15.11, but that it is not sufficiently severe to cause clinical manifestations and its presence can be detected only after the appropriate laboratory tests are performed.

TYPE OF BLEEDING

Bleeding may be localized or generalized. Localized bleeding may take the form of prolonged bleeding from venepuncture sites, excessive bleeding at the site of operation both during operation and post-operatively, and uterine bleeding at the site of placental detachment. The generalized bleeding manifestations include ecchymoses, haematomas, gastrointestinal bleeding, and haematuria. Petechiae are often present because of the associated thrombocytopenia. Serious bleeding due to defibrination occurs most commonly as a complication of obstetrical accidents or surgery, in which it is sometimes catastrophic.

The clinical situations in pregnancy and surgery require special comment, as do the unusual occurrences of snake bite and heatstroke.

Pregnancy

Abruptio placentae is the most common cause of bleeding due to disseminated intravascular coagulation in pregnancy. The bleeding is mainly localized to the placental site; initially, it may be a concealed retroplacental haemorrhage which later becomes manifest as a vaginal bleed; generalized bleeding may also occur. The bleeding is often extensive, but usually stops as the coagulation defect undergoes spontaneous improvement within hours of delivery.

Renal failure may be a serious complication; it is considered to be due to a combination of hypotension and the deposition of fibrin in the small renal vessels.

Amniotic fluid embolism is a rare, but often fatal, condition. In a typical case, the patient develops respiratory distress and shock either during labour and delivery, or immediately after delivery. If the patient survives the initial period of shock, haemorrhagic complications are common. These may take the form of local uterine bleeding and/or generalized bleeding.

Fetal death in utero. Defibrination occurs in approximately 25 per cent of patients in whom fetal death *in utero* has been present for more than one month. In most cases, there is a laboratory defect only or the patient bleeds excessively from venepuncture sites; occasionally, there is a marked coagulation defect with diffuse spontaneous bleeding into skin and mucous membranes.

Surgery

Intravascular coagulation with severe defibrination may develop during or after any surgery, but is more common after thoracic and cardiac surgery. It may be difficult to distinguish from bleeding due to heparin used during cardiopulmonary bypass for cardiac surgery.

With thoracic surgery, intravascular coagulation is possibly due to release of thromboplastin from the lungs during surgical manipulation. *Major trauma* with *massive blood transfusion* may also be complicated by intravascular coagulation, and laboratory assistance may be required to establish the cause of excessive and continuing bleeding.

Heatstroke with hyperpyrexia is an occasional cause of acute intravascular coagulation. This results from extensive tissue damage, and may be associated with collapse and coma and acute renal failure. Cooling, fluid replacement, electrolyte balance, and general support are essential. The bleeding tendency may be treated with plasma and platelet transfusion.

The *venoms* of many different snakes have potent coagulation properties. Some, such as ancrod, the product of the venom of the Malayan pit viper, have a direct thrombin-like action on fibrinogen. They produce fibrin monomer formation in the circulation, which is cleared by fibrinolysis and possibly by the reticulo-endothelial system, resulting in defibrination. The intermediate stages of coagulation are not influenced, and thrombocytopenia does not occur. This state is usually not accompanied by spontaneous bleeding, and ancrod has been shown to be a safe therapeutic agent in a number of thrombotic states. The majority of other venoms, particularly those of Australian snakes, the tiger snake (*Notechis scutatus*) and the taipan (*Pseudechis scutellatus*), act at earlier stages of the coagulation sequence and produce a state of disseminated intravascular coagulation. This can usually be managed with the appropriate antivenom, and recovery occurs rapidly after the remaining venom is neutralized.

Laboratory diagnosis

The abnormalities in coagulation tests result from consumption of clotting factors and platelets, and the presence of circulating fibrin or fibrinogen breakdown products, resulting from the secondary fibrinolytic activity (p. 412). Not all of the clotting factor activities usually consumed during coagulation are necessarily depressed in individual patients with disseminated intravascular coagulation. This is because the initial concentration or turnover rate of these various factors is subject to marked individual variations. Serial testing is therefore important in establishing the diagnosis in most cases.

The useful screening tests include observation of the whole blood clot, the thrombin time, prothrombin time and activated partial thromboplastin time, platelet count, and tests for fibrinogen–fibrin degradation products and fibrin monomers. More extensive investigation of fibrinolysis and clotting factor levels may be done if facilities are available. The major problem is to differentiate between disseminated intravascular coagulation and *primary pathological fibrinolysis*. The former is far more frequently the cause of severe defibrination, and is always accompanied by a detectable degree of fibrinolysis, as shown by the presence of fibrin degradation products. Primary pathological fibrinolysis is a contentious term, and may in reality represent the case in which intravascular coagulation is overwhelmed by an unusually active fibrinolytic response. This occurs in a relatively small number of clinical situations, e.g. disseminated carcinoma of the prostate.

Once the precipitating cause disappears, the clotting factor activities return to normal levels within 24 hours. Fibrinogen may show an increase earlier, although thrombocytopenia may persist for several days. The degradation products of fibrinogen and fibrin remain detectable for 12–24 hours.

Treatment

The principles of treatment are: (a) elimination of the precipitating factor if possible; (b) replacement of coagulation factors and platelets; and (c) inhibition of the clotting process with heparin or other agents.

Elimination of precipitating factor. The precipitating cause is often self-limiting. Thus, the stimulus to disseminated intravascular coagulation usually disappears soon after surgery or after delivery of patients with abruptio placentae. However, some of the underlying causes require specific treatment, e.g. antibiotics for septicaemia, oestrogens for carcinoma of the prostate, radiotherapy and steroids for patients with giant haemangioma.

Replacement of coagulation factors and platelets. Whole blood transfusion is given first to replace blood loss and second to replace the coagulation factors and platelets. If available, blood collected less than 12 hours previously may be used. However, such fresh blood is often not readily obtainable, and platelets and labile coagulation factors V and VIII, as well as fibrinogen and antithrombin, can be replaced with platelet concentrates and fresh frozen plasma. Fibrinogen may also be given in concentrated form, especially when bleeding is severe or does not respond to the above measures, and when the laboratory tests of thrombin time and fibrinogen level indicate severe deficiency. The dose is 5–10 g in 500 ml infused over 2–3 hours. The likelihood of hepatitis after fibrinogen administration is less if the material has been prepared from donor plasma known to be free of hepatitis-associated antigen (Hbs Ag).

Inhibition of the clotting process. The use of heparin or the enzyme inhibitors aprotinin (*Trasylol*) and ε amino-caproic acid (EACA) should be considered in any continuing episode of disseminated intravascular coagulation. Heparin is the agent most widely used, but a place exists for the use of aprotinin and perhaps EACA.

The clear indication for heparin is the occurrence of thrombotic manifestations, which may present as organ failure or as a large vessel occlusion. *Heparin, administered in an attempt to interrupt the underlying coagulation process* per se, *has not been shown to improve the high mortality associated with this condition. On the contrary, the added risk of bleeding is not inconsiderable.*

Treatment should be carefully monitored. The control is best based on the thrombin clotting time, platelet count, fibrinogen level, and activated partial thromboplastin time. When heparin is required, these tests are usually all abnormal, and some further prolongation of clotting times may result after heparin is started. The required dose of heparin is usually less than that necessary to treat patients with overt thrombosis. The average requirement is approximately 1000 units per hour by continuous intravenous infusion, but patients with hepatitis or renal insufficiency, or those in circulatory failure, may be very sensitive to heparin and should be treated initially with a dose of 500 units per hour. When effective, the response to heparin is fairly rapid. The thrombin clotting time and partial thromboplastin time may shorten somewhat, but one of the best guides to successful treatment is a significant increase in fibrinogen levels within 12 hours.

The enzyme inhibitor, aprotinin (*Trasylol*), may also be useful in the treatment of disseminated intravascular coagulation and hyperfibrinolysis. It may be considered as an alternative to heparin or used in combination with the anticoagulant in severe or resistant cases. Similarly, ε amino-caproic acid (EACA) may sometimes be used in combination with heparin and replacement therapy. Care should be taken to establish that fibrinolysis is a major element in the hypofibrinogenaemia when inhibitors are used, as inhibition of *compensatory* local fibrinolysis associated with intravascular coagulation may aggravate the thrombotic tendency.

Haemorrhage and blood transfusion

Haemorrhage resulting from blood transfusion may be caused by: (a) the administration of large amounts of stored blood; (b) haemolytic transfusion reactions (p. 482); and (c) transfusion thrombocytopenia due to platelet allo-antibodies (p. 387). Of these, the first is not uncommon, the second is rare, and the third is very rare.

Bleeding after transfusion of large amounts of stored blood

Platelets and the labile clotting factors V and VIII are unstable in blood stored at 4°C. Thus, when a patient's blood volume is replaced by large amounts of stored blood, or packed red cells and plasma expanders such as albumin solutions, thrombocytopenia and deficiencies of factors V and VIII may develop because of the dilution factor. The severity of the resultant haemostatic defect is related to several factors, including the amount of blood transfused and its rate of transfusion, the period of time that the blood has been stored, and the underlying clinical circumstances.

The amount. Thrombocytopenia regularly occurs when more than 10 units (5000 ml) of stored blood is administered over a 48-hour period. If the blood is given more rapidly, or if larger volumes are given, abnormal bleeding and severe thrombocytopenia may occur. Thrombocytopenia appears to be caused mainly by dilution of the recipient's blood with platelet-poor stored blood, but it is possible that blood loss and other factors may also contribute. The platelets return to normal in about 3–5 days after the last transfusion. The levels of factors V and VIII are variably depressed, commonly to 20–30 per cent of normal.

Age of blood. Blood which is less than 24 hours old still contains significant amounts of factors V and VIII, and some viable platelets. However, the platelet count rapidly falls, and the level of the clotting factors appreciably declines, in blood stored for 24 hours or more. Clearly, plasma expanders and packed red cells are devoid of coagulation factors and platelets.

The circumstances requiring blood transfusion. The severity of the haemostatic defect produced by transfusion with large volumes of stored blood is more marked when the capacity to produce platelets or clotting factors is impaired, e.g. in bone marrow depression, liver disease, and the haemophilias, or when the rate of consumption of platelets or clotting factors is increased, e.g. after major trauma, in chronic idiopathic thrombocytopenic purpura, and in intravascular coagulation.

Citrate overdosage may act as a minor contributing factor to the coagulation defect in massive transfusion. Thus, abnormal *in vitro* clotting tests corrected by the addition of extra calcium have been reported in patients who have bled abnormally after transfusion with large volumes of blood. Patients with liver disease are especially vulnerable to the hypocalcaemic effects of transfusion with citrated blood because citrate is normally metabolized in the liver.

TREATMENT

The coagulation defect produced by transfusion with large volumes can be prevented or minimized if 2 units of fresh blood, or 3–5 units of fresh frozen plasma, are given with every 10 units of packed red cells that is rapidly transfused. Established bleeding caused by transfusion of large amounts of stored blood is treated by administration of fresh frozen plasma, platelet concentrates or fresh whole blood. In addition, hypocalcaemia can be prevented by the injection of calcium gluconate.

Haemorrhagic disorders due to circulating inhibitors of coagulation

Circulating inhibitors are antibodies almost always of the IgG heavy chain class, with activity directed against a coagulation protein. There are two major types of inhibitor: those occurring in the course of haemophilia or other congenital coagulation disorders, and those acquired spontaneously or in the course of some other disease state. The nature of the reaction between inhibitor and clotting factor is complex, but the effect is to inactivate the coagulant protein partially or completely. Thus, inhibitors may be detected because of the property of the patient's plasma to induce a coagulation abnormality in mixtures with normal plasma. The specificity of the reaction can then usually be established by coagulation factor assays.

Inhibitors in haemophilia occur in 5–20 per cent of the patients in different studies. Some are less potent and become undetectable after periods without treatment. Others are very active anticoagulants which persist indefinitely and pose great problems in the treatment of bleeding episodes. Massive doses of factor concentrates may be required; sometimes species specificity is present and a temporarily good response may be obtained with porcine or bovine factor VIII. Immunosuppressive treatment combined with massive factor replacement has been reported to be successful in a small number of cases (Green 1972). An innovation that proved helpful in about 50 per cent of bleeding episodes is the use of concentrates of the *prothrombin complex* in haemophiliacs with inhibitors against factor VIII. These concentrates in some way by-pass the coagulation defect to a degree sufficient to control bleeding (p. 430). Commercial preparations have been produced specifically for this purpose. Immunodepletion by *plasmapheresis* and suppression of antibody activity by *high-dose intravenous gamma globulin* have been reported to be successful in small numbers of patients. The topic is recently reviewed by Bloom (1987).

Acquired inhibitors most commonly occur in disseminated lupus erythematosus. The 'lupus' inhibitor does not normally cause a bleeding tendency. In fact, paradoxically, the condition is not infrequently associated with a thrombotic tendency discussed in detail on p. 459. The inhibitor is detected during routine screening because of prolongation of clotting times in both the activated partial thromboplastin and prothrombin time tests. Further characteristics are discussed on p. 459. Other acquired inhibitors have been described against most of the coagulation factors, but are rare occurrences. The most frequently encountered of these have activity against factor VIII or its von Willebrand factor component, and have been described in association with penicillin reactions, pregnancy, rheumatoid disease, and spontaneously in the elderly, sometimes in association with skin disorders.

Factor VIII inhibitors may result in a bleeding tendency similar to mild or severe haemophilia. Menorrhagia is sometimes severe, and occasionally haemarthrosis, and retroperitoneal or gastrointestinal bleeding occur. When associated with pregnancy, bleeding occurs within a few weeks to several months of childbirth. The inhibitor usually disappears, but has been described to recur with subsequent pregnancies. Passive transfer across the placenta to the fetus has been observed.

Treatment of acquired inhibitors is often unsatisfactory. Remission of the underlying disorder such as lupus usually results in loss of the inhibitor. When bleeding occurs, blood transfusion and large doses of a concentrate of the appropriate factor, together with immunosuppressives, may control haemorrhage.

Investigation of a patient with a bleeding tendency

In the investigation of a patient with abnormal bleeding, three questions must be answered:

1 Is the bleeding due to a local pathological lesion, a haemorrhagic disorder, or a combination of the two?

2 If due to a haemorrhagic disorder, which of the three components of the haemostatic mechanism is affected: the platelets, the blood vessels, or the coagulation mechanism? Is more than one component affected?

3 What is the cause of the haemorrhagic disorder?

The importance of the history and clinical examination must be emphasized because the diagnosis of many haemorrhagic disorders is largely or wholly clinical, and the selection of appropriate laboratory tests required for accurate diagnosis depends on the full clinical assessment.

Table 15.12 summarizes the clinical features that should be sought and the special tests which may be necessary. In most cases, an adequate history and physical examination together with a few relatively simple investigations will establish the cause of the disorder.

Is the bleeding due to a local pathological lesion, a haemorrhagic disorder, or a combination of the two?

This question can often be answered from a consideration of the type of bleeding. Careful questioning about past bleeding and consideration of the existence of predisposing conditions may give valuable information (see Table 15.12). Thus, as pointed out previously, haemorrhagic disorder should be suspected: (a) when there is spontaneous bleeding into the skin, mucous membranes, or interstitial tissues; (b) when there is excessive or prolonged bleeding after minor trauma or minor surgery; and (c) when the bleeding occurs from more than one site. Furthermore, a haemorrhagic disorder may be suspected when there is evidence of a clinical disorder that commonly causes bleeding, or when there is a family history of abnormal bleeding.

It should be realized, however, that although bleeding from more than one site is usual in a haemorrhagic disorder, occasionally an episode of bleeding is localized to one site.

It should also be remembered that abnormal bleeding from a local pathological lesion may be precipitated by an unsuspected haemorrhagic disorder, and that in a patient with a *known* haemorrhagic disorder bleeding may be precipitated by the development of a local pathological lesion.

If due to a haemorrhagic disorder, which of the three components of the haemostatic mechanism is affected?

The affected component can sometimes be suspected from the type of bleeding. Thus, in *platelet disorder*, petechial bleeding is common, ecchymoses tend to be numerous but usually not larger than 2 cm in diameter, and bleeding from mucous membranes is prominent; furthermore, bleeding is commonly spontaneous. When excess bleeding occurs from wounds, it commences immediately, persists for less than 48 hours, and rarely recurs.

In *vascular disorders*, the bleeding is usually confined to the skin and may cause petechiae and ecchymoses. Petechiae tend to be pale and often confluent, and ecchymoses are usually small. Bleeding is not severe in most cases, and is commonly spontaneous. When bleeding occurs from wounds, it is usually immediately excessive, persists for less than 48 hours, and rarely recurs.

In the *coagulation disorders*, petechial hamorrhage is rare. Ecchymoses tend to be larger than in the platelet and vascular disorders, and bleeding more

Table 15.12. *Summary of the investigation of a patient with a haemorrhagic disorder*

History

Full general medical history with special emphasis on the following points:

Age, sex

Present episodes of bleeding

Type of bleeding: petechiae, ecchymoses, haematoma, deep tissue or joint bleeding, wound haemorrhage, menorrhagia, mucous membrane bleeding

Frequency and duration

Apparent cause: spontaneous or following minor trauma or surgery

Co-existing disease

Disorders that may cause vascular bleeding (Table 14.1, p. 364)
Disorders that may cause thrombocytopenia (Table 14.2, p. 377)
Disorders that may cause coagulation defects (Table 15.5, p. 420 and Table 15.9, p. 435)
  Gastrointestinal disease
  Renal disease, particularly advanced
  Liver disease and splenomegaly (hypersplenism)
  Primary haemopoietic disorders
Other possible associations, e.g. pregnancy, allergic reactions, skin disorders

Drug ingestion

Aspirin
Non-steroidal anti-inflammatory agents, e.g. sulphinpyrazone

Anticoagulant administration (p. 439)

Warfarin
Phenindione
Dietary changes or gastrointestinal upsets with vitamin K deficiency
Other drug treatment, e.g. salicylate

Occupation

Exposure to drugs or chemicals
Hazards of trauma

Diet

Ascorbic acid intake

Past history of bleeding and trauma

Especially important in cases of recurrent bleeding and suspected congenital haemostatic defects:
Age at occurrence of first abnormal bleeding and details of incident

Haemorrhagic incidents
Ecchymoses—traumatic and/or spontaneous, size
Haematomas—causes, size, and duration
Petechial haemorrhages
Epistaxis—cause, severity, frequency
Minor wound bleeding—immediate or delayed onset, rate of loss, duration, recurrences, measures required to arrest bleeding
Melaena, haematemesis, haematuria, and haemoptysis—cause and severity
Menstrual bleeding and post-partum bleeding—severity and duration of bleeding, loss of clots, duration of blood staining of lochia, inability to carry out usual occupation during menstruation, haemorrhage associated with delivery

Table 15.12. (*cont'd*)

Bleeding after trauma and surgery
Tooth extraction, tonsillectomy, circumcision, major surgery, and accidents: record all incidents and whether bleeding occurred. Time of onset of bleeding, total duration, severity, and recurrence

Therapeutic measures and response
Blood transfusions, wound-suturing, cautery, pressure bandages, splenectomy, corticosteroids, vitamin K

Family history of bleeding
Draw family tree and enter details; interview older relatives
Bleeding episodes in siblings and children
History in antecedents, both paternal and maternal
Racial and geographic origins
Obtain results of investigations carried out on relatives with a positive history of bleeding

Examination

Complete physical examination with special emphasis on:

General appearance of patient	Cushingoid, myxoedematous, plethoric, icteric, or cachectic appearance. Distribution of skin haemorrhages, contour, and mobility of limbs and trunk
Skin	Telangiectases (spider, cavernous, and punctate), haemangiomas, petechiae, urticaria, ecchymoses. Texture and elasticity of skin, scars. Palms of hands
Mouth	Petechiae, lacerations, telangiectases, superficial vessel bleeding, haematomas
Wounds	Excessive blood clot, degree of healing, nature of scars
Abdomen	Superficial venous engorgement, haematoma in abdominal wall, hepatomegaly, splenomegaly, abdominal masses (intra- and retroperitoneal), ascites
Pelvis	Rectal and vaginal examination (if indicated)
Nervous system	Fundus oculi—retinal haemorrhages, papilloedema Peripheral nerves—sensory and motor
Joints	Swelling, tenderness, and deformity
Urine	Proteinuria, haematuria, and haemoglobinuria

Tourniquet test

Special investigations

Essential investigations for all cases

Full blood examination
Haemoglobin
Red cell morphology
White cell count
Platelet count and examination of a blood film for number, morphology, and presence of platelet clumping

Skin bleeding time

Further investigations that may be required

The further tests that may be indicated vary with disorders suspected after clinical assessment and the screening blood examination.

(a) Screening tests of blood coagulation, including activated partial thromboplastin time and prothrombin time (Table 15.3, p. 414). These detect any of the important congenital or acquired abnormalities in coagulation. More elaborate procedures, such as factor assays and tests for inhibitors, may be necessary.
(b) Tests of platelet function, including adhesiveness and aggregation when a qualitative disorder is suspected (p. 395).

frequently occurs into the deep tissues. Bleeding occurs commonly after minor trauma or surgery, and is less often spontaneous. Wound bleeding tends to commence after a delay of several hours, to persist for more than 48 hours, and to recur after haemostasis has apparently occurred.

Although one may suspect the component involved from the type of bleeding, it can usually be determined with certainty only after blood examination and consideration of the other clinical features. In thrombocytopenia, the platelet count is reduced, the tourniquet test is commonlv positive, and the bleeding time is usually prolonged. In coagulation disorders, one or more of the clotting tests is abnormal. In vascular disorders, the platelet count and clotting tests are normal. Diagnosis of vascular disorders is usually based on clinical association, as there are no constant abnormalities in the special tests; however, in some disorders the tourniquet test is positive and/or the bleeding time is prolonged.

In some haemorrhagic disorders, it is not uncommon for more than one component of the haemostatic mechanism to be involved, e.g. cirrhosis of the liver, in which there may be 'hypoprothrombinaemia' from liver damage and thrombocytopenia due to hypersplenism.

What is cause of the haemorrhagic disorder?

The cause is determined from a consideration of the history and examination, and certain special tests.

The history of bleeding in relation to past trauma is of particular help in determining the cause of the bleeding. A long history of abnormal bleeding, particularly when it commences in childhood, is strong evidence that the disorder is congenital. However, acquired disorders may persist for years before the diagnosis is made. On taking the history, a record should be made of the various traumatic incidents that have been experienced and of abnormal bleeding if this has occurred with any of them (see Table 15.12). Severe tests of haemostatic efficiency are imposed, particularly by tooth extraction and tonsillectomy, and in females by the menstrual cycle. In mild haemorrhagic disorders, abnormal bleeding does not follow every traumatic incident.

References and further reading

Books and monographs

Austen, D.E.G. & Rhymes, I.L. (1975) *A Laboratory Manual of Blood Coagulation*, Blackwell Scientific Publications, Oxford.

Biggs, R. (Ed.) (1978) *The Treatment of Haemophilia A and B and von Willebrand's Disease*, Blackwell Scientific Publications, Oxford.

Bloom, A.L. & Thomas, D.P. (1987) *Haemostasis and Thrombosis*, 2nd Ed., Churchill Livingstone, Edinburgh.

Bloom, A.L. (Ed.) (1982) *The Hemophilias*, Churchill Livingstone, Edinburgh.

Colman, R.W. (Ed.) (1983) *Disorders of Thrombin Function*, Churchill Livingstone, New York.

Colman, R.W., Hirsh, J. & Marder, V. (Eds) (1987) *Hemostasis and Thrombosis*, 2nd Ed., Lippincott, Philadelphia.

Dacie, J.V. & Lewis, S.M. (1984) *Practical Haematology*, 6th Ed., Churchill Livingstone, London.

Mammen, E.F. (Ed.) (1983) Congenital coagulation disorder. *Semin. Thromb. Hemost.* Vol. IX.

Minna, J.D., Robboy, S.J. & Colman, R.W. (1974) *Disseminated Intravascular Coagulation in Man*, C.T. Thomas, Springfield, Illinois.

Ruggeri, Z.M. (Ed.) (1985) Coagulation Disorders, *Clin. Haemat.* vol.14, no.2, W.B. Saunders, London.

Spaet, T.H. (Ed.) (1972, 1974, 1976, 1978, 1980, 1982, 1985) *Progress in Hemostasis and Thrombosis*, Vols 1–7, Grune & Stratton, New York.

Verstraete, M., Vermylen, J., Lijnan, R. & Arnout, J. (Eds) (1987) *Thrombosis and Haemostasis 1987*, Leuven University Press, Belgium.

Physiology and biochemistry of coagulation and fibrinolysis

Berrettini, M., Lammle, B. & Griffin, J.H. (1987) Initiation of coagulation and relationships between intrinsic and extrinsic coagulation pathways. In: Verstraete, M., Vermylen, J., Lijnan, R. & Arnout, J. (Eds) (1987) *Thrombosis and Haemostasis 1987*, p.473, Leuven University Press, Belgium.

Carrell, R.W., Christey, P.B. & Boswell, D.R. (1987) Serpins: antithrombin and other inhibitors of coagulation and fibrinolysis. Evidence from amino acid sequences. In: Verstraete, M., Vermylen, J., Lijnan, R. & Arnout, J. (Eds) *Thrombosis and Haemostasis 1987*, p.1, Leuven University Press, Belgium.

Collen, D. (1980) On the regulation and control of fibrinolysis. *Thromb. Haemostas.* **43**, 77.

de Haen, C., Neurath, H. & Teller, D.C. (1975) The phylogeny of trypsin-related serine proteases and their zymogens. New methods for the investigation of distant evolutionary relationship. *J. Mol. Biol.* **92**, 225.

Doolittle, R.F. (1987) Fibrinogen and fibrin. In: Bloom, AL. & Thomas, D.P. (Eds) *Haemostasis and Thrombosis*, 2nd Ed., p.192, Churchill Livingstone, Edinburgh.

Esmon, C.T. & Owen, W.G. (1981) Identification of an endothelial cell cofactor for thrombin-catalyzed activation of protein C. *Proc. Natl. Acad. Sci. U.S.A.* **78**, 2249.

Hoyer, L.W. (1981) The factor VIII complex: structure and function. *Blood*, **58**, 1.

Lammle, B. & Griffin, J.H. (1985) Formation of the fibrin clot: the balance of procoagulant and inhibitory factors. *Clin. Haemat.* **14**, 281.

Mann, K.G., Tracey, P.B., Krishnaswamy, S. *et al.* (1987) Platelets and coagulation. In: Verstraete, M., Vermylen, J., Lijnan, R. & Arnout, J. (Eds) *Thrombosis and Haemostasis 1987*, p.505, Leuven University Press, Belgium.

Morawitz, P. (1905) Die Chemie der Blutgerinnung. *Ergebn. Physiol.* **4**, 307.

Ratnoff, O.D. & Saito, H. (1979) Surface-mediated reactions. *Curr. Topics Hematol.* **2**, 1.

Rylatt, F.B., Blake, A.S., Cottis, L.E. *et al.* (1983) An immunoassay for human D dimer using monoclonal antibodies. *Thromb. Res.* **31**, 767.

Sadler, J.E. (1987) The molecular biology of von Willebrand factor. In: Verstraete, M., Vermylen, J., Lijnan, R. & Arnout, J. (Eds) *Thrombosis and Haemostasis 1987*, p.61, Leuven University Press, Belgium.

Salem, H.H. (1986) The natural anticoagulants. *Clin. Haemat.* **15**, 371.

Zimmerman, T.S. & Fulcher, C.A. (1985) Factor VIII coagulant protein. *Clin. Haemat.* **14**, 343.

Zimmerman, T.S. & Meyer, D. (1987) Structure and function of factor VIII and von Willebrand factor. In: Bloom, A.L. & Thomas, P.B. (Eds) *Haemostasis and Thrombosis*, 2nd Ed., p.131, Churchill Livingstone, Edinburgh.

Zur, M. & Nemerson, Y. (1987) Tissue factor pathways of blood coagulation. *In*: Bloom, A.L. & Thomas, D.P. (Eds) *Haemostasis and Thrombosis*, 2nd Ed., p. 148, Churchill Livingstone, Edinburgh.

Congenital coagulation defects

Bennet, B. & Ratnoff, O.D. (1973) Detection of the carrier state for classic haemophilia. *New Engl. J. Med.* **288**, 342.

Carr, R., Veitch, S.E., Edmond, E. *et al.* (1984) Abnormalities of circulating lymphocyte subsets in haemophiliacs in an AIDS-free population. *Lancet*, **i**, 1431.

Duckert, F. & Beck, E.A. (1968) Clinical disorders due to deficiency of factor XIII. *Semin. Hematol.* **5**, 83.

Editorial (1983) DDAVP in haemophilia and von Willebrand's disease. *Lancet*, **ii**, 774.

Flute, P. (1977) Disorders of plasma fibrinogen synthesis. *Brit. Med. Bull.* **33**, 253.

Gianelli, F., Anson, D.S., Choo, K.H. *et al.* (1984) Characterisation of an intragenic polymorphic marker for detection of carriers of haemophilia B (factor IX deficiency). *Lancet*, **i**, 239.

Graham, J.B. (1980) Genetic control of factor VIII. *Lancet*, **i**, 340.

Gralnick, H.R. & Rick, M.E. (1983) Danazol increases factor VIII and factor IX in classic hemophilia and Christmas disease. *New Engl. J. Med.* **308**, 1393.

Holmberg, L. & Nilsson, I.M. (1973) Two genetic variants of von Willebrand's disease. *New Engl. J. Med.* **288**, 595.

Howard, M.A. & Firkin, B.G. (1971) Ristocetin: a new tool in the investigation of platelet aggregation. *Thromb. Diath. Haemorrh.* **26**, 362.

Howard, M.A., Salem, H.H., Thomas, V.B. *et al.* (1982) Variant von Willebrand's disease type B—revisited. *Blood*, **60**, 1420.

Kasper, C.K. & Boylen, A.L. (1985) Poor response to danazol in hemophilia. *Blood*, **65**, 211.

Kasper, C.K. & Dietrich, S.L. (1985) Comprehensive management of haemophilia. *Clin. Haemat.* **14**, 489.

Kerr, C.B. (1965) Genetics of human blood coagulation. *J. Med. Genet.* **2**, 221.

Larrieu, M.J., Caen, J.P., Meyer, D.O. *et al.* (1968) Congenital bleeding disorders with long bleeding time and normal platelet count: II. von Willebrand's disease (report of 37 patients). *Am. J. Med.* **45**, 354.

Levine, P.H. & Britten, A.F.H. (1973) Supervised patient management of haemophilia, a study of 45 patients with haemophilia A and B. *Ann. Int. Med.* **78**, 195.

Marlar, R.A. & Griffin, J.H. (1980) Deficiency of protein C inhibitor in combined factor V/VIII deficiency disease. *J. Clin. Invest.* **66**, 1186.

Mannucci, P.M., Aberg, M., Nilsson, I.M. *et al.* (1975) Mechanism of plasminogen activator and factor VIII increase after vasoactive drugs. *Brit. J. Haemat.* **30**, 81.

Mannucci, P.M., Canciani, M.T., Rota, L. *et al.* (1981) Response of factor VIII/von Willebrand factor to DDAVP in healthy subjects and patients with haemophilia A and von Willebrand's disease. *Brit. J. Haemat.* **47**, 283.

Mattison, A. & Gross, S. (1966) Social and behavioural studies on haemophilic children and their families. *J. Pediat.* **68**, 952.

Oberle, I., Camerino, G., Heilig, R. *et al.* (1985) Genetic screening for hemophilia A (classic hemophilia) with a polymorphic DNA probe. *New Engl. J. Med.* **312**, 682.

Ramsey, R.B., Palmer, E.L., McDougal, J.S. *et al.* (1984) Antibody to lymphadenopathy-associated virus in haemophiliacs with and without AIDS. *Lancet*, **ii**, 397.

Rizza, C.R. & Jones, P. (1987) Management of patients with inherited blood coagulation defects. In: Bloom, A.L. & Thomas, D.P. (Eds) *Haemostasis and Thrombosis*, 2nd Ed. p.465, Churchill Livingstone, Edinburgh.

Roberts, H.R. & Macik, B.G. (1987) Factor VIII and IX concentrates: clinical efficacy as related to purity. In: Verstraete, M., Vermylen, J., Lijnan, R. & Arnout, J. (Eds) *Thrombosis and Haemostasis 1987*, p.563, Leuven University Press, Belgium.

Ruggeri, Z.M. (1987) Classification of von Willebrand's disease. In: Verstraete, M., Vermylen, J., Lijnan, R. & Arnout, J. (Eds) *Thrombosis and Haemostasis 1987*, p.419, Leuven University Press, Belgium.

Seligsohn, U. & Ramot, B. (1969) Combined factor V and factor VIII deficiency. Report of four cases. *Brit. J. Haemat.* **16**, 475.

Spero, J.A., Lewis, J.H., van Thiel, D.H. *et al.* (1978) Asymptomatic structural liver disease in hemophilia. *New Engl. J. Med.* **298**, 1373.

Soff, G.A. & Levin, J. (1981) Familial multiple coagulation factor deficiencies. I. Review of the literature: differentiation of single hereditary disorders associated with multiple factor deficiencies from coincidental concurrence of single factor deficiency states. *Sem. Thromb. Hemost.* **7**, 112.

Weiss, A.S., Gallin, J.I. & Kaplan, A.P. (1974) Fletcher factor deficiency. A diminished rate of Hageman factor activation caused by absence of pre-kallikrein with abnormalities of coagulation, fibrinolysis, chemotactic activity and kinin generation. *J. Clin. Invest.* **53**, 622.

Acquired coagulation disorders

Aggeler, P.M. & O'Reilly, R.A. (1966) Pharmacological basis of oral anticoagulant therapy. *Thromb. Diath. Haemorrh.* Supp, **21**, 227.

Aggeler, P.M., Perkins, H.A. & Watkins, H.B. (1967) Hypocalcemia and defective hemostasis after massive blood transfusion. Report of a case. *Transfusion*, **7**, 35.

Bloom, A.L. (1987) The treatment of factor VIII inhibitors. In: Verstraete, M., Vermylen, J., Lijnan, R. & Arnout, J. (Eds) *Thrombosis and Haemostasis 1987*, p.447, Leuven University Press, Belgium.

Cade, J.F., Hunt, D., Stubbs, K.P. *et al.* (1979) Guidelines for the management of oral anticoagulant therapy in patients undergoing surgery. *Med. J. Austr.* **2**, 292.

Chesterman, C.N. (1978) Fibrinolysis and disseminated intravascular coagulation. In: Gaffney, P.J. & Ulutin, S.B. (Eds) *Fibrinolysis. Current Fundamental and Clinical Concepts*, p.157, Academic Press, London.

Collen, D., Rouvier, J. & Verstraete, M. (1972) Metabolism of iodine labelled plasminogen and prothrombin in cirrhosis of the liver. *Clin. Res.* **20**, 483.

Feinstein, D.E. (1982) Diagnosis and management of disseminated intravascular coagulation: the role of heparin therapy. *Blood*, **60**, 284.

Gallus, A.S. & Hirsh, J. (1976) Treatment of venous thromboembolic disease. *Semin. Thromb. Hemost.* **2**, 291.

Green, D. (1972) Circulating anticoagulants. *Med. Clin. N. Am.* **56**, 145.

ICTH/ICSH Report of the expert panel on oral anticoagulant control (1979) *Thromb. Haemostas.* **42**, 1973.

Merskey, C., Johnson, A.J., Kleiner, G.J. *et al.* (1967) The defibrination syndrome: clinical features and laboratory diagnosis. *Brit. J. Haemat.* **13**, 4.

Muller-Berghaus, G. (1987) Septicaemia and the vessel wall. In: Verstraete, M., Vermylen, J., Lijnan, R. & Arnout, J. (Eds) *Thrombosis and Haemostasis 1987*, p. 619, Leuven University Press, Belgium.

Naeye, R.L. (1962) Thrombotic state after a haemorrhagic diathesis, a possible complication of therapy with epsilon-amino-caproic acid. *Blood*, **19**, 694.

O'Reilly, R.A. & Aggeler, P.M. (1966) Surreptitious ingestion of coumarin anticoagulant drugs. *Ann. Int. Med.* **64**, 1034.

Pitney, W.R. (1982) *Venous and Arterial Thrombosis: Evaluation, Prevention and Management*, Churchill Livingstone, Edinburgh.

Poller, L. (1982) Oral anticoagulants reassessed. *Brit. Med. J.* **284**, 1425.

Symposium on the diagnosis and treatment of intravascular coagulation–fibrinolysis (ICF) syndrome with special emphasis on this syndrome in patients cancer. (1974) *Mayo Clin. Proc.* **49**, 635.

Taberner, D.A., Thomson, J.M. & Poller, L. (1976) Comparison of prothrombin complex concentrate and vitamin K_1 in oral anticoagulant reversal. *Brit. Med. J.* **2**, 83.

Chapter 16
Thrombosis: Clinical Features and Management

Thrombosis and atherosclerotic vascular disease are major causes of morbidity and mortality, and increase in incidence with advancing years. There are many contributing factors and predisposing conditions, and the mechanism of thrombus formation itself is complex and only partially understood. Continued investigation is required to provide a rational basis for prevention and treatment. It is the purpose of this section to examine some of the mechanisms involved, the clinical syndromes resulting from thrombosis, and to outline current approaches to their management.

Definition of thrombosis

A thrombus may be defined as a mass of aggregated platelets, adherent to the vessel wall and immobilized with fibrin. There is a variable content of red cells and entrapped leucocytes, and the proportions and arrangement of the various components depend on local and general conditions.

Types of thrombus

The size and constitution of a thrombus depend on general factors (components of the blood), local factors (the blood flow and vessel wall) and the site where thrombus formation occurs, i.e. whether it is within the arterial or venous circulation.

Venous thrombosis is more common when there is sluggish flow or stasis, and endothelial changes are rarely the main causative factor. Such a thrombus is usually composed of abundant fibrin and many red cells. It generally resembles the appearance of clots formed in glass tubes, although the leading, or most proximal, portion often contains prominent platelet masses and is paler than the distal coagulum of red cells and fibrin.

Arterial thrombosis frequently occurs around the orifices of branches and at bifurcations. It is in these areas, where turbulence and sheer stresses are greatest, that endothelial injury and atheromatous changes are most marked, and platelet aggregates are readily formed. Such platelet aggregates may adhere locally and may progressively increase in size as more platelets adhere to the surface. Some coagulation and fibrin formation may occur, and limited red cell entrapment follows. An arterial thrombus thus formed has a pale appearance due to the predominance of platelets.

Effects of thrombosis

Thrombosis may produce both local and distant effects. The local effects depend on the site and the degree of vascular occlusion, and the remote effects are due to embolic phenomena or to the release of vaso-active substances from the evolving thrombus into the passing stream of blood.

Venous thrombosis may result in complete obstruction of major channels such as the popliteal, femoral, or iliac veins with distal oedema, and in exceptional circumstances (such as the mesenteric circulation) may cause tissue infarction. Detachment and embolization of various thrombi may produce obstruction within the pulmonary arterial system (pulmonary emboli).

Local occlusion at the site of initial thrombus formation in *arteries* is nearly always associated with intimal disease or microscopic damage (Jorgensen *et al.* 1972). Such occlusion usually produces marked ischaemic damage and organ dysfunction. The platelet aggregates within an arterial thrombus are often unstable and readily break up, releasing platelet masses into the circulation. Many such aggregates may disperse spontaneously, with return of the platelets to the general circulation. Other platelet masses may produce transient or permanent obstruction in distant small vessels, as is well recognized in the retinal and cerebral circulations.

There is a strong possibility that vascular spasm (for example, of the coronary arteries) may be caused by thromboxane A_2, serotonin, or other vaso-active substances released as a consequence of platelet activation. Such spasm may cause ischaemic symptoms, particularly if the circulation is already compromised by proximal atheroma.

Aetiology of thrombosis

The aetiology of thrombosis is a complex subject, and in most cases is multifactorial. Many associations of clinical thrombosis have, as yet, ill-defined aetiological relationships. Although there are differences between the factors predisposing to arterial and venous thrombosis, considerable areas of overlap exist. Arterial thrombosis and vascular disease are considered first, then the factors predisposing to venous thrombosis, and, finally, the condition of disseminated intravascular coagulation and fibrinolysis.

Vascular disease and arterial thrombosis

There is a close relationship between thrombosis and the development of atherosclerotic vascular disease (Fig. 16.1). There are at least three ways in which blood components may contribute to the development of atherosclerosis and its complications: (a) by haemodynamic factors and platelet–leucocyte interaction with the vessel wall which may lead to endothelial injury and consequent smooth muscle migration and proliferation; (b) by the formation of persistent mural thrombi which are organized and incorporated into the subendothelium, potentiating vessel wall damage; (c) by formation of thrombi in association with advanced atherosclerosis. Vessel wall disease develops through the phases of intimal thickening, medial muscle hypertrophy, lipid accumulation, and later calcification. These result in rigidity, lumen reduction, and disturbed flow, and provide the setting for platelet adherence and thrombus formation.

The early lesions of atherosclerosis, particularly the migration and proliferation of smooth muscle cells, are probably mediated by growth factors released either by platelets or by macrophages attracted to sites of vascular injury. Related mitogens may be released by the vessel wall cells themselves, endothelium and smooth muscle, also as a response to injury. These concepts, developed by Ross and colleagues, are reviewed by Ross *et al.* (1984) and Chesterman & Berndt (1986).

A number of clinical and laboratory parameters have been identified associated with the development of atherosclerotic vascular disease (see Fig. 16.1). Modification of many of these factors may reduce the likelihood of progression of vascular disease and the development of its complications, although it has been surprisingly difficult to prove the value of alterations in dietary habits, for example, in formal clinical studies (Cliff 1987). Mortality statistics, despite their acknowledged deficiencies, suggest a substantial reduction in

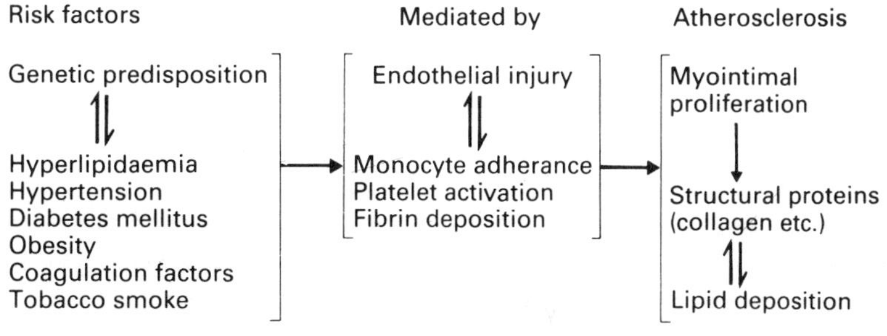

Fig. 16.1. *Links between clinical risk factors, haemostatic components, and the development of atherosclerosis.*

deaths from ischaemic heart disease over the past 20 years in a number of western countries. This is likely to be due, in part, to modifications of the presumed risk factors, particularly reduction in weight, dietary saturated fats, and cigarette smoking, and the earlier treatment of moderate hypertension. Some of the more important 'risk' factors are now briefly discussed.

Hyperlipidaemia. A high level of plasma cholesterol and triglycerides have both been shown to lead to atherosclerotic change in arteries in both experimental animals and humans. Platelets are also susceptible to lipids in their environment and are aggregated by fatty acids, and it is possible that platelet aggregates may form more readily when the lipid pattern of plasma is altered. Hyperlipidaemia and obesity are also associated with decreased plasma fibrinolytic activity, possibly with enhanced coagulation, both of which might aggravate the thrombotic tendency. A high incidence of premature peripheral vascular disease and myocardial infarction is found in persons with hyperlipoproteinaemia (Fredrickson 1971). The Framingham study has also shown a relationship between the total serum cholesterol and risk of coronary artery disease in a normal population studied prospectively (Kannel *et al.* 1971). More recently, it has been suggested that the detrimental effect is associated with the low-density lipoprotein cholesterol fraction. An increased proportion of high-density lipoprotein cholesterol is protective against the development of coronary disease in epidemiological studies.

Diabetes mellitus. Hyperlipidaemia is not uncommon in diabetes, and there is some evidence to suggest enhanced coagulation and increased platelet responsiveness. More striking, however, are functional abnormalities of endothelium that may result in increased tendency to platelet over-reactivity. The topic is reviewed by Banga & Sixma (1986).

Smoking. The increased mortality from ischaemic heart disease, and morbidity from peripheral vascular disease and cerebrovascular disease, associated with cigarette smoking is well documented. The mechanisms underlying the toxicity of tobacco smoke are poorly understood. There is some evidence for increased platelet aggregability due to smoking. Both animal experiments and *in vitro* studies point to toxicity of tobacco products on vascular endothelium. Carbon monoxide and nicotine have been implicated, but the evidence is not overwhelming.

Exercise and body build. The role of exercise and leanness of body as factors that might reduce the incidence of thrombosis have been widely debated. There have been retrospective studies suggesting that myocardial ischaemia is less common in those who exercise regularly, but the relationship remains to be confirmed by properly conducted prospective studies.

Hypertension. Hypertension may produce endothelial injury, and focal increases in endothelial cell replication have been shown in hypertensive animals. At the clinical level, both prospective studies (Welin *et al.* 1987) and the benefit of treatment of mild to moderate hypertension suggest that hypertension is an important risk factor (Australian Therapeutic Trial in Mild Hypertension 1980).

Hypercoagulability. The work of Meade and co-workers (reviewed by Meade 1987) has shown that haemostatic variables, studied prospectively, are important in the risk of subsequent cardiovascular death, principally from ischaemic heart disease. High levels of factor VIIc and fibrinogen are associated with a high incidence of coronary artery disease. Other measurable haemostatic components important in the development of cardiovascular events are platelet aggregability (Tofler *et al.* 1987) and antithrombin III. Lowered antithrombin III levels are associated with oestrogen administration and an increase in cardiovascular events.

Inherited, racial, and dietary factors. These factors must also contribute as the incidence of thrombotic disease is not uniform in different countries. Changes in dietary habits in immigrant racial groups have also been associated with development of thrombotic disorders, suggesting the importance of dietary and environmental factors. Molecular techniques may in the future enable screening for specific genetic characteristics associated with vascular disease, e.g. identifying the genes for apolipoproteins which particularly predispose to lipid accumulation.

Conditions associated with venous thrombosis

CONGENITAL

Antithrombin III deficiency. This is a rare disorder in which there is reduced activity of the natural anticoagulant (inhibitor) against activated factor X (factor Xa) and thrombin (p. 411). Deficiency is inherited as an autosomal dominant and is associated with a high incidence of venous thrombosis and pulmonary embolism, usually presenting in the second or third decade (Marciniak *et al.* 1974). Plasma concentrations 50 per cent of normal are sufficient to predispose to thrombosis. In most cases, the plasma antithrombin III concentration is reduced, but families with dysfunctional molecules have been described.

Protein C deficiency. Recurrent venous thromboembolic disease is associated with reduced plasma levels of the vitamin K-dependent factor, protein C (p. 412) in a small number of heterozygotes in affected families reported since 1981 (Griffin *et al.* 1981). Inheritance is autosomal. Homozygous infants are stillborn or suffer perinatal *purpura fulminans.* It should be noted that in a recent population study of 4723 blood donors reported by Miletich *et al.* (1987), heterozygous protein C deficiency had a prevalence of 1 in 200–300 but was not detectably associated with a risk of thrombosis. Why some families should be affected with thrombosis is thus not explained as yet. A similar deficiency associated with thrombosis has been reported with protein S. These diseases are discussed more fully by Salem (1986).

Plasminogen abnormalities. Rare, functionally deficient plasminogen molecules have been described in association with reduced fibrinolytic activity and a tendency to venous thrombosis (Aoki *et al.* 1978).

Dysfibrinogenaemia. Occasional cases of increased thrombotic tendency have been attributed to functionally abnormal fibrinogen. These are reviewed by Mammen (1983).

ACQUIRED

Surgery and trauma and prolonged recumbency for any reason are associated with a high incidence of venous thrombosis (Table 16.1). Surgery and trauma are characterized by a state of relative hypercoagulability of the blood. When sensitive techniques such as venography and ^{125}I fibrinogen scanning are used, many small areas of thrombosis are found; as many as 50 per cent may not be noticed clinically (Salzman 1975).

During *pregnancy*, and particularly in the *puerperium*, there is also a state of relative hypercoagulability, which may result from increased oestrogen levels in the blood. The activity levels of factors VII, VIII, and X are increased, and there is also a tendency for other clotting factors, particularly fibrinogen, to be elevated and for fibrinolytic activity to be decreased (Castaldi & Hocking 1972). During labour, tissue damage leads to activation of coagulation and readily detectable alterations in a number of factor activities, platelet count, and fibrinolysis, consistent with a state of compensated

Table 16.1. *Conditions associated with venous thrombosis*

Advanced age
Obesity
Surgery
Trauma
Prolonged recumbency
Pregnancy and puerperium
Oral contraceptives*
Myeloproliferative syndromes*
Polycythaemia vera
Essential thrombocythaemia
Malignancy
Varicose veins
Infection
Previous venous thrombosis
Inflammatory diseases
Paroxysmal nocturnal haemoglobinuria*
'Lupus' anticoagulant (antiphospholipid antibody syndrome)*
Conditions associated with disseminated intravascular coagulation*
Hereditary coagulation protein abnormalities

*Predispose to arterial thrombosis as well.

intravascular coagulation. In multiple pregnancies, or when labour is prolonged, these changes are more marked and may lead to overt thrombosis in the puerperium (Kleiner *et al.* 1970). Amniotic fluid embolism, associated with dissemination of fetal material, may also lead to intravascular coagulation.

The use of *oral contraceptive medication* is established as a significant association with thromboembolic disease. The incidence of thromboembolism in women taking oral contraceptives has been shown to be nine times the expected (Vessey & Doll 1968). This includes calf vein thrombosis, cerebral and mesenteric thrombosis, and, in older women, myocardial infarction, although the evidence for the latter is suggestive rather than conclusive (Inman *et al.* 1970). Increased levels of coagulation factors VII and X, and decreased antithrombin III, as well as altered platelet activity, occur during medication with oral contraceptives. Some changes have also been found in factor VIII levels and fibrinolytic activity (Poller *et al.* 1968, McGrath & Castaldi 1975). The incidence of thrombosis is reduced by the use of preparations containing low dosage of oestrogens. It is generally recommended that the oral contraceptives should be discontinued 2–3 months before elective surgery to diminish the risk of post-operative venous thrombosis.

CONDITIONS PREDISPOSING TO BOTH ARTERIAL AND VENOUS THROMBOSIS

Age and sex. There is an increasing incidence of both arterial and venous thrombosis in older individuals. Male sex is associated with a higher incidence of vascular disease and thrombotic incidents.

Thrombocytosis in association with *myeloproliferative disorders* predisposes to thrombosis, which may be venous or arterial. This is the case particularly in *polycythaemia vera*, when erythrocytosis and hyperviscosity (most severe when the PCV is in excess of 0.60) greatly increase the risk of the thrombosis. Myocardial, cerebral, digital, or gastrointestinal infarction may all occur under these conditions.

In *essential thrombocythaemia* (p. 400), bleeding and thrombosis may be present at the same or different times in the one patient. In the thrombocytosis of chronic granulocytic leukaemia (p. 259), thrombosis may occur, especially when the total white blood cell count is elevated above 400×10^9/l and the effective packed cell volume over 0.60, but this is a much less frequent complication than with polycythaemia.

Thrombocytosis may predispose to thrombosis, especially when the platelet count is elevated above 800×10^9/l. The risk of thrombosis is increased in patients with vascular disease and is enhanced by immobilization. The latter situation arises most frequently after splenectomy, when special care must be taken to ensure early ambulation. Thrombocytosis is considered in more detail in Chapter 14.

A number of *malignant disease* states may also lead to thrombosis. This is a well recognized complication of some abdominal malignancies such as carcinoma of the pancreas and some mucin-secreting adenocarcinomas. These may give rise to recumbency-type venous thrombosis or more superficial thrombophlebitis. Extensive investigation has shown some manifestations of intravascular coagulation in many patients with cancer (Mayo Clinic Symposium 1974). Occasionally, a state of overt chronic disseminated intravascular coagulation may develop. This may be responsive to heparin and to treatment directed against the tumour, if localized. In some cases, the mechanism of thrombosis is the release of clot-promoting thromboplastic materials from the tumour. There is some direct evidence to support this possibility, in that some malignant tissues can be shown *in vitro* to contain excessive clot-promoting substances.

It is becoming increasingly recognized also that *inflammatory mediators* such as interleukin-I and tumour necrosis factor produce a number of changes in vascular endothelium that are procoagulant in nature. These changes include the production of tissue factor, release of von Willebrand factor and platelet activating factor, and the secretion of plasminogen activator inhibitor. As the endothelium may provide membrane-associated co-factors for coagulation reactions (p. 400), all the machinery for local fibrin formation is available at sites of tumour metastasis (for a fuller review see Chesterman 1988).

Infections may be associated with an increase in coagulability, and similar mechanisms may pertain. This is seen in some cases of malaria, but it is especially a feature of septicaemia due to Gram-negative organisms. The endotoxins produced are probably responsible for initiating coagulation, possibly because of effects on platelets and endothelium. Associated tissue damage and hypoxia, especially if there is circulatory failure, also contribute. Superficial venous thrombosis may occur, as may disseminated intravascular coagulation. A bleeding tendency results, and may be an important factor in determining the outcome. The thrombocytopenia often observed under these conditions may also result in part from bone marrow suppression due to infection and endotoxinaemia.

Homocystinuria. This metabolic disorder is associated with premature thrombo-embolic complications, both venous and arterial. Abnormally high concentrations of plasma homocystine are believed to injure the endothelium, but the experimental evidence is far from secure. It has also been suggested that heterozygotes may have an increase in the incidence of arterial disease (Wilcken *et al.* 1983).

'Lupus' anticoagulant. A circulating IgG or IgM antibody directed against components of phospholipid is detectable in upward of 15 per cent of patients with *systemic lupus erythematosus*, in patients with other connective diseases, and in association with a wide variety of other disorders. The antibody is termed anticoagulant because it causes prolongation of the *activated partial thromboplastin time* (APTT), and sometimes the *prothrombin time* (PT), which is not corrected by the addition of an equal volume of normal plasma. Both the dilute Russell viper venom test (Thiagarajan *et al.* 1986) and the kaolin clotting time (Exner *et al.* 1978) are sensitive tests to confirm the diagnosis.

The clinical expression is paradoxically a striking tendency to thrombosis and to spontaneous abortion (presumably due to placental insufficiency), and a bleeding tendency, if it occurs, is very uncommon. The thrombosis may be a result of vascular endothelial cell damage, reduced prostacyclin production, or interaction with platelet-activating factors, but is presently not explained.

Lupus anticoagulant and related *antiphospholipid antibodies* can be detected by a recently introduced solid phase immuno-assay using cardiolipin as the antigen (Harris *et al.* 1983). Cardiolipin is representative of the negatively charged phospholipids, and others, such as phosphatidylserine, cross-react in these assays. Some patients with thrombosis have detectable antiphospholipid antibodies without lupus anticoagulant, and *vice versa*, but in many, both tests are positive and it is likely that the assays reflect variability in a family of closely related antibodies.

Corticosteroids may temporarily abolish the lupus anticoagulant and reduce the titre of antiphospholipid antibodies, but if there is a history of thrombo-embolic disease, long-term antithrombotic treatment is indicated either with warfarin (particularly with venous disease) or aspirin (in the case of arterial disease). Recurrent abortion with antiphospholipid antibodies has been successfully treated with a combination of prednisolone and aspirin. Diagnosis and management are discussed further by Boey *et al.* (1983), Harris *et al.* (1983), Vermylen *et al.* (1986), and Lechner (1987).

Paroxysmal nocturnal haemoglobinuria (PNH). Major thrombosis may occur at varying sites as a result of intravascular coagulation associated with severe haemolysis that occurs in the more classic form of this disease. Anticoagulant treatment with vitamin K antagonists has been advocated in PNH.

Disseminated intravascular coagulation

Arterial and venous thrombosis may occur in this condition. Its occurrence has been noted above in association with pregnancy, carcinoma, infection, and PNH, and disseminated intravascular coagulation with thrombotic complications may occur with incompatible blood transfusion and thrombotic thrombocytopenic purpura. It is considered in further detail on p. 442.

Clinical syndromes of thrombosis

Arterial thrombosis

While thrombosis may complicate a variety of diseases and metabolic alterations, there are a

Table 16.2. *Arterial thrombotic syndromes*

Myocardial ischaemia and infarction
Occlusive cerebrovascular disease and transient ischaemia
Peripheral arterial occlusive disease
Homograft rejection
Disorders of uncertain or varied aetiology
Haemolytic uraemic syndrome
Purpura fulminans
Thrombotic thrombocytopenic purpura
Disseminated intravascular coagulation

number of well recognized syndromes that deserve consideration (Table 16.2). Many of these are recognized as disease entities, although in some cases the aetiology is obscure or complex; however, all result from some disturbance in the balance of haemostasis leading to thrombosis and vascular occlusion. For these reasons, they are discussed separately, together with the major laboratory findings when relevant.

Myocardial ischaemia and infarction

Myocardial infarction refers to irreversible ischaemic muscle damage resulting from impaired blood flow in the coronary arterial system. This is usually associated with atherosclerotic changes in these arteries, sufficient to cause narrowing of the lumen, and a thrombus may be found either occluding the lumen or adhering to the vessel wall. However, in some instances, no thrombus can be detected, and full patency is present despite the existence of atheromatous change.

The incidence of autopsy detection of thrombus is related to the care with which it is sought, and it is probable that at the time of onset of a particular ischaemic episode thrombus formation always occurs. Surgical findings and early coronary angiography have confirmed that thrombosis occurs almost invariably with, and is presumably the cause of, full thickness myocardial infarction. However, if the examination of post-mortem specimens is undertaken many hours after the onset of symptoms in fatal episodes, thrombi may have been dislodged or lysed in the natural process of clot dissolution and repair.

Coronary arterial atheroma is the cause of myocardial ischaemia, and may not give rise to infarction. The role of thrombosis in minor ischaemic episodes is difficult to determine. It is probable that platelet aggregation frequently occurs around the orifice of diseased coronary arteries, since this is a region of particular turbulence. Even though such aggregates may be transient and not associated with fibrin formation, local ischaemia could result from their presence, for example by inducing vascular spasm. In such a situation—unstable angina—there is direct evidence that aspirin, an inhibitor of platelet aggregation, reduces the incidence of myocardial infarction (Lewis *et al.* 1983). The accumulation of clinical trial results also suggests that aspirin reduces both the incidence of non-fatal reinfarction and the subsequent mortality after myocardial infarction (reviewed by Gallus 1986). There is similarly convincing evidence to favour the use of anticoagulants, at least during hospitalization after acute myocardial infarction, to prevent venous thrombo-embolism (Chalmers *et al.* 1977, Committee of Principal Investigators 1980).

Occlusive cerebrovascular disease and transient ischaemic attacks

The carotid arteries, particularly at their bifurcation, are important sites of atheroma formation. Intimal thickening and partial occlusion are commonly observed with advancing years. Similar changes may be encountered in intracerebral arteries, and it is only the presence of a rich collateral supply that spares many areas from the effects of ischaemia. Thrombotic episodes causing occlusion may produce a wide range of symptoms, from transient weakness to fully developed stroke resulting from extensive cerebral damage. It is common to detect thrombus after a major episode of cerebral ischaemia. Thrombotic occlusion may involve the carotid system, or may be found in smaller vessels such as the middle cerebral or the vertebrobasilar system. In some cases, major occlusion does not occur, and symptoms arise because of embolism of platelet aggregates or small thrombi from the surface of plaques of atheroma in the carotid vessels. These emboli may produce permanent damage, such as blindness from central retinal artery occlusion, or hemiparesis due to occlusion of the middle cerebral artery or its branches.

Alternatively, only transient ischaemia may occur, giving rise to reversible episodes known as transient ischaemic attacks. Such emboli have been seen by direct retinal observation, strongly supporting their role in these episodes. It is also well recognized that transient ischaemia may progress to major strokes, and this has led to vigorous attempts to deal with the disorder by both medical means and by surgery, chiefly carotid endarterectomy. This operation often has beneficial results in selected patients.

Experience thus far also suggests that inhibitors of platelet aggregation, in particular aspirin (Canadian Cooperative Study Group 1978), may benefit many patients and decrease the incidence of transient ischaemic episodes. Vitamin K antagonists have been shown to be at least as effective, but carry a greater risk of bleeding complications. The topic is reviewed by Kistler *et al.* (1984).

Peripheral arterial occlusive disease

The aorta and its major branches are almost always the sites of atheromatous change with advancing years. A degree of vessel narrowing and rigidity is common, but actual occlusion due to thrombosis is confined to branches such as the mesenteric, renal, and iliac arteries, and embolic blockage may occur with local ischaemia or infarction in more distal vessels. Any of these systems may be blocked by emboli arising more proximally, either from more central areas of atherosclerosis, or from mural thrombus formation in the left ventricle after myocardial infarction.

Claudication or ischaemic limb pain usually results from extensive disease of the large arteries and their major branches. These same vessels are the ones usually involved with major occlusive emboli. However, digital thrombosis with terminal ischaemia may occur in the absence of major vessel disease. Small arterial occlusion of this type is a feature of diabetic atherosclerosis, and is also seen with inflammatory vasculitis, as in scleroderma and other collagen diseases. It may also occur due to hyperviscosity and sluggish flow, as in cold agglutinin disease (with hyperglobulinaemia and red cell agglutination) and in polycythaemia. Small vessel occlusion and digital gangrene may also complicate cryoglobulin syndromes. In these cases, pre-existing atheroma in small vessels may predispose to occlusion, but actual thrombosis is not an essential accompaniment.

Thrombosis within the heart may be a source of peripheral emboli. This may occur with the flow disturbances associated with mitral stenosis and atrial fibrillation. Thrombus formation in the atrium is not uncommon, and may result in embolization when sinus rhythm is restored. Similarly, thrombus formation is a component of the valve deposits occurring in subacute bacterial endocarditis. Prosthetic heart valves are also the site of thrombus formation, and this occurs with such regularity that continuous treatment with oral anticoagulants is required. Thrombus formation within the ventricles may follow myocardial infarction and result in embolization in the periphery or in the pulmonary circulation.

Homograft rejection is associated with thrombosis, well described in the experimental animal and in the transplanted kidney in humans. The immune reaction to foreign tissue mediated by lymphocytes is marked by perivascular inflammation with mononuclear cells predominating, and by intravascular platelet aggregates and thrombus formation. The resultant ischaemia and tissue damage result in rejection. The mechanism of thrombosis under these circumstances is not known. Tissue damage resulting from the action of lymphocytes may be the first event, but antigen–antibody complexes may also be present and contribute to the platelet release reaction and aggregation. Since prevention of rejection and control of threatened rejection depend on immunosuppressive agents and not antiplatelet drugs or anticoagulants, thrombosis must be a secondary event. However, there is evidence that antithrombotic drugs and anticoagulants may prevent the renal vascular lesions associated with graft rejection, so it is likely that the process does depend to a certain degree on thrombus formation (Kincaid-Smith 1970).

Arteriovenous shunts used for chronic haemodialysis suffer from a liability to thrombotic occlusion. This may lead to repeated revision and surgical correction, and any manoeuvre that reduces this requirement is beneficial. The details appear below, but combinations of vitamin K antagonists, heparin during perfusion, and platelet aggregation inhibitors have reduced the incidence of shunt blockage.

Venous thrombosis

Superficial thrombophlebitis is a condition in which tender swellings develop on superficial veins. It is often associated with prolonged infusions with indwelling catheters and the injection of irritant chemicals. Local thrombosis is an accompaniment, but may not extend to deeper veins. Localized tender areas around superficial veins may be difficult to distinguish from thrombophlebitis, and are sometimes called superficial vasculitis. An element of thrombosis in superficial vessels may be involved in this condition, which may also accompany more diffuse small vessel disease in some of the connective tissue disorders. A similar superficial vasculitis may have no discernible underlying basis, but also occurs in association with hyperglobulinaemia of polyclonal type and purpura chiefly affecting females, first described by Waldenström (1952).

Deep venous thrombosis, involving the veins of the soleal system in the calf, characteristically presents with a tender, swollen calf, ankle oedema, distended superficial veins in the foot, and mild fever. However, in as many as 50 per cent of cases it may be asymptomatic and have no superficial accompaniment. More sensitive diagnostic procedures such as ^{125}I fibrinogen scanning and venography may then be required. In addition, a deep venous thrombosis may extend proximally to the popliteal, femoral, and iliac veins, or may arise primarily in pelvic veins. Sometimes major ileofemoral venous thrombosis may give rise to arterial obstruction and the clinical picture known as 'phlegmasia caerulea dolens'. The limb becomes swollen, discoloured and purple with absent pulses, and gangrene may develop. The condition thus has a grave prognosis.

When occurring post-surgery, the clinical onset of lower limb venous thrombosis tends to be delayed for several days, and may occur as late as 10–14 days after operation, even though the initial thrombus formation probably occurred during operation. It is associated with a tendency to increased coagulation, and sometimes elevation of some coagulation factor activities and an increased platelet count. In some studies, platelet aggregability appeared to be increased, but it is not certain that these alterations in coagulation and platelet numbers and function are directly related. There may be other factors of equal importance, such as age, associated disease, and the nature of the predisposing trauma or surgery.

Thrombosis in iliac, pelvic, or peripheral veins results in pulmonary embolism in a significant proportion of patients. There may be little or no clinical evidence of quite large venous thrombi capable of producing a major pulmonary embolus. Indeed, Salzman (1975) indicates that when the triad of local pain, tenderness, and oedema is present, the diagnostic techniques of venography and ^{125}I fibrinogen scan confirm the diagnosis in 80–90 per cent of cases. However, the sensitivity of clinical signs is low, and at least 50 per cent of cases are overlooked.

These facts, together with the serious outcome of many such emboli, have led to increasing efforts to define patients at risk and to offer preventive treatment. According to established criteria, a major pulmonary embolus may be defined as one that produces impairment or abolition of the blood flow to more than one-third of both lungs or two-thirds of one lung. Such acute embolization may be immediately fatal, and almost always produces symptoms; it is detectable by pulmonary angiography and perfusion lung scanning with radioisotopes, and produces changes in cardiopulmonary flow parameters. A similar degree of functional impairment may result from repeated embolization from a chronic peripheral source, but usually without the dramatic picture of acute embolization. Recovery from major pulmonary embolism is followed by gradual resolution of the perfusion defects as fibrinolysis and repair take place. Often some months must elapse before these defects resolve, and indeed they may persist for long periods after full symptomatic recovery and the apparent return of lung function tests to normal.

Microcirculation thrombosis

Haemolytic uraemic syndrome. This is a severe, acute illness of early childhood. It is characterized by the rapid onset of severe anaemia and thrombocytopenia, with renal failure and evidence of small vessel thrombosis, and in some cases intravascular coagulation. The disease is discussed further in Chapter 8 (p. 207).

Thrombotic thrombocytopenic purpura is a severe, uncommon illness of adults, resembling somewhat the haemolytic uraemic syndrome of childhood. In addition to thrombocytopenic bleeding, haemolytic anaemia, and renal failure, this disorder usually includes cerebral involvement, often producing coma. It is discussed in greater depth in Chapter 14 (p. 391).

Disseminated intravascular coagulation (DIC) and pathological fibrinolysis are considered elsewhere (p. 442).

Investigation of thrombotic disorders

The diagnosis and localization of established vascular occlusion is beyond the scope of this chapter, and the reader is referred to texts devoted to thrombosis or vascular disease. Clinicians may, however, avail themselves of haematological investigations for: (a) evidence of established thrombosis; and (b) the diagnosis of a predisposition to thrombosis, be it congenital or acquired.

On the whole, blood tests for *established thrombosis* have proven disappointing because of *lack of specificity*. Fibrin formation and platelet activation accompany the common processes of inflammation, repair following surgery or trauma, and tumour growth and metastasis. If evidence of thrombosis is detected in the blood, all such conditions must be excluded before much weight can be put on such findings.

The transient nature of the thrombotic process and the products of thrombosis in the blood is a further impediment to assays designed to diagnose thrombosis. Finally, technical difficulties in both preparation of plasma samples and the execution of assays for products of thrombosis prevent their widespread acceptance. Thus, much work has gone

Table 16.3. *Screening tests for predispositions to thrombosis*

Important considerations	
Blood count and film	Polycythaemia, thrombocytosis, PNH
Activated partial thromboplastin time Prothrombin time	Lupus anticoagulant, antiphospholipid antibody and DIC
Thrombin clotting time	Dysfibrinogenaemia
Anticardiolipin antibody	Antiphospholipid antibody
Antithrombin III assay	Antithrombin III deficiency
Protein C assay	Protein C deficiency
Protein S assay	Protein S deficiency
Less certain clinical significance	
Euglobulin fibrin plate lysis before and after venous stasis Plasminogen activator inhibitor assay	Abnormalities of plasminogen activator release, or activator inhibitor excess
Platelet aggregation to standardized agonists	Abnormal platelet sensitivity
Extremely rare conditions	
Assays for rare abnormalities of these molecules	Plasminogen, heparin co-factor II, fibrinogen studies

into developing specific assays for products in plasma of thrombin action (fibrinopeptide A and thrombin–antithrombin complexes), platelet activation and release (β thromboglobulin and platelet factor 4), and plasmin action (fibrin/fibrinogen degradation products). Only the tests for fibrin degradation products, either those that non-specifically detect products from fibrinogen or fibrin (Wellco test TM) or those specific for cross-linked fibrin degradation ('Dimertest' TM) are in widespread use, mainly for diagnosis of disseminated intravascular coagulation. As indicated above, the tests have not been found to be sufficiently specific in, for example, the diagnosis of deep venous thrombosis (Tibbutt *et al.* 1975, Rowbotham *et al.* 1986).

In the case of unexplained thrombo-embolism in patients of less than 40–45 years of age, or recurrent thrombo-embolism with a suggestive family history, screening (Table 16.3) for an *inherited* or an *acquired predisposition* is indicated. In general terms, functional assays are preferable, although for convenience immuno-assays are commonly employed. An approach to the diagnosis of inherited thrombotic syndromes has recently been published (Mannucci & Tripodi 1987).

Management of thrombotic disorders

With increasing understanding of the function of platelets and of the processes of blood coagulation and fibrinolysis, the management of thrombotic disorders has become a complex matter. There is now available a large number of compounds active against platelet aggregation and the release reaction (Table 16.4). The use of heparin has undergone extensive re-evaluation since the discovery of the central importance of anti-Xa (antithrombin III) as heparin co-factor (Yin *et al.* 1971). There has been no significant change in the use of vitamin K antagonists, but there is a tendency to use them in combination with antiplatelet agents, dipyridamole in particular, in some situations. Thrombolytic therapy with streptokinase and urokinase has undergone continuing investigation, and the development of more fibrin-selective thrombolytic agents is well advanced. Tissue-type plasminogen activator produced by tissue culture and more recently by recombinant DNA techniques will very likely replace the other plasminogen activators in the future. There is little doubt of their benefit in the treatment of major pulmonary embolism, but cost considerations have tended to restrict their use. The treatment of early acute myocardial infarction with thrombolytic agents has become routine following evidence from early coronary angiography and intracoronary administration of drugs and subsequent large-scale studies of high-dose intravenous administration. The recognition of the involvement of rheological changes and the effects of turbulence and high viscosity have also led to the use of materials such as dextrans which may enhance flow and decrease viscosity.

Table 16.4. *Agents available for the treatment of thrombotic disorders*

Inhibitors of platelet function
Natural: prostacyclin, prostaglandin E_1 (PGE_1)
Chemical: aspirin, sulphinpyrazone, dipyridamole, hydroxychloroquine, ticlopidine
Anticoagulants
Heparin in low and high doses
Low molecular weight heparin and heparinoids
Vitamin K antagonists
Thrombolytic agents
Streptokinase, urokinase and tissue plasminogen activator (t-PA)
Perfusion enhancement
Dextran (antiplatelet effect)
Enhancement of fibrinolysis
Phenformin and ethyloestrenol
Stanozolol

In spite of all these developments, there are persisting areas of uncertainty. There is a continuing need for carefully controlled trials of the use of several of the available agents. It would be helpful if combinations could be avoided before it is shown that there is a real benefit to be derived from them.

Diagnostic criteria must be carefully defined, especially where the treatment commitment is relatively long term, as in the case of peripheral vein thrombosis and cerebral ischaemic episodes, or complex and expensive as in the case of thrombolytic agents. It is the aim in this section to present guidelines for the treatment of various thrombotic states.

Inhibitors of platelet function

Platelet aggregation, as assessed *in vitro*, occurs in two phases. The first is reversible and is not associated with a release reaction (p. 362). The second, an irreversible phase of aggregation, occurs with release of platelet adenosine diphosphate (ADP) and other constituents. A number of natural compounds, including adenosine and prostaglandin E_1 (PGE_1), are potent inhibitors of ADP-induced aggregation, but produce unacceptable side-effects, preventing therapeutic trials. Synthetic prostacyclin, however, has had limited clinical trial, and efforts to produce a more stable analogue may result in a potent antithrombotic drug.

A group of non-steroidal anti-inflammatory agents, including *acetylsalicylic acid* and *phenylbutazone*, and to a lesser extent the uricosuric agent sulphinpyrazone, inhibit platelet cyclo-oxygenase. They thus interfere with the release reaction and secondary aggregation induced by ADP and noradrenaline. They do not inhibit ADP-induced primary aggregation. Aspirin ingestion results in a significant prolongation of the bleeding time (Mielke *et al.* 1969), and a detectable effect on platelet aggregation persists for a number of days due to acetylation and permanent inhibition of platelet cyclo-oxygenase. Any cyclo-oxygenase inhibitor has the inherent disadvantage of inhibiting this enzyme in the vascular endothelium and thus reducing vascular prostacyclin production. This drawback may be more apparent than real, as endothelial enzymes are less affected and, in addition, are being renewed constantly. This is not so in the platelet, which is devoid of synthetic apparatus. Daily doses of 50–100 mg aspirin may provide the desired platelet inhibition without reducing endothelial prostacyclin. The clinical efficacy of such dosage, however, has been demonstrated only in limited studies, in the prevention of renal dialysis shunt and coronary artery bypass graft occlusions.

Dipyridamole, by inhibiting platelet phosphodiesterase, results in accumulation of cyclic adenosine monophosphate (cAMP) with a demonstrable effect *in vitro* on platelet aggregation. *Ticlopidine*, a new drug with unique antiplatelet activity, is showing promise in clinical trials (O'Brien 1983).

A number of large clinical trials has been conducted, mainly in arterial thrombotic disease, and the emerging picture is that aspirin is the only definitely useful agent. In venous thrombosis, antiplatelet agents probably have a very limited therapeutic potential. These drugs and their use have been recently reviewed (Gallus 1986, Fuster *et al.* 1987).

Arterial thrombosis

Many years ago, it was noted that the incidence of fatal myocardial infarction was less in patients with arthritis or other conditions treated by prolonged aspirin ingestion than in an age-matched population (Boston Collaborative Drug Surveillance Group 1972). Whether the two were connected as cause and effect could be established only by large-scale prospective studies, and these have been slow to accumulate convincing answers.

The principal agents which have been subjected to adequate clinical trial are aspirin, dipyridamole, sulphinpyrazone, and hydroxychloroquine. *Dipyridamole* was found to reduce the incidence of experimental thrombosis, and clinical trial suggested that it had an important influence on the incidence of post-operative thrombo-emboli after cardiac valve prosthetic surgery (Sullivan *et al.* 1971), in combination with vitamin K antagonists. Dipyridamole in combination with aspirin was found to prolong the shortened platelet survival seen in patients with cardiac valve prostheses. Similarly, in combination with vitamin K antagonist, Kincaid-Smith (1970) reported a reduction in thrombi in renal allografts in patients receiving dipyridamole. The incidence of *transient cerebral ischaemic attacks* was reduced by dipyridamole in combination with aspirin, although the most convincing demonstration of a therapeutic effect of antiplatelet therapy in this group of patients was achieved by aspirin alone (Canadian Cooperative Study Group, 1978). Overall, the clinical evidence to support the use of dipyridamole as an antithrombotic agent is not convincing (Oates *et al.* 1987).

There have been a number of well-conducted trials which suggest benefit from the use of sulphinpyrazone, aspirin, and hydroxychloroquine in the prevention of shunt thrombosis and blockage of renal dialysis membranes. There are also indications of benefit in elderly patients prone to thrombotic disorders. A series of trials of these drugs given to patients after *acute myocardial infarction* suggest that a modest reduction in mortality in the first few months after the event may be obtained by the administration of sulphinpyrazone (The Anturan Reinfarction Trial Research Group 1980), but more convincingly by aspirin. In addition, the rate of non-fatal reinfarction over the first 12 months is reduced by some 15–20 per cent. Aspirin at a dose of 325 mg daily reduces the mortality and infarction rate in patients with *unstable angina* (Lewis *et al.* 1983), and also substantially reduces the occlusion rate of *CABG* (Gallus *et al.* 1986, Fuster *et al.* 1987).

Anticoagulants

Heparin

This naturally occurring anticoagulant is a mucopolysaccharide which is highly charged and has the ability to bind to proteins. The anticoagulant action of heparin requires the presence of a co-factors, the major component of which has been identified as antithrombin III and the lesser, heparin co-factor II. The major site of action is probably against factor Xa, and the mechanism would appear to be marked potentiation of antithrombin III (also known as anti-Xa). Factor Xa has a potent enzymatic action on prothrombin in the presence of factor V, phospholipid, and calcium ions, and the catalytic effect of factor Xa is to produce quite large amounts of thrombin. The kinetics of these reactions are such that small amounts of heparin in the presence of antithrombin III prevent the formation of large amounts of thrombin. Inhibition of factor Xa by antithrombin III is nearly instantaneous in the presence of heparin, whereas the reaction is much slower in its absence. Once thrombin is formed, however, larger quantities of heparin are required to exert an anticoagulant effect. Heparin has a minor action in inhibiting the activation of factor IX by factor XIa, and the effect of factor IXa.

The principal indications for heparin are:

- post-operative or recumbency stasis thrombosis;
- prophylaxis of deep venous thrombosis with recent myocardial infarction or other predisposing condition;
- treatment of established deep venous thrombosis with or without pulmonary embolism;
- maintenance of anticoagulation in extracorporeal circulations;
- arterial embolization.

The recognition of the inhibitory collaboration between heparin and antithrombin III against factor Xa led to the introduction of *low-dose heparin* as *prophylaxis* against post-operative deep venous thrombosis. Susceptible patients are given a subcutaneous injection of 5000 units of heparin at 8- or 12-hourly intervals. If care is taken with the injection site, local bruising is minimized, and although the systemic effects are variable, sensitive heparin assays show that detectable blood levels occur. Controlled trials have shown that such a regimen commenced before surgery and continued during the risk period of 7–10 days, very favourably influences the incidence of venous thrombosis detected with the ^{125}I fibrinogen scan method, and reduces the number of pulmonary emboli. Other procedures such as calf stimulation during immobilization for surgery, and early ambulation, are important ways of reducing venous thrombosis. Low-dose heparin appears to be superior to dextran in preventing post-operative venous thrombosis. In a large multi-unit controlled trial (1974), positive ^{125}I fibrinogen results were found in 37 per cent of controls, compared with 25 per cent in patients treated with dextran and 12 per cent in heparin-treated patients. Low-dose heparin is therefore more effective than dextran, but does not abolish thrombosis, which emphasizes the need for other physical measures, particularly in the presence of malignant disease or following major hip surgery, when heparin is comparatively ineffective.

Such prophylactic measures should be considered in particular for patients at risk, rather than for all patients. Those most likely to have thrombotic problems are the elderly, those with vascular disease, hypertension or ischaemic heart disease, and malignant disease, and patients with high platelet counts or haematocrits (which should be reduced by venesection wherever possible before surgery). Pregnant women, patients taking oral contraceptives, and those with a past or family history of thrombosis should also be considered to be at risk. The decision to use low- or high-dose heparin depends on individual circumstances. When the indication is truly prophylactic, low-dose heparin usually suffices, but in some patients—for example those with a past history of post-operative thrombosis—a decision may well be taken to change to full doses in the post-operative period.

Side-effects of heparin are uncommon, but include bleeding (p. 439), thrombocytopenia, hypersensitivity, and osteoporosis. Thrombocytopenia due to heparin is described on p. 389.

TREATMENT OF ESTABLISHED THROMBOSIS WITH HEPARIN

Established thrombosis, whether venous or arterial, and embolism, prosthetic heart valves, or vascular surgery, are indications for full heparinization. Heparin is usually given by continuous intravenous infusion in doses adequate to prolong coagulation times, commonly about 30 000 units over 24 hours. Precise levels necessary to achieve adequate anticoagulation are not established, but it is generally accepted that a doubling of the whole blood coagulation time over control levels, and a doubling to tripling in the activated partial thromboplastin time, reflect adequate heparin levels. The thrombin clotting time may also serve as a control test, when the therapeutic range is of the order of 25–50 seconds with a control of 10–15 seconds. However, the dosage required to achieve these levels varies between individuals and at different times in the same patient. The post-operative state, thrombocytosis, infection, and established recent thrombosis all increase the requirement for heparin. High doses of the order of 60 000–70 000 in 24 hours may be required for the initial period of treatment in some patients. Thereafter, the requirement usually diminishes. These variations in requirement for heparin make it important to attempt some form of laboratory control so that appropriate dosage adjustment may be made.

DURATION OF TREATMENT

Individual factors operate to determine the duration of treatment, and in many patients it may be brief and followed by a period of oral anticoagulants. Conventionally, heparin is continued for about one week before oral anticoagulation is introduced. Gallus and colleagues (1986) recently showed that this is probably not necessary, at least in the absence of massive venous thrombo-embolism. There was no difference in efficacy or toxicity if warfarin was begun at the same time as the initial heparin treatment. In uncomplicated cases, there was more than three days' reduction in hospitalization.

Low molecular weight heparin and heparinoid preparations

A number of preparations of low molecular weight heparin and heparinoids (including dermatan and heparan sulphate) have been developed for therapeutic use in the hope that the antithrombotic: haemorrhagic ratio might be better, and the incidence of thrombocytopenia might be lower, than with conventional heparin. A single daily administration was also proposed. A number of clinical studies has been carried out, and it is likely that these agents will be in general use before long. It is still to be proven that the hoped-for advantages will be realized. Recent reviews have been published (Samama & Hemker 1986, Hirsh *et al.* 1987).

Warfarin or vitamin K antagonists

When oral anticoagulants are used after initial treatment with heparin, a sufficient interval of overlap should be allowed before the optimum effect of vitamin K lack is achieved. Although the prothrombin time levels are increased within 24–48 hours of starting warfarin, this is due to an early decrease in factor VII levels. Some days are required before the other vitamin K-dependent factors—II, XI, and X—decrease, and heparin should be continued for the 2–4-day period for these activities to decrease.

Warfarin is definitely preferred to phenindione (*Dindevan*) as the oral anticoagulant of choice, because of the lower incidence of serious side-effects such as skin rashes, liver damage, and bone marrow depression. Because of the interval required for effective decrease in all four coagulation factors, there is probably not much necessity for a 'loading dose' of warfarin. A practical method for the institution of warfarin therapy using the thrombotest as the means of laboratory control has been described by Routledge *et al.* (1977). Warfarin at a dose of 10 mg daily is given on three successive evenings, and the thrombotest is performed on the morning of the fourth day. The predicted maintenance dosage is read from a table, the predictions being accurate if there are no confounding factors such as liver disease or cardiac failure. A similar table has been constructed for the predicted dose depending on the prothrombin ratio providing the basis for a reproducible anticoagulation régime (Fennerty *et al.* 1984). Subsequently, the drug is administered as a single daily dose in the range 1–25 mg, and control maintained with the prothrombin time or thrombotest.

CONTROL OF WARFARIN DOSE

The therapeutic range is the patient: control prothrombin time ratio of 2–4 when the Australian or British comparative thromboplastins are used in the laboratory, and for the thrombotest, an activity of 6–15 per cent. It may be that less intense anticoagulation will be effective (Hull *et al.* 1982). It is helpful if laboratories performing tests to control oral anticoagulants have a standardized approach, so that results are comparable between different centres. This is theoretically attainable if the local prothrombin time measurement is related to what is known as the International Normalized Ratio (INR). In fact, the British (and Australian) ratios are interchangeable with the INR. It is an advantage if results are reported as a ratio rather than a percentage or 'index', regardless of thromboplastin reagent used.

The *duration of treatment* with warfarin needs to be individually planned. In some situations, such as prosthetic heart valves, arteriovenous shunts for haemodialysis, and transient cerebral ischaemic attacks, the need may be indefinite. In others, as after myocardial infarction or post-operative or stasis venous thrombosis and pulmonary embolism, the need may be short lived, and treatment for three months is adequate to allow clot dissolution and revascularization to occur (Coon & Willis 1973). It is advisable that the need for continued oral anticoagulants be regularly reviewed in all patients. The risk of bleeding, sensitivity, and drug interactions are not inconsiderable, and should influence the decision to limit treatment to the minimal effective period.

Drug interaction between warfarin and a large number of other drugs are known to occur, and should be suspected as a cause of any inappropriate result in control tests. Also to be considered are fluctuations in diet with varying vitamin K content and individual vagaries with pill-taking. It is better to ensure that none of these alterations has occurred, and to repeat the test rather than make early adjustments in warfarin dosage. The list of drugs that may interact to enhance or decrease the anticoagulant effect of warfarin is shown in Table 15.10 (p. 440).

Cessation of oral anticoagulants is associated with a temporary increase in coagulation factor levels (especially factor VII) to levels well above the normal. This may be associated with a state of so-called 'rebound' hypercoagulability, and sometimes with re-thrombosis. In the cases reported, such rebound has occurred after the anticoagulants were abruptly stopped because of bleeding, and vitamin K administered. It may be preferable to reduce the dose of warfarin over 1–2 weeks when it is stopped electively, or to avoid vitamin K when warfarin is stopped abruptly because of bleeding, and treat the existing deficiency with a transfusion of fresh frozen plasma or injection of a prothrombin complex such as prothrombinex. On the other hand, Pitney (1982) points out that, because of albumin binding in the plasma, the level of warfarin declines slowly once it is withdrawn, and there is probably little rationale for slow withdrawal.

Thrombolytic therapy with streptokinase and urokinase

In the search for specific treatment for thrombosis, and especially for pulmonary embolism, effective forms of induced fibrinolysis have been developed. The fibrinolytic system is based on the activation of plasminogen to the active enzyme, plasmin (Fig. 16.2). Activation under ordinary conditons probably occurs largely within a formed thrombus, as the plasma contains a potent inhibitory system responsible for localizing the effects of plasmin formation. Vascular endothelium and other tissues contain activators of plasminogen, and urokinase is the activator isolated from human urine. Fibrinolytic activity can be demonstrated in normal blood, but it develops slowly and clot dissolution may take hours to days. In order to hasten this process for more convenient measurement *in vitro*, it is necessary to remove the inhibitory activity by dilution of the plasma or by extraction or fractionation procedures, as in the use of the euglobulin fraction, rich in plasminogen and its substrate, but lacking inhibitors in the euglobulin lysis time test. Extraneous activators, such as tissue plasminogen activator, urokinase, or streptokinase, greatly enhance fibrinolysis in normal plasma and produce clot dissolution within a few minutes in adequate concentration. The effort to reproduce this phenomenon in a therapeutic sense *in vivo*, with safety, has involved a major and expensive effort in clinical and laboratory investigation.

Trials have been conducted on the use of thrombolytic therapy with streptokinase and urokinase in the treatment of myocardial infarction, venous thrombosis, arterial occlusion, and major pulmonary embolism (Fig. 16.3). In the case of *pulmonary embolism*, the most extensive trials have been carried out and comparison made with conventional treatment with heparin in a National Co-operative Study (1974). It is now established beyond reasonable doubt that both streptokinase and urokinase hasten the resolution of major pulmonary emboli, with earlier restoration of the haemodynamic abnormalities compared to heparin. This treatment may therefore be considered as an alternative or addition to heparin or surgical management, and should be considered in patients with embolism affecting more than one-third of the lung. With standard dosage regimens for streptokinase and urokinase, followed by continuous heparin in standard doses, the dissolution of pulmonary emboli is hastened. Trials conducted to date have not shown any difference in mortality in the acute phase or after six months of follow-up in patients treated with heparin or with either thrombolytic agent. In the majority of cases, thrombolytic therapy may not be considered to replace surgery in patients presenting with massive embolism and circulatory collapse, when the facilities are available. If possible, the decision about the alternative

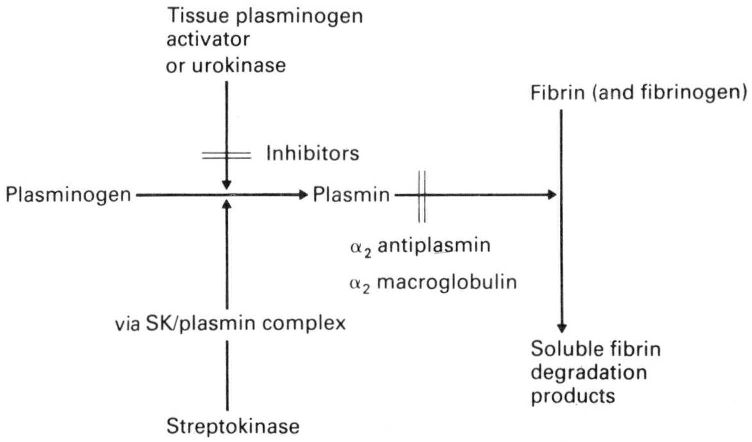

Fig. 16.2. *Relationship of components of the fibrinolytic system with activators used in thrombolytic therapy.*

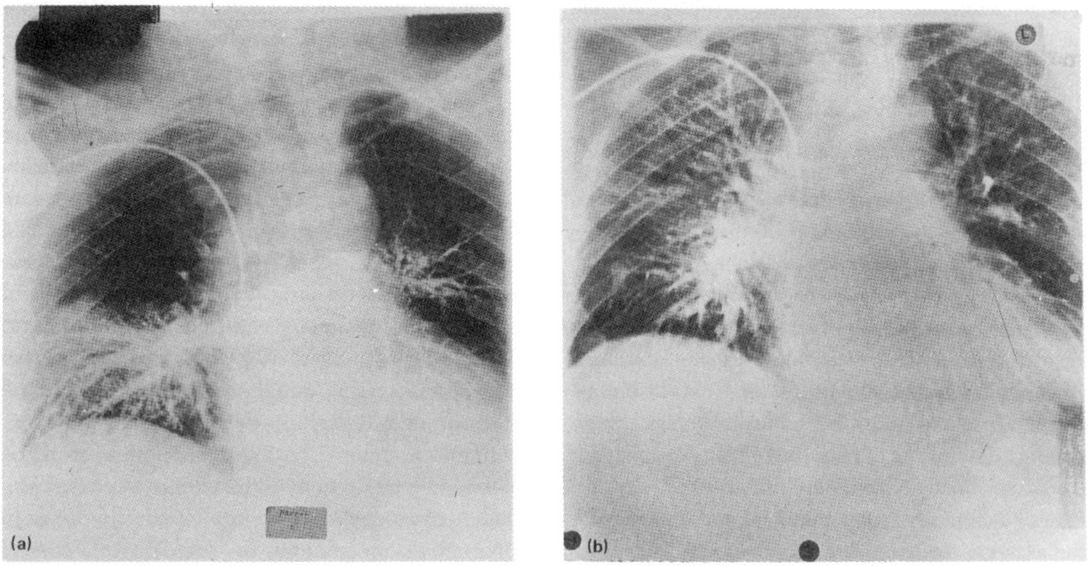

Fig. 16.3. *Pulmonary angiograms in a man of 56 years admitted to hospital with sudden collapse and dyspnoea; plain chest X-ray showed slight shadowing at right costophrenic angle, suggestive of collapse. Pulmonary angiogram shows (a) a thrombus in the right main pulmonary artery with virtual complete obstruction to flow to the right upper zone, as well as marked reduction of flow to all segments on the left. Illustration (b) shows the picture after 48 hours of treatment with streptokinase. The patient was subsequently discharged from hospital, free from cardiovascular symptoms.*

forms of treatment should be made by individuals with the appropriate skills in consultation.

It is now established that thrombolytic therapy confers a significant advantage both in left ventricular function and mortality after acute myocardial infarction. During the 1970s, several large-scale trials of intravenous streptokinase for *acute myocardial infarction* were carried out. The analysis of these trials and pooling of statistics by Stampfer *et al.* (1982) suggested a significant therapeutic effect and mortality reduction of about 20 per cent, but the evidence was not universally accepted. Subsequently, intracoronary administration of thrombolytic agents followed by coronary angiography convincingly demonstrated 70–80 per cent dissolution of coronary thrombus. Further knowledge gained over this period revealed that a much larger bolus dose was more effective and could be safely administered over a short period of time, and that treatment beyond 4–6 hours after onset of symptoms was likely to be ineffective. A massive clinical trial based on these parameters was conducted in Italy (Gruppo Italiano per la studio della streptochinasi 1986). The three-week mortality was 10.7 per cent of 5860 patients treated with 1.5×10^6 units of streptokinase over one hour starting within 12 hours of the onset of symptoms compared to 13 per cent of 5852 untreated control patients. This represents an 18 per cent reduction in mortality, and was highly significant. Further analysis revealed that the benefit of thrombolysis was closely related to the duration of symptoms before treatment, maximum at one hour and insignificant after six hours.

In *deep venous thrombosis*, clot dissolution is hastened and residual venous valve incompetence with dependent oedema may be decreased. These long-term advantages must be weighed against the cost and dangers of thrombolytic therapy and the relative success of treatment with heparin when combined with early ambulation and vascular support. The decision about these alternatives will probably be determined by local expertise and interest.

Streptokinase is antigenic and its use often associated with mild fever. Because of the general presence of antistreptococcal antibodies, a neutralizing dose must be given before effective lytic activity can be achieved.

High doses of streptokinase produce an early state of quite severe lysis of fibrinogen in plasma and depletion of circulating plasminogen. Once plasminogen is depleted, lysis in the plasma is not so severe, and is more localized to sites of clot formation. Urokinase is not antigenic and produces lysis of clots with less systemic effect than streptokinase. However, it is very expensive, and its use is more restricted than that of streptokinase.

New developments in therapeutic plasminogen activators

Biochemical manipulation of streptokinase and plasminogen mixtures have resulted in therapeutic agents that show some promise. In particular, by acylating the active site serine of streptokinase–plasmin complex, a compound, BRL 26921, has been produced (Smith *et al.* 1981) which binds fibrin in inactive form and, thus sited, slowly becomes activated due to de-acylation of the active site.

A more promising approach is the isolation and subsequent cloning of tissue plasminogen activator (Pennica *et al.* 1983). Recombinant tissue plasminogen activator has shown considerable potential in laboratory and animal experiments, and lately in human trials. The advantage of these two products is greater specificity for fibrin, allowing fibrinolysis to take place without the development of a systemic haemorrhagic state. These agents are discussed more fully by Verstraete & Collen (1986).

Control of treatment with these agents can be readily achieved with a limited range of laboratory procedures. The thrombin clotting time is the most useful test, and prolongation reflects the presence of degradation products of fibrin in the circulation and, to a lesser extent, the reduction in the level of circulating fibrinogen. Other tests of lytic activity, such as the euglobulin lysis time, fibrin plate assay, and fibrinogen levels, may also be helpful. Bleeding complications of this treatment are not uncommon, but seldom severe. If vascular catheters are avoided and control confined to venepuncture, bleeding should not occur. Intramuscular injections must not be given. Surgery within the previous two weeks, active peptic ulcer, or an established bleeding tendency are contra-indications. Recent streptococcal infection greatly increases the resistance to streptokinase.

Thrombosis during pregnancy

The treatment of thrombosis during pregnancy must take account of possible fetal damage, which is well documented following warfarin administration. It is advisable to avoid the use of warfarin in the first 12 weeks and in the last 2 weeks before delivery. Some authors (Pitney 1982) are opposed to warfarin at any time during pregnancy. Heparin does not cross the placenta, and can be used in high or low dose without problem. It is the preferred treatment of deep vein thrombosis and pulmonary embolism, and may be continued by low-dose subcutaneous injection if indicated for the rest of the pregnancy.

References and further reading

Books and monographs

Avery, G.S. (Ed.) (1978) *Antithrombotic Drugs,* Adis Press, New York.

Bloom, A.L. & Thomas, D.P. (Eds) (1987) *Haemostasis and Thrombosis.* 2nd Ed., Churchill Livingstone, Edinburgh.

Colman, R.W., Hirsh, J. & Marder, V.J. (Eds) (1987) *Hemostasis and Thrombosis,* 2nd Ed., Lippincott, Philadelphia.

Pitney, W.R. (1982) *Venous and Arterial Thrombosis,* Churchill Livingstone, Edinburgh.

Verstraete, M. & Vermylen, J. (1984) *Thrombosis,* Pergamon Press, Oxford.

Verstraete, M., Vermylen, J., Lijnan, R. & Arnout, J. (Eds) (1987) *Thrombosis and Haemostasis 1987,* Leuven University Press, Belgium.

Thrombosis and vascular disease

Australian Therapeutic Trial in Mild Hypertension: report by the management committee (1980) Lancet, **i**, 1261.

Banga, J.D. & Sixma, J.J. (1986) Diabetes mellitus, vascular disease and thrombosis. *Clin. Haemat.* **15**, 465.

Chesterman, C.N. (1988) Vascular endothelium, haemostasis and thrombosis. *Haemat. Rev.* **2**, 88.

Chesterman, C.N. & Berndt, M.C. (1986) Platelets and vessel wall interaction and the genesis of atherosclerosis. *Clin. Haemat.* 15, 323.

Cliff, W. (1987) Coronary heart disease: animal fat on trial. *Pathology*, **19**, 325.

Frederickson, D.J. (1971) Hyperlipoproteinaemia and coronary artery disease. *Brit. Med. J.* **1**, 187.

Harker, L.A. & Ritchie, J.L. (1980) The role of platelets in acute vascular events. *Circulation*, **62** (Suppl.V), 13.

Jorgensen, L., Packham, M.A.., Roswell, H.C. *et al.* (1972) Deposition of formed elements of blood on the intima and signs of intimal injury in the aorta of rabbit, pig and man. *Lab. Invest.* **27**, 341.

Kannel, W.B., Castelli, W.P., Gordon, T. *et al.* (1971) Serum cholesterol, lipoproteins and the risk of coronary heart disease. The Framingham Study. *Ann. Int. Med.* **74**, 1.

Meade, T.W. (1987) The epidemiology of haemostatic and other variables in coronary artery disease. In: Verstraete, M., Vermylen, J., Lijnen, R. & Arnout, J. (Eds) *Thrombosis and Haemostasis 1987*, p. 37, Leuven University Press, Belgium.

Niewiarowski, A. & Rao, A.K. (1983) Contribution of thrombogenic factors to the pathogenesis of atherosclerosis. *Prog. Card. Dis.* **26**, 197.

Ross, R., Fagiotto, A., Bowen-Pope, D. *et al.* (1984) Role of endothelial injury and platelet and macrophage interactions in atherosclerosis. *Circulation*, **70** (Suppl.III), 77.

Welin, L., Svardsudd, K., Wilhelmsen, L. *et al.* (1987) Analysis of risk factors for stroke in a cohort of men born in 1913. *New Engl. J. Med.* **317**, 521.

Thrombotic disorders

Aoki, N., Moroi, M., Sakata, Y. *et al.* (1978) Abnormal plasminogen. A hereditary molecular abnormality found in a patient with recurrent thrombosis. *J. Clin. Invest.* **61**, 1186.

Boey, M.L., Colaco, C.B., Gharavi, A.E. *et al.* (1983) Thrombosis in systematic lupus erythematosus: striking association with the presence of circulating lupus anticoagulant. *Brit. Med. J.* **2**, 1021.

Carreras, L.O., Defreyn, C., Machin, S.J. *et al.* (1981) Arterial thrombosis, intrauterine death and "lupus" anticoagulant: detection of immunoglobulin interfering with prostacyclin formation. *Lancet*, **i**, 244.

Castaldi, P.A. & Hocking, D.R. (1972) Haemopoiesis and coagulation. In: Shearman, R.P. (Ed.) *Human Reproductive Physiology*, Blackwell Scientific Publications, Oxford.

Editorial (1983) Familial antithrombin III deficiency. *Lancet*, **i**, 1021.

Exner, T., Rickard, K.A. & Kronenberg, H. (1978) A sensitive test demonstrating lupus anticoagulant and its behavioural patterns. *Brit. J. Haemat.* **40**, 143.

Griffin, J.H., Evatt, B., Zimmerman, T.S., *et al.* (1981) Deficiency of protein C in congenital thrombotic disease. *J. Clin. Invest.* **68**, 1370.

Harker, L.A. & Slichter, J. (1970) Studies of platelet and fibrinogen kinetics in patients with prosthetic heart valves. *New Engl. J. Med.* **283**, 1302.

Harris, E.N., Gharavi, A.E., Boey, M.L. *et al.* (1983) Anticardiolipin antibodies: detection by radioimmunoassay and association with thrombosis in systemic lupus erythematosus. *Lancet*, **ii**, 1211.

Inman, W.H.W., Vessey, M.P., Westerholm, B. *et al.* (1970) Thromboembolic disease and the steroidal content of oral contraceptives. A report to the Committee on Safety of Drugs. *Brit. Med. J.* **2**, 203.

Kleiner, G.J., Merskey, C., Johnson, A.L. *et al* (1970) Defibrination in normal and abnormal parturition. *Brit. J. Haemat.* **19**, 159.

Lechner, K. (1987) Lupus anticoagulants and thrombosis. In: Verstraete, M., Vermylin, J., Lijnen, R. & Arnout, J. (Eds) *Thrombosis and Haemostasis 1987*, p. 525, Leuven University Press, Belgium.

Mammen, E.F. (1983) Fibrinogen abnormalities. *Semin. Thromb. Hemost.* **9**, 1.

Marciniak, E., Farley, C.H. & de Simone, P.A. (1974) Familial thrombosis due to antithrombin III deficiency. *Blood*, **43**, 219.

Mannucci, P.M. & Tripodi, A. (1987) Laboratory screening of inherited thrombotic syndromes. *Thromb. Haemostas.* **57**, 247.

McGrath, K.M. & Castaldi, P.A. (1975) Changes in coagulation factors and platelet function in response to progestational agents. *Haemostasis*, **4**, 65.

Miletich, J., Sherman, L. & Broze, G., Jr. (1987) Absence of thrombosis in subjects with heterozygous protein C deficiency. *N. Engl. J. Med.* **317**, 991.

Poller, L., Tablowo, A. & Thompson, J.M. (1968) Effects of low dose oral contraceptives on blood coagulation. *Brit. Med. J.* **2**, 218.

Salem, H.H. (1986) The natural anticoagulants. *Clin. Haemat.* **15**, 371.

Salzman, E.W. (1975) Diagnosis of deep vein thrombosis. *Thromb. Diathes. Haemorrh.* (Stuttg.) **33**, 457.

Schleider, M.A., Nachman, R.L., Jaffe, E.A. *et al.* (1976) A clinical study of the lupus anticoagulant. *Blood*, **48**, 499.

Spicer, T.E. & Rau, J.M. (1976) Purpura fulminans. *Am. J. Med.* **61**, 566.

Thiagarajan, P., Pengo, K. & Shapiro, S. (1986) The use of the dilute Russell viper venom time for the diagnosis of lupus anticoagulants. *Blood*, **68**, 869.

Tibbutt, D.A., Chesterman, C.N., Allington, M.J. *et al.* (1975) Measurement of fibrinogen–fibrin-related antigen in serum as aid to diagnosis of deep vein thrombosis. *Brit. Med. J.* **1**, 367.

Tofler, G.H., Brezinski, D., Schafer, A.I. *et al.* (1987)

Concurrent morning increase in platelet aggregability and the risk of myocardial infarction and sudden death. *New Engl. J. Med.* **316**, 1514.

Vermylen J., Blockmans, D., Spitz, D. *et al.* (1986) Thrombosis and immune disorders. *Clin. Haemat.* **15**, 393.

Vessey, M.P. & Doll, R. (1968) Investigation of relation between use of oral contraceptives and thromboembolic disease. *Brit. Med. J.* **2**, 199.

Waldenström, J. (1952) Three new cases of purpura hyperglobulinaemia. A study in long standing benign increase in serum globulin. *Acta Med. Scand.* Suppl.226, **142**, 931.

Wilcken, D.L., Reddy, S.G. & Gupta, V.J. (1983) Homocysteinemia, ischemic heart disease, and the carrier state for homocystinuria. *Metabolism*, **32**, 363.

Management of thrombosis

Boston Collaborative Drug Surveillance Group (1972) Regular aspirin intake and acute myocardial infarction. *Brit. Med. J.* **1**, 440.

Canadian Cooperative Study Group (1978) A randomized trial of aspirin and sulphinpyrazone in threatened stroke. *New Engl. J. Med.* **299**, 53.

Chalmers, T.C., Matta, R.J. Smith, H. *et al.* (1977) Evidence favouring the use of anticoagulants in the hospital phase of acute myocardial infarction. *New Engl. J. Med.* **297**, 1091.

Committee of Principal Investigators (1980) A double-blind trial to assess long-term anticoagulant therapy in elderly patients after myocardial infarction. *Lancet*, **ii**, 989.

Coon, W.W. & Willis, P.W. (1973) Recurrence of venous thrombo-embolism. *Surgery*, **73**, 823.

EPSIM research group (1982) A controlled comparison of aspirin and anticoagulants in prevention of death after myocardial infarction. *New Engl. J. Med.* **307**, 701.

Feinstein, D.E. (1982) Diagnosis and management of disseminated intravascular coagulation: the role of heparin therapy. *Blood*, **60**, 284.

Fennerty, A., Dolben, J., Thomas, P. *et al.* (1984) Flexible induction dose regimen for warfarin and prediction of maintenance dose. *Brit. Med. J.* **288**, 1268.

Fuster, V., Badimon, L., Badimon, J. *et al.* (1987) Drugs interfering with platelet functions: mechanisms and clinical relevance. In: Verstraete, M., Vermylen, J., Lijnan, R. & Arnout, J. (Eds) *Thrombosis and Haemostasis 1987*, p. 349, Leuven University Press, Belgium.

Fuster, V. & Chesebro, J.H. (1981) Antithrombotic therapy: role of platelet-inhibitor drugs (3 parts). *Mayo Clin. Proc.* **56**, 102, 185, 265.

Gallus, A.S. (1986) The use of antithrombotic drugs in artery disease. *Clin. Haemat.* **15**, 509.

Gallus, A.S., Jackaman, J., Tillett, J. *et al.* (1986) Safety and efficacy of warfarin started early after submassive venous thrombosis or pulmonary embolism. *Lancet*, **ii**, 1293.

Gruppo Italiano per la Studio della Streptochinasi Nell' Infarto Miocardico (GISSI) (1986) Effectiveness of intravenous thrombolytic treatment in acute myocardial infarction. *Lancet*, **i**, 397.

Hirsh, J., Ofosu, F.A. & Levine, M. (1987) Low molecular weight heparins. In: Verstraete, M., Vermylen, J., Lijnen, R. & Arnout, J. (Eds) *Thrombosis and Haemostasis 1987*, p. 325 Leuven University Press, Belgium.

Hull, R., Hirsh, J., Jay, R. *et al.* (1982) Different intensities of oral anticoagulant therapy in the treatment of proximal-vein thrombosis. *New Engl. J. Med.* **307**, 1676.

Kakkar, V.V., Nicolaides, A.M., Field, E.S. *et al.* (1971) Low doses of heparin in prevention of deep-vein thrombosis. *Lancet*, **ii**, 669.

Kakkar, V.V. Spinderl, J., Flute, P.T. (1972) Efficacy of low-dose heparin in prevention of deep-vein thrombosis after major surgery; a double-blind randomized trial. *Lancet*, **ii**, 101.

Kincaid-Smith, P. (1970) The pathogenesis ot the vascular and glomerular lesions of rejection of renal allografts and their modification by antithrombotic and anticoagulant drugs. *Austr. Ann. Med.* **19**, 201.

Kistler, J.P., Ropper, A.H. & Heros, R.D. (1984) Therapy of ischaemic cerebral vascular disease due to atherothrombosis. *New Engl. J. Med.* **311**; part I, 27; part II, 100.

Lewis, H.D., Davis, J.W., Archibold, D.G. *et al.* (1983) Protective effects of aspirin against acute myocordial infarction and death in men with unstable angina. *New Engl. J. Med.* **309**, 396.

Mielke, C.H., Kaneshiro, M.M., Maher, I.A. *et al.* (1969) The standardized normal Ivy bleeding time and its prolongation by aspirin. *Blood*, **34**, 204.

Multi-unit controlled trial (1974) Heparin versus dextran in the prevention of deep-vein thrombosis. *Lancet*, **ii**, 118.

National Co-operative Study (1974) The urokinase-streptokinase embolism trial: phase 2 results. *J. Am. Med. Ass.* **229**, 1606.

Nilsson, I.M. (1975) Phenformin and ethylestrenol in recurrent venous thrombosis. In: Davidson, J.F., Samama, M.M. & Desnoyers, P.C. (Eds) *Progress in Chemical Fibrinolysis and Thrombolysis*, Vol. 1, Raven Press, New York.

Oates, J.A. & Wood, A.J.J. (1987) Dipyridamole. *New Engl. J. Med.* **316**, 1247.

O'Brien, J. (Ed.) (1983) Ticlopidine. A promise for the prevention of thrombosis and its complications. *Haemostasis*, **13**, suppl. 1.

Pennica, D., Holmes, W.E., Kohr, W.J. *et al.* (1983) Cloning and expression of human tissue-type plasminogen activator cDNA in E. coli. *Nature*, **301**, 214.

Persantin–Aspirin reinfarction study research group (1980) *Circulation*, **62**, 449.

Renney, J.T.G., Kakkar, V.V. & Nicolaides, A.N. (1970)

The prevention of post-operative deep-vein thrombosis comparing dextran 70 and intensive physiotherapy (abstr.) *Brit. J. Surg.* **57**, 388.

Routledge, P.A., Davies, D.M., Bell, S.M. *et al.* (1977) Predicting patients' warfarin requirements. *Lancet*, **ii**, 854.

Rowbotham, B., Carrole, P., Whitaker, A.N. *et al.* (1987) Measurement of cross-linked fibirin derivatives—use in the diagnosis of venous thrombosis. *Thromb. Haemost*, **57**, 59.

Samama, M. & Hemker, H.C. (Eds) (1986) Low molecular weight heparin and its clinical use. *Haemostasis*, **16**, 69.

Smalling, R.W., Fuentes, F., Matthews, M.W. *et al.* (1983) Sustained improvement in the left ventricular function and mortality by intracoronary streptokinase administration during evolving myocardial infarction. *Circulation*, **68**, 131.

Smith, R.A.G., Dupe, R.J., English, P.D. *et al.* (1981) Fibrinolysis with acyl-enzymes: a new approach to thrombolytic therapy. *Nature*, **290**, 505.

Stampfer, M.J. Goldhaber, S.Z., Yusuf, S. *et al.* (1982) Effect of intravenous streptokinase on acute myocardial infarction: pooled results from randomized trials. *New Engl. J. Med.* **307**, 1180.

Sullivan, J., Harken, D.E. & Gorlin, R. (1971) Pharmacologic control of thromboembolic complications of cardiac-valve replacement *New Engl. J. Med.* **284**, 1391.

Symposium on the diagnosis and treatment of intravascular coagulation (1974) Fibrinolysis (ICF) syndrome with special emphasis on this syndrome in patients with cancer. *Mayo Clin. Proc.* **48**, 635.

The Anturan reinfarction trial research group (1980) *New Engl. J. Med.* **302**, 250.

Tonascia, J., Gordis, L. & Schmerler, H. (1975) Retrospective evidence favouring use of anticoagulants for myocardial infarctions. *New Engl. J. Med.* **292**, 1362.

Verstraete, M. & Collen, D. (1986) Thrombolytic therapy in the eighties. *Blood*, **67**, 1529.

Verstraete, M. & Kienast, J. (1986) Pharmacology of the interaction between platelets and vessel wall. *Clin. Haemat.* **15**, 493.

Weksler, B.B., Pett, S.B., Alonso, D. *et al.* (1983) Differential inhibition by aspirin of vascular and platelet prostaglandin synthesis in atherosclerotic patients. *New Engl. J. Med.* **308**, 800.

Yin, E.T., Wessler, S. & Stoll, P.J. (1971) Biological properties of the naturally occurring plasma inhibitor to activated factor X. *J. Biol. Chem.* **246**, 3703.

Chapter 17
Blood Groups; Blood Transfusion; Acquired Immune Deficiency Syndrome

This chapter opens with a brief account of some of the basic facts about blood groups and their importance in clinical medicine. This is followed by a discussion of the complications of blood transfusion. For a detailed account of blood groups, the reader is referred to the monographs of Mollison, Engelfriet & Contreras (1987), and Issitt (1985).

Blood groups: red cell groups

Antigens

Human red blood cells contain on their surface a series of glycoproteins and glycolipids which constitute the blood group antigens. The development of these antigens is genetically controlled; they appear early in fetal life and remain unchanged until death. On the basis of these antigens, at least 15 well-defined red cell blood group systems of wide distribution in most racial groups have been described. They are the ABO, MNSs, P, Rh, Lutheran, Kell, Lewis, Duffy, Kidd, Diego, Yt, Xg, Ii, Dombrock, and Colton systems; of these only two are of major importance in clinical practice—the ABO and Rh systems. Inheritance of all these blood group systems is determined by autosomal genes, with the exception of the Xg system which is determined by genes on the X chromosome.

Some antigens, such as the Diego and Sutter antigens, are found only in certain racial groups. There are also a relatively large number of 'private' antigens found in a very small proportion of people; some may be confined to single families.

Antibodies

CLASSIFICATION

The antibodies to the red cell antigens are of two types: naturally occurring, and immune.

Naturally occurring antibodies occur without any obvious antigenic stimulus in the serum of individuals lacking the corresponding red cell antigen. The iso-agglutinins of the ABO system are the main example. In the other blood group systems, naturally occurring antibodies are encountered only occasionally or rarely.

Immune or acquired antibodies are produced in individuals as a result of stimulation by a red cell antigen which is not present on their own red cells or in their body fluids. This antigenic stimulation may arise from blood transfusion or as the result of pregnancy (p. 479). All red cell antigens have the power of stimulating the production of their corresponding antibody, but some are much stronger antigens than others. Certain antibodies may also result from the injection of substances that are chemically closely related to a red cell antigen. For example, some biological products, such as tetanus toxoid, contain substances closely related to A and B antigens. Thus the sera of persons who have received injections of such biological products may contain immune anti-A or anti-B antibodies, particularly the former.

Complement-binding antibodies. Both naturally occurring and immune antibodies may or may not bind complement, the majority doing so. All the main blood group antibodies bind complement, with the exception of Rh and MN antibodies.

IMMUNOCHEMISTRY

Naturally occurring red cell antibodies are either wholly or partly IgM, and generally react better with their corresponding antigens at temperatures below 37°C. Immune antibodies, most of which react best at 37°C, may be either IgG or IgM, usually the former. Antibodies produced early in immunization tend to be IgM, and those produced later IgG. A difference of clinical importance between IgM and IgG antibodies is that the latter readily transfer across the placenta while the former do not.

LABORATORY DETECTION OF ANTIBODIES

There are four main methods of detecting red cell antibodies: (a) the saline agglutination test; (b) tests using cells suspended in colloid media, e.g. albumin; (c) tests using enzyme-treated cells; and (d) the indirect antiglobulin (Coombs') test. Details are given by Dacie & Lewis (1984). On the basis of their reactions in these tests, antibodies may be classified as either complete or incomplete antibodies. Most complete antibodies are of the IgM type, and most incomplete of the IgG type.

Complete antibodies are detected by the saline agglutination test, i.e. they cause agglutination of cells containing the corresponding antigen, when the cells are suspended in a saline medium.

Incomplete antibodies combine with cells containing the corresponding antigen when the cells are suspended in saline, but do not cause them to agglutinate. However, most of them cause the cells to agglutinate when they are suspended in a colloid medium. They can also be detected by the indirect antiglobulin test and tests using enzyme-treated red cells.

Most incomplete antibodies can be detected by these three methods, but some react with only one or two methods, and fail to react with the others; this fact is of particular importance in the cross-matching of blood for patients who have been previously transfused. In general, the indirect antiglobulin test has the widest spectrum and detects some antibodies not detected by enzyme-treated cells, such as anti-Duffy and some anti-Kell antibodies. On the other hand, the method using enzyme-treated cells is more sensitive for the Rh system, and occasional antibodies are detected by this method but not by the indirect antiglobulin test.

The ABO blood groups

The ABO system consists of four main groups, AB, A, B, and O, which are determined by the presence or absence on the red cell of two antigens, A and B. The antigens are under the control of three allelic genes, *A*, *B*, and *O*, situated on the long arm of chromosome 9. The *A* and *B* genes are co-dominant, and the *O* gene is an amorph, i.e. it has no effect on antigenic structure. Group AB red cells possess both antigens, group A cells possess the A antigen, group B cells possess the B antigen, and group O cells possess neither A nor B. The serum of an individual contains antibodies against the antigens lacking in the person's red cells. Thus, as a group A person lacks the B antigen, the serum contains anti-B agglutinins. Similarly, a group B person lacks the A antigen and the serum contains anti-A, while the serum of a group O person, who lacks both A and B antigens, contains anti-A and anti-B. Group AB persons have neither antibody in their serum. These relationships are set out in Table 17.1.

The A subgroups. Several subgroups of A exist, the

Table 17.1. *The ABO blood groups*

Name of blood group	Antigens present in red cells	Antibodies normally present in serum	Approximate frequency in British persons (%)
AB	AB	nil	3
A	A	anti-B	42
B	B	anti-A	8
O	O	anti-B and anti-A	47

most important being A_1 and A_2. Group AB has similar subgroups—A_1B and A_2B. Approximately 20 per cent of group A and group AB subjects belong to group A_2 and A_2B respectively; the remainder belong to group A_1 and A_1B. The subgroups are of some practical importance in that A_2 cells react less strongly with anti-A sera. Thus, no anti-A serum is considered suitable for blood grouping until it has been shown to give strong reactions with group A_2 cells as well as with group A_1 cells, as weak agglutination by A_2 cells could be overlooked and cause blood to be wrongly grouped.

Further, in rare cases, patients of subgroup A_2 have an anti-A_1 antibody, active at 37°C, which can destroy transfused A_1 cells.

Naturally occurring and immune antibodies. Naturally occurring anti-A and anti-B agglutinins are IgM saline agglutinating antibodies; they are most active at 20°C, but are also active at 37°C. They agglutinate red cells bearing the corresponding antigen, and the great majority are also haemolytic, although to a lesser degree than the immune type.

Anti-A and anti-B may also exist in an IgG immune form, which react at 20°C but better at 37°C. Immune anti-A and anti-B are most commonly seen in persons who have received injections of pneumococcal or TAB vaccine, tetanus toxoid, or horse serum, but may also occur in persons who have been transfused with blood of incompatible ABO group, and in pregnancy where the mother is group O and the fetus group A or group B. IgG immune antibodies readily bind complement, and are potent haemolysins. They are readily transferred across the placenta.

The Rhesus (Rh) blood groups

The Rhesus (Rh) blood group system was first demonstrated in human red cells by the use of an antiserum prepared by immunizing rabbits with red cells from a Rhesus monkey. It was found that some human red cells were agglutinated by the serum—Rh-positive cells—while others were not agglutinated—Rh-negative cells. It is now known that the originally demonstrated Rh antigen is not the same as the clinically important D antigen. However, this fact is of genetic rather than practical clinical importance.

Antigens. According to the Fisher–Race theory, inheritance of Rh antigens (C, c, D, E, e) is determined by three pairs of closely linked allelic genes located on chromosome 1, *C or c, D or d, E or e*. One set of the three genes is inherited from each parent, giving rise to various combinations of genotypes, e.g. *CDe* from one parent and *CDe* from the other, with the resulting genotype *CDe/CDe*. The antigens produced by the genes are given similar notations; the gene *d* is thought to be an amorph, and there is no *d* antigen. The theory of Weiner postulates a series of allelic genes at a single locus rather than three linked genes. D is a strong antigen, and is by far the most important. In clinical practice, Rh grouping is performed with an *anti-D antiserum*; persons who are D positive are referred to as Rh positive, and those who are D negative as Rh negative. Approximately 83 per cent of the British population is Rh positive, and 17 per cent is Rh negative.

Antibodies. Practically all Rh antibodies result from immunization; naturally occurring Rh antibodies, with the exception of anti-E, are rare. Immunization may result from the transfusion of Rh-positive blood into an Rh-negative person, or from the passage of Rh-positive cells from a fetus into the circulation of an Rh-negative mother during pregnancy. When an Rh-negative person has been immunized either by a transfusion or pregnancy, the transfusion of Rh-positive blood can result in a haemolytic transfusion reaction, which may be fatal.

D is a strong antigen, and thus a large proportion of Rh-negative persons exposed to Rh-positive cells become immunized. Transfusion constitutes a more effective stimulus than pregnancy (p. 479). The antibody to the D antigen (anti-D) may occur in two forms: as a saline agglutinating antibody (usually IgM), and as an incomplete antibody (usually IgG); the latter is the more common.

The other antigens of the Rh system are much less antigenic than D, and thus are of less clinical importance. However, occasionally anti-E, anti-C, anti-c, and rarely anti-e develop as a result of transfusion or pregnancy; they may develop in

D-positive patients. Their presence can be detected by careful cross-matching; their identification requires special laboratory investigation.

White cell groups

The most readily recognized antigens on the surface of granulocytes and lymphocytes belong to the HLA (Human Leucocyte Antigen) system. This system has assumed great clinical importance in recent years with the demonstration that the same antigens are present on the nucleated cells of many body tissues and act as transplantation antigens. ABO antigens are present on lymphocytes, and possibly granulocytes, but in much smaller amounts than on red cells. Non-HLA granulocyte-specific antigens have also been identified, and are of clinical importance in a rare type of neonatal neutropenia.

The HLA system

The antigens of the HLA system (Bodmer 1987) are determined by allelomorphic genes at six closely linked loci, designated HLA-A, HLA-B, HLA-C, HLA-DR, HLA-DQ, and HLA-DP, situated along a segment of chromosome 6 referred to as the HLA region. An individual has a maximum of two alleles for each locus, one contributed by the paternal and the other by the maternal chromosome, so that the theoretical total number of HLA antigens is 12. The antigenic determinants inherited from each parent are called haplotypes, and together the two haplotypes constitute the genotype. Clearly defined antigens are written with an A, B, or C followed by an Arabic numeral, e.g. HLA-A1, HLA-B5. The letter w preceding the numeral indicates that the antigen is less clearly defined, e.g. HLA-Aw25. HLA-D antigens, unlike A, B, and C, have a restricted tissue distribution, being found only on B lymphocytes, macrophages, and activated T lymphocytes.

Antibodies against HLA antigens on leucocytes do not occur naturally, but immune antibodies are frequently found in the sera of multiparous females, and after blood transfusion or allogeneic tissue grafting. They are capable of causing febrile transfusion reactions (p. 481), and may be involved in early graft rejection. They are IgG or IgM, those with cytotoxic properties usually being IgG.

DETECTION OF HLA ANTIGENS/ANTIBODIES

Microlymphocytotoxicity tests are the most common means employed in the laboratory for HLA-A, HLA-B, HLA-C, and HLA-DR typing and antibody detection. Cytotoxicity tests involve complement-dependent lysis of lymphocytes by antibody, the injury to the cell being indicated by loss of ability to prevent the entrance of certain dyes into the cytoplasm. Antisera for antigen identification are obtained from recipients of multiple blood transfusions, multiparous women, or deliberately immunized volunteers. Antibodies from these sources are usually multispecific.

HLA-D determinants are also defined by a functional test, the mixed lymphocyte reaction, in which test lymphocytes are co-cultured with lymphocytes of known HLA-D antigenic status. Absence of a cellular proliferative response implies antigenic identity. The most widely used methods for identification of granulocyte-specific antigens and antibodies are based on reactions employing fluorescein-labelled antibodies.

Platelet groups

ABO and HLA-A, HLA-B, and HLA-C antigens are found on the surface of platelets, and a number of platelet-specific antigens have also been demonstrated. Platelet antibodies may be detected in patients who have received multiple blood or platelet transfusions, and in multiparous females. The majority of the antibodies have HLA specificity, and their presence is demonstrated by lymphocyte cytotoxicity testing. The incidence of allo-immunization in leukaemic patients receiving prophylactic platelet transfusions reaches 50 per cent in some series, and the resulting shortening of the survival time of the transfused platelets may cause considerable management problems (p. 257). Platelet-specific antigens and antibodies are usually defined by tests using fluorescein-labelled anti-immunoglobulin serum.

Clinical significance of blood group antigens

The importance of blood groups in clinical medicine lies in the fact that an antigen may, in certain circumstances, react with its corresponding antibody and cause harmful clinical effects.

Of the many red cell blood group systems, only two are of major clinical importance—the ABO and Rh systems. The other systems are of much less clinical importance since: (a) naturally occurring antibodies are found only occasionally and when present, usually react only at low temperatures; and (b) immune antibodies are formed only occasionally because many of the antigens are of low antigenicity. Some are strongly antigenic (e.g. Kell), but are of low frequency, and therefore the chances of immunization are relatively small. The harmful clinical effects of red cell antigen–antibody reactions are haemolytic transfusion reactions, and haemolytic disease of the newborn.

Haemolytic transfusion reactions are most often due to incompatibilities involving the ABO and Rh systems, and only rarely the other systems (p. 482).

Haemolytic disease of the newborn

Haemolytic disease of the newborn results from the passage of IgG antibodies from the maternal circulation across the placenta into the circulation of the fetus where they react with and damage the fetal red cells, causing their premature destruction. The majority of cases of haemolytic disease of the newborn are due to ABO incompatibility. Cases due to Rh incompatibility are clinically more important because of their severity. They occur when an Rh-negative mother immunized to the Rh antigen becomes pregnant with an Rh-positive fetus. Most often, immunization results from a previous pregnancy, but in some cases it is due to a previous transfusion of Rh-positive blood. Immunization due to pregnancy results from the passage of red cells from an Rh-positive fetus across the placenta into the circulation of an Rh-negative woman. Very small numbers of fetal red cells cross the placenta throughout pregnancy, but significant haemorrhage leading to immunization generally occurs at delivery or in association with other intrapartum episodes such as amniocentesis, external version, or abortion.

It must be emphasized that when an Rh-negative woman is married to an Rh-positive man, the chance of her becoming sensitized to the Rh antigen and thus having children affected with haemolytic disease of the newborn is initially relatively small. If anti-D immunoglobulin prophylaxis (see below) is not given, the risk of developing antibodies increases with succeeding pregnancies. It has been estimated that one pregnancy with an ABO-compatible, Rh-positive infant will immunize 17 per cent of Rh-negative women without such prophylactic intervention. Half will have antibody detectable six months after delivery, and half will have antibody detectable during the second Rh-positive pregnancy. Before the introduction of anti-D prophylaxis, the overall incidence of haemolytic disease of the newborn due to anti-Rh(D) was about 1 in 200 of all pregnancies. Sensitization due to pregnancy practically never results in haemolytic disease of the first-born child; on the other hand, sensitization due to previous blood transfusion may cause the first child to be affected. Most cases of Rh haemolytic disease of the newborn are due to anti-D and mixtures of anti-D with anti-C or anti-E, but cases due to anti-C, anti-E, and anti-c alone occur occasionally.

Important determinants of maternal sensitization are the Rh genotype of her male partner and ABO incompatibility between mother and infant. If the partner is homozygous for the Rh(D) antigen, all the infants will be Rh(D) positive but if he is heterozygous any pregnancy has a 50 per cent chance of producing an Rh(D)-negative child which will not be affected by antibodies to the Rh(D) antigen. If the Rh(D)-positive infant is ABO incompatible with the mother, Rh(D) immunization is much less likely.

Haemolytic disease of the newborn due to ABO incompatibility is now being recognized with increased frequency. It can occur only in the 20 per cent of pregnancies in which there is ABO incompatibility between the mother and fetus, i.e. when the pregnancy is heterospecific. Thus, if the mother is group O (which is usually the case) and the fetus is group A or group B, the anti-A or anti-B antibodies may pass across the placenta into the fetal circulation and damage the fetal red cells. The placenta is relatively impermeable to naturally occurring IgM anti-A and anti-B antibodies; however, immune anti-A and anti-B of the IgG type will cross the placenta and may thus cause haemolytic disease. ABO haemolytic disease of the newborn shows certain general differences from Rh haemolytic disease: (a) it commonly occurs with the first pregnancy; (b) positive results with the direct antiglobulin test are often not obtained; and (c) it tends to be less severe, and the great majority do not require therapy.

Haemolytic disease of the newborn due to other blood group antibodies is rare, but cases due to anti-Kell, anti-S, and anti-s have been reported.

Discussion of the clinical features, diagnosis, and treatment of haemolytic disease of the newborn is beyond the scope of this work; for details the reader is referred to Mollison, Engelfriet & Contreras (1987) or standard textbooks of paediatrics.

PREVENTION OF HAEMOLYTIC DISEASE OF THE NEWBORN DUE TO ANTI-Rh(D)

Prevention of Rh(D) immunization in pregnancy by the administration of anti-D immunoglobulin to Rh(D)-negative mothers within 72 hours after delivery has been a major advance, and widespread application of the procedure has led to a reduction in maternal Rh(D) sensitization and in the incidence and mortality of haemolytic disease of the newborn.

Failure of prophylaxis when anti-D is given immediately after delivery has become a rare event, occurring in 1–2 per cent of women at risk (Bowman & Pollock 1987). Causes of failure include an inadequate dose of anti-D due to underestimation of the volume of transplacental haemorrhage, and primary immunization early in pregnancy. Antenatal administration of anti-D at 28 and 34 weeks prevents most cases of early immunization, and recent trials have confirmed the efficacy of such treatment. Clarke *et al.* (1985) have estimated that one-third of recent deaths due to haemolytic disease in the UK could have been prevented by giving antenatal as well as postnatal anti-D. Cost constraints have prevented universal application, and it has recently been suggested that maximum cost–benefit would be achieved by limiting antenatal prophylaxis to the first pregnancy.

Blood transfusion

The indications for transfusion in individual haematological disorders have been considered in the discussion of these disorders. Transfusion of granulocytes is discussed in Chapter 9, p. 228, and of platelets in Chapter 14, p. 393. Description of the technique of transfusion is beyond the scope of this work. The remainder of this chapter is devoted to a discussion of the complications of transfusion.

The complications of blood transfusion

In the majority of carefully prepared and properly supervised transfusions, there are no untoward effects. Nevertheless, complications occur in a small percentage (5–6 per cent) of transfusions; while these complications are often of only minor severity, they are sometimes serious and occasionally cause death. The frequency of occurrence of complications is inversely proportional to the care exercised in preparing for and supervising the transfusion. However, even when all precautions are taken, complications occur in a certain number of cases. Thus, blood transfusion carries a slight but definite risk, and is not a procedure to be undertaken lightly. *No transfusion should be administered unless the benefits to be gained outweigh the risks involved, and until simpler and safer therapy has proved ineffective or impossible under the circumstances.*

The complications of transfusion may be listed as follows:

febrile reactions;
allergic reactions;
circulatory overload;
haemolytic reactions;

reactions due to infected blood;
thrombophlebitis;
air embolism;
transmission of disease;
transfusion haemosiderosis;
complications of massive transfusion;
post-transfusion purpura (p. 387).

Febrile reactions

A slight rise in temperature is not uncommon during or after transfusion. In a few cases, probably two per cent, there is a greater rise, commonly accompanied by chills and other symptoms.

Febrile reactions are usually seen in multiparous females or in previously transfused patients who have developed antibodies to leucocytes or platelets. They are relatively common in patients who have received repeated transfusions, e.g. persons with aplastic anaemia, and in general the liability to develop reactions tends to be greater as the number of transfusions increases. The antibodies are generally directed against HLA antigens, and react with the leucocytes of the transfused blood. Granulocyte-specific and platelet antibodies may contribute; however, in general, platelet antibodies alone cause only mild reactions (p. 478). The serology of febrile transfusion reactions is reviewed by de Rie *et al.* (1985).

In a person who develops a febrile reaction for the first time, slowing of the drip rate, a warm drink, aspirin, and if necessary a sedative may bring symptomatic relief and permit cautious continuation of the transfusion. In persons with a history of previous reactions, if not severe, the prior administration of aspirin and a slow drip rate may prevent or minimize the reaction. If this strategy is unsuccessful, several techniques for the depletion of leucocytes from whole blood are available. Centrifugation of the blood pack and removal of the plasma and buffy coat is the simplest, but if this is not effective, methods such as washing, filtration, or freeze–thawing followed by washing may be used (Hughes & Brozovic 1982). A serum sample from the patient should be sent to a reference laboratory to confirm the presence of leucocyte and/or platelet antibodies.

Allergic reactions

Allergic reactions occur in about one per cent of all transfusions. They range in severity from small urticarial wheals of little consequence, to life-threatening circulatory collapse. In most cases, they are characterized by the sudden onset of wheals surrounded by areas of erythema, usually shortly after the commencement of the transfusion. Headache, nausea, vomiting, dyspnoea, oedema of the face, and swelling of mucous membranes may also occur. Laryngeal oedema is an uncommon but important complication. Rarely, an anaphylactic type of reaction occurs; the clinical picture is that of shock with acute peripheral circulatory failure, tachycardia, hypotension, and respiratory distress. In most cases, the patient gives a history of previous transfusions of blood or plasma.

Some allergic reactions are due to anti-IgA antibodies in the patient's circulation which react with IgA in the transfused plasma. Two types of antibody are recognized. The more common is occasionally found in untransfused normal subjects but occurs more frequently in multitransfused patients and women who have had one or more pregnancies. It is of limited specificity and reacts with some, but not all, IgA idiotypes. The titre of the antibody, which is usually IgG, is low, and sensitive haemagglutination techniques are required for detection. Reactions are mild and generally take the form of urticaria. The second type of antibody, which is class specific and reacts with all IgA idiotypes, is found in subjects who lack IgA in their serum and who usually have no previous history of transfusion. The antibody titre is high, and it may be detected by the use of immune precipitation techniques. Reactions are usually severe. Both types of anti-IgA antibody are IgG and bind complement.

In some allergic reactions, no specific aetiological mechanism can be defined. Antibody reactions against uncharacterized plasma protein constituents are presumed in these cases (Rivat *et al.* 1977).

Treatment. When the allergic reaction is mild and

is limited to only a few wheals, the transfusion is slowed, and an antihistamine drug administered. With more severe reactions, the transfusion is stopped and adrenalin given subcutaneously or, if necessary, intravenously.

Reactions in patients with a history of allergic episodes after transfusion may often be prevented by using washed red cells and administering antihistamines and corticosteroids before transfusion. Patients with high titres of anti-IgA and a history of severe reactions should receive blood from IgA-deficient donors.

Circulatory overload

Circulatory overload resulting in pulmonary congestion and acute heart failure is a most important complication of transfusion, and is probably the most common cause of death following transfusion. The risk of circulatory overload is particularly high in patients with chronic anaemia, and in the elderly, the very young, and in those with cardiac or pulmonary disease. It is important to minimize circulatory overload by giving packed red cells rather than whole blood whenever possible. Partial exchange transfusion and continuous monitoring of venous pressure may be necessary in particularly severe cases.

Most often, the clinical picture is that of acute pulmonary oedema. Less commonly, there is a more insidious onset of cardiac failure with progressive dyspnoea, cyanosis, and the development of crepitations at the lung bases over 12–24 hours. Such cases are sometimes complicated by a terminal bronchopneumonia.

Treatment. The transfusion is immediately discontinued and the patient is propped up in bed. Digoxin, a rapidly acting diuretic, e.g. frusemide, and morphine are given intravenously; oxygen is administered. If there is no response, rotating tourniquets or venesection are used, and in desperate cases intubation and positive pressure respiration may bring relief.

Haemolytic reactions

A haemolytic transfusion reaction has been defined by Mollison as 'the occurrence of signs of red cell destruction following transfusion, the most obvious of these signs being haemoglobinuria and jaundice'. Haemolytic reaction is the most important complication of blood transfusion, and together with circulatory overload is responsible for most fatalities.

AETIOLOGY

Most haemolytic reactions are due to blood group incompatibility. However, a haemolytic type of reaction may also result from the transfusion of blood that has been improperly stored or stored for too long, or from the transfusion of blood that is already haemolysed, e.g. by overheating or freezing. Rarely, increased destruction of donor red cells in blood which has been properly stored occurs in the absence of demonstrable antibodies.

Incompatibility

Incompatibility may be due to destruction of donor cells or of the recipient's cells.

Destruction of donor cells. Most incompatibility reactions are due to destruction of donor cells by specific allo-antibodies in the recipient's plasma. The majority of serious incompatibilities result from ABO or Rh incompatibility. Incompatibility due to one of the rare allo-antibodies of other blood group systems sometimes occurs, and is most likely to occur in persons who have received multiple transfusions. In general, ABO incompatibility results in a more severe reaction than does Rh incompatibility or incompatibility due to one of the other systems.

The mechanism of the red cell destruction varies with the type of antibody involved. By virtue of their ability to activate complement to the C8 and C9 stage, most IgM anti-A and anti-B antibodies have lytic properties and produce intravascular haemolysis. In contrast, IgG Rh antibodies are not complement binding, and antibody-coated cells are phagocytosed by cells of the reticulo-endothelial system, principally in the spleen (p. 194). Although lifespan is considerably reduced, frank intravascular haemolysis does not occur (Greenwalt 1981).

The administration of incompatible blood may be due to an error in blood grouping or cross-matching, or to an error in identification of the blood, so that the wrong blood is administered to the patient; this may result from inadequate or incorrect labelling of blood containers, failure to check the labels on the container before administration, or confusion of identity of patients with the same or similar names. Many fatal reactions have arisen from this cause.

Destruction of the recipient's cells. This is much less common and less important than destruction of donor cells. It is classically seen when group O blood containing immune anti-A and/or anti-B is transfused to a recipient other than group O. Reactions are seldom as marked as in destruction of donor cells in ABO incompatibility, but fatal cases have been reported.

CLINICAL FEATURES

Although there is considerable variation in the clinical picture, the course of a *severe immediate haemolytic reaction* is typically characterized by four phases: the phase of haemolytic shock, the post-shock phase in which the clinical features of increased blood destruction become obvious, the oliguric phase, and the diuretic phase.

The phase of haemolytic shock

The time of onset of symptoms varies with the rapidity of destruction. Sometimes symptoms occur when as little as 50 ml, or even less, has been transfused; for this reason, it is wise to administer the first 50–100 ml of a transfusion slowly. In other cases, symptoms do not appear until 1–2 hours after cessation of transfusion, whilst in some they do not occur at all.

The severity of the clinical features is influenced significantly by the amount and nature of the antibody. Severe reactions occur particularly when the causative antibody is of high titre and activates complement, causing marked intravascular red cell destruction. Typical symptoms (most of which are due to the action of liberated complement fragments C3a and C5a) are an aching pain in the lumbar region, sometimes in the thighs and down the legs, flushing of the face, throbbing in the head, anxiety, precordial pain or constriction, breathlessness, nausea, vomiting, chills, a rise in temperature, tachycardia, and a fall in blood pressure. Occasionally, the picture resembles anaphylactic shock with profound hypotension and peripheral circulatory failure. There is sometimes a feeling of heat along the vein into which the blood is being transfused.

In about 50 per cent of cases, a *haemorrhagic diathesis* develops, and in fact may be the first manifestation of a haemolytic reaction. It is typically characterized by persistent oozing from the surgical field and from venepunctures; it commonly lasts for several days, and sometimes reaches serious or even fatal proportions. The abnormal bleeding is due to disseminated intravascular coagulation, which is probably initiated by a combination of red cell stroma-derived procoagulant material and interaction of complement components with the early stages of the coagulation cascade.

In *patients under anaesthesia*, the haemolytic reaction is masked; however, the possibility of such a reaction in a transfused anaesthetized patient should be considered if one or more of the following develop without obvious reason—a sharp rise in pulse rate, a fall in blood pressure, flushing, sweating, or bleeding which is difficult to control. *Morphine* may also modify or mask a haemolytic reaction.

The post-shock phase

In this phase, the two clinical features that indicate increased blood destruction, namely haemoglobinuria and jaundice, become obvious; however, neither sign is invariable. *Haemoglobinuria*, when present, is usually obvious in the first specimen of urine passed. As it is sometimes transient and present only in the first specimen it may be missed. *Jaundice* develops in about 12 hours, and persists for several days, commonly being deepest on the day after transfusion. If the reaction is mild, jaundice on the day after transfusion may be the only sign of incompatibility, and the symptoms characteristic of the first stage may be absent. The haemoglobin value falls in proportion to the amount of blood destroyed. Red cell agglutination may be present on the blood film, and a moderate leucocytosis, e.g. $15–20 \times 10^9/l$, is usual.

The oliguric phase

In many, but not all, patients with haemolytic reactions, the kidneys are damaged due to the development of acute tubular necrosis. It is not possible to predict the occurrence of renal damage in the individual patient with a haemolytic reaction. Nevertheless, it appears that the incidence bears a relationship to the rapidity with which the haemolysis occurs and the condition of the patient at the time of transfusion, and that shock and pre-existing renal damage act as predisposing factors.

The pathophysiologic mechanisms responsible for renal damage are not well defined, but factors of importance include haemodynamic alterations in the renal microcirculation leading to stasis and activation of the coagulation system with resulting deposition of fibrin thrombi in small vessels (Goldfinger 1977).

Oliguria is the first sign of renal failure; thus an accurate record of fluid intake and urinary output should be commenced immediately, as fluid balance is critical in this situation. The oliguria is accompanied by progressive azotaemia and the clinical picture of acute renal failure. The oliguric phase usually lasts for 6–12 days, but may persist for up to three weeks or even longer. Complete anuria may develop, but is uncommon.

The diuretic phase

The end of the oliguric phase is marked by a spontaneous diuresis; occasionally, there is a sudden massive diuresis, but more commonly there is a gradual increase of urinary output by 200–300 ml per day. The diuretic phase usually heralds recovery; the clinical and biochemical features of the oliguric phase persist for several days, but then gradually and progressively disappear. However, the diuretic phase is attended by excess loss of sodium, potassium, and water, which if uncorrected may cause the death of the patient.

Delayed haemolytic transfusion reactions occur three days to three weeks after the administration of apparently compatible blood. In such cases, the amount of antibody in the patient's pretransfusion serum is so low that no incompatibility is detected by the usual serological tests and there is no immediate haemolysis after transfusion of incompatible red cells. Over the following days, a secondary immune response occurs, with the production of large amounts of antibody and gradually increasing, predominantly extravascular, destruction of the transfused red cells. Symptoms are often mild or absent, and the first indication of the reaction may be the onset of fever or the development of jaundice or an unexplained fall in haemoglobin. Impairment of renal function is unusual, but may occur. Antibodies most frequently involved are Rh and Kidd.

DIAGNOSIS

In the case of a suspected haemolytic reaction, the transfusion must immediately be stopped, and the following should be collected:

1 The pretransfusion blood sample taken from the patient for grouping and cross-matching.

2 Samples from the pilot bottles or plastic pack tubing used for cross-matching.

3 Samples from the units, which should always be retained for 24 hours after transfusion. These samples allow re-checking of the blood groups and cross-matching.

4 A sample of venous blood collected from a vein well away from the transfusion site. Part is delivered into collection tubes containing heparin and EDTA, and part is placed in a plain tube and allowed to clot.

5 Urine specimens from the patient, which are examined for haemoglobin. As haemoglobinuria is often transient, examination of the first specimen is particularly important.

The laboratory investigations necessary to establish the diagnosis of a haemolytic reaction and to determine its cause are given by Dacie & Lewis (1984). Direct proof of intravascular haemolysis requires demonstration of one or more of the following: haemoglobinaemia, methaemalbuminaemia, or haemoglobinuria. A raised serum bilirubin in a patient with a previously normal bilirubin is strong presumptive evidence of haemolysis. If the supernatant of the centrifuged heparinized specimen does not show evidence of free haemoglobin, or of any obvious increase in bilirubin, it is not likely that there has been any serious degree of haemolysis.

MANAGEMENT

The immediate steps consist of: (a) cessation of the transfusion; (b) administration of 80–120 mg frusemide, intravenously; (c) transfusion of compatible *red cells* and infusion of a plasma volume expander and intravenous hydrocortisone; and (d) when abnormal bleeding occurs, measures to treat disseminated intravascular coagulation (p. 445).

Management of the oliguric and diuretic phases is that of acute renal failure. Fluid balance is critical. Peritoneal or haemodialysis may be needed in severe cases. Details are given in standard medical texts.

Reactions due to infected blood

Bacterial infection of stored blood is a potential hazard in blood transfusions, but fortunately it seldom occurs. Nevertheless, it is a most important complication, as the administration of even small amounts of badly infected blood may result in severe shock with peripheral circulatory failure and rapid progression to death. Gram-negative organisms are usually responsible, and they produce severe endotoxic shock.

Despite the most careful collecting technique, a small percentage of blood units becomes contaminated by organisms from either the skin or air. As fresh blood is bactericidal, these contaminants usually die; even if they do persist they very rarely grow at refrigeration temperature. Therefore, when blood is taken with the usual sterile precautions and is immediately and continuously refrigerated, it rarely becomes clinically infected. However, if the blood is taken from the refrigerator and left at room temperature, any organisms present may multiply; thus all blood must be kept refrigerated until immediately before use. Rare cases have been reported in which the blood has become infected by psychrophilic organisms which grow at refrigeration temperature.

Contamination may be suggested by the appearance of the residue of the donor blood, but haemolysis does not invariably occur; further, when it is present, the free haemoglobin may be limited to the plasma trapped amongst the sedimented blood cells and may not be obvious in the supernatant plasma. A slight smell of hydrogen sulphide is sometimes noted on opening a bottle of infected blood.

Clinical features. The administration of heavily infected blood is followed within a short time by high fever, rigors, prostration, peripheral circulatory failure with persistent hypotension and tachycardia, vomiting, diarrhoea, and melaena. Commonly, the patient complains of a burning pain along the vein into which the blood is infused. Death usually occurs within a matter of hours. The diagnosis is suggested by this clinical picture and is confirmed by bacteriological examination of the blood, including culture at 4°C and 20°C; the organisms may be sufficiently numerous to be seen in a 'hanging drop' preparation or on a direct smear. Cultures from the blood unit and from the patient should be taken.

Treatment. Treatment consists of *vigorous measures to combat shock*, e.g. the administration of plasma volume expanders, pressor agents, hydrocortisone, and an antibiotic regimen effective against both Gram-positive and Gram-negative organisms, using large doses.

Thrombophlebitis

Thrombophlebitis, in some instances associated with septicaemia, is an important complication of blood transfusion, especially when dextrose or saline is used in addition to the blood. It occurs more commonly after cutting down and cannulation than when the vein is needled; it is also more common in the saphenous vein of the ankle than in the veins of the arm. The most important causative factor appears to be the length of the transfusion, the incidence of thrombophlebitis increasing significantly when transfusion at one site lasts longer than 12 hours. Thus, it tends to be seen more often with plastic cannulae than with steel needles, because the former are frequently left in for longer periods. This point is of particular importance in people who 'live by their veins', e.g. haemophiliacs and patients with aplastic anaemia, in whom the practice of leaving in plastic cannulae for long periods of time must be strictly avoided (Goldman *et al.* 1973).

Air embolism

Although in healthy persons the entry of a small amount of air into the circulation may not cause a significant disturbance, in sick patients small amounts, e.g. 10–40 ml, may cause alarming symptoms and even death, especially in patients with ventricular septal defects. Thus, strict precautions must always be taken to prevent any air from entering the vein. Air embolism results from the entry of air into the veins from the transfusion tubing. It arises most commonly when air is blown into the transfusion bottle under pressure by a Higginson's syringe and the bottle becomes empty unnoticed. Thus, when transfusions need to be hastened, it is preferable to use some other method, such as a pump on the tubing. With the increasing use of plastic packs for blood collection, the problem of air embolism with blood under pressure has largely been solved. Pressure can be applied externally to the packs, either manually or by the application of a sphygmomanometer cuff, or by means of a special cuff. This method of external pressure does not involve the risk of air embolism. Air may also be introduced at the beginning of a transfusion or when bottles or packs are being changed. Before commencing a transfusion, air should be driven out of the tubing by running blood through it, and, when changing bottles or packs, a very small amount of blood should be left in one container before changing to the next, so that the tubing remains full of blood.

Clinically, air embolism results in the sudden onset of severe dyspnoea and cyanosis; there is a fall of blood pressure, the pulse becomes rapid and thready, and syncope may occur from cerebral ischaemia. These features may subside fairly quickly, but in some cases death results. When the diagnosis is suspected, the patient should be placed on their left side in a head-down position; the air is then displaced away from the outflow tract of the right ventricle.

Transmission of disease

A number of diseases carried by blood may be transmitted in blood transfusion, and rigorous procedures must always be observed to minimize this risk. Historically, syphilis, malaria and 'serum hepatitis' were the three principal problems recognized, and every blood donor is questioned prior to acceptance as to any known association with the latter two; serological screening of blood for syphilis has been a part of transfusion practice in western countries for more than 40 years. Whilst screening for hepatitis B has greatly reduced the frequency of transmission of this disease, it is now recognized that other forms of viral infection can cause hepatitis—non-A, non-B hepatitis and cytomegalovirus in particular—and, since 1981, Acquired Immune Deficiency Syndrome (AIDS) has emerged as an even more serious problem. Transmission of the AIDS virus, its spread through blood transfusion and plasma products, and antibody development to its antigenic components are included in a fuller description of the disease in the final section of this chapter (p. 488).

Hepatitis B varies greatly in incidence in different parts of the world, ranging from approximately 0.1 per cent of blood donors in countries such as Australia up to figures as high as 2 per cent in some South-East Asian and Polynesian countries.

The major advance in eliminating the risk of transmission of hepatitis B was the recognition by Blumberg *et al.* (1965) of a specific antigen in the serum of carriers. This is now known as the 'surface' antigen of HBsAg. It consists of lipoprotein, which forms part of the shell of the virus; it is synthesized in hepatocytes and shed into the blood as very large numbers of small spherical particles or filaments. The infective virion is a larger body known as the Dane particle, in which a core is surrounded by a double shell. Core antigen (HBcAg) and a specific component of that core termed 'e' antigen (HBeAg) are present in the liver during the long incubation period (60–180 days) in active disease. Antibodies to these antigens can be detected during the period of active viral replication. Surface antigen usually appears in the blood during the incubation period and the clinical illness. It may be absent during the late acute stage or early convalescence, so that screening of blood which ordinarily is based on detection of HBsAg must be supplemented by clinical assessment of donors. HBsAg returns during the convalescent phase, and may be detectable for several years thereafter; the presence of antibody to this antigen usually indicates the development of immunity (Krugman *et al.* 1979).

Screening of every blood donation for HBsAg is now uniform in most western countries, the most sensitive tests depending upon radio-immunoassay or enzyme-linked immunosorbent assay (ELISA). Whilst the incidence of transmission of hepatitis B in transfusion practice has been greatly reduced by these procedures, occasional transmission of the virus inevitably occurs, and the risk of such transmission is much greater with blood products in which plasma from many donations is pooled, such as in the preparation of concentrates of factor VIII. The virus is resistant to the concentrations of ethanol used in plasma fractionation and to freezing, but the introduction of heat treatment of such plasma products to inactivate the virus has further greatly reduced this hazard. Products such as stabilized plasma protein solution are safe in this regard because of pasteurization, and procedures generally used in the production of gamma globulin for immunization also inactivate the virus.

With control of hepatitis B, the principal cause of post-transfusion hepatitis, it has now become clear that a number of other agents can also cause this disease.

Non-A, non-B hepatitis is a term applied to the disorder found in a group of patients with anicteric or icteric hepatitis due to a transmissable agent as yet poorly identified; it is very probably caused by more than one virus. It shows a shorter incubation period than hepatitis B, and some two-thirds of cases are non-icteric but may proceed to prolonged chronic active hepatitis (Tabor & Gerety 1979). Until screening for these agents can be introduced, prevention must depend on careful clinical assessment of donors.

Cytomegalovirus was first recognized as a cause of post-transfusion pyrexia and hepatitis in patients undergoing open heart surgery (Kaarianen *et al.* 1966) and is now recognized as a significant problem, particularly in recipients not previously exposed to CMV infection. In most, clinical and haematological manifestations are similar to infectious mononucleosis (p. 231), but heterophile antibodies are not detected. Significant CMV-induced disease is much more common in recipients who are immunosuppressed, such as transplant cases and patients on cytotoxic therapy. Rising titres of antibody to CMV are generally found with active infection, and it must be borne in mind that in western communities the incidence of complement-fixing antibodies to CMV in adults is 40–80 per cent (Krech 1973).

Epstein–Barr virus is the common cause of infectious mononucleosis (p. 231) and may also be transmitted by blood transfusion. In Australia, and probably in most western countries, it is a less common cause of post-transfusion hepatitis than hepatitis B, non-A, non-B hepatitis, or CMV (Cossart *et al.* 1982).

Malaria may be transmitted in blood from a donor who carries the infection. In temperate regions, donors should always be questioned as to exposure during travel.

Syphilis is a rare disease to be transmitted by transfusion, both because of screening procedures and the fact that the spirochaete does not survive for more than 72 hours in blood stored at 4°C.

Other protozoal and bacterial infections occasionally transmitted by transfusion include *toxoplasmosis* and *brucellosis* (Lang & Valeri 1977).

Transfusion haemosiderosis

The term 'transfusion haemosiderosis' is used to describe the increased deposition of iron in the tissues which occurs after repeated transfusion in cases of chronic anaemia not due to blood loss. The body has no mechanism for iron excretion except in very small amounts — 1 mg or less per day (p. 41). Haemorrhage is the only method by which significant quantities of iron can be lost from the body. Thus, it is obvious that in a patient who is not bleeding the iron released by the breakdown of the transfused red cells at the end of their lifespan must be retained in the tissues. The haemoglobin in 500 ml of blood contains approximately 250 mg iron. In patients who have been extensively transfused, the amount of iron in the body becomes greatly increased and may equal that found in haemochromatosis, i.e. 20 g or more. In some reported cases, the amount of iron found in the tissues at necropsy exceeded the calculated amount of iron present in the transfused blood. This is due to the fact that chronic anaemia, particularly when associated with ineffective erythropoiesis, modifies the regulation of absorption of iron, with the result that a greater than normal amount of iron is absorbed from the alimentary tract. The iron is deposited chiefly in the liver and spleen, but smaller amounts may occur in other tissues, such as lymph nodes, bone marrow, pancreas, heart, kidneys, and adrenal glands.

Usually, the iron deposits are not associated with any functional disturbance of the organs in which they occur, and thus do not produce any clinical manifestations, except pigmentation of the skin. Nevertheless, occasionally there is severe hepatic fibrosis, and the histological appearance is indistinguishable from idiopathic haemochromatosis. Hepatomegaly, sometimes with impairment of liver function, glycosuria, gonadal atrophy, and cardiac failure, may ensue.

Transfusion haemosiderosis is seen most commonly in patients with thalassaemia major, aplastic anaemia, sideroblastic anaemia, or chronic haemolytic anaemia who require repeated transfusions over periods of months or years. It does not occur in patients requiring repeated transfusion for blood loss. There is marked variation in the number of transfusions required to produce impairment of organ function in haemosiderosis. Thus, although in general the incidence is greater in much transfused patients, i.e. those who have received 30–50 litres or more, it is often absent in such patients. Rarely, it is seen in patients who have received only relatively small amounts of blood, possibly because they have been given large amounts of oral iron.

The administration of desferrioxamine, a chelating agent with a high affinity for iron, will lessen iron overload. It is now widely used in the management of transfusion-dependent subjects with thalassaemia (p. 160), and should be considered in all patients in whom transfusions over a period of years are anticipated, especially if there is evidence of impairment of liver function.

Complications of massive transfusion

Patients receiving massive transfusions (e.g. 5 litres over 24 hours or less) are liable to certain special complications, the most important of which are cardiac arrhythmias, which may proceed to ventricular fibrillation and cardiac arrest. A number of factors are considered to contribute to this complication, but the relative significance of each of these is yet to be precisely defined. These factors are excess of citrate, which may cause a fall in ionized serum calcium, a rise in serum potassium, a fall in blood pH, and cold blood; the effect of these factors may be aggravated by impairment of liver function. Measures to prevent cardiac arrest include the maintenance of adequate perfusion, careful warming of the blood to body temperature (with strict precautions to prevent haemolysis from overheating), and the administration of calcium gluconate (e.g. 10 ml of 10 per cent calcium gluconate solution per litre of blood after the first two litres), when the rate of blood administration is very rapid.

Acquired immune deficiency syndrome (AIDS)

Definition of the disease

The first reports of AIDS were of cases of *Pneumocystis carinii* pneumonia and Kaposi's sarcoma in previously healthy young male homosexuals, associated with a selective disturbance of cellular immunity, particularly a striking decrease in T helper or T4 lymphocytes (Centers for Disease Control 1981a, 1981b, 1982a, 1982b). The definition of the syndrome, established for surveillance purposes, required laboratory proof of infection by one of a number of pathogens recognized as commonly occurring in this condition, including a number of specific protozoal, helminthic, fungal, bacterial, and viral infections, or the presence either of histologically confirmed Kaposi's sarcoma or of lymphoma limited to the brain. This definition was subsequently extended to include a broader range of opportunistic infections, and chronic lymphoid interstitial pneumonitis in children. It was further extended to include non-Hodgkin's lymphoma in other sites in persons with antibody to the virus causative of AIDS, human immunodeficiency virus (HIV) (Centers for Disease Control 1985), and patients with antibody proof of infection with the virus, together with massive weight loss or cerebral complications (Centers for Disease Control 1987a).

It must be emphasized that AIDS, as so defined, represents the late stage of a disease which has many other manifestations and in which the natural history of infection by the causative virus is still unfolding.

The human immunodeficiency virus (HIV)

Recognition of the disease in male homosexuals in the first instance, followed by its occurrence in intravenous drug abusers and Haitians, led to much speculation as to its aetiology and means of spread. However, the finding of AIDS amongst recipients of blood transfusion and blood products pointed clearly to the likelihood of causation by an agent transmissible in blood or semen. Theories abounded concerning the possibility of mutation in known agents such as the Epstein–Barr virus or cytomegalovirus, but a novel virus was identified as the cause in three independent laboratories (Barre-Sinoussi *et al.* 1983, Gallo *et al.* 1984, Levy *et al.* 1984). The three laboratories initially gave different names to the virus: lymphadenopathy associated virus (LAV) from the Pasteur Institute, human T cell lymphotrophic virus III (HTLV-III) from the National Cancer Institute in Washington, and AIDS-related virus (ARV) from California.

Collaborative research established that the three viruses were one and the same. It is an RNA retrovirus, containing reverse transcriptase, and attaches particularly to T4 lymphocytes. The enzyme reads the message for reproduction of the virus into the genetic material of the cell, and subsequently such cells are capable of elaborating vast numbers of viral particles. International agreement was reached through the International Committee on the Taxonomy of Viruses that the term 'human immunodeficiency virus' (HIV) be used to describe the virus in all of its variants. Since 1986, this convention has been followed.

Retroviruses belong to three subfamilies: oncovirinae, lentivirinae, and spumivirinae. HTLV-I and HTLV-II, previously discovered by Gallo, both cause lymphoid tumours and resemble other oncogenic retroviruses. HIV, on the other hand, causes lysis of lymphocytes and resembles lentiviruses of the animal kingdom in many respects. Lentiviruses cause a variety of protracted neurological, haematological, musculoskeletal, and respiratory diseases in hooved animals; even more closely related retroviruses have now been termed STLV-III or simian immunodeficiency virus (SIV) (Kanki *et al.* 1985). Spumiviruses are syncytial viruses which differ substantially from lentiviruses in their effects at the cellular level *in vivo*.

In retrospect, the disease AIDS appeared in epidemic form in Africa at a similar time to its emergence in North America and the Caribbean. This lends particular significance to the finding of a closely related virus in the African green monkey (Kanki *et al.* 1985). It is probable that the disease originated in central Africa in its present virulent form. The epidemic is likely then to have spread through interchange of workers between Africa and the Caribbean islands and also to Europe and North America, either directly or through Caribbean migrants and vacationers.

The structure of the virus comprises the RNA genome with its genetic message, surrounded by a protein core and then an external lipid–glycoprotein envelope (Fig. 17.1). The characteristics of each of its components have been the subject of intense study, with application of the full armamentarium of molecular virology, including molecular cloning and nucleotide analysis.

The RNA genome includes the three characteristic viral genes present in all previously known retroviruses — *gag*, *pol*, and *env* (Weiss *et al.* 1985) (Fig. 17.2). The *gag* gene encodes the proteins which make up the internal core of the virus, the *pol* gene delivers the enzyme reverse transcriptase, and the *env* gene codes for the membrane glycoproteins which play a critical part in binding of the virus to receptors on the target cells, and are also important as antigens. In the DNA form of the retroviral genome, the terminus at either end is provided by a sequence known as *long terminal repeats* (*LTRs*) which play the role of controlling viral expression and integration. In addition to these, however, critical gene formations have been identified,

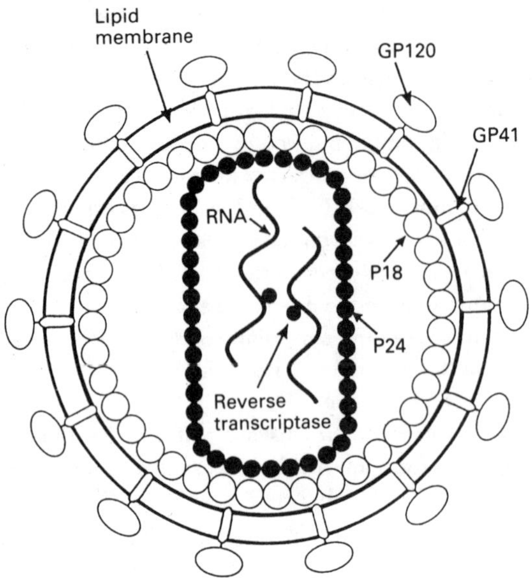

Fig. 17.1 *Schematic representation of the human immunodeficiency virus (HIV).*

known as *tat* and *art*, which serve a trans-acting or regulating function of the other genes, and two further genes known as *sor* and *orf* which are believed to have important functions *in vivo*, although less critical to replication in tissue culture cells (Fisher *et al.* 1986, Sodroski *et al.* 1986).

The core proteins include the enzyme reverse transcriptase, which transfers the genetic information contained in the single-stranded RNA genome to a full-length, double-stranded, linear DNA intermediate, which is transported to the nucleus. It is there circularized and integrated with the DNA of the host cell. Once integrated in the host genome, the retroviral sequence is termed a *provirus* and acts as the template for subsequent production of new virus by a complex pattern of transcription of the full-length RNA, together with production of mRNAs encoding for the protein products of the *sor*, *tat*, *art*, and *orf* proteins, many of which are subsequently synthesized in the cytoplasm of the cell, assembled in proximity to the plasma membrane, and formed into virus particles which incorporate the full-length viral RNA genome. The lipid component of the viral membrane is provided from the parent cell but incorporates glycoprotein products of the *env* gene (Meusing *et al.* 1985).

Antibodies to HIV

Detection of antibody to the AIDS retrovirus (Brun-Vezinet *et al.* 1984, Safai *et al.* 1984) was a most important step in the unfolding of the AIDS story. It permitted identification of those carrying infection prior to their developing AIDS, and thus the study of the natural history of the infection. The type of test most widely employed in screening for antibodies was that developed specifically for testing of blood donated for the purposes of transfusion and depended on *enzyme linked immunosorbent assay* (ELISA) technology. The test involves the use of antigen prepared from culture of virus in lymphocytes. Inevitably, such antigen is contaminated with traces of protein derived from lymphocytes. Whilst such tests are very sensitive to the presence of IgG antibody in persons carrying the infection (higher than 99.9 per cent sensitivity), IgG antibody appears only some 2–4 months after infection, so that in early infection the test is negative (Salahuddin *et al.* 1984). A positive test to mixed antigen derived from HIV cultures can, in fact, also be due to antibodies to lymphocyte antigens, commonly present in multiparous women or persons who have received multiple blood transfusions. These *false positive* tests are found particularly when persons at little risk of infection, such as blood transfusion donors, are screened. Demonstration of antibodies to specific HIV antigens depends on a more precise presentation of the antigen. The *Western Blot*

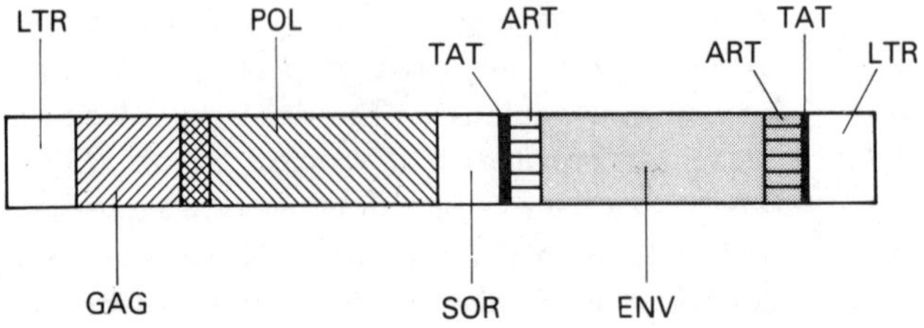

Fig. 17.2. *Genetic constitution of HIV. The genes gag, pol, and env code for structural proteins, and the genes sor, tat, and art code for regulatory proteins. LTR = long terminal repeat.*

technique is generally the reference test for confirmation in sera detected as repeatedly positive by the ELISA technique. Alternatives for detection of antibody to HIV include the use of *radio-immuno-precipitation assays* (RIPA), *competitive inhibitory radio-immuno-assay*, and a variety of assays dependent on detection of antibody to selective antigens prepared by the application of recombinant DNA genetic engineering techniques.

Antibody develops to a variety of different antigenic components, including both the core proteins and the glycoprotein coat. The principal glycoprotein is heavily glycosylated, and has a molecular weight of around 160 kd (see Fig. 17.1). It subsequently gives rise to one glycoprotein of 120 kd and another of 41 kd. The gp120–gp41 complex is a particularly important antigenic structure, gp120 being primarily on the outer surface of the virus, and gp41 more deeply embedded in the membrane. Portions of gp120 are known to be very variable in amino-acid composition, giving rise to 'antigenic drift' from isolate to isolate. These proteins are the product of the *env* gene. Most antibodies are not 'neutralizing' in the sense of inhibiting viral growth, but antibodies to some portions of gp120 appear to have this property (Coffin 1986). Of the products of the *gag* gene, the p24 protein is a readily detected antigen, and antibody is frequently present in the early stages of infection.

Natural history of HIV infection

Following infection, some patients develop a minor clinical illness associated with fever, headaches, widespread aches and pains, lymph node enlargement, and commonly a macular skin eruption. The illness subsides spontaneously in 1–2 weeks, but is characterized by the presence of atypical mononuclear cells in the peripheral blood, resembling those of infectious mononucleosis. This occurs several weeks after infection, and tests for antibody to HIV are negative at this stage (Cooper *et al.* 1985).

After a period of 2–4 months, in most individuals the antibody test becomes positive but the person remains free of symptoms. The proportion that subsequently develops complications has varied greatly from report to report. In those followed for a period of 5–7 years, it appears that 30–40 per cent, whilst not developing AIDS, will have either generalized lymph node enlargement or more serious symptoms, which may include weight loss, recurrent episodes of fever, diarrhoea, or chest infections, haemopoietic disturbance with either thrombocytopenia or neutropenia, peripheral neuropathy, or central nervous system disability commonly associated with major psychiatric disturbance (Melbye *et al.* 1986, Rutherford *et al.* 1986). Lymphadenopathy syndrome does not necessarily progress to more serious consequences, but the other group of symptoms, known as *AIDS-related complex* (ARC), is generally associated with significant and progressive immunodeficiency, and is likely to go on to AIDS.

The proportion of patients presenting with AIDS 5–7 years after infection is variable, but falls in the range of 20–30 per cent or more. Half to two-thirds have preceding symptoms of AIDS-related complex, whereas the others present without prior warning. Average survival from the date of the diagnosis of AIDS, without the use of effective antiviral agents, is substantially less than 18 months, and is shorter in those with opportunistic infections than in those presenting with Kaposi's sarcoma, even though in the earlier stages, opportunistic infections and the neoplastic diseases are commonly responsive to therapy in their own right.

As experience of the clinical manifestations of HIV infection increases, it has become clear that the early clinical classifications and earlier surveillance definitions are inadequate as a basis for studying the disease (Centers for Disease Control 1986d, 1987a). Continued evolution in terminology and classification can be anticipated.

In children, AIDS follows a similar but usually more rapidly progressive pattern; lymphocytic interstitial pneumonitis and encephalitis are relatively common (Bernstein *et al.* 1986, Centers for Disease Control 1987d).

Modes of transmission of the infection

The virus has been recovered from peripheral blood, cell free plasma, semen, cervical and vaginal secretions, lymph nodes, brain and cerebrospinal fluid, saliva, and tears (Salahuddin *et al.* 1985, Shaw *et al.* 1985, Gartner *et al.* 1986). However, with very few exceptions, transmission, as documented in careful epidemiological studies, is confined to:

sexual transmission;

blood from an infected person entering the circulation of a second individual;

transmission from an infected mother to baby during pregnancy, at the time of delivery, or in the early postnatal phase.

Sexual transmission is undoubtedly the principal basis of spread worldwide. Anal intercourse appears to transmit the infection far more readily than vaginal intercourse, hence accounting for the predominant appearance of disease in the male homosexual community in western countries. In Africa, however, the high incidence of untreated sexually transmissible diseases and the common occurrence of genital ulceration appear to be major contributory factors to widespread heterosexual disease seen in that continent (Biggar 1987). Heterosexual transmission to women from bisexual men, and from those infected through intravenous drug abuse, blood, or blood products to sexual partners of either sex, undoubtedly occurs in western countries. Whilst in industrial societies with good health services, sexual transmission will remain mainly associated with the male homosexual community, slow but increasing heterosexual spread will undoubtedly occur (Penington 1987).

Spread through blood transfusion and plasma products was extensive in most western countries before the introduction of antibody screening for blood donations (Jaffe *et al.* 1985, Johnson *et al.* 1985). In Australia, the further safeguard of a signed declaration form at every blood donation, backed by legislation providing significant penalties for a false declaration, resulted in an incidence of confirmed positive tests of less than 0.0004 per cent in 1986 compared with 0.0021 per cent in the UK in that year, and 0.04 per cent in the United States in 1985 (Crofts & Gust 1987). In countries not enforcing strict use of donor declaration forms, spread of the virus by transfusion will still occur because of the delay in development of antibody detectable with screening tests in the early months of infection.

Spread through intravenous drug abuse remains a major problem on the eastern seaboard of the United States, in many European cities, and increasingly elsewhere. Sharing of syringes and needles between drug abusers, where the dead-space of the syringe and hub of the needle may be filled with blood, is a potent means by which infection is spread. There is then further spread of the virus from those individuals to sexual partners of either sex, and from infected mothers to infants. As many young women addicted to opiates engage in prostitution to earn money to purchase drugs, this group represents a major avenue for heterosexual spread of the infection in western communities (Centers for Disease Control 1986a).

Parenteral spread through accidental needle-stick injury is rare, but a small number of cases of such transmission has been recorded. In others, infection has been acquired through accidental spillage or spattering of blood on damaged or diseased skin (Centers for Disease Control 1987b). The low but definite risk from exposure in health care workers (McCray 1986) indicates the need to observe strict precautions in the handling of blood and body fluids of infected persons. This applies in all health care situations, including wards and laboratories, and in procedures such as haemodialysis or cytapheresis where accidental spillage of blood may occur (Peterman *et al.* 1986). Laboratory centrifuges should permit sealing of tubes, gloves should be worn when handling blood and other body fluids from persons who may carry the infection, and eye protection should be employed where there is a danger of aerosols or of spattering.

Maternal–infant transmission is known to occur with infected mothers. The rate is unknown, and may vary depending on the immune status of the mother. With mothers who are intravenous drug abusers, the incidence of infection in infants is in the range of 30–50 per cent. Infection may occur in the baby during pregnancy, at the time of delivery, or in the early neonatal period, when it appears likely that transmission is through breast feeding (Ziegler *et al.* 1985). In some women, deterioration of immune status has been observed during pregnancy, and termination may be considered to be advisable (Centers for Disease Control 1986b).

Other forms of transmission are exceedingly rare. Extensive studies of families where one member carries the infection have established that HIV is not transmitted through close casual contact, even that which may include sharing of accommodation, eating utensils, toilet facilities, and even toothbrushes (Friedland *et al.* 1986). Spread through casual association as in the workplace is, therefore, not a matter for concern.

Survival of the virus outside the body

The virus survives at room temperature outside the body for a matter of days (Spire *et al.* 1985, Resnik *et al.* 1986), but it is readily destroyed by moist or dry heat (autoclaving for 15 minutes at 121°C, 1 hour at 170°C in a dry oven, or boiling for 10–30 minutes, depending upon the extent of contamination). Chemical disinfection may be readily achieved using 2 per cent freshly prepared glutaraldehyde solution; 0.5 per cent sodium hypochlorite (5000 ppm available chlorine) for heavily contaminated surfaces or one-tenth this concentration for general cleaning of benches; or 70 per cent ethanol for 1 hour (Centers for Disease Control 1986c, 1987b).

The future course of AIDS

The future course of the epidemic remains difficult to predict with any precision, as does the evolving pattern of late manifestations of disease in those carrying the human immunodeficiency virus. Sadly, it is clear that the virus will take a terrible toll of suffering and death, particularly in central Africa and some Carribean islands and amongst those principally at risk in western communities (Institute of Medicine, National Academy of Sciences 1986). No attempt has been made to review the fast developing field of antiviral drugs or strategies for reconstitution of the immune system which offer hope to those already carrying the infection. Similarly, no review is provided of the early attempts to develop a vaccine aimed at halting the epidemic.

Until an effective vaccine becomes available, every possible endeavour must be made to curb spread of the infection through the routes that have now been clearly identified. These include measures to minimize sexual spread and spread through intravenous drug abuse (Centers for Disease Control 1986a, 1987c, Penington 1987) and in health care settings (Centers for Disease Control 1987b).

References and further reading

Blood transfusion

Alter, H.J., Holland, P.V., Morrow, A.G. *et al.* (1975) Clinical and serological analysis of transfusion-associated hepatitis. *Lancet*, **ii**, 838.

Bailey, D.N. & Bove, J.R. (1975) Chemical and hematological changes in stored CPD blood. *Transfusion*, **15**, 244.

Barbara, J.A.J. & Tedder, R.S. (1984) Viral infections transmitted by blood and its products. *Clin. Haemat.* **13**, 693.

Barton, J.C. (1981) Nonhemolytic, noninfectious transfusion reactions. *Semin. Hematol.* **18**, 95.

Bayer, W.L., Tegtmeier, G.E. & Barbara, J.A.J. (1984) The significance of non-A, non-B hepatitis, cytomegalovirus and the acquired immune deficiency syndrome in transfusion practice. *Clin. Haemat.* **13**, 253.

Beal, R.W. & Isbister, J.P. (1985) *Blood Component Therapy in Clinical Practice*, Blackwell Scientific Publications, Oxford.

Blumberg, B.S., Alter H.J. & Vismich, S. (1965) A new antigen in leukemia serum. *J. Am. Med. Ass.* **191**, 541.

Bodmer, W.F. (1987) The HLA system: structure and function. *J. Clin. Pathol.* **40**, 948.

Bowman, J.M. & Pollock, J.M. (1987) Failures of intravenous Rh immune globulin prophylaxis: an analysis of the reasons for such failures. *Transfus. Med. Rev.* **1**, 101.

Clarke, Sir Cyril (1982) Rhesus haemolytic disease of the newborn and its prevention. *Brit. J. Haemat.* **52**, 525.

Clarke, C.A., Mollison, P.L. & Whitfield, A.G.W. (1985) Death from rhesus haemolytic disease in England and Wales in 1982 and 1983. *Brit. Med. J.* **291**, 17.

Collins, J.A. (1976) Massive blood transfusion. *Clin. Haemat.* **5**, 201.

Conrad, M.E. (1981) Diseases transmissible by blood transfusion: viral hepatitis and other infectious disorders. *Semin. Hematol.* **18**, 122.

Cossart, Y.E., Kirsch, S. & Ismay, S.L. (1982) Post-transfusion hepatitis in Australia. Report of the Australian Red Cross study. *Lancet*, **i**, 208.

Dacie, J.V. & Lewis, S.M. (1984) *Practical Haematology*, 6th Ed., Churchill Livingstone, London.

Decary, F., Ferner, P., Giavedoni, L. *et al.* (1984) An investigation of nonhemolytic transfusion reactions. *Vox Sang*, **46**, 277.

de Rie, M.A., van den Plas-van Dalen, C.M., Engelfriet, C.P. *et al.* (1985) The serology of febrile transfusion reactions. *Vox Sang*, **49**, 126.

Dutcher, J.P., Schiffer, C.A., Acaner, J. *et al.* (1981) Long-term follow up of patients with leukemia receiving platelet transfusion: Identification of a large group of patients who do not become alloimmunized. *Blood*, **58**, 1007.

Feinstone, S.M., Kapikian, A.Z., Purcell, R.H. *et al.* (1975) Transfusion-associated hepatitis was due to viral hepatitis type A or B. *New Engl. J. Med.* **292**, 767.

Gitnick, G. (1984) Non-A, non-B hepatitis: etiology and clinical course. *Ann. Rev. Med.* **35**, 265.

Gocke, D.J. (1972) A prospective study of post transfusion hepatitis. The role of Australia antigen. *J. Am. Med. Ass.* **219**, 1165.

Goldfinger, D. (1977) Acute hemolytic transfusion reaction—a fresh look at pathogenesis and considerations regarding therapy. *Transfusion*, **17**, 85.

Goldman, D.A., Maki, D.G., Rhame, F.S. *et al.* (1973) Guidelines for infection control in intravenous therapy. *Ann. Int. Med.* **79**, 848.

Greenwalt, T.J. (1981) Pathogenesis and management of hemolytic transfusion reactions. *Semin. Hematol.* **18**, 84.

Hughes, A.S.B. & Brozovic, B. (1982) Leucocyte depleted blood: an appraisal of available techniques. *Brit. J. Haemat.* **50**, 381.

Issitt, P.D. (1985) *Applied Blood Group Serology*, 3rd Ed., Montgomery Scientific Publications, Florida.

Kaariainen, L., Klemola, E. & Palo Leimo, J. (1966) Rise of cytomegalovirus antibodies in an infectious mononucleosis-like syndrome after transfusion. *Brit. Med. J.* **1**, 1270.

Kay, A.B. (1976) Some complications associated with the administration of blood and blood products. *Clin. Haemat.* **5**, 165.

Kelton, J.G. & Ali, A.M. (1983) Platelet transfusion—a critical appraisal. *Clin. Oncol.* **2**, 549.

Koistinen, J. & Leikola, J. (1977) Weak anti-IgA antibodies with limited specificity and non-hemolytic transfusion reactions. *Vox Sang*, **32**, 77.

Koretz, R.L. & Gitnick, G.L. (1975) Prevention of post-transfusion hepatitis. Role of sensitive Hepatitis B antigen screening tests, source of blood and volume of transfusion. *Am. J. Med.* **59**, 754.

Krech, U. (1973) Complement-fixing antibodies against cytomegalovirus in different parts of the world. *Bull. Wld. Hlth. Org.* **49**, 103.

Krugman, S., Overby, L.R., Mushahwar, I.K. *et al.* (1979) Viral hepatitis type B: Studies on the natural history and prevention re-examined. *New Engl. J. Med.* **300**, 101.

Lang, D.J. & Valeri, C.R. (1977) Hazards of blood transfusion. *Adv. Paediat.* **24**, 311.

Menitove, J.E., McElligott, M.C. & Aster, R.H. (1982) Febrile transfusion reaction: what blood component should be given next? *Vox Sang*, **42**, 318.

Meryman, H.T., Bross, J. & Lebovitz, R. (1980) Preparation of leukocyte-poor red blood cells: a comparative study. *Transfusion*, **20**, 285.

Minchinton, R.M. & Waters, A.H. (1984) The occurrence and significance of neutrophil antibodies. *Brit. J. Haemat.* **56**, 521.

Mollison, P.L., Engelfriet, C.P. & Contreras, M. (1987) *Blood Transfusion in Clinical Medicine*, 8th Ed., Blackwell Scientific Publications, Oxford.

Mollison, P.L. (1970) The role of complement in antibody-mediated red-cell destruction. *Brit. J. Haemat.* **18**, 249.

Murphy, M.F. & Waters, A.H. (1985) Immunological aspects of platelet transfusions. *Brit. J. Haemat.* **60**, 409.

National Blood Transfusion Committee of the Australian Red Cross (1971) The care of blood during transport and in hospitals. *Med. J. Austr.* **2**, 108.

Petz, L.D. & Swisher, S.N. (1981) *Clinical Practice of Blood Transfusion*, Churchill Livingstone, New York.

Pineda, A.A. & Taswell, H.F. (1975) Transfusion reactions associated with anti-IgA antibodies: report of four cases and review of the literature. *Transfusion*, **15**, 10.

Pineda, A.A., Brzica, S.M., Jr., & Taswell, H.F. (1978) Hemolytic transfusion reaction: recent experience in a large blood bank. *Mayo Clin. Proc.* **53**, 378.

Polesky, H.F. (1982) Diagnosis, prevention, and therapy in hemolytic disease of the newborn. *Clin. Lab. Med.* **2**, 107.

Popovsky, M.A., Abel, M.D. & Moore, S.B. (1983) Transfusion related acute lung injury associated with passive transfer of antileucocyte antibodies. *Am. Rev. Resp. Dis.* **128**, 185.

Race, R.R. & Sanger, R. (1975) *Blood Groups in Man*, 6th Ed., Blackwell Scientific Publications, Oxford.

Rivat, L., Rivat, C., Daveau, M. *et al.* (1977) Comparative frequencies of anti-IgA antibodies among patients with anaphylactic transfusion reactions and among normal blood donors. *Clin. Immunol. Immunopathol.* **7**, 340.

Robinson, E.A.E. (1984) Single donor granulocytes and platelets. *Clin. Haemat.* **13**, 185.

Sander, S.G. & Grumet, F.C. (1982) Post transfusion cytomegalovirus infection. *Pediatrics*, **69**, 650.

Schmidt, P.J. (1982) Transfusion reactions: status in 1982. *Clin. Lab. Med.* **2**, 221.

Seef, L.B. & Hoofnagle, J.H. (1979) Immuno-prophylaxis of viral hepatitis. *Gastroenterol.* **77**, 161.

Shafritz, D.A. & Lieberman, H.M. (1984) The molecular biology of hepatitis B virus. *Ann. Rev. Med.* **35**, 219.

Sohmer, P.R. & Scott, R.L. (1982) Massive transfusion. *Clin. Lab. Med.* **2**, 21.

Strauss, R.G. (1983) Granulocyte transfusion therapy. *Clin. Oncol.* **2**, 635.

Szmuness, W., Stevens, C.E. & Harley, E.J. (1980) Hepatitis B vaccine: demonstration of efficacy in a controlled clinical trial in a high risk population in the United States. *New Engl. J. Med.* **303**, 833.

Tabor, E. (1985) The three viruses of non-A, non-B hepatitis. *Lancet*, **i**, 743.

Tabor, E. & Geraty, R.J. (1979) Non-A, non-B hepatitis: New findings and prospectus for prevention. *Transfusion*, **19**, 669.

Tovey, G.H. & Gillespie, W.A. (1974) The investigation of blood transfusion reactions. Association of Clinical Pathologists, Broadsheet 54.

Tovey, L.A.D., Stevenson, B.J., Townley, A. *et al.* (1983)

The Yorkshire antenatal anti-B immunoglobulin trial in primagravidae. *Lancet*, **ii**, 244.

Urbaniak, S.J. (1984) Therapeutic plasma and cellular aphoresis. *Clin. Haemat.* **13**, 217.

Urbaniak, S.J. (1985) Rh(D) haemolytic disease of the newborn: the changing scene. *Brit. Med. J.* **291**, 4.

Wolf, C.F.W. & Canale, V.C. (1976) Fatal pulmonary hypersensitivity reaction to HL-A incompatible blood transfusion: report of a case and review of the literature. *Transfusion*, **16**, 135.

Acquired immune deficiency syndrome

Barre-Sinoussi, F., Chermann, J.C., Rey, F. *et al.* (1983) Isolation of a T-lymphotrophic retrovirus from a patient at risk for AIDS. *Science*, **220**, 868.

Bernstein, L.J., Krieger, B.Z., Novick, B. et al. (1985) Bacterial infection in the acquired immunodeficiency syndrome of children. *Pediat. Infect. Dis.* **4**, 472.

Biggar, R.J. (1987) Epidemiology of human retrovirus and related clinical conditions in AIDS. In: Broder, S. (Ed.) *Modern Concepts and Therapeutic Challenges*, p. 91, Marcel Dekkar, New York.

Brun-Vezinet, F., Rouzioux, C., Barre-Sinoussi, F. *et al* (1984) Detection of IgG antibodies to lymphadenopathy-associated virus in patients with AIDS or lymphadenopathy syndrome. *Lancet*, **i**, 1253.

Centers for Disease Control (1981a) Pneumocystis pneumonia—Los Angeles. *Morbid. Mortal. Weekly Rep.* **30**, 260.

Centers for Disease Control (1981b) Kaposi's sarcoma and pneumocystis pneumonia among homosexual men—New York City and California. *Morbid. Mortal. Weekly Rep.* **30**, 305.

Centres for Disease Control (1982a) Persistent generalised lymphadenopathy among homosexual males. *Morbid. Mortal. Weekly Rep.* **31**, 249.

Centers for Disease Control (1982b) Update on acquired immune deficiency syndrome (AIDS)—United States. *Morbid. Mortal. Weekly Rep.* **31**, 507.

Centers for Disease Control (1985) Revision of the case definition of AIDS for national reporting—United States. *Morbid. Mortal. Weekly Rep.* **34**, 373.

Centers for Disease Control (1986a) Additional recommendations to reduce sexual and drug abuse related transmission of HTLV-III/LAV. *Morbid. Mortal. Weekly Rep.* **35**, 152.

Centers for Disease Control (1986b) Recommendations for assisting in the prevention of perinatal transmission of human T-lymphotropic virus type III/lymphadenopathy associated virus and the acquired immunodeficiency syndrome. *Morbid. Mortal. Weekly Rep.* **34**, 721, 731.

Centers for Disease Control (1986c) HTLV-III/LAV agent summary statement. *Morbid. Mortal. Weekly Rep.* **35**, 540.

Centers for Disease Control (1986d) Classification system of human T-lymphotropic virus type III/lymphadenopathy associated virus infections. *Morbid. Mortal. Weekly Rep.* **35**, 334.

Centers for Disease Control (1987a) Revision of the CDC surveillance case definition for Acquired Immunodeficiency Syndrome. *Morbid. Mortal. Weekly Rep.* **36**, (Suppl.1S) 3S.

Centers for Disease Control (1987b) Recommendations for prevention of HIV transmission in health care settings. *Morbid. Mortal. Weekly Rep.* **36**, (Suppl.2S) 3S.

Centers for Disease Control (1987c) Public Health Service guidelines for counseling and antibody testing to prevent HIV Infection and AIDS. *Morbid. Mortal. Weekly Rep.* **36**, 509.

Centers for Disease Control (1987d) Classification system for human immunodeficiency virus (HIV) infection in children under 13 years of age. *Morbid. Mortal. Weekly Rep.* **36**, 225.

Coffin, J.M. (1986) Genetic variations in AIDS viruses. Background paper, Committee on a national strategy for AIDS. Cited in: Institute of Medicine, National Academy of Sciences. *Confronting AIDS*, p. 225, National Academy Press, Washington D.C.

Cooper, D.A., Gold, J., MacLean, P. *et al.* (1985) Acute AIDS retrovirus infection: definition of a clinical illness associated with seroconversion. *Lancet*, **i**, 537.

Crofts, N. & Gust, I.D. (1987) Screening test for anti-HIV in Australian Blood Banks in 1986. *Med. J. Aust.* **146**, 556.

Curran, J.W., Lawrence, D.N., Jaffe, H. *et al.* (1984) Acquired immunodeficiency syndrome (AIDS) associated with transfusion. *New Engl. J. Med.* **310**, 69.

Fisher, A.G., Feinberg, M.B., Josephs, S.F. *et al.* (1986). The transactivator gene of HTLV-III is essential for virus replication. *Nature*, **320**, 367.

Friedland, G.H., Saltzman, B.R., Rogers, M.F. *et al.* (1986) Lack of transmission of HTLV-III/LAV infection to household contacts of patients with AIDS or AIDS-related complex with oral candidiasis. *New Engl. J. Med.* **314**, 344.

Gallo, R.C., Salahuddin, S.Z. & Popovic, M. (1984) Frequent detection and isolation of cytopathic retroviruses (HTLV-III) from patients with AIDS and at risk for AIDS. *Science*, **224**, 500.

Gartner, S., Markovitz, P., Markovitz, D.M. *et al.* (1986) The role of mononuclear phagocytes in HTLV-III/LAV infection. *Science*, **233**, 215.

Institute of Medicine, National Academy of Sciences (1986) Confronting AIDS. Directions for Public Health, Health Care and Research. National Academy Press, Washington D.C.

Jaffe, H.W., Sarngadharan, M.G., de Vico, A.L. *et al.* (1985) Infection with HTLV-III/LAV and transfusion associated immunodeficiency syndrome. Serologic evidence of an association. *J. Am. Med. Ass.* **254**, 770.

Johnson, R.E., Lawrence, D.N., Evatt, B.L. *et al.* (1985) Acquired immunodeficiency syndrome among patients attending hemophilia treatment centers and mortality experience of hemophiliacs in the United States. *Am. J. Epidemiol.* **121**, 797.

Kanki, P.J., Alroy, J. & Essex, M. (1985) Isolation of a T-lymphotropic retrovirus related to HTLV-III LAV from wild-caught African green monkeys. *Science*, **230**, 951.

Kreiss, J.K., Kitchen, L.W., Prince, H.E. *et al.* (1985) Antibody to human T-lymphotropic virus type III in wives of hemophiliacs: evidence of sexual transmission. *Ann. Int. Med.* **102**, 623.

Levy, J.A., Hoffman, A.D., Kramer, S.M. *et al.* (1984) Isolation of lymphocytopathic retroviruses from San Francisco patients with AIDS. *Science*, **225**, 840.

McCray, E. (1986) Occupational risk of the acquired immunodeficiency syndrome among health care workers. *New Engl. J. Med.* **314**, 1127.

Melbye, M., Biggar, R., Ebbesen, P. *et al.* (1986) Long-term sero-positivity for human T-lymphotropic virus type III in homosexual men without the acquired immunodeficiency syndrome: Development of immunological and clinical abnormalities. *Ann. Int. Med.* **104**, 496.

Meusing, M.A., Smith, D.H., Cabrabdilla, C.D. *et al.* (1985) Nucleic acid structure and expression of the human AIDS/lymphadenopathy retrovirus. *Nature*, **313**, 450.

Penington, D.G. (1987) The AIDS epidemic—where are we going? *Med. J. Austr.* **147**, 265.

Peterman, T.A., Lang, G.R., Mikos, N.J. *et al.* (1986) HTLV-III/LAV infection in hemodialysis units. *J. Am. Med. Assoc.* **225**, 2324.

Resnik, L., Veren, K., Salahuddin, S.Z. *et al.* (1986) Stability and inactivation of HTLV-III/LAV under clinical and laboratory environment. *J. Am. Med. Assoc.* **55**, 1887.

Rutherford, G.W., Echenberg, D.F., O'Malley, P.M. *et al.* (1986) The natural history of LAV/HTLV-III infection and viraemia in homosexual and bisexual men on a 6-year follow-up study. In: Abstracts of Second International Conference on AIDS, Paris, June 23–25 1986, p. 99.

Safai, B., Sarngadharan, M.G., Groopman, J.E. *et al.* (1984) Sero-epidemiological studies of human T-lymphotropic retrovirus type III in acquired immunodeficiency syndrome. *Lancet*, **i**, 1438.

Salahuddin, S.Z., Markham, P.D., Popovic, M. *et al.* (1985) Isolation of infectious human T-cell leukemia/lymphotropic virus type III (HTLV-III) from patients with acquired immunodeficiency syndrome (AIDS) or AIDS-related complex (ARC) and from healthy carriers: A study of risk groups and tissue sources. *Proc. Natl. Acad. Sci. U.S.A.* **82**, 5530.

Salahuddin, S.Z., Markham, P.D., Redfield, R.R. *et al.* (1984) HTLV-III in symptom-free seronegative persons. *Lancet*, **ii**, 1418.

Sarngadharan, M.G., Popovic, M., Bruch, J. (1984) Antibodies reactive with human T-lymphotropic retroviruses (HTLA-III) in the serum of patients with AIDS. *Science*, **224**, 506.

Shaw, G.M., Harper, M.E., Hahn, B.H. *et al.* (1985) HTLV-III infection in brains of children and adults with AIDS encephalopathy. *Science*, **227**, 177.

Sodroski, J.G., Goh, W.C., Rosen, C. *et al.* (1986) Replicative and cytopathic potential of HTLV-III/LAV with *sor* gene deletions. *Science*, **231**, 1549.

Spire, B., Barre-Sinoussi, F., Dormont, D. *et al.* (1985) Inactivation of lymphadenopathy-associated virus by heat, gamma rays and ultraviolet light. *Lancet*, **i**, 188.

Weiss, R.A., Clapham, P.R., Cheingson-Popov, R. *et al.* (1985) Neutralisation of human T-lymphotropic virus type III by sera of AIDS and AIDS-risk patients. *Nature*, **316**, 69.

Ziegler, J.B., Cooper, D.A., Johnson, R.O. *et al.* (1985) Postnatal transmission of AIDS-associated retrovirus from mother to infant. *Lancet*, **i**, 896.

Index

Page numbers in *italics* refer to figures and page numbers in **bold** type refer to tables.